The Massachusetts Eye and Ear Infirmary Illustrated Manual of Ophthalmology

NEIL J. FRIEDMAN, MD
Private Practice
Palo Alto, California;
Adjunct Clinical Associate Professor, Department of Ophthalmology
Stanford University School of Medicine
Stanford, California

PETER K. KAISER, MD
Director, Digital OCT Reading Center
Staff Surgeon, Vitreoretinal Service
Cole Eye Institute, The Cleveland Clinic Foundation
Cleveland, Ohio

Associate author
Roberto Pineda II, MD
Assistant Professor of Ophthalmology
Harvard Medical School
Cornea and Refractive Surgery Service
Massachusetts Eye and Ear Infirmary
Boston, Massachusetts

3rd EDITION

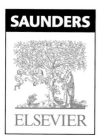

SAUNDERS

ELSEVIER

SAUNDERS
ELSEVIER

First edition © 1998
Second edition © 2004
© 2009, Elsevier Inc. All rights reserved.

13 digit ISBN: 978-1-4377-0908-7

British Library Cataloguing in Publication Data
A catalogue record for this book is available from the British Library

Library of Congress Cataloging in Publication Data
A catalog record for this book is available from the Library of Congress

Printed in China

Last digit is the print number: 9 8 7 6 5 4 3 2 1

The Massachusetts Eye and Ear Infirmary Illustrated Manual of Ophthalmology

Commissioning Editor: Russell Gabbedy
Development Editor: Ben Davie
Project Manager: Elouise Ball
Design: Charles Gray
Marketing Manager(s) (UK/USA): John Canelon/William Veltre

Preface

We are delighted to present the 3rd edition of this book. Our original goal, to produce a concise manual that covered a broad variety of ophthalmic disorders and present it in a user friendly diagnostic atlas, has not changed. In fact, improvements to this edition, we believe, better achieve that goal.

We have updated and expanded the format of this comprehensive ophthalmology manual to make it even more accessible, instructive and useful. Specifically, new diagnoses have been added throughout the book, and existing sections have been updated to reflect the most current diagnostic and treatment options. Numerous sections have been completely revised. Once again, current residents, fellows, and attending physicians have reviewed and contributed to various chapters to ensure that the text remains relevant to a wide audience of ophthalmologists. Moreover, we have added many new figures, including images of various tests (i.e., CT/MRI scans, fluorescein angiography, spectral domain optical coherence tomography (OCT), fundus autoflourescence, HRT, and visual field tests), improved the quality of existing images, and converted all the figures to color.

In this edition, we have expanded the appendix by adding brand new tables and lists. The existing sections, in particular the exam and medication sections, have been thoroughly updated. The index has also been improved to make it easier to navigate the book.

We believe that this new edition retains all of its previous attributes and also incorporates important improvements to keep pace with our ever-changing field of medicine. The book will continue to provide the type of information you are accustomed to obtaining when referring to previous editions, and we hope it will surpass your expectations.

Neil J. Friedman, MD
Peter K. Kaiser, MD
Roberto Pineda II, MD

Contributors

The contribution of the following colleagues, who have reviewed and edited various chapters of this text, is greatly appreciated:

Mehran Taban, MD, Sumit Sharma
Cole Eye Institute
Cleveland Clinic Foundation
Cleveland, Ohio

Jason Ehrlich, MD, ATul Jain, MD, Christopher Zoumalan, MD
Department of Ophthalmology
Stanford University School of Medicine
Stanford, California

Thomas N. Hwang, MD, PhD, Timothy J. McCulley, MD (Chapters 2, 3, 4, 7, 11)
Department of Ophthalmology
University of California at San Francisco
San Francisco, California

Acknowledgments

There are many people we must thank for their involvement with this project. We are particularly grateful to the faculty, staff, fellows, residents, colleagues, and peers at our various training programs including the Bascom Palmer Eye Institute, the Cole Eye Institute, the Cullen Eye Institute, the Massachusetts Eye and Ear Infirmary, the New York Eye and Ear Infirmary, and Stanford University for their guidance, instruction, and support of this book. We are indebted to those individuals who contributed valuable suggestions and revisions to the text.

We especially acknowledge our editorial and publishing staff at Elsevier: Russell Gabbedy, Ben Davie, and the members of their department, for their expertise and assistance in producing this work. In addition, we are indebted to Tami Fecko, Nicole Brugnoni, Sumit Sharma, Kaori Sayanagi, Shawn Perry, Louise Carr-Holden, Ditte Hesse, Kit Johnson, Bob Masini, Audrey Melacan, Jim Shigley, and Huynh Van, as well as the dedicated staff of their photography departments for all the wonderful pictures without which this book would not be possible. We would also like to thank the many physicians whose photographs complete the vast collection of ophthalmic disorders represented in the book.

Finally, a special heartfelt thank you to our families, including Mae, Jake, Alan, Diane, Lisa, Maureen, Peter (PJ), Stephanie, Peter, Anafu, Christine, Roberto, Anne, Gabriela, and Nicole, for their love, support, and encouragement.

Neil J. Friedman, MD
Peter K. Kaiser, MD
Roberto Pineda II, MD

Contents

Introduction, 1

1 ORBIT, 3
Trauma, 3
  Blunt Trauma, 3
    Orbital Contusion, 3
    Orbital Hemorrhage/Orbital
      Compartment Syndrome, 4
    Orbital Fractures, 5
  Penetrating Trauma, 8
    Intraorbital Foreign Body, 8
Globe Subluxation, 9
Carotid-Cavernous and Dural Sinus
  Fistulas, 10
Infections, 12
  Preseptal Cellulitis, 12
  Orbital Cellulitis, 13
Inflammation, 15
  Thyroid-Related
    Ophthalmopathy, 15
  Idiopathic Orbital Inflammation
    (Orbital Pseudotumor), 18
Congenital Anomalies, 19
  Congenital Anophthalmia, 19
  Microphthalmos, 20
  Microphthalmos with Cyst, 20
  Nanophthalmos, 20
  Craniofacial Disorders, 20
Pediatric Orbital Tumors, 21
  Benign Pediatric Orbital Tumors, 21
    Orbital Dermoid (Dermoid
      Cyst), 21

Lymphangioma, 21
Juvenile Xanthogranuloma, 22
Histiocytic Tumors, 23
Malignant Pediatric Orbital
  Tumors, 23
  Rhabdomyosarcoma, 23
  Neuroblastoma, 24
  Leukemia, 24
Adult Orbital Tumors, 26
  Benign Adult Orbital
    Tumors, 26
    Cavernous Hemangioma, 26
    Mucocele, 26
    Neurilemoma (Schwannoma), 27
    Meningioma, 28
    Fibrous Histiocytoma, 28
    Fibro-Osseous Tumors, 29
    Cholesterol Granuloma, 29
    Aneurysmal Bone Cyst, 29
  Malignant Adult Orbital
    Tumors, 29
    Lymphoid Tumors, 29
    Fibro-Osseous Tumors, 30
    Metastatic Tumors, 31
Acquired Anophthalmia, 31
Atrophia Bulbi and Phthisis
  Bulbi, 32
  Atrophia Bulbi Without
    Shrinkage, 32
  Atrophia Bulbi With Shrinkage, 32
  Atrophia Bulbi With Disorgani-
    zation (Phthisis Bulbi), 32

2   OCULAR MOTILITY AND
    CRANIAL NERVES, 35
Strabismus, 35
    Phoria, 35
    Tropia, 35
Horizontal Strabismus, 37
    Esotropia, 37
        Infantile Esotropia, 37
        Accommodative Esotropia, 38
        Acquired Nonaccommodative
            Esotropia and Other Forms
            of Esotropia, 39
    Exotropia, 40
        Basic Exotropia, 40
        Convergence Insufficiency, 40
        Pseudodivergence Excess, 41
        True Divergence Excess, 41
    A-, V-, and X-Patterns, 41
        A-pattern, 41
        V-pattern, 42
        X-pattern, 42
Vertical Strabismus, 42
    Brown's Syndrome (Superior Oblique
        Tendon Sheath Syndrome), 42
        Dissociated Strabismus Complex:
            Dissociated Vertical Deviation,
            Dissociated Horizontal
            Deviation, Dissociated
            Torsional Deviation, 43
    Monocular Elevation
        Deficiency (Double Elevator
        Palsy), 44
        Type 1, 44
        Type 2, 44
        Type 3, 44
Miscellaneous Strabismus, 45
    Duane's Retraction Syndrome, 45
        Type 1, 45
        Type 2, 45
        Type 3, 45
    Möbius' Syndrome, 46
    Restrictive Strabismus, 46
    Congenital Fibrosis Syndrome, 46
        Generalized Fibrosis (Autosomal
            Dominant [AD] > Autosomal
            Recessive [AR] > Idiopathic), 46
        Congenital Fibrosis of Inferior
            Rectus (Sporadic or Familial), 46

Strabismus Fixus (Sporadic), 47
Vertical Retraction Syndrome, 47
Congenital Unilateral Fibrosis
    (Sporadic), 47
Nystagmus, 47
    Congenital Nystagmus, 47
    Acquired Nystagmus, 48
    Physiologic Nystagmus, 49
Third Cranial Nerve Palsy, 50
    Nuclear, 51
    Fascicular, 51
    Subarachnoid Space, 51
    Intracavernous Space, 51
    Orbital Space, 51
Fourth Cranial Nerve Palsy, 53
    Nuclear, 54
    Fascicular, 54
    Subarachnoid Space, 54
    Intracavernous Space, 54
Sixth Cranial Nerve Palsy, 56
    Nuclear, 56
    Fascicular, 56
    Subarachnoid Space, 57
    Petrous Space, 57
    Intracavernous Space, 57
Multiple Cranial Nerve Palsies, 58
    Brain Stem, 58
    Subarachnoid Space, 58
    Cavernous Sinus Syndrome, 59
    Orbital Apex Syndrome, 59
Chronic Progressive External
    Ophthalmoplegia, 61
        Kearns–Sayre Syndrome, 61
        Mitochondrial Encephalopathy,
            Lactic Acidosis, and Stroke-
            like Episodes, 61
        Myoclonic Epilepsy and Ragged
            Red Fibers, 61
        Myotonic Dystrophy, 61
        Oculopharyngeal Muscular
            Dystrophy, 61
Horizontal Motility Disorders, 63
    Internuclear Ophthalmoplegia, 63
    One-and-a-Half Syndrome, 63
Vertical Motility Disorders, 65
    Progressive Supranuclear Palsy
        (Steele–Richardson–Olszewski
        Syndrome), 65

Dorsal Midbrain (Parinaud's)
Syndrome, 65
Skew Deviation, 65
Myasthenia Gravis, 67

3   LIDS, LASHES, AND LACRIMAL
SYSTEM, 69
Eyelid Trauma, 69
Contusion, 69
Abrasion, 70
Avulsion, 70
Laceration, 71
Eyelid Infections, 73
Blepharitis and Meibomitis, 73
Herpes Simplex Virus, 75
Herpes Zoster Virus, 76
Molluscum Contagiosum, 77
Demodicosis, 78
Phthiriasis or Pediculosis, 78
Leprosy, 79
Eyelid Inflammations, 79
Chalazion or Hordeolum
(Stye), 79
Contact Dermatitis, 80
Blepharochalasis, 82
Madarosis, 82
Vitiligo and Poliosis, 83
Acne Rosacea, 84
Eyelid Malpositions, 85
Ptosis, 85
Aponeurotic (Involutional), 85
Mechanical, 85
Myogenic, 85
Neurogenic, 86
Congenital, 86
Dermatochalasis, 88
Ectropion, 89
Cicatricial, 89
Congenital, 89
Inflammatory, 89
Involutional, 89
Mechanical, 89
Paralytic, 89
Entropion, 91
Cicatricial, 91
Congenital, 91
Involutional, 92
Spastic, 92

Blepharospasm, 93
Essential Blepharospasm, 93
Meige's Syndrome, 93
Bell's Palsy, 94
Floppy Eyelid Syndrome, 96
Trichiasis, 97
Congenital Eyelid Anomalies, 99
Ankyloblepharon, 99
Blepharophimosis, 99
Coloboma, 99
Cryptophthalmos, 100
Distichiasis, 100
Epiblepharon, 101
Epicanthus, 101
Euryblepharon, 102
Microblepharon, 102
Telecanthus, 102
Benign Eyelid Tumors, 103
Pigmented Benign Eyelid
Tumors, 103
Acquired Nevus, 103
Ephelis (Freckle), 103
Oculodermal Melanocytosis
(Nevus of Ota), 104
Seborrheic Keratosis, 104
Squamous Papilloma, 105
Verruca Vulgaris (Viral
Papilloma), 105
Nonpigmented Benign Eyelid
Tumors, 106
Xanthelasma, 106
Moll's Gland Cyst (Hidrocystoma,
Sudoriferous Cyst), 107
Epidermal Inclusion Cyst, 107
Inverted Follicular Keratosis, 108
Milia, 108
Sebaceous (Pilar) Cyst, 108
Pilomatrixoma (Calcifying
Epithelioma of Malherbe), 109
Vascular Benign Eyelid Tumors, 109
Capillary Hemangioma, 109
Lymphangioma, 110
Port Wine Stain (Nevus
Flammeus), 110
Malignant Eyelid Tumors, 110
Basal Cell Carcinoma, 110
Squamous Cell Carcinoma, 111
Actinic Keratosis, 112

Keratoacanthoma, 112
Sebaceous Cell Carcinoma, 113
Malignant Melanoma, 114
Merkel Cell Tumor, 115
Metastatic Tumors, 115
Kaposi's Sarcoma, 116
Systemic Diseases, 116
Neurofibromatosis, 116
Sarcoidosis, 118
Amyloidosis, 119
Canaliculitis, 120
Dacryocystitis, 121
Nasolacrimal Duct Obstruction, 123
Dacryoadenitis, 125
Lacrimal Gland Tumors, 128
Benign Mixed Cell Tumor
(Pleomorphic Adenoma), 128
Malignant Mixed Cell Tumor
(Pleomorphic Adenocarcinoma),
129
Adenoid Cystic Carcinoma
(Cylindroma), 129

4 CONJUNCTIVA AND
SCLERA, 131
Trauma, 131
Foreign Body, 131
Laceration, 131
Open Globe, 131
Subconjunctival Hemorrhage, 134
Telangiectasia, 135
Microaneurysm, 136
Dry Eye Disease (Dry Eye Syndrome,
Keratoconjunctivitis Sicca), 136
Aqueous-deficient dry eye, 137
Evaporative dry eye, 137
Inflammation, 141
Chemosis, 141
Follicles, 141
Granuloma, 142
Hyperemia, 142
Membranes, 142
Papillae, 142
Phlyctenule, 143
Conjunctivitis, 144
Acute Conjunctivitis, 144
Infectious, 144
Gonococcal, 144
Nongonococcal Bacterial, 144

Adenoviral, 145
Herpes Simplex Virus, 145
Herpes Zoster Virus, 146
Pediculosis, 146
Allergic, 146
Seasonal, 146
Atopic Keratoconjunctivitis, 146
Vernal Keratoconjunctivitis, 147
Toxic, 147
Chronic Conjunctivitis, 148
Infectious, 148
Chlamydial, 148
Molluscum Contagiosum, 148
Allergic, 148
Perennial, 148
Giant Papillary Conjunctivitis,
149
Toxic, 149
Other, 149
Superior Limbic
Keratoconjunctivitis, 149
Kawasaki's Disease, 150
Ligneous, 150
Parinaud's Oculoglandular
Syndrome, 150
Ophthalmia Neonatorum, 150
Degenerations, 153
Amyloidosis, 154
Concretions, 154
Pinguecula, 154
Pterygium, 154
Ocular Cicatricial Pemphigoid, 156
Stevens–Johnson Syndrome
(Erythema Multiforme Major), 157
Tumors, 158
Congenital, 158
Hamartoma, 158
Choristoma, 159
Epithelial, 159
Cysts, 159
Papilloma, 159
Conjunctival Intraepithelial
Neoplasia, 160
Squamous Cell Carcinoma, 161
Melanocytic, 161
Nevus, 161
Ocular Melanocytosis, 162
Oculodermal Melanocytosis
(Nevus of Ota), 163

Primary Acquired Melanosis, 163
Secondary Acquired
    Melanosis, 163
Malignant Melanoma, 164
Stromal, 165
    Cavernous Hemangioma, 165
    Juvenile Xanthogranuloma, 165
    Kaposi's Sarcoma, 165
    Lymphangiectasis, 166
    Lymphoid, 166
    Pyogenic Granuloma, 167
Caruncle, 167
Episcleritis, 168
Scleritis, 169
Scleral Discoloration, 171
    Alkaptonuria (Ochronosis), 171
    Ectasia (Staphyloma), 172
    Osteogenesis Imperfecta, 172
    Scleral Icterus, 172
    Senile Scleral Plaque, 172

5 CORNEA, 175
Trauma, 175
    Abrasion, 175
    Birth Trauma, 176
    Burn, 177
    Foreign Body, 178
    Laceration, 179
    Recurrent Erosion, 180
Peripheral Ulcerative Keratitis, 180
    Marginal Keratolysis, 180
    Mooren's Ulcer, 180
    Staphylococcal Marginal
        Keratitis, 180
    Marginal Keratolysis, 181
    Mooren's Ulcer, 181
    Staphylococcal Marginal
        Keratitis, 182
Contact Lens-Related
    Problems, 183
    Rigid Lenses, 183
    Soft Lenses, 184
    Corneal Abrasion, 185
    Corneal Hypoxia, 185
    Contact Lens-Related Dendritic
        Keratitis, 185
    Contact Lens Solution
        Hypersensitivity or Toxicity, 185
    Corneal Neovascularization, 185

Corneal Warpage, 186
Damaged Contact Lens, 187
Deposits on Contact Lens, 187
Giant Papillary Conjunctivitis, 187
Infectious Keratitis, 188
Sterile Corneal Infiltrates, 188
Poor Fit (Loose), 188
Poor Fit (Tight), 188
Superior Limbic
    Keratoconjunctivitis, 188
Superficial Punctate Keratitis, 188
Miscellaneous, 189
Delle, 189
Exposure Keratopathy, 189
Filamentary Keratitis, 190
Keratic Precipitates, 190
Superficial Punctate Keratitis, 191
Thygeson's Superficial Punctate
    Keratitis, 191
Corneal Edema, 193
Graft Rejection or Failure, 194
Infectious Keratitis (Corneal
    Ulcer), 196
    Bacterial, 196
    Fungal, 197
    Parasitic, 197
    Viral, 198
Interstitial Keratitis, 203
Pannus, 205
Degenerations, 206
    Arcus Senilis, 206
    Band Keratopathy, 207
    Crocodile Shagreen, 207
    Furrow Degeneration, 208
    Lipid Keratopathy, 208
    Spheroidal Degeneration (Actinic
        Degeneration, Labrador
        Keratopathy, Climatic Droplet
        Keratopathy, Bietti's Nodular
        Dystrophy), 208
    Salzmann's Nodular
        Degeneration, 208
    Terrien's Marginal
        Degeneration, 209
    White Limbal Girdle
        of Vogt, 209
Ectasias, 211
    Keratoconus, 211
    Keratoglobus, 212

Pellucid Marginal
Degeneration, 212
Congenital Anomalies, 214
Cornea Plana, 214
Dermoid, 214
Haab's Striae, 215
Megalocornea, 215
Microcornea, 216
Sclerocornea, 216
Dystrophies, 218
Anterior (Epithelial and Bowman's
Membrane), 218
Anterior Basement Membrane
Dystrophy (Epithelial
Basement Membrane
Dystrophy, Map-Dot-
Fingerprint Dystrophy, Cogan's
Microcystic Dystrophy), 218
Gelatinous Droplike
Dystrophy, 218
Reis-Bückler Dystrophy
(Honeycomb Dystrophy,
Thiel-Behnke Dystrophy),
219
Stromal, 219
Avellino Dystrophy, 219
Central Cloudy Dystrophy of
François, 219
Schnyder's Central Crystalline
Dystrophy, 220
Congenital Hereditary Stromal
Dystrophy, 220
François-Neetans Fleck
(Mouchetée) Dystrophy, 221
Granular Dystrophy, 221
Lattice Dystrophy, 221
Macular Dystrophy, 222
Pre-Descemet's Dystrophy (Deep
Filiform Dystrophy), 223
Posterior (Endothelial), 223
Congenital Hereditary
Endothelial Dystrophy, 223
Fuchs' Endothelial
Dystrophy, 223
Posterior Polymorphous
Dystrophy, 224
Metabolic Diseases, 225
Deposits, 226
Calcium, 226

Copper, 226
Cysteine (Cystinosis), 227
Drugs, 227
Immunoglobulin (Multiple
Myeloma), 228
Iron, 228
Lipid or Cholesterol
(Dyslipoproteinemias), 228
Melanin, 229
Tyrosine (Tyrosinemia)
Type II, 229
Urate (Gout), 229
Verticillata (Vortex Keratopathy),
229
Enlarged Corneal Nerves, 230
Tumors, 231

6 ANTERIOR CHAMBER, 233
Primary Angle-Closure
Glaucoma, 233
Secondary Angle-Closure Glaucoma,
236
Hypotony, 238
Hyphema, 240
Cells and Flare, 241
Hypopyon, 243
Endophthalmitis, 244
Postoperative, 244
Posttraumatic, 244
Endogenous, 245
Anterior Uveitis (Iritis,
Iridocyclitis), 248
Infectious Anterior Uveitis, 248
Herpes Simplex and Herpes
Zoster Ophthalmicus, 248
Lyme Disease, 248
Syphilis, 248
Tuberculosis, 248
Noninfectious Anterior
Uveitis, 249
Nongranulomatous, 249
Granulomatous, 251
Uveitis-Glaucoma-Hyphema
Syndrome, 255

7 IRIS AND PUPILS, 257
Trauma, 257
Angle Recession, 258
Cyclodialysis, 258

Iridodialysis, 258
Sphincter Tears, 259
Corectopia, 261
Seclusio Pupillae, 262
Peripheral Anterior Synechiae, 263
Rubeosis Iridis, 264
Neovascular Glaucoma, 265
Pigment Dispersion Syndrome, 266
Pigmentary Glaucoma, 268
Iris Heterochromia, 269
　Heterochromia Iridis, 269
　Heterochromia Iridum, 269
　Congenital, 269
　Acquired, 270
Anisocoria, 271
　Greater Anisocoria in Dark
　　(Abnormal Pupil is
　　Smaller), 271
　Greater Anisocoria in Light
　　(Abnormal Pupil is Larger),
　　271
　Anisocoria Equal in Light and
　　Dark, 271
Adie's Tonic Pupil, 272
Argyll Robertson Pupil, 274
Horner's Syndrome, 275
　Central (first-order neuron), 275
　Preganglionic (second-order
　　neuron), 275
　Postganglionic (third-order
　　neuron), 275
Relative Afferent Pupillary Defect
　(Marcus Gunn Pupil), 277
Leukocoria, 279
Congenital Anomalies, 280
　Aniridia, 280
　Coloboma, 281
　Persistent Pupillary
　　Membrane, 281
Mesodermal Dysgenesis
　Syndromes, 282
　Axenfeld's Anomaly, 283
　Alagille's Syndrome, 283
　Rieger's Anomaly, 283
　Rieger's Syndrome, 283
Iridocorneal Endothelial
　Syndromes, 285
　　Essential Iris Atrophy
　　　(Progressive Iris Atrophy), 285

Chandler's Syndrome, 285
Iris Nevus (Cogan-Reese)
　Syndrome, 286
Tumors, 287
　Cyst, 287
　Nevus, 288
　Nodules, 288
　Iris Pigment Epithelium
　　Tumors, 290
　Juvenile Xanthogranuloma, 290
　Malignant Melanoma, 290
　Metastatic Tumors, 291

8　LENS, 293
Congenital Anomalies, 293
　Coloboma, 293
　Lenticonus, 294
　Lentiglobus, 294
　Microspherophakia, 294
　Mittendorf Dot, 295
Congenital Cataract, 296
　Capsular, 296
　Lamellar or Zonular, 296
　Lenticular or Nuclear, 296
　Polar, 297
　Sutural, 297
　Hereditary or Syndromes, 297
　Intrauterine Infections, 298
　Metabolic, 298
　Ocular Disorders, 298
　Other, 299
Acquired Cataract, 300
　Cortical Degeneration, 300
　Nuclear Sclerosis, 301
　Subcapsular Cataract, 302
　Senile, 303
　Systemic Disease, 303
　Other Eye Diseases, 304
　Toxic, 305
　Trauma, 305
Posterior Capsular Opacification
　(Secondary Cataract), 306
Aphakia, 308
Pseudophakia, 309
Exfoliation, 310
Pseudoexfoliation Syndrome, 311
Pseudoexfoliation Glaucoma, 312
Lens-Induced Glaucoma, 314
　Lens Particle, 314

Phacolytic, 314
Phacomorphic, 314
Dislocated Lens (Ectopia Lentis), 316
Ectopia Lentis et Pupillae
(Autosomal Recessive), 316
Homocystinuria (Autosomal
Recessive), 316
Hyperlysinemia, 316
Marfan's Syndrome (Autosomal
Dominant), 316
Microspherophakia, 317
Simple Ectopia Lentis (Autosomal
Dominant), 317
Sulfite Oxidase Deficiency
(Autosomal Recessive), 317
Other, 317

9   VITREOUS, 319
Amyloidosis, 319
Asteroid Hyalosis, 320
Persistent Hyperplastic Primary
Vitreous (Persistent Fetal
Vasculature Syndrome), 321
Posterior Vitreous Detachment, 323
Synchesis Scintillans, 324
Vitreous Hemorrhage, 324
Vitritis, 326

10   RETINA AND CHOROID, 327
Trauma, 328
Choroidal Rupture, 328
Commotio Retinae (Berlin's
Edema), 328
Purtscher's Retinopathy, 329
Traumatic Retinal Breaks, 330
Chorioretinitis Sclopetaria, 331
Hemorrhages, 331
Preretinal Hemorrhage, 331
Intraretinal Hemorrhage, 331
Subretinal Hemorrhage, 333
Cotton-Wool Spot, 333
Branch Retinal Artery Occlusion, 334
Central Retinal Artery Occlusion, 336
Ophthalmic Artery Occlusion, 339
Branch Retinal Vein Occlusion, 340
Central/Hemiretinal Vein
Occlusion, 342
Venous Stasis Retinopathy, 346

Ocular Ischemic Syndrome, 346
Retinopathy of Prematurity, 348
Coats' Disease/Leber's Miliary
Aneurysms, 350
Eales' Disease, 352
Idiopathic Juxtafoveal Retinal
Telangiectasia, 352
Type 1A (Unilateral Congenital
Parafoveal Telangiectasia), 353
Type 1B (Unilateral Idiopathic
Parafoveal Telangiectasia), 353
Type 2 (Bilateral Acquired
Parafoveal Telangiectasia), 353
Type 3 (Bilateral Perifoveal
Telangiectasis with Capillary
Obliteration), 354
Retinopathies Associated with Blood
Abnormalities, 354
Retinopathy of Anemia, 354
Leukemic Retinopathy, 355
Sickle Cell Retinopathy, 356
Diabetic Retinopathy, 357
Insulin-Dependent Diabetes
(Type I), 357
Non-Insulin-Dependent Diabetes
(Type II), 358
Non-Proliferative Diabetic
Retinopathy, 358
Proliferative Diabetic
Retinopathy, 360
Hypertensive Retinopathy, 363
Toxemia of Pregnancy, 364
Acquired Retinal Arterial
Macroaneurysm, 365
Radiation Retinopathy, 366
Age-Related Macular
Degeneration, 367
Non-exudative (Dry) Macular
Degeneration, 368
Exudative (Wet) Macular
Degeneration, 370
Retinal Angiomatous
Proliferation, 374
Polypoidal Choroidal
Vasculopathy, 375
Myopic Degeneration/Pathologic
Myopia, 377
Angioid Streaks, 379

Central Serous Chorioretinopathy
(Idiopathic Central Serous
Choroidopathy), 381
Cystoid Macular Edema, 383
Macular Hole, 385
Epiretinal Membrane/Macular
Pucker, 388
Myelinated Nerve Fibers, 390
Solar/Photic Retinopathy, 391
Toxic (Drug) Maculopathies, 392
Aminoglycosides (Gentamicin/
Tobramicin/Amikacin), 392
Canthaxanthine
(Orobronze), 392
Chloroquine (Aralen)/
Hydroxychloroquine
(Plaquenil), 392
Chlorpromazine (Thorazine), 394
Deferoxamine (Desferal), 394
Interferon-alpha, 394
Methoxyflurane (Penthrane), 394
Niacin, 395
Quinine (Quinamm), 395
Sildenafil (Viagra), 396
Tadalafil (Cialis)/Vardenafil
(Levitra), 396
Talc, 396
Tamoxifen (Nolvadex), 396
Thioridazine (Mellaril), 397
Lipid Storage Diseases, 397
Farber's Disease (Glycolipid), 398
Mucolipidosis
(Mucopolysaccharidoses), 398
Niemann–Pick Disease (Ceramide
Phosphatidyl Choline), 398
Sandhoff's Disease (Gangliosidosis
Type II), 398
Tay–Sachs Disease (Gangliosidosis
Type I), 398
Peripheral Retinal Degenerations, 398
Lattice Degeneration, 398
Pavingstone (Cobblestone)
Degeneration, 399
Peripheral Cystoid Degeneration,
400
Snail Track Degeneration, 400
Retinoschisis, 400
Retinal Detachment, 403

Rhegmatogenous Retinal
Detachment, 403
Serous (Exudative) Retinal
Detachment, 404
Traction Retinal Detachment, 405
Choroidal Detachment, 407
Choroidal Effusion, 407
Choroidal Hemorrhage, 407
Chorioretinal Folds, 408
Chorioretinal Coloboma, 409
Proliferative Vitreoretinopathy, 410
Intermediate Uveitis/Pars Planitis, 411
Neuroretinitis (Leber's Idiopathic
Stellate Neuroretinitis), 412
Posterior Uveitis: Infections, 414
Acute Retinal Necrosis, 414
Candidiasis, 415
Cysticercosis, 416
Cytomegalovirus, 416
Diffuse Unilateral Subacute
Neuroretinitis, 418
Human Immunodeficiency Virus, 419
Pneumocystis carinii
Choroidopathy, 419
Presumed Ocular Histoplasmosis
Syndrome, 420
Progressive Outer Retinal Necrosis
Syndrome, 421
Rubella, 422
Syphilis (Luetic
Chorioretinitis), 422
Toxocariasis, 423
Toxoplasmosis, 424
Tuberculosis, 426
Posterior Uveitis: White Dot
Syndromes, 426
Acute Macular Neuroretinopathy,
426
Acute Posterior Multifocal Placoid
Pigment Epitheliopathy, 426
Acute Retinal Pigment Epitheliitis
(Krill's Disease), 428
Birdshot Choroidopathy
(Vitiliginous
Chorioretinitis), 429
Multifocal Choroiditis and
Panuveitis/Subretinal Fibrosis
and Uveitis Syndrome, 430

Punctate Inner
Choroidopathy, 430
Multiple Evanescent White Dot
Syndrome, 431
Acute Idiopathic Blind Spot
Enlargement Syndrome, 432
Posterior Uveitis: Other
Inflammatory Disorders, 432
Behçet's Disease, 432
Idiopathic Uveal Effusion
Syndrome, 433
Masquerade Syndromes, 434
Posterior Scleritis, 435
Sarcoidosis, 436
Serpiginous Choroidopathy
(Geographic Helicoid
Peripapillary Choroidopathy), 437
Sympathetic Ophthalmia, 438
Vogt–Koyanagi–Harada
Syndrome/Harada's Disease, 439
Posterior Uveitis: Evaluation/
Management, 440
Hereditary Chorioretinal
Dystrophies, 442
Central Areolar Choroidal
Dystrophy, 442
Choroideremia, 443
Congenital Stationary Night
Blindness, 444
Crystalline Retinopathy of
Bietti, 446
Gyrate Atrophy, 446
Progressive Cone Dystrophy, 447
Rod Monochromatism
(Achromatopsia), 448
Hereditary Macular Dystrophies, 448
Adult Foveomacular Vitelliform
Dystrophy, 448
Best's Disease, 448
Butterfly Pattern Dystrophy, 451
Dominant Drusen (Doyne's
Honeycomb Dystrophy, Malattia
Leventinese), 451
North Carolina Macular Dystrophy
(Lefler-Wadsworth-Sidbury
Dystrophy), 452
Pseudoinflammatory Macular
Dystrophy (Sorsby's Dystrophy),
453

Sjögren Reticular Pigment
Dystrophy, 453
Stargardt's Disease/Fundus
Flavimaculatus, 453
Hereditary Vitreoretinal
Degenerations, 454
Familial Exudative
Vitreoretinopathy, 454
Enhanced S-cone Syndrome/
Goldmann–Favre Syndrome, 456
Marshall Syndrome, 456
Snowflake Degeneration, 456
Wagner/Jansen/Stickler
Vitreoretinal Dystrophies, 456
Leber's Congenital Amaurosis, 458
Retinitis Pigmentosa, 459
Atypical forms, 459
Retinitis Pigmentosa Inversus, 459
Retinitis Pigmentosa Sine
Pigmento, 459
Retinitis Punctata Albescens,
459
Sector Retinitis Pigmentosa, 459
Forms Associated with Systemic
Abnormalities, 459
Abetalipoproteinemia (Bassen-
Kornzweig Syndrome), 459
Alstrom's Disease, 459
Cockayne's Syndrome, 460
Kearns–Sayre Syndrome, 460
Laurence–Moon/Bardet–Biedl
Syndromes, 460
Neuronal Ceroid Lipofuscinosis
(Batten Disease), 461
Refsum's Disease, 461
Usher's Syndrome, 461
Albinism, 464
Ocular Albinism, 464
Oculocutaneous Albinism, 464
Phakomatoses, 465
Angiomatosis Retinae (von
Hippel-Lindau Disease), 465
Ataxia Telangiectasia (Louis-Bar
Syndrome), 465
Encephalotrigeminal
Angiomatosis (Sturge–Weber
Syndrome), 466
Neurofibromatosis (von
Recklinghausen's Disease), 466

Racemose Hemangiomatosis
(Wyburn–Mason
Syndrome), 467
Tuberous Sclerosis (Bourneville's
Disease), 467
Tumors, 468
Benign Choroidal Tumors, 468
Choroidal Hemangioma, 468
Choroidal Nevus, 470
Choroidal Osteoma, 470
Benign Retinal Tumors, 471
Astrocytic Hamartoma, 471
Capillary Hemangioma, 471
Cavernous Hemangioma, 472
Congenital Hypertrophy of the
Retinal Pigment
Epithelium, 473
Bear Tracks, 474
Combined Hamartoma of
Retinal Pigment Epithelium
and Retina, 475
Malignant Tumors, 475
Choroidal Malignant
Melanoma, 475
Choroidal Metastasis, 477
Primary Intraocular Lymphoma
(Reticulum Cell Sarcoma), 479
Retinoblastoma, 479
Paraneoplastic Syndromes, 480
Bilateral Diffuse Uveal
Melanocytic Proliferation
Syndrome, 480
Carcinoma-Associated
Retinopathy, 480
Cutaneous Melanoma-Associated
Retinopathy, 481

11 **OPTIC NERVE AND
GLAUCOMA, 483**
Papilledema, 483
Idiopathic Intracranial Hypertension
(Pseudotumor Cerebri), 485
Optic Neuritis, 486
Papillitis, 486
Retrobulbar, 486
Devic's Syndrome, 487
Anterior Ischemic Optic
Neuropathy, 488
Arteritic, 488

Nonarteritic, 488
Traumatic Optic Neuropathy, 491
Other Optic Neuropathies, 493
Compressive, 493
Hereditary, 493
Infectious, 494
Infiltrative, 494
Ischemic, 494
Nutritional, 494
Toxic, 495
Congenital Anomalies, 496
Aplasia, 497
Dysplasias, 497
Coloboma, 497
Hypoplasia, 497
Morning Glory
Syndrome, 498
Optic Nerve Drusen, 498
Pit, 499
Septo-Optic Dysplasia
(De Morsier Syndrome), 500
Tilted Optic Disc, 500
Tumors, 501
Angioma (von Hippel Lesion), 501
Astrocytic Hamartoma, 501
Combined Hamartoma of
Retina and Retinal Pigment
Epithelium, 501
Glioma, 502
Melanocytoma, 502
Meningioma, 503
Chiasmal Syndromes, 505
Congenital Glaucoma, 508
Primary Open-Angle Glaucoma, 509
Secondary Open-Angle
Glaucoma, 517
Drug Induced, 517
Intraocular Tumor, 518
Traumatic, 518
Uveitic, 518
Normal (Low) Tension Glaucoma, 520

12 **VISUAL ACUITY, REFRACTIVE
PROCEDURES, AND SUDDEN
VISION LOSS, 523**
Refractive Error, 523
Ametropia, 523
Anisometropia, 523
Astigmatism, 523

Emmetropia, 524
Hyperopia (Farsightedness), 524
Myopia (Nearsightedness), 524
Presbyopia, 524
Refractive Surgery Complications, 526
Intraocular Refractive
Procedures, 526
Clear Lens Extraction (Refractive
Lens Exchange), 526
Phakic Intraocular Lens, 526
Corneal Refractive Procedures, 527
Incisional, 527
Excimer Laser, 528
Implants, 532
Thermokeratoplasty, 533
Refractive Surgery Complications:
Evaluation/Management, 533
Vertebrobasilar Insufficiency
(Vertebrobasilar Atherothrombotic
Disease), 535
Migraine, 536
Migraine without Aura, 536
Migraine with Aura, 536
Childhood Periodic
Syndromes, 537
Retinal Migraine, 537
Complications of Migraine, 537
Convergence Insufficiency, 538
Accommodative Excess
(Accommodative Spasm), 539
Functional Visual Loss, 540
Malingering, 540
Hysteria, 540
Transient Visual Loss (Amaurosis
Fugax), 541
Amblyopia, 542
Strabismic, 542
Anisometropic, 542
Isoametropic, 543
Deprivation, 543
Occlusion, 543
Cortical Blindness (Cortical Visual
Impairment), 544
Visual Pathway Lesions, 544

APPENDIX, 549
Ophthalmic History and
Examination, 549
History, 549

Ocular Examination, 549
Vision, 549
Refraction, 552
Retinoscopy, 553
Lensometer, 553
Potential Acuity Meter, 554
Contrast Sensitivity, 554
Color Vision, 555
Stereopsis, 555
4D Base Out Prism Test, 556
Worth 4Dot Test, 556
Ocular Motility, 556
Cover Tests, 557
Corneal Light Reflex
Tests, 559
Forced Ductions, 560
Optokinetic Testing, 560
Pupils, 561
Visual Fields, 561
Amsler Grid, 562
Tangent Screen, 562
Goldmann Visual Field, 562
Humphrey Visual Field, 563
External Examination, 563
Exophthalmometry, 563
Schirmer's Test, 564
Jones' Dye Tests, 564
Other Cranial Nerve
Examination, 564
Slit Lamp Examination, 565
Dyes, 566
Gonioscopy, 566
Fundus Contact and
Noncontact Lenses, 567
Tonometry, 567
Specialized Tests, 568
Pachymetry, 568
Keratometry, 569
Corneal Topography, 570
Wavefront Aberrometry, 570
Specular Microscopy, 570
Fundus Examination, 571
Specialized Tests, 573
Ultrasonography, 573
Partial Coherence Laser
Interferometry
(IOLMaster), 574
Optical Coherence
Tomography, 574

AAO Suggested Routine Eye
    Examination Guidelines, 575
Differential Diagnosis of Common
    Ocular Symptoms, 575
    Blurred vision, 575
    Eye Pain, 577
    Tearing, 577
    Discharge, 577
    Flashes of light, 577
    Red eye, 577
Common Ophthalmic
    Medications, 577
    Anti-infectives, 577
        Antibiotics, 577
        Antiamoebics, 580
        Antifungals, 580
        Antivirals, 581
    Antiinflammatories, 581
        NSAIDs, 581
        Immunomodulator, 581
        Steroids, 581
    Ocular Hypotensive (Glaucoma)
        Medications, 582
        Alpha-Adrenergic Receptor
            Agonists, 582
        Beta-Blockers, 582

Cholinergic Agonists (Miotics), 582
Carbonic Anhydrase
    Inhibitors, 583
Prostaglandin Analogues, 583
Hyperosmotics, 583
Combinations, 583
Allergy Medications, 583
Mydriatics/Cycloplegics, 584
Anesthetics, 584
Miscellaneous, 585
Artificial Tear Gel Formulations, 585
Artificial Tear Solution
    Formulations, 585
Color Codes for Topical Ocular
    Medication Caps, 586
Ocular Toxicology, 586
List of Important Ocular
    Measurements, 587
List of Eponyms, 588
Common Ophthalmic
    Abbreviations, 591
Common Spanish Phrases, 593
    Suggested Readings, 595

INDEX, 597

Figure Courtesy Lines

The following figures are reproduced from Essentials of Ophthalmology, Friedman and Kaiser, 2007, Saunders: 2-3, 2-15, 2-22, 4-1, 4-2, 4-31, 4-44, 7-17, 7-18, 7-19, 10-128, 11-29, 12-15, A-7, A-10, A-19, A-20, A-23, A-27, A-28, A-30, A-31, A-32, A-43. Table A-2, and Table A-3.

The following figures are reproduced from Review of Ophthalmology, Friedman, Kaiser, and Trattler, 2007, Saunders: 2-25, 2-26, 7-1, 7-5, A-14, A-16, A-17, A-21, and A-29.

The following figures are courtesy of the Bascom Palmer Eye Institute:
3-10, 4-3, 4-42, 4-52, 4-65, 5-8, 5-12, 5-25, 5-31, 5-36, 5-43, 5-60, 5-61, 5-67, 5-72, 5-74, 5-79, 6-10, 6-11, 6-12, 7-7, 7-13, 7-20, 7-21, 8-6, 8-19, 8-33, 8-35, 8-37, 9-7, 10-1, 10-5, 10-6, 10-11, 10-29, 10-31, 10-38, 10-39, 10-40, 10-44, 10-52, 10-53, 10-59, 10-61, 10-86, 10-89, 10-90, 10-99, 10-106, 10-118, 10-132, 10-133, 10-136, 10-137, 10-138, 10-139, 10-146, 10-152, 10-181, 10-182, 10-185, 10-187, 10-198, 10-199, 10-213, 10-215, 10-220, 10-222, 10-223, 10-196, 10-224, 10-227, 10-233, 10-235, 10-236, 10-237, 10-238, 10-239, 10-240, 10-241, 10-245, 10-246, 10-247, 11-15, 11-18, and 11-21.

The following figures are courtesy of the Cole Eye Institute:
1-3, 1-28, 1-32, 1-33, 1-34, 1-35, 3-3, 3-11, 3-14, 3-19, 3-22, 3-23, 3-37, 3-49, 3-52, 3-56, 3-65, 4-8, 4-19, 4-25, 4-29, 4-32, 4-39, 4-40, 4-43, 4-49, 4-54, 4-55, 4-57, 4-64, 4-67, 4-68, 5-5, 5-6, 5-11, 5-20, 5-24, 5-34, 5-35, 5-38, 5-39, 5-47, 5-53, 5-57, 5-64, 5-85, 5-90, 5-91, 5-92, 5-93, 6-13, 6-14, 7-29, 7-43, 8-4, 8-8, 8-9, 8-10, 8-11, 8-21, 8-24, 9-2, 9-6, 10-2, 10-12, 10-16, 10-17, 10-18, 10-19, 10-20, 10-22, 10-25, 10-27, 10-28, 10-32, 10-33, 10-34, 10-35, 10-41, 10-43, 10-45, 10-46, 10-47, 10-39, 10-54, 10-55, 10-56, 10-57, 10-62, 10-66, 10-67, 10-70, 10-71, 10-72, 10-73, 10-83, 10-85, 10-87, 10-88, 10-92, 10-93, 10-95, 10-96, 10-104, 10-111, 10-115, 10-116, 10-119, 10-121, 10-122, 10-123, 10-124, 10-125, 10-129, 10-130, 10-131, 10-135, 10-141, 10-143, 10-144, 10-145, 10-147, 10-148, 10-149, 10-150, 10-151, 10-158, 10-159, 10-160, 10-166, 10-167, 10-168, 10-169, 10-170, 10-171, 10-174, 10-175, 10-176, 10-177, 10-178, 10-179, 10-180, 10-184, 10-188, 10-190, 10-191, 10-193, 10-194, 10-195, 10-196, 10-197, 10-202, 10-203, 10-204, 10-206, 10-207, 10-208, 10-212, 10-217, 10-225, 10-228, 10-229, 10-234, 10-242, 10-243, 10-244, 10-248, 11-1, 11-2, 11-3, 11-4, 11-12, 11-16, 11-17, 11-22, 11-3, 11-33, 11-35, 12-3, 12-5, 12-6, 12-9, 12-10, and 12-11.

The following figures are courtesy of the Massachusetts Eye and Ear Infirmary:
1-2, 1-11, 1-8, 1-9, 1-10, 1-11, 1-12, 1-13, 1-14, 1-15, 1-16, 1-21, 1-36, 2-1, 2-2, 2-4, 2-7, 2-10, 2-11, 2-12, 2-20, 2-23, 2-24, 3-5, 3-8, 3-12, 3-13, 3-17, 3-20, 3-21, 3-24, 3-29, 3-41, 3-47, 3-48, 3-57, 3-63, 3-64, 3-68, 4-4, 4-5, 4-6, 4-9, 4-11, 4-12, 4-14, 4-15, 4-16, 4-17, 4-18, 4-20, 4-26, 4-27, 4-30, 4-33, 4-34, 4-36, 4-37, 4-38, 4-48, 4-50, 4-51, 4-56, 4-58, 4-60, 4-61, 4-62, 5-2, 5-7, 5-14, 5-15, 5-16, 5-17, 5-19, 5-21, 5-22, 5-26, 5-27, 5-28, 5-32, 5-33, 5-37, 5-40, 5-41, 5-48, 5-51, 5-52, 5-56, 5-58, 5-68, 5-70, 5-71, 5-73, 5-78, 5-80, 5-82, 5-83, 5-84, 5-86, 6-1, 6-2, 6-5, 6-8, 6-15, 7-2, 7-4, 7-6, 7-9, 7-11, 7-15, 7-22, 7-25, 7-27, 7-28, 7-31, 7-34, 7-35, 7-36, 7-37, 7-39, 7-40, 7-41, 7-42, 7-44, 8-1, 8-3, 8-5, 8-7, 8-12, 8-13, 8-15, 8-16, 8-17, 8-18, 8-22, 8-23, 8-26, 8-36, 8-38, 8-41, 9-1, 9-3, 10-4, 10-26, 10-42, 10-60, 10-63, 10-64, 10-65, 10-105, 10-112, 10-113, 10-114, 10-117, 10-126, 10-134, 10-142, 10-153, 10-154, 10-155, 10-156, 10-157, 10-161, 10-162, 10-165, 10-173, 10-183, 10-186, 10-201, 10-205, 10-214, 10-216, 10-218, 10-219, 10-221, 10-226, 11-5, 11-6, 11-7, 11-10, 11-25, 11-28, 11-34, and 12-4.

The following figures are courtesy of the New York Eye and Ear Infirmary:
3-16, 3-34, 3-39, 3-59, 4-13, 4-21, 4-35, 4-45, 4-46, 4-47, 4-53, 4-59, 4-63, 5-13, 5-42, 5-44, 5-46, 5-45, 5-49, 5-50, 5-55, 5-69, 5-88, 5-89, 7-3, 7-8, 7-10, 7-12, 7-24, 8-14, 8-25, 8-27, 8-32, 8-34, 8-40, 9-5, 9-9, 10-3, 10-8, 10-9, 10-10, 10-15, 10-21, 10-27, 10-30, 10-48, 10-58, 10-82, 10-103, 10-140, 10- 163, 10-164, 10-172, 10-183, 10-189, 10-200, 10-209, 10-210, 10-211, 11-11, and 11-20.

The following figures are courtesy of Warren Chang, MD: 2-8 and 2-9.

The following figures are courtesy of Cullen Eye Institute: 1-7, 5-76, and 11-14.

The following figure is courtesy of Eric D. Donnenfeld, MD: 3-6.

The following figure is courtesy of Chris Engelman, MD: 11-36.

The following figures are courtesy of Neil J. Friedman, MD: 1-6, 5-3, 5-4, 5-29, 5-62, 5-63, 5-75, 6-3, 7-14, 10-7, 11-26, 11-30, 11-31, 11-32, 12-12, 12-16, Appendix-34, Appendix-35, Appendix-42, Appendix-44, and Appendix-45.

The following figures are courtesy of Ronald L. Gross, MD: 5-66, 6-4, 6-9, 7-23, 7-26, 7-32, and 11-22.

The following figures are courtesy of M. Bowes Hamill, MD: 4-7, 4-26, 4-28, 4-41, 4-66, 5-9, 5-10, 5-81, 7-30, and 7-33.

The following figure is courtesy of Thomas N. Hwang, MD, PhD: 11-9.

The following figures are courtesy of ATul Jain, MD: 6-6, 9-4, 10-13, and 10-14.

The following figures are courtesy of Peter K. Kaiser, MD: 2-13, 2-16, 2-19, 2-21, 9-8, 10-23, 10-24, 10-36, 10-37, 10-50, 10-51, 10-68, 10-69, 10-74, 10-75, 10-76, 10-77, 10-78, 10-79, 10-80, 10-81, 10-84, 10-91, 10-94, 10-97, 10-98, 10-100, 10-101, 10-102, 10-105, 10-107, 10-108, 10-120, 10-192, 11-16, Appendix-1, Appendix-2, Appendix-3, Appendix-4, Appendix-6, Appendix-8, Appendix-9, Appendix-11, Appendix-12, Appendix-13, Appendix-15, Appendix-18, Appendix-22, Appendix-24, Appendix-25, Appendix-26, Appendix-38, Appendix-39, Appendix-40, and Appendix-41.

The following figures are courtesy of Robert Kersten, MD: 3-51, 3-62, 3-66.

The following figures are courtesy of Jonathan W. Kim, MD: 1-25, 1-26, and 3-43.

The following figures are courtesy of Douglas D. Koch, MD: 5-30, 5-65, 8-2, 8-20, 8-28, 8-29, 8-30, 8-31, 8-39, 12-8, and 12-14.

The following figures are courtesy of Andrew G. Lee, MD: 2-14, 2-17, 2-27, 7-16, 11-1, and 11-8.

The following figures are courtesy of Peter S. Levin, MD: 1-23, 3-9, 3-30, 3-38, 3-58, 3-60, 3-61, and 3-67.

The following figure is courtesy of Thomas Loarie: 12-13.

The following figure is courtesy of Edward E. Manche, MD: 12-7.

The following figures are courtesy of Timothy J. McCulley, MD: 1-1, 1-5, 1-18, 1-20, 1-21, 1-22, 1-24, 1-30, 1-31, 3-2, 3-4, 3-25, 3-44, 3-45, and 11-24.

The following figure is courtesy of George J. Nakano, MD: 5-87.

The following figures are courtesy of James R. Patrinely, MD: 1-17, 1-27, 3-18, 3-28, 3-31, 3-32, 3-33, 3-35, 3-36, 3-40, 3-42, 3-50, 3-53, 3-54, and 3-55.

The following figures are courtesy of Julian Perry, MD: 3-1 and 3-46.

The following figure is courtesy of Roberto Pineda II, MD: 5-18, Appendix-33, Appendix-36, and Appendix-37.

The following figures are courtesy of David Sarraf, MD and ATul Jain, MD: 10-109, 10-110, 10-230, 10-231, and 10-232.

The following figures are courtesy of Paul G. Steinkuller, MD: 1-19, 2-5, 2-6, and 12-1.

The following figures are courtesy of Christopher N. Ta, MD: 3-15, 3-26, 3-27, 4-10, 4-22, 4-23, 4-24, 5-1, 5-23, 5-54, 5-59, 5-77, 7-38, and 12-2.

Introduction

I am pleased to write an introduction to the 3rd edition of the *MEEI Illustrated Manual of Ophthalmology*. This edition continues the tradition of excellence forged by its authors in the first two editions. Drs. Friedman, Kaiser, and Pineda have provided us with an accessible, portable, yet comprehensive compendium that optimizes its availability for use by the practitioner.

The new edition takes advantage of the growing importance of our most sophisticated technologies, such as optical coherence tomography (OCT), computed tomography (CT), and magnetic resonance imaging (MRI) while maintaining its logical organization and clarity of description. It serves as both a valuable teaching tool and a standard reference for the practicing clinician.

The authors, all of whom trained at Harvard Medical School as students or residents and fellows, embody the best of the clinician–teacher paradigm. While research – basic, translation, and clinical – moves our practice forward, the skill to imbue this knowledge to successive generations of ophthalmologists is critical. We are grateful for their erudition, judgment, and, above all, hard work in updating this classic text.

Joan W. Miller, MD
Henry Willard Williams Professor of Ophthalmology and Chair
Harvard Medical School
Chief of Ophthalmology, Massachusetts Eye and Ear Infirmary

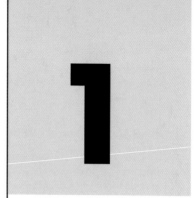

Trauma	3
Globe Subluxation	9
Carotid-Cavernous and Dural Sinus Fistulas	10
Infections	12
Inflammation	15
Congenital Anomalies	19
Pediatric Orbital Tumors	21
Adult Orbital Tumors	26
Acquired Anophthalmia	31
Atrophia Bulbi and Phthisis Bulbi	32

Orbit

Trauma

Blunt Trauma

Orbital Contusion

Periocular bruising caused by blunt trauma; often with injury to the globe, paranasal sinuses, and bony socket; traumatic optic neuropathy or orbital hemorrhage may be present. Patients report pain and may have decreased vision. Signs include lid edema and ecchymosis, and ptosis. Isolated contusion is a preseptal (eyelid) injury and typically resolves without sequelae. Traumatic ptosis secondary to levator muscle contusion may take up to 3 months to resolve; most oculoplastic surgeons observe for 6 months prior to surgical repair.

Figure 1-1 • Orbit contusion demonstrating severe eyelid ecchymosis and edema, subconjunctival hemorrhage and conjunctival chemosis.

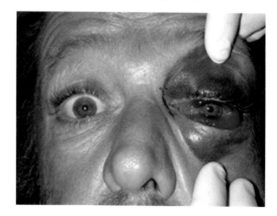

- In the absence of orbital signs (afferent pupillary defect, visual field defect, limited extraocular motility, and proptosis) imaging studies are not necessarily required, but should be considered with more serious mechanisms of injury (e.g., motor vehicle accident [MVA], massive trauma, or loss of consciousness) even in the absence of orbital signs. When indicated, orbital computed tomography (CT) scan is the imaging study of choice.

- When the globe is intact and vision unaffected, ice compresses can be used every hour for 20 minutes during the first 48 hours to decrease swelling.
- Concomitant injuries should be treated accordingly.

Orbital Hemorrhage/Orbital Compartment Syndrome

Accumulation of blood throughout the intraorbital tissues due to surgery or trauma (retrobulbar hemorrhage) may cause proptosis, distortion of the globe, and optic nerve stretching and compression (orbital compartment syndrome). Patients may report pain and decreased vision. Signs include bullous, subconjunctival hemorrhage, tense orbit, proptosis, resistance to retropulsion of globe, limitation of ocular movements, lid ecchymosis, and increased intraocular pressure. Immediate recognition and treatment is critical in determining outcome. Urgent treatment measures may include canthotomy and cantholysis. Evacuation of focal hematomas or bony decompression is reserved for the most severe cases with an associated optic neuropathy.

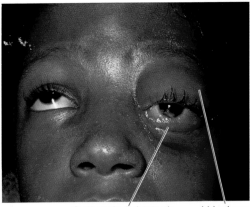

Figure 1-2 • Retrobulbar hemorrhage of the left eye demonstrating proptosis, lid swelling, chemosis, and restricted extraocular motility on upgaze.

Conjunctival chemosis   Lid edema

OPHTHALMIC EMERGENCY

- If orbital compartment syndrome is suspected, lateral canthotomy and cantholysis should be performed emergently.
- **Lateral canthotomy:** This procedure is performed by compressing the lateral canthus with a hemostat, and Stevens scissors are then used to make a full-thickness incision from the lateral commissure (lateral angle of the eyelids) posterolaterally to the lateral orbital rim. Some advocate compression of the lateral canthal tendon prior to incision. The inferior crus of the lateral canthal tendon is then transected by elevating the lateral lower lid margin away from the face, placing the scissors between the cut edges of lower lid conjunctiva and lower lid skin, palpating the tendon with the tips of the scissors, and transecting it. If the inferior eyelid is not extremely mobile, the inferior crus has not been transected adequately and the procedure should be repeated. If the intraocular pressure remains elevated and the orbit remains tense, the superior crus of the lateral canthal tendon may be cut. Septolysis, blunt dissection through the orbital

septum at the base of the cantholysis incision, may be performed when pressure is not adequately relieved with lysis of the canthal tendon.

- Emergent inferior orbital floor fracture, while advocated by some, is fraught with complications and is not advised for surgeons with little experience in orbital surgery; however, it should be considered in emergent situations with risk of blindness.

- Canthoplasty can be scheduled electively approximately 1 week after the hemorrhage.

- Orbital CT scan (without contrast, direct coronal and axial views, 3-mm slices) once visual status has been determined and emergent treatment (if necessary) administered (i.e., after canthotomy and cantholysis). Magnetic resonance imaging (MRI) is *contraindicated* in acute trauma.

- If vision is stable and intraocular pressure is elevated (>25 mmHg), topical hypotensive agents may be administered (brimonidine 0.15% [Alphagan P] 1 gtt tid, timolol 0.5% 1 gtt bid, and/or dorzolamide 2% [Trusopt] 1 gtt tid).

Orbital Fractures

Fracture of the orbital walls may occur in isolation (e.g., blow-out fracture) or with displaced or nondisplaced orbital-rim fractures. There may be concomitant ocular, optic nerve, maxillary, mandibular, or intracranial injuries.

Orbital floor (blow-out) fracture

This is the most common orbital fracture requiring repair and usually involves the maxillary bone in the posterior medial floor (weakest point), and may extend laterally to the infraorbital canal. Orbital contents may prolapse or become entrapped in maxillary sinus. Signs and symptoms include diplopia on upgaze (anterior fracture) or downgaze (posterior fracture), enophthalmos, globe ptosis, and infraorbital nerve hypesthesia. Orbital and lid emphysema is often present and may become extensive with nose blowing.

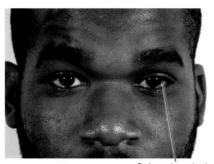
Subconjunctival hemorrhage

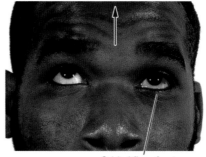
Orbital floor fracture with entrapment

Figure 1-3 • Orbital floor blow-out fracture with enophthalmos and globe dystopia and ptosis of the left eye.

Figure 1-4 • Same patient as Figure 1-3 demonstrating entrapment of the left inferior rectus and inability to look up.

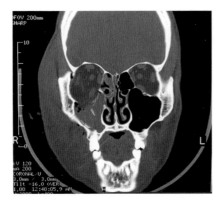

Figure 1-5 • Orbital CT demonstrating large right orbital floor fracture.

- For mild trauma, orbital CT scan need not be obtained in the absence of orbital signs.
- Orbital surgery consultation should be considered especially in the setting of diplopia, large floor fractures that are prone to enophthalmos, trismus, facial asymmetry, inferior rectus entrapment, and enophthalmos. Consider surgical repair after 1 week to allow for reduction of swelling, except in cases of pediatric trapdoor type fractures with extraocular muscle entrapment where emergent repair is advocated.

Pediatric floor fracture

This differs significantly from an adult fracture because the bones are pliable rather than brittle. A "trapdoor" phenomenon is created where the inferior rectus muscle or perimuscular tissue can be entrapped in the fracture site. In this case, enophthalmos is unlikely, but ocular motility is limited dramatically. The globe halts abruptly with ductions opposite the entrapped muscle (most often on upgaze with inferior rectus involvement) as if it is "tethered." Forced ductions are positive; nausea and bradycardia (oculocardiac reflex) are common. Despite the severity of the underlying injury, the eye is typically quiet, hence the nickname "white eyed blowout fracture."

- Urgent surgery (<24 hours) is indicated in pediatric cases with entrapment.

Medial wall (nasoethmoidal) fracture

This involves the lacrimal and ethmoid (lamina papyracea) bones. It is occasionally associated with depressed nasal fracture, traumatic telecanthus (in severe cases), and orbital floor fracture. Complications include nasolacrimal duct injury, severe epistaxis due to anterior ethmoidal artery damage, and orbit and lid emphysema. Medial rectus entrapment is rare, and enophthalmos due to isolated medial wall fractures is extremely uncommon.

- Fractures extending through the nasolacrimal duct should be reduced with stenting of the drainage system. If not repaired primarily, persistent obstruction requiring dacryocystorhinostomy may result.
- Otolaryngology consultation is indicated in the presence of nasal fractures.

Orbital roof fracture

This is an uncommon fracture usually secondary to blunt or projectile injuries. It may involve the frontal sinus, cribriform plate, and brain. It may be associated with cerebrospinal fluid (CSF) rhinorrhea or pneumocephalus.

* Neurosurgery and otolaryngology consultations are advised, especially in the presence of CSF rhinorrhea or pneumocephalus.

Orbital apex fracture

This may be associated with other facial fractures and involve optic canal and superior orbital fissure. Direct traumatic optic neuropathy is likely. Complications include carotid-cavernous fistula and fragments impinging on optic nerve. These are difficult to manage due to proximity of multiple cranial nerves and vessels.

* Obvious impingement by a displaced fracture on the optic nerve may require immediate surgical intervention by an oculoplastic surgeon or neurosurgeon. High-dose systemic steroids may be given for traumatic optic neuropathy (see Chapter 11).

Tripod fracture

This involves three fracture sites: the inferior orbital rim (maxilla), lateral orbital rim (often at the zygomaticofrontal suture), and zygomatic arch. The fracture invariably extends through the orbit floor. Patients may report pain, tenderness, binocular diplopia, and trismus (pain on open-ing mouth or chewing). Signs include orbital rim discontinuity or palpable "step off", malar flattening, enophthalmos, infraorbital nerve hypesthesia, orbital, conjunctival or lid emphysema, limitation of ocular movements, epistaxis, rhinorrhea, ecchymosis, and ptosis. Enophthalmos may not be appreciated on exophthalmometry due to retrodisplaced lateral orbital rim.

Le Fort fractures

These are severe maxillary fractures with the common feature of extension through the pterygoid plates:

Le Fort I low transverse maxillary bone; no orbital involvement.

Le Fort II nasal, lacrimal, and maxillary bones (medial orbital wall), as well as bones of the orbital floor and rim; may involve nasolacrimal duct.

Le Fort III extends through the medial wall, traverses the orbital floor, and through the lateral wall (craniofacial dysjunction); may involve optic canal.

* Orbital CT scan (without contrast, direct axial and coronal views, 3-mm slices) is indicated in the presence of orbital signs (afferent papillary defect, diplopia, limited extraocular motil-ity, proptosis, and enophthalmos) or ominous mechanism of injury (e.g., MVA, massive facial trauma). MRI is of limited usefulness in the evaluation of fractures as bones appear dark.

* Otolaryngology consultation is indicated in the presence of mandibular fracture.

* Orbital surgery consultation is indicated in the presence of isolated orbital and trimalar fractures.

* Instruct patient to avoid blowing nose. "Suck-and-spit" technique should be used to clear nasal secretions.

* Nasal decongestant (oxymetazoline hydrochloride [Afrin nasal spray] bid as needed for 3 days; Note: may cause urinary retention in men with prostatic hypertrophy).

- Ice compresses for first 48 hours.
- Systemic oral antibiotic (amoxicillin-clavulanate [Augmentin] 250–500 mg po tid for 10 days) are advocated by some.
- Nondisplaced zygomatic fractures may become displaced after initial evaluation due to masseter and temporalis contraction. Orbital or otolaryngology consultation is indicated for evaluation of such patients.

Penetrating Trauma

These may result from either a projectile (e.g., pellet gun) or stab (e.g., knife, tree branch) injury. Foreign body should be suspected even in the absence of significant external wounds.

Intraorbital Foreign Body

Retained orbital foreign body with or without associated ocular and optic nerve involvement. Inert foreign body (FB) (e.g., glass, lead, BB, plastics) may be well tolerated, and should be evaluated by an oculoplastic surgeon in a controlled setting. Organic matter carries significant risk of infection and should be removed surgically. Long-standing iron FB can produce iron toxicity (siderosis) including retinopathy.

Patients may be asymptomatic or may report pain or decreased vision. Critical signs include eyelid or conjunctival laceration. Other signs may include ecchymosis, lid edema and erythema, conjunctival hemorrhage or chemosis, proptosis, limitation of ocular movements, and chorioretinitis sclopetaria (see Fig. 10.7). A relative afferent pupillary defect (RAPD) may be present. Prognosis is generally good if the globe and optic nerve are not affected.

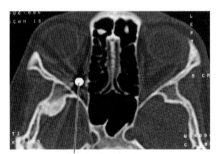

Intraorbital foreign body

Figure 1-6 • Orbital CT demonstrating foreign body (BB) at the orbital apex.

- Precise history (may be necessary to isolate a minor child from the parents while obtaining history) is critical in determining the nature of any potential FB.
- Orbital CT scan (without contrast, direct coronal and axial views, 1.5-mm to 3-mm slices depending on suspected FB) to determine character and position of foreign body. MRI is *contraindicated* if foreign body is metallic.
- **Lab tests**: Culture entry wound for bacteria and fungus. Serum lead levels should be monitored in patients with a retained lead foreign body.
- If there is no ocular or optic nerve injury, small inert foreign bodies posterior to the equator of the globe usually are not removed but observed.
- Patients are placed on systemic oral antibiotic (amoxicillin-clavulanate [Augmentin] 500 mg po tid for 10 days) and are followed up the next day.

- Tetanus booster (tetanus toxoid 0.5 mL IM) if necessary for prophylaxis (>7 years since last tetanus shot or if status is unknown).
- Indications for surgical removal include fistula formation, infection, optic nerve compression, large foreign body, or easily removable foreign body (usually anterior to the equator of the globe). Surgery should be performed by an orbital surgeon. Organic material should be removed more urgently.

Globe Subluxation

Definition Spontaneous forward displacement of the eye so that the equator of the globe protrudes in front of the eyelids, which retract behind the eye.

Etiology Most often spontaneous in patients with proptosis (e.g., Graves' disease), but may be voluntary or traumatic.

Mechanism Pressure against the globe, typically from spreading the eyelids, causes the eye to move forward, and then when a blink occurs, the eyelids contract behind the eye locking the globe in a subluxed position.

Epidemiology Occurs in individuals of any age (range 11 months to 73 years) and has no sex or race predilection. Risk factors include eyelid manipulation, exophthalmos, severe eyelid retraction, floppy eyelid syndrome, thyroid-related ophthalmopathy, and shallow orbits (i.e., Crouzon's syndrome).

Symptoms Asymptomatic; may have pain, blurred vision, and anxiety.

Signs Dramatic proptosis of the eye beyond the eyelids. Depending on the length of time the globe has been subluxed, may have exposure keratopathy, corneal abrasions, blepharospasm, and optic neuropathy.

Figure 1-7 • Globe subluxation with equator of globe and lacrimal gland in front of the eyelids.

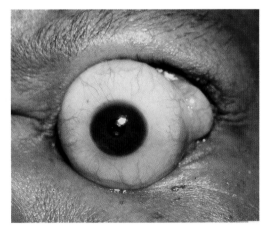

Evaluation
- Complete ophthalmic history with attention to previous episodes and potential triggers.
- Complete eye exam (after the eye has been repositioned) with attention to visual acuity, pupils, motility, exophthalmometry, lids, cornea, and ophthalmoscopy.

Management

- Immediately reposition the globe. Relax the patient, instill topical anesthetic, and digitally reduce the subluxation by one of the following methods:
    (1) While patient looks down, pull the upper eyelid up and depress the globe.
    (2) Place a retractor under the center of the upper eyelid, push the globe downward and advance the eyelid forward, once the eyelid is past the equator of the globe, have the patient look up to pull the eyelid over the eye.
- May require a facial nerve block, sedation, or general anesthesia.
- Instruct the patient to avoid triggers and how to reduce a subluxation.
- Treat any underlying condition.
- Surgical options include partial tarsorrhaphy and orbital decompression.

Prognosis   Good unless complications develop.

Carotid-Cavernous and Dural Sinus Fistulas

Definition   Arterial venous connection between the carotid artery and cavernous sinus; there are two types:

High-Flow Fistula

Between the cavernous sinus and internal carotid artery (carotid-cavernous fistula)

Low-Flow Fistula

Between small meningeal arterial branches and the dural walls of the cavernous sinus (dural sinus fistula).

Etiology

High-Flow Fistula

Spontaneous; occurs in patients with atherosclerosis and hypertension with carotid aneurysms that rupture within the sinus, or secondary to closed head trauma (basal skull fracture).

Low-Flow Fistula

Slower onset compared with the carotid-cavernous variant; dural sinus fistula is more likely to present spontaneously.

Symptoms   May hear a "swishing" noise (venous souffle); may have red "bulging" eye.

Signs

High-Flow Fistula

May have orbital bruit, pulsating proptosis, chemosis, epibulbar injection and vascular tortuosity (conjunctival corkscrew vessels), congested retinal vessels, and increased intraocular pressure.

Low-Flow Fistula

Mild proptosis and orbital congestion. However, in more severe cases findings similar to those described for carotid-cavernous fistula may occur.

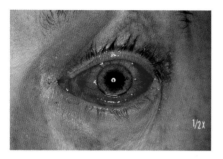

Figure 1-8 • Carotid-cavernous fistula with conjunctival injection and chemosis.

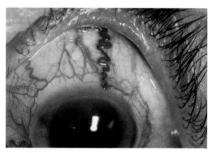

Figure 1-9 • Carotid-cavernous fistula with dilated, corkscrew, episcleral, and conjunctival vessels.

Differential Diagnosis Orbital varices that expand in a dependent position or during Valsalva maneuvers and may produce hemorrhage with minimal trauma. Carotid-cavernous fistula may also be mistaken for orbital inflammatory syndrome and occasionally uveitis.

Evaluation
- Complete history with attention to onset and duration of symptoms, and history of trauma and systemic diseases (atherosclerosis, hypertension).
- Complete eye exam with attention to orbital auscultation, exophthalmometry, conjunctiva, tonometry, and ophthalmoscopy.
- Orbital CT scan or MRI: Enlargement of superior ophthalmic vein.
- Arteriography usually is required to identify the fistula; CTA and MRA have largely replaced conventional angiography.

Management

- Consider treatment with selective embolization or ligation for severely symptomatic patients (uncontrolled increase in intraocular pressure, severe proptosis, retinal ischemia, optic neuropathy, severe bruit, involvement of the cortical veins).
- Treatment for all cases of carotid-cavernous fistula has been advocated but is controversial.

Prognosis Up to 70% of dural sinus fistulas may resolve spontaneously.

| Infections

Preseptal Cellulitis

Definition Infection of the eyelids not extending posterior to the orbital septum. The globe and orbit are not involved.

Etiology Usually follows periorbital trauma or dermal infection. Suspect *Staphylococcus aureus* in traumatic cases. *Haemophilus influenzae* in children less than 5 years old is uncommon now that they receive *H. influenzae* vaccination.

Symptoms Eyelid swelling, redness, ptosis, and pain; low-grade fever.

Signs Eyelid erythema, edema, ptosis, and warmth (may be quite dramatic); visual acuity is normal; full ocular motility without pain; no proptosis; the conjunctiva and sclera appear uninflamed; an inconspicuous lid wound may be visible; an abscess may be present.

Differential Diagnosis Orbital cellulitis, idiopathic orbital inflammation, dacryoadenitis,

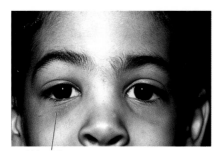

Lid erythema

Figure 1-10 • Mild preseptal cellulitis with right eyelid erythema in a young child.

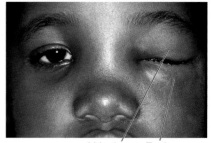

Lid edema   Erythema

Figure 1-11 • Moderate preseptal cellulitis with left eyelid edema and erythema.

dacryocystitis, conjunctivitis, and trauma.

Evaluation
- Complete ophthalmic history with attention to trauma, sinus disease, recent dental work or infections, history of diabetes or immunosuppression.
- Complete eye exam with attention to visual acuity, color vision, pupils, motility, exophthalmometry, lids, conjunctiva, and sclera.
- Check vital signs, head and neck lymph nodes, meningeal signs (nuchal rigidity), and sensorium.
- Orbital and sinus CT scan in the absence of trauma or in the presence of orbital signs to look for orbital extension and paranasal sinus opacification.
- **Lab tests**: Complete blood count (CBC) with differential, blood cultures; wound culture if present.

Management

MILD PRESEPTAL CELLULITIS

- Systemic oral antibiotic:
  - Amoxicillin-clavulanate (Augmentin) 250–500 mg po tid or
  - Cefaclor (Ceclor) 250–500 mg po tid or
  - Trimethoprim-sulfamethoxazole (Bactrim) 1 double-strength tablet po bid, in penicillin-allergic patients.
- Topical antibiotic (bacitracin or erythromycin ointment qid) for concurrent conjunctivitis.
- Eyelid abscess should be drained (avoid injury to the orbital septum and levator aponeurosis).

MODERATE-TO-SEVERE PRESEPTAL CELLULITIS

- Systemic intravenous antibiotic:
  - Cefuroxime 1 g IV q8h or
  - Ampicillin-sulbactam (Unasyn) 1.5–3.0 g IV q6h.
- Systemic intravenous treatment also indicated for septic patients, outpatient noncompliant patients, children less than 5 years old, and patients who fail oral antibiotic treatment after 48 hours.
- Daily follow-up in all cases until improvement noted.

Prognosis Usually good when treated early.

Orbital Cellulitis

Definition Infection extending posterior to the orbital septum. May occur in combination with preseptal cellulitis.

Etiology Most commonly secondary to ethmoid sinusitis. May also result from frontal, maxillary, or sphenoid infection. Other causes include dacryocystitis, dental caries, intracranial infections, trauma, and orbital surgery. *Streptococcus* and *Staphylococcus* species are most common isolates. *Haemophilus influenzae* is uncommon in children under 5 years old now that they receive *H. influenzae* vaccination. Fungi in the group *Phycomycetes* (*Absidia*, *Mucor*, or *Rhizopus*) are the most common causes of fungal orbital infection causing necrosis, vascular thrombosis, and orbital invasion. Fungal infections usually occur in immunocompromised patients (e.g., those with diabetes mellitus, metabolic acidosis, malignancy, or iatrogenic immunosuppression); and can be fatal due to intracranial spread.

Symptoms Decreased vision, pain, red eye, headache, diplopia, "bulging" eye, lid swelling, and fever.

Signs Decreased visual acuity, fever, lid edema, erythema, and tenderness, limitation of or pain on extraocular movements, proptosis, relative afferent pupillary defect, conjunctival injection and chemosis; may have optic disc swelling; fungal infection usually manifests with proptosis and orbital apex syndrome (see Chapter 2). The involvement of multiple cranial nerves suggests extension posteriorly to the orbital apex and/or cavernous sinus.

Lid edema/erythema

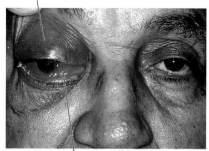

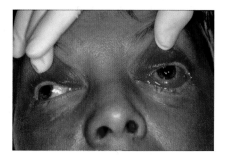

Conjunctival chemosis/injection

Figure 1-12 • Orbital cellulitis with right-sided proptosis, lid edema and erythema, conjunctival injection and chemosis, and right exotropia (note decentered right corneal light reflex at the limbus).

Figure 1-13 • Mucormycosis of the left orbit with eyelid edema, conjunctival injection, chemosis, and gaze restriction.

Differential Diagnosis Thyroid-related ophthalmopathy (adults), idiopathic orbital inflammation, subperiosteal abscess, orbital neoplasm (e.g., rhabdomyosarcoma, lymphoproliferative disease, ruptured dermoid cyst), orbital vasculitis, trauma, carotid-cavernous fistula, and cavernous sinus thrombosis.

Evaluation
- Complete ophthalmic history with attention to trauma, sinus disease, recent dental work or infections, history of diabetes or immunosuppression.
- Complete eye exam with attention to visual acuity, color vision, pupils, motility, exophthalmometry, lids, conjunctiva, cornea (including corneal sensitivity), CN V sensation, and ophthalmoscopy.
- Check vital signs, head and neck lymph nodes, meningeal signs (nuchal rigidity), and sensorium. Look in the mouth for evidence of fungal involvement.
- CT scan of orbits and paranasal sinuses (with contrast, direct coronal and axial views, 3-mm slices) to look for sinus opacification or abscess.
- **Lab tests:** CBC with differential, blood cultures (results usually negative in phycomycosis); culture wound, if present.

Management

- Systemic intravenous antibiotic (1-week course):
  - Nafcillin 1–2 g IV q4h and ceftriaxone 1–2 g IV q12–24h *or*
  - Ampicillin-sulbactam (Unasyn) 1.5–3.0 g IV q6h.
- Topical antibiotic (bacitracin or erythromycin ointment qid) for conjunctivitis or corneal exposure.
- Daily follow-up required to monitor visual acuity, color vision (red desaturation), ocular movements, proptosis, intraocular pressure, cornea, and optic nerve.
- Systemic oral antibiotic (10-day course) after improvement on intravenous therapy:
  - Amoxicillin-clavulanate (Augmentin) 250–500 mg po tid *or*
  - Cefaclor (Ceclor) 250–500 mg po tid *or*
  - Trimethoprim-sulfamethoxazole (Bactrim) 1 double-strength tablet po bid in penicillin-allergic patients.
- Subperiosteal abscess requires urgent referral to an oculoplastic surgeon for close observation and possible surgical drainage.
- Otolaryngology consultation is indicated to obtain tissue diagnosis for opacified sinuses and if phycomycosis suspected.
- Diabetic or immunocompromised patients are at high risk for phycomycosis (mucormycosis). Given the very high mortality rate, the patients require emergent debridement and biopsy, systemic intravenous antifungal (amphotericin B 0.25–1.0 mg/kg IV divided equally q6h), and management of underlying medical disorders.

Prognosis Depends on organism and extent of disease at the time of presentation. May develop orbital apex syndrome, cavernous sinus thrombosis, meningitis, or permanent neurologic deficits. Mucormycosis in particular may be fatal.

Inflammation

Thyroid-Related Ophthalmopathy

Definition An immune-mediated disorder usually occurring in conjunction with Graves' disease that causes a spectrum of ocular abnormalities. Also called dysthyroid orbitopathy or ophthalmopathy or Graves' ophthalmopathy.

Epidemiology Most common cause of unilateral or bilateral proptosis in adults; female predilection (8:1); >90% of patients have abnormal thyroid function test results; hyperthyroidism is most common (93%), although patients may be hypothyroid (6%) or euthyroid (1%); 1% of patients have or will develop myasthenia gravis. Cigarette smoking is a risk factor for thyroid disease and greatly increases the incidence of thyroid-related ophthalmopathy (TRO) in patients with Graves' disease.

Symptoms

Note: Signs and symptoms reflect four clinical components of this disease process as follows: eyelid disorders, eye surface disorders, ocular motility disorders, and optic neuropathy.

May have red eye, foreign-body sensation, tearing, decreased vision, dyschromatopsia, binocular diplopia, or prominent ("bulging") eyes.

Signs Eyelid retraction, edema, lagophthalmos, lid lag (von Graefe's sign), reduced blinking, superficial keratopathy, conjunctival injection, exophthalmos, limitation of extraocular movements (supraduction most common reflecting inferior rectus involvement), positive forced ductions, resistance to retropulsion of globe, decreased visual acuity and color vision, relative afferent papillary defect, and visual field defect. A minority of cases may have acute congestion of the socket and periocular tissues.

The Werner Classification of Eye Findings in Graves' Disease ("NO SPECS") is:

No signs or symptoms

Only signs

Soft tissue involvement (signs and symptoms)

Proptosis

Extraocular muscle involvement

Corneal involvement

Sight loss (optic nerve compression).

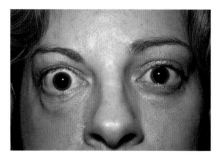

Figure 1-14 • Thyroid ophthalmopathy with proptosis, lid retraction, and superior and inferior scleral show of the right eye.

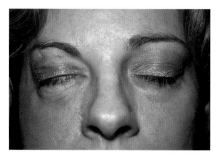

Figure 1-15 • Same patient as Figure 1-14, demonstrating lagophthalmos on the right side with eyelid closure (note the small incomplete closure of the right eyelids).

Differential Diagnosis Idiopathic orbital inflammation, orbital and lacrimal gland tumors, orbital vasculitis, trauma, cellulitis, arteriovenous fistula, cavernous sinus thrombosis, gaze palsy, cranial nerve palsy, and physiologic exophthalmos.

Evaluation

- Complete ophthalmic history with attention to history of thyroid disease, autoimmune disease, or cancer; history of hyperthyroid symptoms such as heat intolerance, weight loss, palpitations, sweating, and irritability.
- Complete eye exam with attention to cranial nerves, visual acuity, color vision, pupils, motility, forced ductions, exophthalmometry, lids, cornea, tonometry, and ophthalmoscopy.
- Check visual fields as a baseline study in early cases and to rule out optic neuropathy in advanced cases.

- **Lab tests**: Thyroid function tests (thyroid stimulating hormone [TSH], thyroxine [total and free T4], and triiodothyronine [T3], and thyroid stimulating immunoglobulin [TSI]).
- Orbital CT scan (with contrast, direct coronal and axial views, 3-mm slices): Extraocular muscle enlargement with sparing of the tendons; inferior rectus is most commonly involved, followed by medial, superior, and lateral.
- Endocrinology consultation.

Management

- Surgical interventions are deferred until a 9–12-month stable interval is recorded, except in cases of optic neuropathy or extreme proptosis causing severe exposure keratopathy.
- After an adequate quiescent interval, surgery proceeds in a stepwise fashion, moving posteriorly to anteriorly: orbital bony decompression, strabismus surgery, then eyelid reconstruction as indicated.
- Underlying thyroid disease should be managed by an endocrinologist.

EXPOSURE
- Topical lubrication with artificial tears (see Appendix) up to q1h while awake and ointment (Refresh PM) qhs.
- Consider lid taping or moisture chamber goggles at bedtime.
- Punctal occlusion for more severe dry eye symptoms.
- Permanent lateral tarsorrhaphy or canthorrhaphy is useful in cases of lateral chemosis or widened lateral palpebral fissure.

EYELID RETRACTION
- Surgical eyelid recession (lengthening) after an adequate stable interval.

DIPLOPIA
- Oral steroids (prednisone 80–100 mg po qd for 1–2 weeks, then taper over 1 month) are controversial.
- Fresnel (temporary) prisms.
- Strabismus surgery (rectus muscle recessions) considered after a 6-month stable interval and after orbital surgery completed.

OPTIC NEUROPATHY
- Immediate treatment with oral steroids (prednisone 100 mg po qd for 2–14 days).
- The use of external beam irradiation (15–30 Gy) is controversial and falling out of favor.
- Orbital decompression for compressive optic neuropathy should be performed by an oculoplastic surgeon. A balanced approach with decompression of the medial and lateral orbital walls is most commonly employed. Removal of the inferior wall is avoided if possible due to higher incidence of induced diplopia.

Prognosis Diplopia and ocular surface disease are common; 6% develop optic nerve disease. Despite surgical rehabilitation, which may require multiple procedures, patients are often left with functional and cosmetic deficits.

Idiopathic Orbital Inflammation (Orbital Pseudotumor)

Definition Acute or chronic idiopathic inflammatory disorder of the orbital tissues sometimes collectively termed orbital pseudotumor. Any of the orbital tissues may be involved: lacrimal gland (dacryoadenitis), extraocular muscles (myositis), sclera (scleritis), optic nerve sheath (optic perineuritis), and orbital fat.

Tolosa–Hunt syndrome is a form of idiopathic orbital inflammation (IOI) involving the orbital apex and/or anterior cavernous sinus that produces painful external ophthalmoplegia.

Epidemiology Occurs in all age groups; usually unilateral, although bilateral disease is more common in children; adults require evaluation for systemic vasculitis (e.g., Wegener's granulomatosis, polyarteritis nodosa) or lymphoproliferative disorders.

Symptoms Acute onset of orbital pain, decreased vision, binocular diplopia, red eye, headaches, and constitutional symptoms. (Constitutional symptoms including fever, nausea, and vomiting are present in 50% of children.)

Signs Marked tenderness of involved region, lid edema and erythema, lacrimal gland enlargement, limitation of and pain on extraocular movements (myositis), positive forced ductions, proptosis, resistance to retropulsion of globe, induced hyperopia, conjunctival chemosis, reduced corneal sensation (due to CN V_1 involvement), increased intraocular pressure; papillitis or iritis may occur and are more common in children.

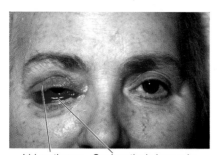

Lid erythema   Conjunctival chemosis

Figure 1-16 • Idiopathic orbital inflammation of the right orbit with lid edema, ptosis, and chemosis.

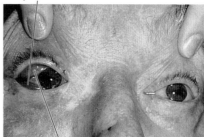

Conjunctival chemosis

Lacrimal gland enlargement

Figure 1-17 • Idiopathic orbital inflammation of the right orbit with lacrimal gland involvement. Note the swollen, prolapsed, lacrimal gland superiorly.

Differential Diagnosis Thyroid-related ophthalmopathy, orbital cellulitis, orbital tumors, lacrimal gland tumors, orbital vasculitis, trauma, cavernous sinus thrombosis, cranial nerve palsy, and herpes zoster ophthalmicus.

Evaluation

- Complete ophthalmic history with attention to previous episodes and history of cancer or other systemic disease.
- Complete eye exam with attention to eyelid and orbital palpation, pupils, motility, forced ductions, exophthalmometry, lids, cornea, tonometry, and ophthalmoscopy.
- **Lab tests** for bilateral or unusual cases (vasculitis suspected): CBC with differential, erythrocyte sedimentation rate (ESR), antinuclear antibodies (ANA), blood urea nitrogen (BUN), creatinine, fasting blood glucose, antineutrophil cytoplasmic antibodies (ANCA), angiotensin converting enzyme (ACE), and urinalysis.
- Orbital CT scan: Thickened, enhancing sclera (ring sign), extraocular muscle enlargement with involvement of the tendons, and/or lacrimal gland involvement, diffuse inflammation with streaking of orbital fat.
- Consider orbital biopsy for steroid-unresponsive, recurrent, or unusual cases.

Management

- Oral steroids (prednisone 80–100 mg po qd for 1 week, then taper slowly over 6 weeks); check purified protein derivative (PPD) and controls, blood glucose, and chest radiographs before starting systemic steroids.
- Add H_2-blocker (ranitidine HCl [Zantac] 150 mg po bid) or proton pump inhibitor when administering systemic steroids.
- Topical steroid (prednisolone acetate 1% up to q2h initially, then taper over 3–4 weeks) if iritis present.
- Patients should respond dramatically to systemic corticosteroids within 24–48 hours. Failure to do so strongly suggests another diagnosis.

Prognosis Generally good for acute disease, although recurrences are common. The sclerosing form of this disorder has a more insidious onset and is often less responsive to treatment.

Congenital Anomalies

Usually occur in developmental syndromes, rarely in isolation.

Congenital Anophthalmia

Absence of globe with normal-appearing eyelids due to failure of optic vesicle formation; extraocular muscles are present and insert abnormally into orbital soft tissue. Extremely rare condition that produces a hypoplastic orbit that becomes accentuated with contralateral hemifacial maturation. Usually bilateral and sporadic. Characteristic "purse stringing" of the orbital rim. Orbital CT, ultrasonography, and examination under anesthesia are required to make the diagnosis. In most cases, a rudimentary globe is present but not identifiable short of post-mortem sectioning of the orbital contents.

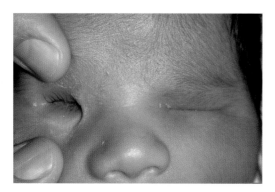

Figure 1-18 • Congenital anophthalmia demonstrating absence of globe with normal eyelids and lashes.

Microphthalmos

Small, malformed eye due to disruption of development after optic vesicle forms. More common than anophthalmos and presents similar orbital challenges. Usually unilateral and recessive. Associated with cataract, glaucoma, aniridia, coloboma, and systemic abnormalities including polydactyly, syndactyly, clubfoot, polycystic kidneys, cystic liver, cleft palate, and meningoencephalocele. True anophthalmia and severe microphthalmia can be differentiated only on histologic examination.

Microphthalmos with Cyst

Disorganized, cystic eye due to failure of embryonic fissure to close. Appears as blue mass in lower eyelid. Associated with various conditions including rubella, toxoplasmosis, maternal vitamin A deficiency, maternal thalidomide ingestion, trisomy 13, trisomy 15, and chromosome 18 deletion.

• Treatment is aimed at progressive orbital expansion for facial symmetry and includes serial orbital implants requiring multiple orbitotomies over the first several years of life, expandable orbital implants, and serial conjunctival conformers. Avoid enucleation in cases of microphthalmos.

• Age of orbital maturation is not known, but elective enucleation should be deferred in early childhood. Enucleation before the age of 9 years old may produce significant orbital asymmetry (radiographically estimated deficiency up to 15%), while enucleation after 9 years old leads to no appreciable asymmetry.

• Reconstructive surgery can be undertaken after the first decade of life.

Nanophthalmos

Small eye (axial length <20.5 mm) with normal structures; lens is normal in size but sclera is thickened. Associated with hyperopia and angle-closure glaucoma, and increased risk of choroidal effusion during intraocular surgery.

Craniofacial Disorders

Midfacial clefting syndromes can involve the medial superior or medial inferior orbit (sometimes with meningoencephalocele) and can produce hypertelorism (increased bony expanse between the medial walls of the orbit). Hypertelorism also occurs in craniosynostoses such as Crouzon's syndrome (craniofacial dysostosis) and Apert's syndrome (arachnoencephalo-dactyly) in which there is premature closure of cranial sutures. Exorbitism and lateral canthal dystopia are also found in these syndromes.

- Craniofacial surgery by an experienced oculoplastic surgeon.

Pediatric Orbital Tumors

Benign Pediatric Orbital Tumors
Orbital Dermoid (Dermoid Cyst)

Common, benign, palpable, smooth, painless choristoma composed of connective tissue and containing dermal adnexal structures including sebaceous glands and hair follicles. Most common pediatric orbital tumor. Usually manifests in childhood (90% in first decade) and may enlarge slowly. Most common location is superotemporal at the zygomatico-frontal suture. Symptoms include ptosis, proptosis, and diplopia. There may be components external or internal to the orbit, or both ("dumb-bell" dermoid).

Figure 1-19 • Dermoid cyst of the right orbit appearing as a mass at the lateral orbital rim. Also note the epicanthus causing pseudostrabismus.

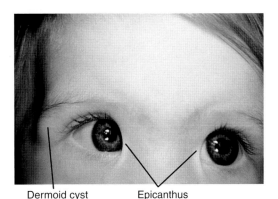

Dermoid cyst   Epicanthus

- Orbital CT scan (with contrast, direct coronal and axial views, 3-mm slices): Well-circumscribed, cystic mass with bony molding.
- Complete surgical excision; preserve capsule and avoid rupturing cyst to avoid recurrence and prevent an acute inflammatory process should be performed by an oculoplastic surgeon.

Lymphangioma

Low-flow malformations misnamed lymphangioma. Benign, nonpigmented choristoma characterized by lymphatic fluid-filled spaces lined by flattened endothelial cells; vascular channels do not contain red blood cells; patients do not produce true lymphatic vessels. May appear blue through the skin. May be associated with head and neck components. Becomes apparent in first decade with an infiltrative growth pattern or with abrupt onset due to hemorrhage within the tumor ("chocolate cyst"). May enlarge during upper respiratory tract infections. Strabismus and amblyopia are common complications. Slow, relentless progression is common; may regress spontaneously.

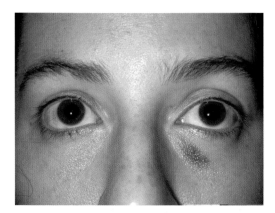

Figure 1-20 • Lymphangioma with subcutaneous hemorrhage of the left lower eyelid.

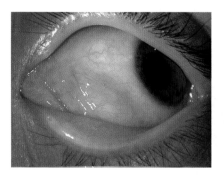

Figure 1-21 • Lymphangioma with anterior component visible as vascular subconjunctival mass at the medial canthus.

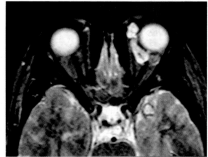

Figure 1-22 • MRI (T2) of same patient as Figure 1-21 demonstrating the irregular cystic appearance of the left orbital lymphangioma.

- CT scan of orbit, paranasal sinuses, and pharynx with contrast: Nonencapsulated, irregular mass with cystic spaces; infiltrative growth pattern.
- Orbital needle aspiration of hemorrhage ("chocolate cysts") or surgical exploration for acute orbital hemorrhage with compressive optic neuropathy.
- Complete surgical excision is usually not possible. Limited excision indicated for ocular damage or severe cosmetic deformities; should be performed by an oculoplastic surgeon. Children should undergo pediatric otolaryngologic examination to rule out airway compromise.

Juvenile Xanthogranuloma

Nevoxanthoendothelioma, composed of histiocytes and Touton giant cells that rarely involve the orbit. Appears between birth and 1 year of age. Associated with yellow–orange cutaneous lesions, and may cause destruction of bone. Spontaneous resolution often occurs.

- Most cases can be observed with frequent spontaneous regression.
- Consider local steroid injection (controversial).
- Surgical excision in the rare case of visual compromise.

Histiocytic Tumors

Initially designated *Histiocytosis X,* the Langerhans' cell histiocytoses comprise a spectrum of related granulomatous diseases that occur most frequently in children aged 1–4 years. Immunohistochemical staining and electron microscopy reveals atypical (Langerhans') histiocytes with characteristic Birbeck's (cytoplasmic) granules.

Hand–Schüller–Christian disease

Chronic, recurrent form. Classic triad of proptosis, lytic skull lesions, and diabetes insipidus.

* Treatment is with systemic glucocorticoids and chemotherapy.

Letterer–Siwe disease

Acute, systemic form. Occurs during infancy with hepatosplenomegaly, thrombocytopenia, and fever, and with very poor prognosis for survival.

* Treatment is with systemic glucocorticoids and chemotherapy.

Eosinophilic granuloma

Localized form. Most likely to involve the orbit. Bony lesion with soft-tissue involvement that typically produces proptosis and more often is located in the superior orbit as a result of frontal bone disease.

* Treatment is with local incision and curettage, intralesional steroid injection, or radiotherapy.

Malignant Pediatric Orbital Tumors

Rhabdomyosarcoma

Most common primary pediatric orbital malignancy and most common pediatric soft-tissue malignancy; mean age 7–8 years old; 90% of cases occur in patients under 15 years old; male predilection (5:3). Presents with rapid onset, progressive, unilateral proptosis, eyelid edema, and discoloration. Epistaxis, sinusitis, and headaches indicate sinus involvement. History of trauma may be misleading. Predilection for superonasal orbit. CT scan commonly demonstrates bony orbital destruction. Arises from primitive mesenchyme, not extraocular muscles. Urgent biopsy necessary for diagnosis. Four histologic forms:

Embryonal

Most common (70%); cross striations found in 50% of cells.

Alveolar

Most malignant, worst prognosis, inferior orbit, second most common (20–30%); few cross-striations.

Botryoid

Grapelike, originates within paranasal sinuses or conjunctiva; rare.

Pleomorphic

Rarest (<10%), most differentiated, occurs in older patients, best prognosis; 90–95% 5-year survival rate if limited to orbit; cross-striations in most cells.

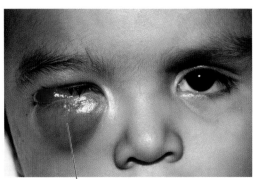

Figure 1-23 • Rhabdomyosarcoma of the right orbit with marked lower eyelid edema, discoloration, and chemosis.

Eyelid edema/discoloration

- Emergent diagnostic biopsy with immunohistochemical staining in all cases.
- Pediatric oncology consultation for systemic evaluation including abdominal and thoracic CT, bone marrow biopsy, and lumbar puncture.
- Treatment involves combinations of surgery, systemic chemotherapy, and radiotherapy.

Neuroblastoma

Most common pediatric orbital metastatic tumor (second most common orbital malignancy after rhabdomyosarcoma). Occurs in first decade. Usually arises from a primary tumor in the abdomen (adrenals in 50%), mediastinum, or neck from undifferentiated embryonic cells of neural crest origin. Patients typically have sudden proptosis with eyelid ecchymosis ("raccoon eyes") that may be bilateral; may develop ipsilateral Horner's syndrome and opsoclonus (saccadomania). Prognosis is poor.

- Orbital CT scan: Poorly defined mass with bony erosion (most commonly the lateral wall).
- Pediatric oncology consultation for systemic evaluation.
- Treatment is with local radiotherapy and systemic chemotherapy.

Leukemia

Advanced leukemia, particularly the acute lymphocytic type, may appear with proptosis; granulocytic sarcoma (chloroma), an uncommon subtype of myelogenous leukemia, may also produce orbital proptosis, often prior to hematogenous or bone marrow signs. Both forms usually occur during first decade.

- Pediatric oncology consultation.
- Treatment is with systemic chemotherapy.

Figure 1-24 • (A) Neuroblastoma presenting with bilateral eyelid ecchymosis and right-upper-eyelid swelling. (B) CT scan demonstrates the orbital metastases.

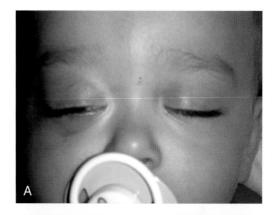

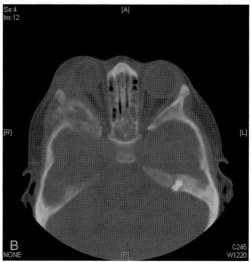

Figure 1-25 • Orbital neuroblastoma demonstrating bilateral eyelid ecchymosis ("raccoon eyes").

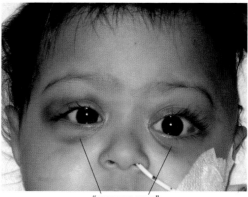

"raccoon eyes"

Adult Orbital Tumors

Benign Adult Orbital Tumors

Cavernous Hemangioma

This misnamed tumor is a vascular hamartoma and the most common adult orbital tumor. Probably present from birth, but typically appears in fourth to sixth decades. It is one of the four periocular tumors that are more common in females (meningioma, sebaceous carcinoma, and choroidal osteoma). Patients usually have painless, decreased visual acuity or diplopia. Signs include slowly progressive proptosis and compressive optic neuropathy. May have induced hyperopia and choroidal folds due to posterior pressure on the globe. May enlarge during pregnancy.

- Orbital CT scan (in cases of suspected tumor, CT scans are ordered with contrast): Well-circumscribed intraconal or extraconal lesion; no bony erosion (remodeling is possible); adjacent structures may be displaced, but are not invaded or destroyed.

- Orbital MRI: Tumor appears hypointense on T1-weighted images and hyperintense on T2-weighted images with heterogenous internal signal density.

- A-scan ultrasonography: High internal reflectivity.

- Complete surgical excision (usually requires lateral orbitotomy with bone removal) indicated for severe corneal exposure, compressive optic neuropathy, intractable diplopia, or exophthalmos; should be performed by an oculoplastic surgeon.

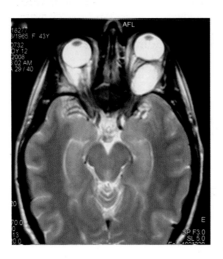

Figure 1-26 • MRI (T2) demonstrating cavernous hemangioma of the left orbit as a hyperintense mass displacing the globe and optic nerve.

Mucocele

Cystic sinus mass due to the combination of an orbital wall fracture and obstructed sinus excretory ducts, lined by pseudostratified ciliated columnar epithelium and filled with mucoid material. Patients usually have a history of chronic sinusitis (frontal and ethmoidal sinuses). Associated with cystic fibrosis; usually occurs in the superonasal orbit; must be differentiated from encephalocele and meningocele.

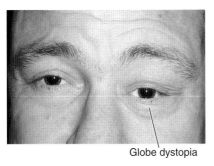

Globe dystopia

Figure 1-27 • Mucocele of the orbit with left globe dystopia.

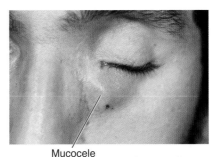

Mucocele

Figure 1-28 • Mucocele of the left eye.

- Head and orbital CT scan: Orbital lesion and orbital wall defect with sinus opacification.
- Complete surgical excision should be performed by an oculoplastic or otolaryngology plastic surgeon. May require obliteration of frontal sinus; preoperative and postoperative systemic antibiotics (ampicillin-sulbactam [Unasyn] 1.5–3.0 g IV q6h).

Neurilemoma (Schwannoma)

Rare, benign tumor (1% of all orbital tumors) that occurs in young to middle-aged individuals. Patients have gradual, painless proptosis and globe displacement. May be associated with neurofibromatosis type 1. One of two truly encapsulated orbital tumors. Histologic examination demonstrates two patterns of Schwann cell proliferation enveloped by perineurium: Antoni A (solid, nuclear palisading, Verocay bodies) and Antoni B (loose, myxoid areas). Recurrence and malignant transformation are rare.

Figure 1-29 • Neurilemoma (Schwannoma) producing proptosis of the left eye.

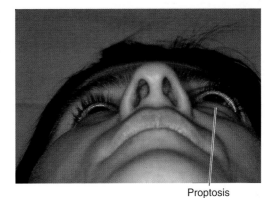

Proptosis

- Orbital CT scan: Well-circumscribed lesion; virtually indistinguishable from "cavernous hemangioma"; may have cystic areas.
- A-scan ultrasonography: Low internal reflectivity.
- Complete surgical excision should be performed by an oculoplastic surgeon.

Meningioma

Symptoms relate to specific location, but proptosis, globe displacement, diplopia, and optic neuropathy are common manifestations. Median age at diagnosis is 38 years old with female predilection (3:1). See Chapter 11 for complete discussion.

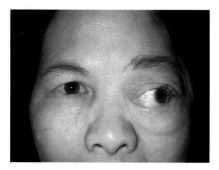

Figure 1-30 • Sphenoid wing meningioma producing proptosis and exotropia of the left eye.

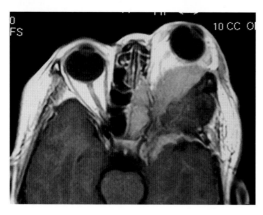

Figure 1-31 • MRI (T1) of same patient as Figure 1-30 demonstrating the orbital mass and globe displacement.

Primary orbital meningioma

Typically arises from the optic nerve (see Chapter 11).

Sphenoid meningioma

Usually arises intracranially with expansion into the orbit.

- Optic nerve meningiomas are generally observed. Radiation is considered first-line therapy for progressive tumors. Excision is reserved for the most aggressive lesions when no useful vision remains, because complete excision usually involves injury or transection of the optic nerve.

Fibrous Histiocytoma

Most common mesenchymal orbital tumor, but extremely rare. Firm, well-defined lesion that is usually located in the superonasal quadrant. Occurs in middle-aged adults. Less than 10% have metastatic potential. Histologically, cells have a cartwheel or storiform pattern. Recurrence is often more aggressive, with possible malignant transformation.

- Complete surgical excision should be performed by an oculoplastic surgeon.

Fibro-Osseous Tumors

Fibrous dysplasia

Nonmalignant, painless, bony proliferation often involving single (monostotic) or multiple (polyostotic) facial and orbital bones, occurs in Albright's syndrome. Most appear in first decade, with rapid growth during puberty and little growth during adulthood. Most patients will have pathologic long-bone fractures.

- Orbital radiographs: Diffuse bony sclerosis with ground glass appearance, radiolucent lesions, thickened occiput.

Osteoma

Rare, slow-growing, benign bony tumor frequently involving frontal and ethmoid sinuses. Causes globe displacement away from tumor. Surgical intervention is usually palliative and clinical cure almost impossible. However, many are found incidentally, most are nonprogressive, and surgical excision/debridement is rarely indicated.

- Orbital CT scan: Well-circumscribed lesion with calcifications.
- Osteoma usually can be excised completely if visual function threatened or intracranial extension.
- Should be evaluated by an oculoplastic surgeon.
- Consider otolaryngology consultation.

Cholesterol Granuloma

Idiopathic hemorrhagic lesion of orbital frontal bone, usually occurring in males. Causes proptosis, blurred vision, diplopia, and a palpable mass. Surgical excision is curative.

- Orbital CT scan: Well-defined superotemporal mass with bony erosion.

Aneurysmal Bone Cyst

Idiopathic, osteolytic, expansile mass typically found in long bones of the extremities or less commonly in the superior orbit. Occurs during adolescence. Intralesional hemorrhage produces proptosis, diplopia, and cranial nerve palsies.

- Orbital CT scan: Well-defined soft-tissue mass with bony lysis.

Malignant Adult Orbital Tumors

Lymphoid Tumors

Lymphoid infiltrates account for 10% of orbital tumors. The noninflammatory orbital lymphoid infiltrates are classified as reactive lymphoid hyperplasia and malignant lymphoma. Often clinically indistinguishable, the diagnosis is made by microscopic morphology and immunophenotyping. Most common in patients 50–70 years old; extremely rare in children; more common in women than in men (3:2). Patients have painless proptosis, diplopia, decreased visual acuity (induced hyperopia), or a combination of these symptoms. Lesions may be intraconal, extraconal, or both. Fifty percent of patients with orbital lymphoma eventually develop systemic involvement; risk of systemic disease is lower in cases of mucosa-associated lymphoid tissue (MALT) lymphomas. Radiation adequately controls local disease in nearly 100% of cases. Systemic disease is usually treated with chemotherapy. Good prognosis with 90% 5-year survival.

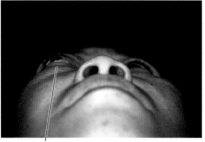

Proptosis

Figure 1-32 • Right proptosis from orbital lymphoid tumor.

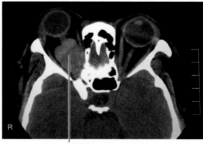

Orbital tumor

Figure 1-33 • Orbital CT of same patient as Figure 1-32 demonstrating the orbital lymphoid tumor and proptosis.

- Orbital CT scan: Unencapsulated solid tumor that molds to surrounding structures; bony changes are usually absent.
- Tissue biopsy and immunohistochemical studies on fresh (not preserved) specimens required for diagnosis.
- Reactive infiltrates demonstrate follicular hyperplasia without a clonal population of cells.
- Lymphoma is diagnosed in the presence of monoclonality, specific gene rearrangements assessed with PCR, or sufficient cytologic and architectural atypia; nearly always extranodal B-cell non-Hodgkin's lymphomas; greater than 50% are MALT-type lymphomas.
- Multiclonal infiltrates not fulfilling the criteria to be diagnosed as lymphoma may progress to malignant lymphoma.
- Systemic evaluation by internist or oncologist in the presence of biopsy-proven orbital lymphoma: includes thoracic, abdominal, and pelvic CT scan, whole body positron emission tomography (PET) scan, complete blood count (CBC) with differential, serum protein electrophoresis, erythrocyte sedimentation rate, and possibly bone scan; bone marrow biopsy is reserved by select cases.
- Low-dose, fractionated radiotherapy for localized orbital lesions (15–20 Gy for benign lesions; 20–30 Gy for malignancy) and chemotherapy with or without adjunctive ocular radiotherapy for systemic disease.

Fibro-Osseous Tumors

Chondrosarcoma

Usually occurs after age 20 years old with slight female predilection; often bilateral with temporal globe displacement. Intracranial extension is often fatal.

- Orbital CT scan: Irregular lesion with bony erosion.

Osteosarcoma

Common primary bony malignancy; usually occurs before age 20 years old.
- Orbital CT scan: Lytic lesion with calcifications.

Metastatic Tumors

Metastases account for 10% of all orbital tumors but are the most common orbital malignancy. Most common primary sources are breast, lung (bronchogenic), prostate, and gastrointestinal tract. Symptoms include rapid-onset, painful proptosis, limitation of extraocular movements, and diplopia. Visual acuity may be normal. Scirrhous breast cancer characteristically causes enophthalmos from orbital fibrosis.

- Orbital CT scan: Bony erosion and destruction of adjacent structures.
- Local radiotherapy for palliation should be performed by a radiation oncologist experienced in orbital processes.
- Palliative surgical debulking/excision may be considered in cases with intractable pain.
- Hematology and oncology consultation.

Acquired Anophthalmia

Absence of the eye resulting from enucleation or evisceration of the globe due to malignancy, trauma, or pain and blindness; more common in men than women. Inflammation or infection of the socket or implant may present with copious mucopurulent discharge, pain greater in one direction of eye movement, or serosanguinous tears; pain is qualitatively different from preenucleation pain; signs may include inflamed conjunctiva, dehiscence or erosion of conjunctiva with exposure of implant, blepharitis, or cellulitis.

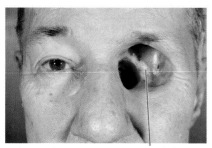

Anophthalmia

Figure 1-34 • Acquired anophthalmia of the left eye secondary to evisceration for orbital tumor.

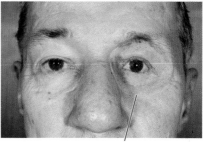

Prosthesis

Figure 1-35 • Same patient as Figure 1-34 with prosthesis in place.

- Eyelids should be observed for cellulitis, ptosis, or retraction.
- Superior tarsal conjunctiva must be examined for giant papillae (see Chapter 4).
- In the absence of conjunctival defect or lesion, treat with broad spectrum topical antibiotic (gentamicin or polymyxin B sulfate [Polytrim] 1 gtt qid).
- If conjunctival defect is observed, refer to an oculoplastic surgeon for evaluation. Treatment may include removal of avascular portion of porous implant, secondary implant, dermis fat graft placement, or other techniques.

- Exposed implant is at risk for orbital cellulitis and should be treated with systemic oral antibiotic, surgically, or both:
  - Cephalexin 250–500 mg po qid or
  - Amoxicillin-clavulanate [Augmentin] 250–500 mg po tid.
- Orbital prosthesis should be replaced with orbital conformer during period of infection. If conjunctival defect is present, the prosthesis must be reconstructed by ocularist postoperatively while conformer is used for 1 month.
- Socket should not be left without prosthesis or conformer for longer than 24 hours (controversial) due to conjunctival cicatrization, forniceal foreshortening, and socket contracture.

Atrophia Bulbi and Phthisis Bulbi

Progressive functional ocular decompensation, after either accidental or surgical trauma, the end stage of which is called phthisis bulbi. Three stages exist.

Atrophia Bulbi Without Shrinkage

Globe shape and size are normal, but with cataract, retinal detachment, synechiae, or cyclitic membranes.

Atrophia Bulbi With Shrinkage

Soft and smaller globe with decreased intraocular pressure; collapse of the anterior chamber; edematous cornea with vascularization, fibrosis, and opacification.

Atrophia Bulbi With Disorganization (Phthisis Bulbi)

Globe approximately two-thirds normal size with thickened sclera, intraocular disorganization, and calcification of cornea, lens, and retina; spontaneous hemorrhages or inflammation can occur, and bone may be present in the uveal tract. These eyes usually have no vision, and they carry an increased risk of intraocular malignancies.

Figure 1-36 • Phthisis bulbi demonstrating shrunken globe. The cornea is opaque, edematous, and thickened, and the anterior chamber is shallow.

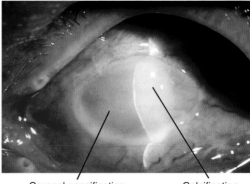

Corneal opacification   Calcification

- B-scan ultrasonography should be performed annually to rule out intraocular malignancies.
- Blind, painful eyes are first treated with topical steroid (prednisolone acetate 1% qid) and a cycloplegic (atropine 1% tid). Consider retrobulbar alcohol or chlorpromazine (Thorazine) injection for severe ocular pain.
- Cosmetic shell can be created by an ocularist and is worn over the phthisical eye to improve appearance and support the eyelid.
- Enucleation typically relieves pain permanently and can improve cosmesis in many cases. Modern enucleation techniques involve porous orbital implants with extraocular muscles attached, allowing for natural-appearing movement of the prosthesis.

Strabismus 35
Horizontal Strabismus 37
Vertical Strabismus 42
Miscellaneous Strabismus 45
Nystagmus 47
Third Cranial Nerve Palsy 50
Fourth Cranial Nerve Palsy 53
Sixth Cranial Nerve Palsy 56
Multiple Cranial Nerve Palsies 58
Chronic Progressive External Ophthalmoplegia 61
Horizontal Motility Disorders 63
Vertical Motility Disorders 65
Myasthenia Gravis 67

2

Ocular Motility and Cranial Nerves

Strabismus

Definition Ocular misalignment that may be horizontal or vertical; comitant (same angle of deviation in all positions of gaze) or incomitant (angle of deviation varies in different positions of gaze); latent, manifest, or intermittent.

Phoria

Latent deviation.

Tropia

Manifest deviation.

Esotropia

Inward deviation.

Exotropia

Outward deviation.

Hypertropia

Upward deviation.

Hypotropia

Downward deviation (vertical deviations usually are designated by the hypertropic eye, but if the process clearly is causing one eye to turn downward, this eye is designated hypotropic).

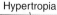
Hypertropia

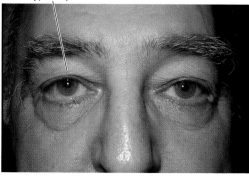

Figure 2-1 • Hypertropia of the right eye. Note the increased amount of scleral show inferiorly.

Etiology Congenital or acquired local or systemic muscle, nerve, or neuromuscular abnormality; childhood forms are usually idiopathic. See below for full description of the various types of strabismus (horizontal, vertical, miscellaneous forms). See also cranial nerve palsy, chronic progressive external ophthalmoplegia (CPEO), and myasthenia gravis.

Symptoms Asymptomatic; may have eye turn, head turn, head tilt, decreased vision, binocular diplopia (in older children and adults), headaches, asthenopia, and eye fatigue.

Signs Normal or decreased visual acuity (amblyopia), strabismus, limitation of ocular movements, reduced stereopsis; may have other ocular pathology (i.e., corneal opacity, cataract, aphakia, retinal detachment, optic atrophy, macular scar, phthisis) causing a secondary sensory deprivation strabismus (usually esotropia in children <6 years old, exotropia in older children and adults).

Differential Diagnosis See above; pseudostrabismus (epicanthal fold), negative angle kappa (pseudoesotropia), positive angle kappa (pseudoexotropia), dragged macula (e.g., retinopathy of prematurity, toxocariasis).

Evaluation

- Complete ophthalmic history with attention to age of onset, direction and frequency of deviation, family history of strabismus, neurologic symptoms, trauma, and systemic disease.
- Complete eye exam with attention to visual acuity, refraction, cycloplegic refraction, pupils, motility (versions, ductions, cover and alternate cover test), measure deviation (Hirschberg, Krimsky, or prism cover tests), measure torsional component (double Maddox rod test), Parks–Bielschowsky three-step test (identifies isolated cyclovertical muscle palsy [see Fourth Cranial Nerve Palsy section]), head posture, stereopsis (Titmus stereoacuity test, Randot stereotest), suppression/anomalous retinal correspondence (Worth 4-dot, 4 prism diopter [PD] base-out prism, Maddox rod, red glass, Bagolini's

striated lens, or after-image tests), fusion (amblyoscope, Hess screen tests), forced ductions, and ophthalmoscopy.

- Orbital computed tomography (CT) or magnetic resonance imaging (MRI) in select cases.
- **Lab tests**: Thyroid function tests (triiodothyronine [T3], thyroxine [T4], thyrotropin [TSH]) in cases of muscle restriction, and antiacetylcholine (anti-ACh) receptor antibody titers if myasthenia gravis is suspected.
- Electrocardiogram in patients with chronic progressive external ophthalmoplegia (CPEO) to rule out heart block in Kearns–Sayre syndrome.
- Consider edrophonium chloride (Tensilon) test to rule out myasthenia gravis.
- Neurology consultation and brain MRI if cranial nerves are involved.
- Medical consultation for dysthyroid and myasthenia patients.

Management

- Treat underlying etiology.
- Correct any refractive component.
- In children, patching or occlusion therapy for amblyopia (see Chapter 12); initially patch dominant or fixating eye; part-time patching can be used at any age. If full-time patching is used (during all waking hours, then taper as amblyopia improves), do not occlude one eye for more than 1 week per year of age. Atropine penalization, one drop in the better-seeing eye every day or every other day, is a good substitute to patching in children who are not compliant with occlusion.
- Timing of reexamination is based on patient's age (1 week per each year of age; e.g., 2 weeks for 2 year old, 4 weeks for 4 year old).
- Consider muscle surgery depending on the type and degree of strabismus (see below).

Prognosis Usually good; depends on etiology.

Horizontal Strabismus

Esotropia

Eye turns inward; most common ocular deviation (>50%).

Infantile Esotropia

Appears by age 6 months with a large, constant angle of deviation (80% >35 PD); often cross-fixate; normal refractive error; positive family history is common; may be associated with inferior oblique overaction (70%), dissociated vertical deviation (DVD) (70%), latent nystagmus, and persistent smooth pursuit asymmetry.

Esotropia

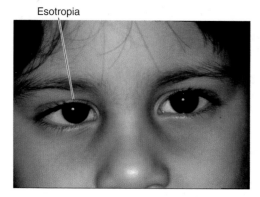

Figure 2-2 • Esotropia (inward turn) of the right eye. The corneal light reflex in the deviated eye is at the temporal edge of the pupil rather than the center.

- Treat amblyopia with occlusive therapy of fixating or dominant eye before performing surgery.
- Correct any hyperopia greater than +2.00 diopters (D).
- Muscle surgery should be performed early (6 months to 2 years): bilateral medial rectus recession or unilateral recession of medial rectus and resection of lateral rectus; additional surgery for inferior oblique overaction, dissociated vertical deviation (DVD), and over-correction and undercorrection is necessary in a large percentage of cases.

Accommodative Esotropia

Develops between age 6 months and 6 years, usually around age 2 years, with variable angle of deviation (eyes usually straight as infant); initially intermittent when child is tired or sick. There are three types:

Refractive

Usually hyperopic (average +4.75D), normal accommodative convergence-to-accommodation (AC/A) ratio (3:1PD to 5:1PD per diopter of accommodation), esotropia at distance (ET) similar to that at near (ET').

Nonrefractive

High AC/A ratio; esotropia at near greater than at distance (ET' > ET).
- Methods of calculating AC/A ratio
  (1) *Heterophoria method*: AC/A = IPD + [(N − D) / Diopter]
      IPD, interpupillary distance (cm); N, near deviation; D, distance deviation; Diopter, accommodative demand at fixation distance
  (2) *Lens gradient method*: AC/A = (WL − NL) / D
      WL, deviation with lens in front of eye; NL, deviation with no lens in front of eye; D, dioptric power of lens used

Mixed

Not completely correctable with single vision or bifocal glasses.
- Give full cycloplegic refraction if child is under 6 years old, and as much as tolerated if over 6 years old; if esotropia corrects to within 8PD, then no further treatment necessary.

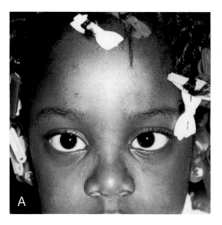
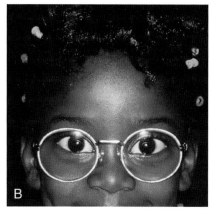

Figure 2-3 • (A) Accommodative esotropia that improves when the child wears full hyperopic correction (B).

- With high AC/A ratio and residual ET', prescribe executive-style, flat-top bifocal segment that bisects the pupil (+2.50D to +3.00D) or try miotic agents, especially in infant too young for glasses (echothiophate iodide 0.125% qd; be careful not to use with succinylcholine for general anesthesia); a combination of both can be used in refractory cases.
- Muscle surgery as above should be performed if residual esotropia greater than 10PD.

Acquired Nonaccommodative Esotropia and Other Forms of Esotropia

Due to stress, sensory deprivation, divergence insufficiency (ET ≥ ET'), spasm of near reflex, consecutive (after exotropia surgery), or cranial nerve (CN) VI palsy.

- Muscle surgery can be considered either in symptomatic cases or if angle of deviation is large.
- If no evident cause, MRI indicated to rule out Arnold–Chiari malformation.

Table 2-1 Surgical Numbers for Horizontal Strabismus Surgery — Esotropia

Prism Diopters (PD)	Bilateral MR Recession (mm)	Bilateral LR Resection (mm)	RECESSION & RESECTION (R & R)	
			MR Recess (mm)	LR Resect (mm)
15	3	3.5	3	3.5
20	3.5	4.5	3.5	4.5
25	4	5.5	4	5.5
30	4.5	6	4.5	6
35	5	6.5	5	6.5
40	5.5	7	5.5	7
50	6	8	6	7.5
60	6.5	–	6.5	8
70	7	–	–	–

MR, Medial rectus; LR, lateral rectus.

Cyclical Esotropia

Very rare form of nonaccommodative ET (1:3000); occurs between 2 and 6 years of age; child is usually orthophoric (eyes straight) but develops esotropia for 24-hour to 48-hour periods; can progress to constant esotropia.

- Correct any hyperopia greater than +3.00D.
- Muscle surgery as above can be performed when deviation stabilizes.

Exotropia

Eye turns outward; may be intermittent (usually at age 2 years, amblyopia rare) or constant (rarely congenital, consecutive [after esotropia surgery], due to decompensated intermittent exotropia [XT] or from sensory deprivation [in children >5 years of age]); amblyopia rare due to alternate fixation or formation of anomalous retinal correspondence.

Basic Exotropia

Exotropia at distance (XT) equal to that at near (XT′); normal AC/A ratio, normal fusional convergence.

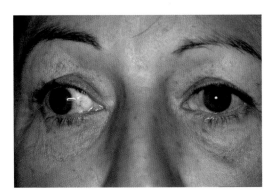

Figure 2-4 • Exotropia (outward turn) of the right eye. The corneal light reflex in the deviated eye is at the nasal edge of the iris rather than the center of the pupil.

Convergence Insufficiency

Inability to adequately converge while fixating on an object as it moves from distance to near (increased near point of convergence); exotropia at near greater than at distance (XT′ > XT); reduced fusional convergence amplitudes. Rare before 10 years of age; slight female predilection. Symptoms often begin during teen years with asthenopia, difficulty reading, blurred near vision, diplopia, and fatigue. Common in neurodegenerative disorders, such as Parkinson's disease, and with traumatic brain injury; may rarely be associated with accommodative insufficiency and ciliary body dysfunction.

- Treatment consists of prismatic correction (often ineffective) or monocular occlusion. Bifocals can be more difficult for patients with convergence insufficiency to use and should probably be avoided.
- Consider muscle surgery: bilateral medial rectus resection should be used with caution due to the risk of disrupting alignment at distance.

- Orthoptic exercises are controversial: near-point pencil push-ups (bring pencil in slowly from distance until breakpoint reached, then repeat 10–15 times) is the most common but is minimally effective; saccadic exercises or prism convergence exercises (increase amount of base-out prism until breakpoint reached, then repeat starting with low prism power 10–15 times) are more effective.

Pseudodivergence Excess

XT > XT' except after prolonged patching (patch test) when near deviation increases (full latent deviation); near deviation also increases with +3.00D lens; may have high AC/A ratio.

True Divergence Excess

XT > XT' even after patch test; may have high AC/A ratio.

- Correct any refractive error and give additional minus (to stimulate convergence), especially with high AC/A ratio.
- Consider base-in prism lenses to help with convergence.
- Muscle surgery if the patient manifests exotropia over 50% of the time and is older than 4 years old: bilateral lateral rectus recession; consecutive esotropia (postoperative diplopia) can be managed with prisms or miotics unless it lasts more than 8 weeks, then reoperate.

Table 2-2 Surgical Numbers for Horizontal Strabismus Surgery — Exotropia

| Prism Diopters (PD) | Bilateral LR Recession (mm) | Bilateral MR Resection (mm) | RECESSION & RESECTION (R & R) | |
			LR Recess (mm)	MR Resect (mm)
15	4	3	4	3
20	5	4	5	4
25	6	5	6	5
30	7	5.5	7	5.5
35	7.5	6	7.5	6
40	8	6.5	8	6.5
50	9	–	9	7

MR, Medial rectus; LR, lateral rectus.

A-, V-, and X-Patterns

Amount of horizontal deviation varies from upgaze to downgaze; occurs in up to 50% of strabismus.

A-pattern

Amount of horizontal deviation changes between upgaze (larger esotropia in upgaze) and downgaze (larger exotropia in downgaze); more common with exotropia; clinically significant if difference is 10PD or greater; associated with superior oblique muscle overaction; patients may have chin-up position.

- Muscle surgery if deviation is clinically significant: weakening of oblique muscles if over-action exists or transposition of horizontal muscles (medial recti moved up, lateral recti moved down) if no oblique overaction.
- Absolutely no superior oblique tenotomies if patient is bifixator with 40 seconds of arc of stereoacuity.

V-pattern

Amount of horizontal deviation changes between upgaze (larger exotropia in upgaze) and downgaze (larger esotropia in downgaze); more common with esotropia; clinically signifi-cant if difference is 15PD or greater; associated with inferior oblique muscle overaction, increased lateral rectus muscle innervation, underaction of superior rectus muscle, Apert's syndrome, and Crouzon's syndrome; patients may have chin-down position.

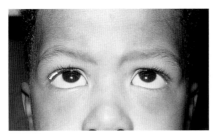

Figure 2-5 • V-pattern esotropia demonstrating reduced esotropia in upgaze.

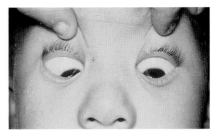

Figure 2-6 • Same patient as shown in Figure 2-5, demonstrating increased esotropia in downgaze.

- Muscle surgery if deviation is clinically significant: weakening of oblique muscles if over-action exists or transposition of horizontal muscles (medial recti moved down, lateral recti moved up) if no oblique overaction.

X-pattern

Larger exotropia in upgaze and downgaze than in primary position; due to secondary con-tracture of the oblique muscles or the lateral recti, causing a tethering effect in upgaze and downgaze.

- Muscle surgery if deviation is clinically significant: staged surgery if due to oblique muscles or lateral rectus recessions if due to tether effect.

Vertical Strabismus

Brown's Syndrome (Superior Oblique Tendon Sheath Syndrome)

Congenital or acquired anomaly of the superior oblique tendon sheath, causing an inability to elevate the affected eye especially in adduction. Elevation in abduction is normal or slightly decreased; may have hypotropia in primary gaze causing a chin-up position, positive forced duction testing that is worse on retropulsion and when moving eye up and in (differentiates from inferior rectus restriction, which is worse with proptosing eye); V-pattern (differentiates from superior oblique overaction, which is A-pattern), no superior oblique overaction, down-shoot in adduction, and widened palpebral fissures on adduction in severe cases; 10% bilateral, female predilection (3:2), and affects right eye more often than left eye; acquired forms are associated with rheumatoid arthritis, juvenile rheumatoid arthritis, sinusitis, surgery (sinus, orbital, strabismus, or retinal detachment), scleroderma, hypogammaglobulinemia, postpartum, and trauma.

Figure 2-7 • Brown's syndrome, demonstrating inability to elevate left eye in adduction.

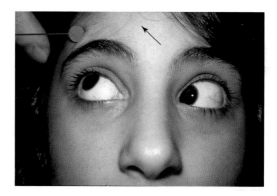

- No treatment usually required, especially for acquired forms, which may improve spontaneously depending on the etiology.
- Consider injection of steroids near trochlea or oral steroids if inflammatory etiology exists.
- Muscle surgery for abnormal head position or large hypotropia in primary position: superior oblique muscle tenotomy or tenectomy or silicon band expander, with or without ipsilateral inferior oblique muscle recession.

Dissociated Strabismus Complex: Dissociated Vertical Deviation, Dissociated Horizontal Deviation, Dissociated Torsional Deviation

Updrift, horizontal, oblique, or torsional movement of nonfixating eye with occlusion or visual inattention. Often bilateral, asymmetric, and asymptomatic; does not obey Hering's law (equal innervation to yoke muscles). Demonstrates Bielschowsky phenomenon (downdrift of occluded eye as increasing neutral density filters are placed over fixating eye), red lens phenomenon (when red lens held over either eye while fixating on light and the red image is always seen below the white image); associated with congenital esotropia (75%), latent nystagmus, inferior oblique overaction, and after esotropia surgery.

- No treatment usually required.
- Muscle surgery for abnormal head position or if deviation is large and constant or very frequent: bilateral superior rectus recession, inferior rectus resection, or inferior oblique weakening.

Table 2-3 Surgical Numbers for Vertical Strabismus Surgery

DISSOCIATED VERTICAL DEVIATION	
Magnitude	*Recess SR*
Mild	5 mm
Moderate	7 mm
Severe	10 mm
INFERIOR OBLIQUE OVERACTION	
Magnitude	*Recess IO*
Mild	10 mm
Moderate	15 mm
Severe	Myectomy

SR, superior rectus; IO, inferior oblique.

Monocular Elevation Deficiency (Double Elevator Palsy)

Sporadic, unilateral defect causing total inability to elevate one eye (may have good Bell's reflex); hypotropia in primary position and increases on upgaze, ipsilateral ptosis common, may have chin-up head position to fuse; may be supranuclear, congenital, or acquired (due to cerebrovascular disease, tumor, or infection). Three types:

Type 1

Inferior rectus muscle restriction-unilateral fibrosis syndrome.

Type 2

Elevator weakness (superior rectus, inferior oblique) – true double elevator palsy.

Type 3

Combination (inferior rectus restriction and weak elevators).

Ptosis/hypotropia

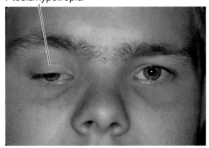

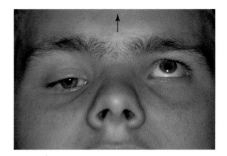

Figure 2-8 • Monocular elevation deficiency (double elevator palsy) demonstrating ptosis and hypotropia of the right eye.

Figure 2-9 • Same patient as shown in Figure 2-8, demonstrating inability to elevate right eye.

- Muscle surgery for chin-up head position, large hypotropia in primary position, or poor fusion: inferior rectus recession for inferior rectus muscle restriction; Knapp procedure (elevation and transposition of medial and lateral recti to the side of superior rectus) for superior rectus muscle weakness.
- May require surgery to correct residual ptosis.

Miscellaneous Strabismus

Duane's Retraction Syndrome

Congenital agenesis or hypoplasia of the abducens nerve (CN VI) with variable dysinnervation of the lateral rectus muscle; 20% bilateral, female predilection (3:2), affects left eye more often than right eye (3:1). Three types (type 1 more common than type 3, and type 3 more common than type 2):

Type 1

Limited abduction; esotropia in primary position.

Type 2

Limited adduction; exotropia in primary position.

Type 3

Limited abduction and adduction.

Co-contraction of medial and lateral rectus muscles causes globe retraction and narrowing of palpebral fissure; narrowing of palpebral fissure on adduction and widening on abduction in all three types; upshoots and downshoots (leash phenomenon) common; may have head turn to fuse; amblyopia rare; rarely associated with deafness and less commonly with other ocular or systemic conditions.

Upshoot/limited adduction/
narrowing of palpebral fissure

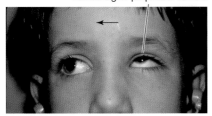

Limited abduction/widened PF

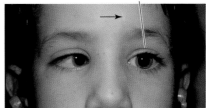

Figure 2-10 • Duane's retraction syndrome type 3, demonstrating limited adduction, upshoot (leash phenomenon) and narrowing of the palpebral fissure of the left eye.

Figure 2-11 • Same patient as shown in Figure 2-10, demonstrating limited abduction and widening of the palpebral fissure of the left eye.

- No treatment usually required.
- Correct any refractive error.
- Treat amblyopia.

- Muscle surgery if there is significant ocular misalignment in primary position, abnormal head position, or significant upshoot or downshoot: medial rectus muscle recession in type 1 or lateral rectus muscle recession in type 2; never perform lateral rectus muscle resection. Recess medial and lateral rectus muscles in type 3 with severe retraction.

Möbius' Syndrome

Congenital bilateral aplasia of CN VI and VII nuclei (CN V, IX, and XII may also be affected); inability to abduct either eye past midline; associated with esotropia, epiphora, exposure keratitis, and mask-like facies; patient may have limb deformities or absence of pectoralis muscle (Poland anomaly).

- Muscle surgery for esotropia: bilateral medial rectus recession.
- Treat exposure keratopathy due to facial nerve palsy (see Chapters 3 and 5).

Restrictive Strabismus

Various disorders that cause tethering of one or more extraocular muscles; restriction of eye movement in the direction of action of the affected muscle (these processes cause incomitant strabismus); positive forced ductions. Most commonly occurs in thyroid-related ophthalmopathy (see Chapter 1), also in orbital fractures (see Chapter 1), and congenital fibrosis syndrome.

Limited elevation/enophthalmos

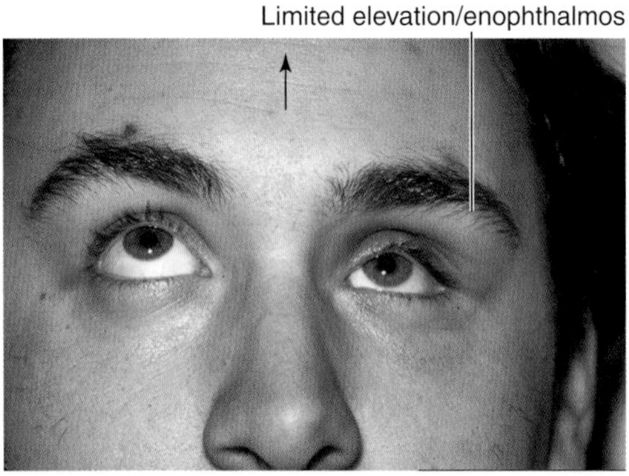

Figure 2-12 • Restrictive strabismus due to an orbital fracture of the left eye with inferior rectus entrapment, demonstrating limited elevation of the left eye; also note enophthalmos (sunken appearance of left eye).

Congenital Fibrosis Syndrome

Variable muscle restriction and fibrosis. Five types:

Generalized Fibrosis (Autosomal Dominant [AD] > Autosomal Recessive [AR] > Idiopathic)

Most severe form; all muscles in both eyes affected including levator (ptosis), inferior rectus usually affected the worst.

Congenital Fibrosis of Inferior Rectus (Sporadic or Familial)

Only inferior rectus affected.

Strabismus Fixus (Sporadic)

Horizontal muscles affected in both eyes; medial rectus more often than lateral rectus causing severe esotropia.

Vertical Retraction Syndrome

Vertical muscles affected in both eyes; superior rectus more often than inferior rectus causing restriction of downgaze.

Congenital Unilateral Fibrosis (sporadic)

All muscles affected in one eye causing enophthalmos and ptosis.

Nystagmus

Definition Involuntary, rhythmic oscillation of eyes; may be horizontal, vertical, rotary, or a combination; fast or slow; symmetric or asymmetric; pendular (equal speed in both directions) or jerk (direction designated by the fast phase component).

Etiology

Congenital Nystagmus

Nystagmus is different depending on gaze; may have null point (nystagmus slows or stops in certain eye positions; usually 15° off center); one dominant locus; most cases occur independent of vision.

Afferent or sensory deprivation

Pendular or jerk nystagmus; due to visual dysfunction from ocular albinism, aniridia, achromatopsia, congenital stationary night blindness, congenital optic nerve anomaly, Leber's congenital amaurosis, and congenital cataracts.

Efferent or motor

Usually horizontal nystagmus, but can be vertical, torsional or any combination; due to ocular motor disturbance; present at or shortly after birth, may be hereditary; mapped to chromosome 6p. Usually horizontal; may have null point and head turn (to move eyes to the null point); decreases with convergence and stops during sleep; no oscillopsia; may have head oscillations, a latent component, and inversion with horizontal optokinetic (OKN) testing (60%); associated with strabismus (33%).

Latent

Bilateral jerk nystagmus when one eye is covered (jerk component away from covered eye) that resolves when eye is uncovered; may be associated with congenital esotropia and DVD; only present under monocular viewing conditions; therefore, binocular visual acuity is better than when each eye is tested separately; normal OKN response; may have a null point.

Spasmus nutans

Triad of nystagmus (monocular or asymmetric, fine, very rapid, horizontal, and variable), head nodding, and torticollis (head turning). Benign condition that develops between 4 and 12 months of age, disappears by 5 years of age; otherwise neurologically intact. Similar eye movements can occur with chiasmal gliomas and parasellar tumors; therefore, check pupils for relative afferent pupillary defect and optic nerve carefully and perform neuroimaging; spasmus nutans is a diagnosis of exclusion; monitor for amblyopia.

Acquired Nystagmus

Various types of nystagmus are localizing.

Convergence–retraction

Co-contraction of horizontal recti muscles causes jerk convergence–retraction of eyes on attempted upward saccade; occurs in dorsal midbrain syndrome; classically associated with a pinealoma, but also with other neoplasms, trauma, stroke or demyelination (multiple sclerosis).

Dissociated or dysconjugate

Unilateral or asymmetric nystagmus; most commonly occurs in internuclear ophthalmoplegia (INO).

Downbeat

Jerk nystagmus with rapid downbeat and slow upbeat; seen most easily in lateral and down-gaze; null point is usually in upgaze. Associated with cervicomedullary junctional lesions including Arnold–Chiari malformation, syringomyelia, multiple sclerosis, cerebrovascular accidents, and drug intoxication (lithium); may respond to clonazepam treatment.

Drug-induced

Associated with use of anticonvulsants (phenytoin, carbamazepine), barbiturates, tranquilizers, and phenothiazines; often gaze-evoked; may be absent in downgaze.

Gaze-evoked

Jerk nystagmus in direction of gaze, no nystagmus in primary position; can be physiologic (fatigable with prolonged eccentric gaze, symmetric) or pathologic (prolonged, asymmetric); often due to medications (anticonvulsants, sedatives) or brain stem or posterior fossa lesions.

Opsoclonus (saccadomania)

Rapid, unpredictable, multidirectional saccades; absent during sleep. Associated with neuroblastoma or after postviral encephalopathies in children; occurs with visceral carcinomas in adults; called flutter if restricted to horizontal meridian.

Periodic alternating

Very rare, horizontal jerk nystagmus present in primary gaze with spontaneous direction changes every 60 to 90 seconds, with periods as long as 10 to 15 seconds of no nystagmus;

cycling persists despite fixating on targets. May be congenital or due to vestibulocerebellar disease; also associated with cervicomedullary junction lesions; may respond to treatment with baclofen.

See-saw

One eye rises and incyclotorts while other eye falls and excyclotorts, then the process alternates; may have INO. Most commonly occurs in conjunction with a suprasellar mass; also diencephalon lesions, after cerebrovascular accidents or trauma, or congenital.

Upbeat

Nystagmus occurs in primary position, and worsens in upgaze. Non-localizing, usually due to anterior vermis and lower brain stem lesion; also associated with Wernicke's syndrome or drug intoxication.

Vestibular

Usually horizontal with rotary component (fast component toward normal side, slow component toward abnormal side); may have associated vertigo, tinnitus, and deafness; due to lesion of end organ, peripheral nerve (fixation dampens nystagmus), or central (fixation does not inhibit nystagmus).

Voluntary

Usually hysterical or malingering; unable to sustain nystagmus longer than 30 seconds; typically in horizontal plane with rapid back-to-back saccades; lid fluttering may be present.

Physiologic Nystagmus

Occurs normally in a variety of situations including end gaze, optokinetic nystagmus (OKN), caloric, and rotational (VOR; vestibuloocular reflex).

Symptoms Asymptomatic, may have decreased vision, oscillopsia (in acquired nystagmus), and other neurologic deficits depending on etiology (e.g., reduced hearing, tinnitus, vertigo with vestibular nystagmus).

Signs Variable decreased visual acuity, ocular oscillations; may have better near than distance visual acuity, head turn, other ocular or systemic pathology (e.g., aniridia, bilateral media opacities, macular scars, optic atrophy, foveal hypoplasia, and albinism).

Differential Diagnosis See above; multiple sclerosis.

Evaluation

- Complete ophthalmic history with attention to drug or toxin ingestion, and eye exam with attention to monocular and binocular visual acuity, retinoscopy, pupils, motility, head posture, and ophthalmoscopy.
- May require head CT scan or MRI to rule out intracranial process.
- May require neurology or neuro-ophthalmology consultation.

Management

- No effective treatment for most forms.
- Consider base-out prism lenses for congenital nystagmus (dampens nystagmus by stimulating convergence).
- Consider baclofen (5–80 mg po tid) for periodic alternating nystagmus.
- Consider muscle surgery with Kestenbaum's procedure for congenital nystagmus if patient has head turn to keep eyes in null point.
- Discontinue inciting agent if condition is due to drug or toxin ingestion.

Prognosis Usually benign; depends on etiology.

Third Cranial Nerve Palsy

Definition Paresis of CN III (oculomotor) caused by a variety of processes anywhere along its course from the midbrain to the orbit; can be complete or partial (superior division innervates superior rectus and levator; inferior division innervates medial rectus, inferior rectus, inferior oblique, and parasympathetic fibers to iris sphincter and ciliary muscle); can be isolated with or without pupil involvement.

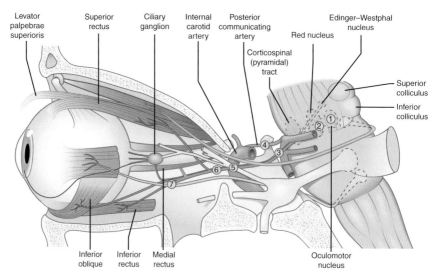

Figure 2-13 • Seven syndromes of third cranial nerve palsy. 1, Nuclear palsy; 2, fascicular syndromes; 3, uncal herniation; 4, posterior communicating artey aneurysm; 5, cavernous sinus syndrome; 6, orbital syndrome; 7, pupil-sparing isolated palsy.

Etiology Depends on age: congenital due to birth trauma or neurologic syndrome; in children due to infection, postviral illness, trauma, or tumors (pontine glioma); in adults, most commonly due to ischemia or microvascular problems (20–45% hypertension or diabetes mellitus); also associated with aneurysm (15–20%), trauma (10–15%), and tumors (10–15%); 10–30% are of undetermined cause; rarely associated with ophthalmoplegic migraine. Aberrant regeneration suggests a compressive lesion such as an intracavernous aneurysm or tumor, but can also occur after trauma, but never after ischemic or microvascular causes; pupil sparing usually microvascular or ischemic (80% are pupil sparing); 95% of compressive lesions involve the pupil. Important to localize level of pathology:

Nuclear

Almost never occurs in isolation; usually due to microvascular infarctions; signs include bilateral ptosis and contralateral superior rectus involvement; also caused by more diffuse brainstem lesions (neoplasm, post-surgical), and other abnormalities are present.

Fascicular

Usually due to demyelinating vascular, or metastatic lesions; associated with several syndromes including Benedikt's syndrome (CN III palsy with contralateral hemitremor, hemiballismus, and loss of sensation), Nothnagel's syndrome (CN III palsy and ipsilateral cerebellar ataxia and dysmetria), Claude's syndrome (combination of Benedikt's and Nothnagel's syndromes), and Weber's syndrome (CN III palsy and contralateral hemiparesis).

Subarachnoid Space

Usually due to aneurysms (notably posterior communicating artery aneurysm), trauma, or uncal herniation; rarely microvascular disease or infections; pupil usually involved.

Intracavernous Space

Usually due to cavernous sinus fistula, aneurysms, tumors (e.g., lymphoproliferative), inflammation (e.g., Tolosa–Hunt syndrome, sarcoidosis), infections (e.g., herpes zoster, tuberculosis), or pituitary apoplexy; often associated with CN IV, V, and VI findings and sympathetic abnormalities (see Multiple Cranial Nerve Palsies section); pupil usually spared (90%).

Orbital Space

Rare but may be due to neoplasm, trauma, or infections; often associated with CN II, IV, V, and VI findings (see Multiple Cranial Nerve Palsies section); CN III splits before superior orbital fissure, so partial (superior or inferior division) palsies may occur (however, partial CN III palsies from fascicular and subarachnoid lesions may resemble divisional injury clinically).

Symptoms Binocular diplopia (disappears with one eye closed), eye turn; may have pain, headache, ipsilateral droopy eyelid.

Signs Ptosis, ophthalmoplegia except lateral gaze, torsion with attempted infraduction due to action of the trochlear nerve, negative forced ductions, exotropia and hypotropia in primary gaze (eye is down and out); may have mid-dilated nonreactive pupil ("blown" pupil, efferent defect); in cases of aberrant regeneration: lid-gaze dyskinesis (inferior rectus or medial rectus fibers to levator causing upper lid retraction on downgaze [pseudo-von Graefe's sign] or on adduction), pupil-gaze dyskinesis (inferior rectus or medial rectus fibers to iris sphincter causing pupil constriction on downgaze or on adduction); may have other neurologic deficits or cranial nerve palsies.

Ptosis   Dilated pupil

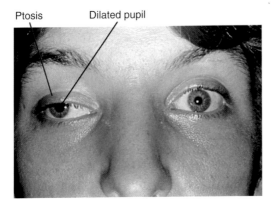

Figure 2-14 • Third cranial nerve palsy with right ptosis, pupillary dilation, exotropia, and hypotropia. This is the typical appearance of the "down and out" eye with a droopy lid and large pupil.

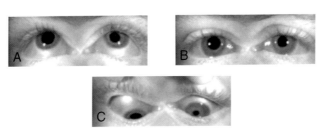

A   B

C

Figure 2-15 • (A–C) Primary abberant regeneration of the left third nerve. The left pupil constricts on downgaze because the nerves that normally supply the inferior rectus are now innervating the iris sphincter muscle.

Differential Diagnosis Myasthenia gravis, thyroid-related ophthalmopathy, CPEO.

Evaluation

- Complete ophthalmic history, neurologic exam with attention to cranial nerves, and eye exam with attention to pupils, lids, proptosis, motility, and forced ductions.
- MRI or magnetic resonance or computed tomography angiography (MRA, CTA), or both, if pupil involved in any patient, if associated with other neurologic abnormalities, if pupil spared in patients <50 years old, if signs of aberrant regeneration are present, or if no improvement of isolated pupil-sparing microvascular cases after 3 months.
- **Lab tests**: Fasting blood glucose, complete blood count (CBC), erythrocyte sedimentation rate (ESR), venereal disease research laboratory (VDRL), fluorescent treponemal antibody absorption (FTA-ABS), and antinuclear antibody (ANA).
- Check blood pressure.
- Consider conventional angiography to rule out aneurysm (neurosurgical emergency) if pupil involved and MRI-MRA/CTA results inconclusive.
- Consider lumbar puncture to assess for infection, cytology, or evidence of subarachnoid hemorrhage.
- Consider edrophonium chloride (Tensilon) test to rule out myasthenia gravis.
- Neuro-ophthalmology or interventional neuroradiology consultation (especially if pupil involved).

Management

- Treatment depends on etiology.
- Follow isolated pupil-sparing lesions closely for pupil involvement during first week.
- Occlusion with Transpore clear surgical tape or clear nail polish across one spectacle lens to help alleviate diplopia in adults.
- May require neurosurgery for aneurysms, tumors, and trauma.
- Treat underlying medical condition.

Prognosis Depends on etiology; complete or near complete recovery expected with microvascular palsies, which tend to resolve within 2–3 months (6 months maximum). Worse for palsies due to trauma or compressive lesions in which aberrant regeneration may develop.

Fourth Cranial Nerve Palsy

Definition Paresis of CN IV (trochlear) caused by a variety of processes anywhere along its course from the midbrain to the orbit.

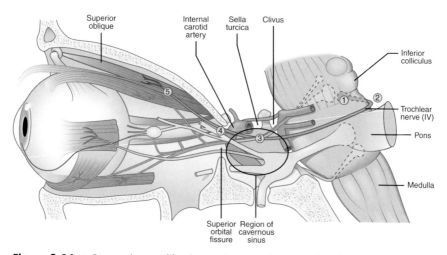

Figure 2-16 • Five syndromes of fourth cranial nerve palsy. 1, Nuclear/fascicular syndrome; 2, subarachnoid space syndrome; 3, cavernous sinus syndrome; 4, orbital syndrome; 5, isolated palsy.

Etiology Common causes include trauma (especially closed head trauma with contrecoup forces), microvascular disease (e.g., hypertension or diabetes mellitus), congenital (may or may not have head tilt), cavernous sinus disease (inflammatory, infectious, neoplastic), brainstem pathology (stroke, neoplasm); rarely aneurysm. In roughly 30% no cause is identified; bilateral injury can occur with severe head trauma. Important to localize level of pathology:

Nuclear

Most often due to stroke, less often neoplasm, and almost never isolated; other causes include demyelinative disease and trauma.

Fascicular

Rare, same associations as nuclear; may get contralateral Horner's syndrome; trauma (especially near anterior medullary velum) may cause bilateral CN IV palsies.

Subarachnoid Space

Usually due to closed head trauma; rarely tumor, infection, or aneurysm.

Intracavernous Space

Due to cavernous sinus disease from inflammation (sarcoidosis), infection (fungal), or neoplasm (lymphoproliferative, meningioma, pituitary macroadenoma); usually associated with CN III, V, and VI findings and sympathetic abnormalities (see Multiple Cranial Nerve Palsies section).

Symptoms Binocular vertical or oblique diplopia; may have torsional component, blurred vision, contralateral head tilt.

Signs Superior oblique palsy with positive Parks–Bielschowsky three-step test (see below), ipsilateral hypertropia (greatest on contralateral gaze and ipsilateral head tilt), excyclotorsion (if >10°, likely bilateral), large vertical fusional amplitude in congenital cases (>4PD); chin-down position; negative forced ductions; bilateral cases have V-pattern esotropia, left hypertropia on right gaze, and right hypertropia on left gaze; other neurologic deficits if CN IV paresis is not isolated.

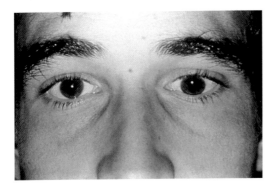

Figure 2-17 • Fourth cranial nerve palsy with right hypertropia.

Differential Diagnosis Myasthenia gravis, thyroid-related ophthalmopathy, orbital disease, CN III palsy, Brown's syndrome, and skew deviation.

Evaluation
- Complete ophthalmic history, neurologic exam with attention to cranial nerves, and eye exam with attention to motility, head posture (check old photographs for longstanding head tilt in congenital cases), vertical fusion, double Maddox rod test (measure torsional component), and forced ductions.

Figure 2-18 • Parks–Bielschowsky 3-step test revealing a right superior oblique (RSO) palsy. Circle the pair of muscles at each step and the paretic muscle will have three circles around it.

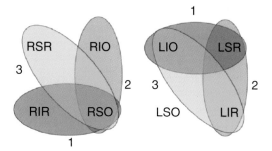

- Perform Parks–Bielschowsky three-step test to determine paretic muscle:
  - Step 1: Identify hypertropic eye in primary gaze (e.g., if right hypertropia then problem is with right inferior rectus/superior oblique or left superior rectus/inferior oblique).
  - Step 2: Identify horizontal direction of gaze that makes the hypertropia worse (e.g., if left gaze then problem is with right superior oblique/inferior oblique or left superior rectus/inferior rectus).
  - Step 3: Bielschowsky head-tilt test: identify direction of head tilt that makes the hypertropia worse (e.g., if right head tilt, then problem is with right superior oblique/superior rectus or left inferior oblique/inferior rectus).

  After three steps, the paretic muscle will be identified (e.g., right hypertropia in primary position, worse on left gaze, and right head tilt indicates right superior oblique).

- Observation for isolated cases in a patient with known vascular risk factors. If not resolved in 3 months individualized assessment is warranted; considerations include:
  - **Lab tests**: Fasting blood glucose, CBC, cholesterol and lipid panels, angiotensin-converting enzyme (ACE), VDRL, FTA-ABS, ANA; consider ESR and C-reactive protein (CRP) if giant cell arteritis (GCA) is suspected.
  - Check blood pressure.
  - Consider neuroimaging in nonresolving cases and those with associated findings. CT scan may suffice if there is evidence of orbital disease; MRI for suspected intracranial pathology, and angiography (conventional, MRA or CTA) to assess for an aneurysm.

Management

- Treatment depends on etiology.
- Occlusion with Transpore clear surgical tape or clear nail polish across one spectacle lens, or prism glasses to help alleviate diplopia in adults.
- Consider muscle surgery in longstanding, stable cases: Knapp classification for management of superior oblique palsy offers guidance, consider Harado Ito procedure (lateral transposition of superior oblique tendon) to correct torsional component.
- May require neurosurgery for aneurysms, tumors, and trauma.
- Treat underlying medical condition.

- Consider lumbar puncture.
- Consider edrophonium chloride (Tensilon) test to rule out myasthenia gravis.
- Neuro-ophthalmology consultation.

Prognosis Depends on etiology; complete or near complete recovery is expected with microvascular palsies.

Sixth Cranial Nerve Palsy

Definition Paresis of CN VI (abducens) caused by a variety of processes anywhere along its course from the pons to the orbit.

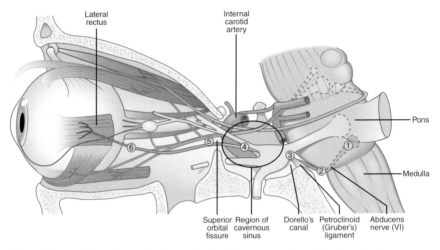

Figure 2-19 • Six syndromes of sixth cranial palsy. 1, Brainstem syndrome; 2, subarachnoid syndrome; 3, petrous apex syndrome; 4, cavernous sinus syndrome; 5, orbital syndrome; 6, islolated palsy.

Etiology Depends on age: in children (<15 years old) most commonly tumors (e.g., pontine glioma) or postviral; in young adults (15–40 years old) usually miscellaneous or undetermined (8–30%); in adults (>40 years old) usually due to trauma or microvascular disease (e.g., hypertension, diabetes mellitus [most common isolated cranial nerve palsy in diabetes: CN VI>III>IV]); also associated with multiple sclerosis, cerebrovascular accidents, increased intracranial pressure, and, rarely, tumors (e.g., nasopharyngeal carcinoma). Important to localize level of pathology:

Nuclear

Due to pontine infarcts, pontine gliomas, cerebellar tumors, microvascular disease, or Wernicke–Korsakoff syndrome; causes an ipsilateral, horizontal gaze palsy (cannot look to side of lesion).

Fascicular

Usually due to tumors, microvascular disease, or demyelinating disease; can cause Foville's syndrome (dorsal pons lesions with horizontal gaze palsy, ipsilateral CN V, VI, VII, VIII palsies, and ipsilateral Horner's syndrome) and Millard–Gubler syndrome (ventral pons lesion with ipsilateral CN VI and VII palsies and contralateral hemiparesis).

Subarachnoid Space

Usually due to elevated intracranial pressure (30% of patients with idiopathic intracranial hypertension have CN VI palsy); also basilar tumors (e.g., acoustic neuroma, chordomas), basilar artery aneurysm, hemorrhage, inflammations, or meningeal infections.

Petrous Space

Due to trauma (e.g., basal skull fracture) or infections; Gradenigo's syndrome (infection of petrous bone secondary to otitis media causing ipsilateral CN VI and VII paresis, ipsilateral Horner's syndrome, ipsilateral trigeminal pain, and ipsilateral deafness; occurs in children) or pseudo-Gradenigo's syndrome (nasopharyngeal carcinoma may cause severe otitis media with findings similar to those of Gradenigo's syndrome).

Intracavernous Space

Due to cavernous sinus disease from inflammation (sarcoidosis), infection (fungal), or neoplasm (lymphoproliferative, meningioma, pituitary macroadenoma); usually associated with CN III, V, and VI findings and sympathetic abnormalities (see Multiple Cranial Nerve Palsies section).

Symptoms Horizontal binocular diplopia (worse at distance than near, and in direction of gaze of paretic muscle); may have eye turn.

Signs Lateral rectus muscle palsy with esotropia and inability to abduct eye fully or slow abducting saccades; negative forced ductions; other neurologic deficits if CN VI paresis is not isolated.

Figure 2-20 • Sixth cranial nerve palsy demonstrating the inability to abduct the left eye on left gaze.

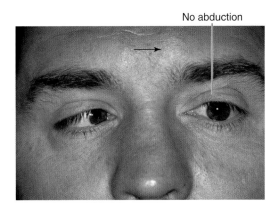

No abduction

Differential Diagnosis Thyroid-related ophthalmopathy, myasthenia gravis, orbital inflammatory pseudotumor, Duane's retraction syndrome type I, Möbius' syndrome (CN VI and VII palsy), orbital fracture with medial rectus entrapment, spasm of near reflex.

Evaluation
- Complete ophthalmic history, neurologic exam with attention to cranial nerves, and eye exam with attention to motility, forced ductions, and ophthalmoscopy.
- Observation for isolated cases in a patient with known vascular risk factors. If not resolved in 3 months individualized assessment is warranted; considerations include:
  - **Lab tests**: Fasting blood glucose, CBC, cholesterol and lipid panels, ACE, VDRL, FTA-ABS, ANA; consider ESR and CRP if GCA is suspected.
  - Check blood pressure.
  - Consider neuroimaging in nonresolving cases and those with associated findings. CT scan may suffice if there is evidence of orbital disease; MRI for suspected intracranial pathology, and angiography (conventional, MRA or CTA) to assess for an aneurysm.
  - Consider lumbar puncture.
  - Consider edrophonium chloride (Tensilon) test to rule out myasthenia gravis.
  - Neuro-ophthalmology consultation.

Management

- Treatment depends on etiology.
- Occlusion with Transpore clear surgical tape or clear nail polish across one spectacle lens, or prism glasses to help alleviate diplopia in adults.
- Consider muscle surgery in longstanding, stable cases.
- May require neurosurgery for aneurysms, tumors, and trauma.
- Treat underlying medical condition.

Prognosis Depends on etiology; microvascular palsies tend to resolve within 3 months.

Multiple Cranial Nerve Palsies

Definition Paresis of multiple cranial nerves appearing simultaneously; caused by a variety of processes anywhere along their courses from the brain stem to the orbits.

Etiology Myasthenia gravis, Guillain–Barré syndrome (especially Miller–Fisher variant), Wernicke's encephalopathy, chronic progressive external ophthalmoplegia, stroke, multiple sclerosis, cavernous sinus/orbital apex or orbital disease.

Brain Stem

Due to midbrain or pons vascular lesions or tumors involving cranial nerve nuclei that are in close proximity.

Subarachnoid Space

Usually due to infiltrations, infections, or neoplasms.

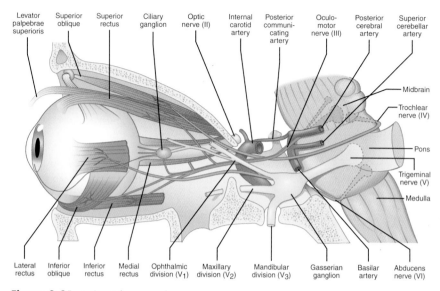

Levator palpebrae superioris — Superior oblique — Superior rectus — Ciliary ganglion — Optic nerve (II) — Internal carotid artery — Posterior communicating artery — Oculo-motor nerve (III) — Posterior cerebral artery — Superior cerebellar artery

Midbrain
Trochlear nerve (IV)
Pons
Trigeminal nerve (V)
Medulla

Lateral rectus — Inferior oblique — Inferior rectus — Medial rectus — Ophthalmic division (V₁) — Maxillary division (V₂) — Mandibular division (V₃) — Gasserian ganglion — Basilar artery — Abducens nerve (VI)

Figure 2-21 • Cranial nerve pathways.

Cavernous Sinus Syndrome

Multiple cranial nerve pareses (CN III, IV, V_1, V_2, VI) and sympathetic involvement due to parasellar lesions, which affect these motor nerves in various combinations in the sinus or superior orbital fissure; may have Horner's syndrome due to oculosympathetic paresis; caused by aneurysms (e.g., intracavernous carotid artery), arteriovenous fistulas (e.g., carotid-cavernous fistula, dural sinus fistula), tumors (e.g., leukemia, lymphoma, meningioma, pituitary adenoma, chordoma), inflammations (e.g., Wegener's granulomatosis, sarcoidosis, Tolosa–Hunt syndrome), or infections (e.g., cavernous sinus thrombosis, herpes zoster, tuberculosis, syphilis, mucormycosis); lesions of the cavernous sinus do not necessarily affect all the cranial nerves in it.

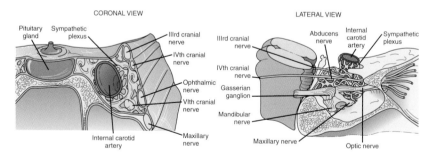

CORONAL VIEW

Pituitary gland — Sympathetic plexus — IIIrd cranial nerve — IVth cranial nerve — Ophthalmic nerve — VIth cranial nerve — Internal carotid artery — Maxillary nerve

LATERAL VIEW

IIIrd cranial nerve — IVth cranial nerve — Gasserian ganglion — Mandibular nerve — Abducens nerve — Internal carotid artery — Sympathetic plexus — Maxillary nerve — Optic nerve

Figure 2-22 • Anatomy of the cavernous sinus.

Orbital Apex Syndrome

Multiple motor cranial nerve palsies and optic nerve (CN II) dysfunction; etiologies similar to those mentioned above.

Symptoms Pain, diplopia; may have eye turn, droopy eyelid, variable decreased vision, and dyschromatopsia.

Signs Normal or decreased visual acuity and color vision (orbital apex syndrome), ptosis, strabismus, limitation of ocular motility, negative forced ductions, decreased facial sensation in CN V_1-V_2 distribution, relative afferent pupillary defect, miosis (Horner's syndrome), and trigeminal (facial) pain; may have proptosis, conjunctival injection, chemosis, increased intraocular pressure, bruit, and retinopathy in cases of high-flow arteriovenous fistulas; fever, lid edema, and signs of facial infection in cases of cavernous sinus thrombosis.

Differential Diagnosis Thyroid-related ophthalmopathy, myasthenia gravis, giant cell arteritis, Miller–Fisher variant of Guillain–Barré syndrome, chronic progressive external ophthalmoplegia, orbital disease (see Chapter 1).

Evaluation
- Complete ophthalmic history, neurologic exam with attention to cranial nerves, and eye exam with attention to facial sensation, ocular auscultation, visual acuity, color vision, pupils, motility, forced ductions, exophthalmometry, tonometry, and ophthalmoscopy.
- **Lab tests**: Fasting blood glucose, CBC with differential, ESR, VDRL, FTA-ABS, ANA; consider blood cultures if infectious etiology suspected.
- Head, orbital, and sinus CT scan or MRI-MRA or both.
- Consider lumbar puncture.
- Consider cerebral angiography to rule out aneurysm or arteriovenous fistula.
- Consider edrophonium chloride (Tensilon) test to rule out myasthenia gravis.
- Neuro-ophthalmology, otolaryngology, or medical consultations as needed.

Management

- Treatment depends on etiology.
- May require neurosurgery for aneurysms, tumors, and trauma.
- Oral steroids (prednisone 60–100 mg po qd) for Tolosa–Hunt syndrome; check purified protein derivative, blood glucose, and chest radiographs before starting systemic steroids.
- Add H_2-blocker (ranitidine [Zantac] 150 mg po bid) or proton pump inhibitor when administering systemic steroids.
- Systemic antibiotics (vancomycin 1 g IV q12h and ceftazidime 1 g IV q8h for staphylococcus and streptococcus) for cavernous sinus thrombosis; penicillin G (2.4 million U IV q4h for 10–14 days, then 2.4 million U IM q week for 3 weeks) for syphilis.
- Systemic antifungal (amphotericin B 0.25–1.0 mg/kg IV over 6 hours) for mucormycosis.
- Treat underlying medical condition.

Prognosis Depends on etiology; usually poor.

Chronic Progressive External Ophthalmoplegia

Definition Slowly progressive, bilateral, external ophthalmoplegia affecting all directions of gaze.

Etiology Isolated or hereditary myopathy; several rare syndromes.

Kearns–Sayre Syndrome (Mitochondrial DNA)

Triad of CPEO, pigmentary retinopathy (see Chapter 10), and cardiac conduction defects (arrhythmias, heart block, cardiomyopathy); also associated with mental retardation, short stature, deafness, vestibular problems, and elevated cerebrospinal fluid protein.

Mitochondrial Encephalopathy, Lactic Acidosis, and Stroke-like Episodes (Mitochondrial DNA)

Mitochondrial encephalomyopathy with lactic acidosis and stroke-like episodes (MELAS) beginning at a young age; may also have vomiting, seizures, hemiparesis, hearing loss, dementia, short stature, hemianopia, CPEO, optic neuropathy, pigmentary retinopathy, and cortical blindness.

Myoclonic Epilepsy and Ragged Red Fibers (Mitochondrial DNA)

Encephalomyopathy with myoclonus, seizures, ataxia, spasticity, dementia, and ragged red fibers on muscle biopsy (Gomori trichrome stain) (MERRF) may also have dysarthria, optic neuropathy, nystagmus, short stature, and hearing loss.

Myotonic Dystrophy (Autosomal Dominant)

CPEO, bilateral ptosis, lid lag, orbicularis oculi weakness, miotic pupils, "Christmas tree" (polychromic) cataracts, and pigmentary retinopathy with associated muscular dystrophy (worse in morning), cardiomyopathy, frontal baldness, temporalis muscle wasting, testicular atrophy, and mental retardation.

- **Genetics:** Mapped to chromosome 19q.

Oculopharyngeal Muscular Dystrophy (Autosomal Dominant)

CPEO with dysphagia; usually French-Canadian lineage.

- **Genetics:** Mapped to chromosome 14q.

Symptoms Variable decreased vision (if associated with a syndrome with retinal or optic nerve abnormality), droopy eyelids, foreign body sensation, tearing. Usually no diplopia, even with ocular misalignment.

Signs Normal or decreased visual acuity, limitation of eye movements (even with doll's head maneuvers and caloric stimulation), absent Bell's phenomenon, often orthophoric (may develop strabismus, usually exotropia), negative forced ductions, ptosis, orbicularis oculi weakness, superficial punctate keratitis (especially inferiorly), cataracts, retinal pigment epithelial changes or pigmentary retinopathy (see Chapter 10); pupils usually spared.

Differential Diagnosis Downgaze palsy (lesion of rostral interstitial nucleus of the medial longitudinal fasciculus [riMLF]), upgaze palsy, progressive supranuclear palsy, dorsal midbrain syndrome, myasthenia gravis.

Ptosis

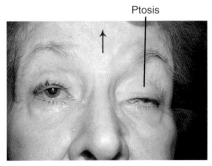

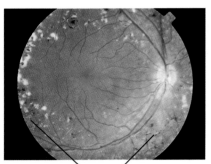

Pigmentary changes

Figure 2-23 • Chronic progressive external ophthalmoplegia, demonstrating ptosis and limited elevation of both eyes. The patient is attempting to look upward (note raised brows), yet the eyes remain in primary position (note the corneal light reflex centered over the pupil of the right eye) and the lids remain ptotic (markedly on the left side).

Figure 2-24 • Retinal pigmentary changes in a patient with Kearns–Sayre syndrome. Areas of retinal pigment epithelial hyperpigmentation, as well as atrophy, are apparent around the optic nerve and vascular arcades.

Evaluation
- Complete ophthalmic history, neurologic exam with attention to cranial nerves, and eye exam with attention to visual acuity, motility, doll's head maneuvers, Bell's phenomenon, forced ductions, lids, pupils, and ophthalmoscopy.
- Consider muscle biopsy (deltoid) to check for abnormal "ragged red" muscle fibers or electromyography for definitive diagnosis.
- Consider edrophonium chloride (Tensilon) test to rule out myasthenia gravis.
- Consider lumbar puncture.
- Medical consultation for complete cardiac evaluation including electrocardiogram (Kearns–Sayre syndrome, myotonic dystrophy) and swallowing studies (oculopharyngeal dystrophy).
- Mitochondrial DNA analysis for deletions (Kearns–Sayre syndrome).

Management

- No treatment effective.
- Topical lubrication with nonpreserved artificial tears (see Appendix) up to q1h and ointment (Refresh PM) qhs if signs of exposure keratopathy exist.
- Kearns–Sayre syndrome requires a cardiology consultation; may require pacemaker.
- Ptosis surgery can be considered but risks corneal exposure.

Prognosis Depends on syndrome; usually poor.

Horizontal Motility Disorders

Definition

Internuclear Ophthalmoplegia

Lesion of the medial longitudinal fasciculus (MLF), which traverses between the contralateral CN VI nucleus and the ipsilateral CN III subnucleus, serving the medial rectus muscle; results in an ipsilateral deficiency of adduction and contralateral abducting nystagmus; convergence can be absent (mesencephalic lesion; anterior lesion) but is usually intact (lesion posterior in the MLF); may be unilateral or bilateral (appears exotropic; WEBINO, "wall-eyed" bilateral INO).

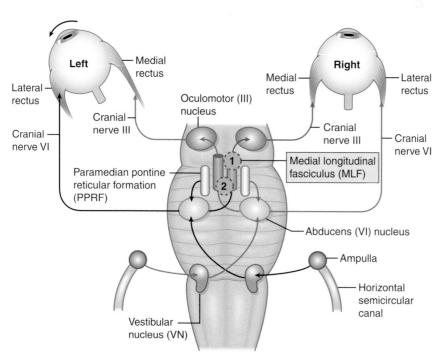

Figure 2-25 • Right internuclear ophthalmoplegia (INO) 2- Bilateral INO (reproduced with permission from Bajandas FJ, Kline LB: Neuro-Ophthalmology Review Manual. Thorofare, NJ, Slack, 1988).

One-and-a-Half Syndrome

So-called internuclear ophthalmoplegia (INO) plus with lesion of paramedian pontine reticular formation (PPRF; the horizontal gaze center) or CN VI nucleus, and the ipsilateral MLF causing conjugate gaze palsy to ipsilateral side (one) and INO or inability to adduct on gaze to contralateral side (half).

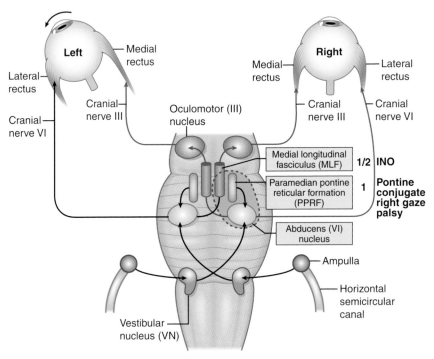

Figure 2-26 • Right acute one-and-a-half syndrome (paralytic pontine exotropia) (reproduced with permission from Bajandas FJ, Kline LB: Neuro-Ophthalmology Review Manual. Thorofare, NJ, Slack, 1988).

Etiology   Depends on age: less than 50 years old usually demyelinative (unilateral or bilateral INO) or tumor (pontine glioma for one-and-a-half syndrome); bilateral in children, often due to brain stem glioma; over 50 years old usually vascular disease; other causes include arteriovenous malformation, aneurysm, basilar artery occlusion, multiple sclerosis, or tumor (pontine metastasis).

Symptoms   Binocular horizontal diplopia worse in contralateral gaze.

Signs   Limitation of eye movements (cannot adduct on side of lesion in INO; can abduct only on side contralateral to lesion in one-and-a-half syndrome); nystagmus in abducting contralateral eye (INO); doll's head maneuvers and caloric stimulation absent, negative forced ductions; may have upbeat nystagmus or skew deviation (involvement of nuclei rostral to the MLF).

Differential Diagnosis   Medial rectus palsy, myasthenia gravis.

Evaluation
- Complete ophthalmic history, neurologic exam with attention to cranial nerves, and eye exam with attention to motility, doll's head maneuvers (caloric stimulation and forced duction testing are not necessary to make the diagnosis).
- MRI with attention to brain stem and midbrain.

- Consider edrophonium chloride (Tensilon) test to rule out myasthenia gravis.
- Consider neurology or neurosurgery consultation.

Management

- Treatment depends on etiology.
- Aneurysms, tumors, and trauma may require neurosurgery.
- Treat underlying neurologic or medical condition.

Prognosis Usually good, with complete recovery in patients with a vascular lesion or demyelination. Permanent deficits develop in multiple sclerosis from repeated insults.

Vertical Motility Disorders

Definition

Progressive Supranuclear Palsy (Steele–Richardson–Olszewski Syndrome)

Degenerative neurologic disorder with Parkinsonian features that causes progressive, bilateral, external ophthalmoplegia affecting all directions of gaze; usually starts with vertical gaze (downgaze first).

Dorsal Midbrain (Parinaud's) Syndrome

Supranuclear palsy of vertical gaze (upgaze first) due to lesions of the dorsal midbrain.

Skew Deviation

Comitant or incomitant acquired vertical misalignment of the eyes due to supranuclear dysfunction from posterior fossa process; hypotropic eye is ipsilateral to lesion; typically have other brainstem-related signs and symptoms.

Etiology

Dorsal Midbrain (Parinaud's) Syndrome

Classically described with pineal tumors (in young men), also occurs with cerebrovascular accidents, hydrocephalus, arteriovenous malformation, trauma, multiple sclerosis, or syphilis.

Skew Deviation

Non-localizing but occurs most often with brainstem or cerebellar lesions.

Symptoms Blurred vision, binocular diplopia (at near with dorsal midbrain syndrome); may have trouble reading, foreign body sensation, tearing, or dementia (progressive supranuclear palsy [PSP]), or other neurologic symptoms (skew deviation).

Progressive Supranuclear Palsy (Steele–Richardson–Olszewski Syndrome)

Progressive limitation of voluntary eye movements (but doll's head maneuvers give full range of motion), negative forced ductions; may have nuchal rigidity and seborrhea, progressive dementia, dysarthria, and hypometric saccades.

Dorsal Midbrain (Parinaud's) Syndrome

Supranuclear paresis of upgaze (therefore vestibular, doll's head maneuver, and Bell's phenomenon intact), negative forced ductions, light-near dissociation; may have papilledema, convergence-retraction nystagmus (on attempted upgaze or downward OKN drum), lid retraction (Collier's sign), spasm of convergence and accommodation (causing induced myopia), skew deviation, superficial punctate keratitis (especially inferiorly).

Skew Deviation

Vertical ocular misalignment (comitant or incomitant), hypotropic eye is ipsilateral to lesion, hypertropic eye is extorted and hypotropic eye is intorted (evident on fundoscopic examination); may have other neurologic signs.

Differential Diagnosis Downgaze palsy (lesion of riMLF), upgaze palsy, CPEO, myasthenia gravis, oculogyric crisis (transient bilateral tonic supraduction of eyes and neck hyperextension; occurs in phenothiazine overdose and more rarely in Parkinson's disease).

Evaluation
- Complete ophthalmic history, neurologic exam with attention to cranial nerves, and eye exam with attention to motility, doll's head maneuvers, forced ductions, lids, accommodation, pupils, cornea, and ophthalmoscopy.
- Head and orbital CT scan or MRI-MRA, or both, with attention to brain stem and midbrain.
- Consider edrophonium chloride (Tensilon) test to rule out myasthenia gravis.
- Consider neurology or neurosurgery consultation.

Management

- Treatment depends on etiology.
- Topical lubrication with nonpreserved artificial tears (see Appendix) up to q1h and ointment (Refresh PM) qhs if signs of exposure keratopathy exist.
- Aneurysms, tumors, and trauma may require neurosurgery.
- Treat underlying neurologic or medical condition.

Prognosis Depends on etiology.

Myasthenia Gravis

Definition Autoimmune disease of the neuromuscular junction causing muscle weakness; hallmark is variability and fatigability.

Etiology Autoantibodies to acetylcholine receptors of striated muscles found in 70–90% of patients with generalized myasthenia, but is as low as 50% in purely ocular myasthenia; does not affect pupils or ciliary muscle.

Epidemiology Female predilection; positive family history in 5%; 90% have eye involvement (levator, orbicularis oculi, and extraocular muscles), 75% as initial manifestation, 20% ocular only; increased incidence of autoimmune thyroid disease, thymoma (10% with systemic and probably less in purely ocular myasthenia), scleroderma, systemic lupus erythematosus, rheumatoid arthritis, Hashimoto's thyroiditis, multiple sclerosis, and thyroid-related ophthalmopathy.

Symptoms Binocular diplopia, droopy eyelids, dysarthria, dysphagia; all symptoms are more severe when tired or fatigued.

Signs Variable, asymmetric ptosis (worse with fatigue, sustained upgaze, and at end of day), variable limitation of extraocular movements (mimics any motility disturbance), negative forced ductions, strabismus, orbicularis oculi weakness; Cogan's lid twitch (upper eyelid twitch when patient looks up to primary position after looking down for 10–15 seconds); rarely gaze-evoked nystagmus; very rarely may resemble an INO.

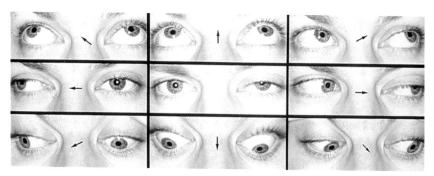

Figure 2-27 • Myasthenia gravis with left ptosis and adduction deficit. The left ptosis is most evident in primary gaze and gaze to the left; the left adduction deficit is apparent in all right gaze positions.

Differential Diagnosis Gaze palsy, multiple sclerosis, CN III, IV, or VI palsy, INO, thyroid-related ophthalmopathy, CPEO, idiopathic orbital inflammation, and levator dehiscence.

Evaluation

- Complete ophthalmic history, neurologic exam with attention to cranial nerves, and eye exam with attention to motility, forced ductions, lids, pupils, and cornea.
- **Lab tests**: Anti-ACh receptor antibodies, thyroid function tests (T3, T4, TSH, TSI).
- **Edrophonium chloride (Tensilon) test:** Test dose of edrophonium chloride 2 mg IV with 1 mL saline flush, then observe for improvement in diplopia and lid signs over next minute; if no improvement, increase edrophonium chloride dose to 4 mg IV with 1 mL saline flush and observe for improvement in diplopia and lid signs; repeat two times; if no improvement in diplopia and lid signs after 3 to 4 minutes, the test result is negative; a negative test result does not rule out myasthenia gravis. Note: consider cardiac monitoring in at-risk patients because of cardiovascular effects of edrophonium chloride; if bradycardia, angina, or bronchospasm develop, inject atropine (0.4 mg IV) immediately; consider pretreating with atropine 0.4 mg IV.
- Consider single-fiber electromyography of peripheral or orbicularis muscles for definitive diagnosis.
- Chest CT scan to rule out thymoma.
- Neurology or medical consultation or both.

Management

- No treatment required if symptoms are mild.
- Oral anticholinesterase (pyridostigmine 60–120 mg po qid) for moderate symptoms.
- Consider oral steroids (prednisone 20–100 mg po qd); check purified protein derivative, blood glucose, and chest radiographs before starting systemic steroids.
- Add H_2-blocker (ranitidine [Zantac] 150 mg po bid) or proton pump inhibitor when administering systemic steroids.
- Occlusion with Transpore clear surgical tape or clear nail polish across one spectacle lens to help alleviate diplopia in adults.
- Surgery for thymoma if present.
- Treat underlying medical condition.

Prognosis   Variable, chronic, progressive; good if ocular only.

Eyelid Trauma	69
Eyelid Infections	73
Eyelid Inflammations	79
Eyelid Malpositions	85
Blepharospasm	93
Bell's Palsy	94
Floppy Eyelid Syndrome	96
Trichiasis	97
Congenital Eyelid Anomalies	99
Benign Eyelid Tumors	103
Malignant Eyelid Tumors	110
Systemic Diseases	116
Canaliculitis	120
Dacryocystitis	121
Nasolacrimal Duct Obstruction	123
Dacryoadenitis	125
Lacrimal Gland Tumors	128

3

Lids, Lashes, and Lacrimal System

Eyelid Trauma

Eyelid trauma must be evaluated thoroughly, because seemingly trivial trauma may threaten the viability of the globe. Embedded foreign bodies, incomplete eyelid closure, or lacrimal system damage all can have lasting effects beyond any obvious cosmetic consequences. Trauma can be blunt or sharp, with common examples including fist, motor vehicle accidents, or athletic injury. Ominous mechanism of injury, orbital signs, or massive periocular injury may warrant orbital evaluation including computed tomography (CT) scan.

Contusion

Bruising of eyelid with edema and ecchymosis, usually secondary to blunt injury. Hematomas are often not discrete but infiltrative, involving multiple layers. Unless there is a focal collection of blood, hematomas cannot be effectively evacuated surgically, so the goal of treatment is to reduce further bleeding. Posterior extension into the orbit should be evaluated and, when present, managed accordingly. Ocular involvement is common; traumatic ptosis may occur (mechanical from edema and hematoma, or direct levator injury) and can take up to 6 months to resolve. Usually excellent prognosis if no ocular or bony injuries.

- Cold compresses for up to 45 minutes per hour while awake for 24–48 hours.
- Rule out and treat open globe (see Chapter 4) or other associated ocular trauma.
- Preseptal hematoma (absent orbital signs) is not an indication for canthotomy. Orbital compartment syndrome does not result from preseptal edema/hemorrhage.

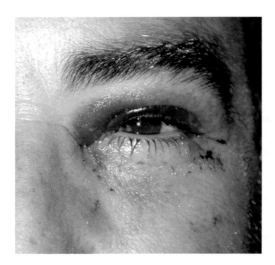

Figure 3-1 • Eyelid contusion with prominent ecchymosis of the upper lid and eyelid swelling nasally.

Abrasion

Superficial abrasions or mild dermal epithelial abrasions usually heal by secondary intention; rarely require skin grafting.

- Antibiotic ointment (erythromycin or bacitracin) lubrication can be used for superficial wounds. With deeper (full thickness dermis) defects consider systemic antibiotics.

Avulsion

Tearing or shearing injury to the eyelid resulting in partial or complete severance of eyelid tissue. Surgical repair of eyelid defect depends upon the degree of tissue loss and damage; entirely avulsed remnant should be sought and surgically replaced. Lid-sharing procedures should be avoided in young children due to the risk of occlusion amblyopia.

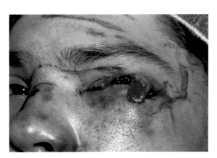

Figure 3-2 • Eyelid avulsion demonstrating large tissue defect and fragment of upper lid dangling.

When tissue loss is encountered, the approach is individually tailored. Factors such as horizontal eyelid laxity are considered in procedure selection. For example, in an older patient with advanced involutional changes, a defect of up to 30% might be repaired with direct closure, whereas in a younger patient a defect as small as 10% might not be amenable to direct closure without cantholysis. Below are some general treatment guidelines based on defect size.

Upper Lid Defects

- Small (<33%): Direct closure with or without lateral canthotomy and superior cantholysis.
- Moderate (33–50%): Tenzel semicircular flap advancement, or adjacent tarsoconjunctival flap and full-thickness skin graft.
- Large (>50%): Lower eyelid bridge flap reconstruction (Cutler–Beard procedure), free tarsoconjunctival graft and skin flap, median forehead flap, or full-thickness lower eyelid switch flap advancement.

Lower Lid Defects

- Small (<33%): Direct closure with or without lateral canthotomy and inferior cantholysis.
- Moderate (33–50%): Tenzel semicircular flap advancement, or full adjacent tarsoconjunctival flap and full-thickness skin graft.
- Large (>50%): Upper eyelid tarsoconjunctival pedicle flap with full-thickness skin graft (Hughes procedure), free tarsoconjunctival graft and skin flap, Mustarde's rotational cheek flap, or anterior lamella reconstruction with retroauricular free skin graft or skin flap advancement.

Laceration

Cut in the eyelid involving skin and deeper structures (muscle and fat), usually due to penetrating trauma. Lid lacerations are divided into: (1) no lid margin involvement, (2) lid margin involvement, and (3) canthal angle involvement (tendon and lacrimal gland system). Early, clean wounds usually are repaired successfully but can be complicated by lid notching, entropion, ectropion, or cicatrix; dirty wounds are also at risk for infection.

Lacerations involving the canaliculus (tear duct) at the nasal lid margin between the punctum and the medial canthus of either eyelid can result from a number of mechanisms. Penetrating injury such as that which occurs with a dog bite may involve the canaliculus directly. Alternately, they often result from shearing at the eyelid's weakest point. This may occur in conjunction with lacerations located more laterally on the eyelid and due to their relatively small size are often overlooked. They can be identified on slit lamp examination of the medial eyelid and confirmed with probing and irrigation. Prognosis is good if repaired early over a stent.

Figure 3-3 • Full-thickness upper eyelid laceration involving the lid margin.

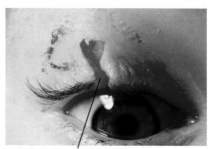

Full thickness lid laceration

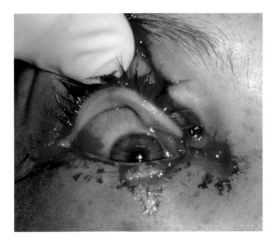

Figure 3-4 • Full-thickness upper eyelid laceration with canalicular laceration.

- Tetanus booster (tetanus toxoid 0.5 mL IM) if necessary for tetanus prophylaxis (>10 years since last tetanus shot or if status is unknown); consider rabies with animal bites.
- Fat prolapse into wound suggests orbital septum violation.
- For dirty wounds, systemic antibiotic (dicloxacillin 250–500 mg po qid or cephalexin 250–500 mg po qid for 7–10 days; consider penicillin V 500 mg po qid for animal or human bites).
- **Surgical repair of eyelid laceration not involving lid margin:** The area around the wound is infiltrated with 2% lidocaine with epinephrine 1:100,000. The area is prepped and draped using povidone-iodine (Betadine) solution. The wound is inspected carefully for the presence of foreign bodies. Deep portions are probed to the base of the wound and any septal penetration noted. (Wounds involving levator muscle or levator aponeurosis require layered closure, usually with an extended incision along the major lid crease, and external repair.) Copiously irrigate with saline or bacitracin solution. All tissue should be preserved if possible; only severely necrotic tissue must be excised. Horizontal or arcuate wounds oriented along orbicularis typically are closed in a single layer that includes skin only; gaping wounds or wounds which are oriented transverse to orbicularis are closed in two layers. 6-0 polyglactin interrupted, buried sutures are used to close orbicularis; skin can be closed separately. Some advocate interrupted sutures whereas others prefer a running stitch. If permanent sutures are used, such as a 6-0 prolene or nylon, they should be removed 5 or 6 days later. Alternatively, an absorbable suture (6-0 fast absorbing gut) can be used. This is particularly advantageous in children in whom suture removal is challenging or in patients felt unlikely to reliably return for suture removal. Topical and, in most cases of trauma, systemic antibiotics should be prescribed.
- **Surgical repair of eyelid laceration involving lid margin, sparing canaliculus:** The area around the wound is infiltrated with 2% lidocaine with epinephrine 1:100,000. The area is prepped and draped using povidone-iodine (Betadine) solution. The wound is inspected carefully for the presence of foreign bodies. Canalicular involvement is assessed via lacrimal probing and irrigation. All tissue should be preserved, if possible; only severely necrotic tissue must be excised. The lid margin is reapproximated using two to three interrupted 6-0 nylon or 7-0 Vicryl sutures. The initial suture is passed through the meibomian gland orifices, usually in a vertical mattress fashion, to align the tarsus,

with one to two additional interrupted sutures to align the lash line. For each suture, it is important that the bites on the two sides are equidistant from the wound margin. It is important to cinch the tarsal suture tightly to evert the reapproximated wound edges slightly; otherwise, as the wound heals and stretches, a notch may form at the lid margin. These sutures are left long. The margin sutures can be placed untied on Steri-Strips temporarily to allow better exposure for tarsal closure. The remaining tarsus is closed using interrupted lamellar 6-0 polyglactin sutures with the knot on the anterior tarsal surface to avoid erosion to the ocular surface. Attention must be paid to the distance from the lid margin each suture is placed to ensure even reapproximation of the tarsus. In the upper lid it is important to avoid full-thickness bites onto the conjunctival surface, although this is safely tolerated in the lower eyelid. If left untied, the lid margin sutures are now tied. Orbicularis is closed using interrupted, buried 6-0 polyglactin sutures. Skin is closed using interrupted 6-0 nylon or fast-absorbing gut sutures. The long ends of the lid margin sutures are incorporated into a skin suture to keep them away from the cornea. The wound is dressed with antibiotic ointment. Skin sutures can be removed in 7–10 days, but the lid margin sutures should remain for 10–14 days to avoid dehiscence of the margin with resultant notching.

- **Surgical repair of eyelid laceration involving lid margin and canaliculus:** The area around the wound is infiltrated with 2% lidocaine with epinephrine 1:100,000. The area is prepped and draped using povidone-iodine (Betadine) solution and inspected carefully with minimal manipulation. Small (0.3-mm) forceps and cotton-tipped applicators are helpful in locating the nasal end of the transected canaliculus. The punctum of the involved canaliculus is dilated and then intubated with a silicone stent with nasolacrimal probes on each end. The first probe is passed through the puncta and the lateral portion of the lacerated canaliculus. It is then inserted into the medial portion of the canaliculus and advanced into the nasolacrimal sac to a hard stop against the lacrimal sac fossa. The nasolacrimal duct is then intubated by slowly rotating the probe in a superior-inferior orientation with slight downward pressure until a path of low resistance is found, which will be the probe passing through the opening of the nasolacrimal duct. The probe is then retrieved from under the inferior turbinate in the nose by using a straight hemostat, groove director, or hook inserted through the naris. The second arm of the tube is advanced through the opposite puncta and retrieved in the same manner, and the tubes are secured at the external naris. The canalicular tear is closed using two to three interrupted 7-0 polyglactin sutures, which are passed through the canalicular walls. Pericanalicular sutures are added as needed. The lid margin is repaired as described above except that there is no tarsus medial to the puncta. The stent is removed after 3 months.

Eyelid Infections

Blepharitis and Meibomitis

Definition Inflammation of the eyelid margins (blepharitis) and inspissation of the oil-producing sebaceous glands of the lids (meibomitis); often occur together. Blepharitis is classified by location (anterior [infectious], posterior [meibomitis], angular [at lateral canthus]) or etiology.

Etiology Chronic *Staphylococcus* or *Demodex* infection, seborrhea (alone, with staphylococcal superinfection, with meibomian seborrhea, with secondary meibomitis), primary meibomitis, atopic dermatitis, psoriasis, and fungal; angular blepharitis is associated with *Moraxella* infection. Ocular surface disease results from disruption of the tear film (from bacterial lipolytic exoenzymes and abnormal meibum), epithelial cell death, and inflammation.

Epidemiology Very common in adult population, prevalence estimated at 12% for anterior blepharitis and 24% for posterior blepharitis; often coexists with dry eye disease (see Chapter 4); also associated with staphylococcal marginal keratitis (see Chapter 5) and acne rosacea (see below).

Symptoms Itching, red eye, burning, tearing, mild pain, foreign body sensation, filmy vision; often worse on awakening and late in the day.

Signs

Anterior blepharitis

Crusting/scales along eyelashes ("scurf" and "collarettes"), loss of eyelashes (madarosis); may develop pannus, phlyctenules, corneal infiltrates, and ulceration.

Meibomitis

Thickened and erythematous eyelid margins with telangiectatic blood vessels; atrophic, swollen, pitted, or blocked meibomian glands; turbid, thickened meibum (may have "toothpaste sign": gentle pressure on lids expresses columns of thick, white sebaceous material); may have Meiobomian gland inclusions (visible under the tarsal conjunctiva as yellow bumps), decreased tear break-up time, tear film debris and foam, conjunctival injection, corneal staining (typically inferiorly); may also develop recurrent chalazia/hordeola.

Flakes/collarettes   Telangiectatic vessels

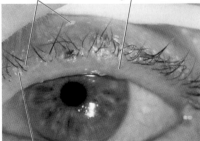
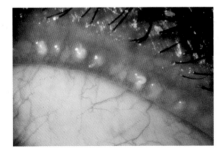

Thickened lid margins

Figure 3-5 • Anterior blepharitis with thickened eyelid margins, flakes, and collarettes.

Figure 3-6 • Meibomitis demonstrating inspissated meibomian glands with obstructed, pouting orifices, thickened sebum, and telangiectasia of the lid margin.

Differential Diagnosis Dry eye disease, primary herpes simplex virus infection, allergic or infectious conjunctivitis, corneal foreign body, sebaceous cell carcinoma, squamous or basal cell carcinoma, discoid lupus, medicamentosa, ocular cicatricial pemphigoid.

Evaluation
- Complete history with attention to history of skin cancer, sexually transmitted diseases, cold sores, allergies, eye medications, and chronic recurrent disease; unilateral, chronic, or refractory symptoms suggest malignancy.

- Complete eye exam with attention to facial skin, lids, meibomian gland orifices, lashes, tear film, conjunctiva, and cornea.
- Biopsy if lesions are suspicious for malignancy (ulcerated, yellow, chronic, scarred, or unilateral lid lesions, often with concomitant corneal pathology).
- **Lab tests**: Chlamydia cultures (if there is associated chronic follicular conjunctivitis or suspicion of sexually transmitted disease).

Management

- Lid hygiene: Daily application of hot compresses to the eyelids followed by massage and cleansing of the lid margins with commercial lid scrub pads, or face cloth or cotton-tipped applicator soaked in dilute baby shampoo or tea tree shampoo solution. In addition, consider weekly application of 50% tea tree oil followed by topical steroid drop tid for 2 days.
- Topical antibiotic ointment (bacitracin or erythromycin qhs for 2–4 weeks).
- Consider short course (1–2 weeks) of topical antibiotic-steroid (Tobradex drops qid or ointment bid).
- Nutritional supplements (i.e., oral flaxseed/fish oils [omega-3 fatty acids]).
- Consider oral antibiotic (doxycycline 50 mg po bid or minocycline 50 mg po qd for 2 weeks, then doxycyline 20 mg po qd) for recalcitrant or rosacea associated cases. Tetracycline 250 mg is also effective but requires more frequent dosing and is associated with more frequent gastrointestinal side effects. These agents are not offered to women in their childbearing years or to children with deciduous dentition. Alternatively, erythromycin 250 mg po bid then qd may be used.
- Consider azithromycin (Azasite) bid for 2 days, then qd for 2–4 weeks.
- Consider topical cyclosporine 0.05% (Restasis) bid for 3 months.
- Treat associated pathology such as rosacea and dry eye.

Prognosis Good; flare-ups and remissions are common; maintenance treatment often required indefinitely.

Herpes Simplex Virus

Primary infection due to herpes simplex virus; often mild and unrecognized. Patients may note pain, itching, and redness. Appears as small crops of seropurulent vesicles on the eyelid that eventually rupture and crust over; marginal ulcerative blepharitis, follicular conjunctivitis, punctate or dendritic keratitis, and preauricular lymphadenopathy may also occur.

- Cold compresses bid to qid to affected skin area.
- Systemic antiviral (acyclovir [Zovirax] 400 mg po 5 times/day or famciclovir [Famvir] 500 mg po or valacyclovir [Valtrex] 1 g po tid for 7–10 days).
- Topical antiviral (trifluridine 0.1% 9 times/day or vidarabine 3% 5 times/day for 14 days) for patients with blepharoconjunctivitis or corneal involvement.

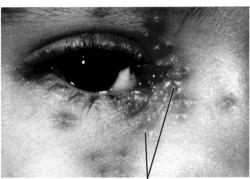

Figure 3-7 • Primary herpes simplex virus infection with eyelid vesicles.

Seropurulent vesicles

Herpes Zoster Virus

Reactivation of latent varicella zoster virus in the first division of cranial nerve V (herpes zoster ophthalmicus, HZO) usually involving the upper eyelid. Herpes zoster affects 20–30% of the population and increases in incidence and severity with age >60 years (50% in 85 year old), 10–20% of these patients have HZO. Appears as an acute, painful, unilateral, dermatomal maculopapular skin eruption, followed by vesicular ulceration and crusting; new lesions develop for up to 1 week and then resolve in 2–6 weeks. Patients have a prodrome of fever, headache, malaise, and pain (tingling, paresthesias, itching, burning) over the affected cranial nerve V_1 dermatome, which may occur without the rash (*zoster sine herpete*); involvement of the tip or side of the nose (Hutchinson's sign) is an indicator of ocular involvement (nasociliary branch of the ophthalmic nerve). Ocular involvement occurs in 50% if no antiviral treatment is given; lid scarring may result with entropion, ectropion, trichiasis, lash loss (madarosis), canalicular and punctal stenosis, necrosis, and lid retraction with lagophthalmos and exposure keratitis. 50% develop complications, most common is postherpetic neuralgia (PHN), a neuropathic pain syndrome that continues or occurs after resolution of the rash. PHN also increases in incidence and severity with increasing age (37% in those >60 years old, 48% in those >70 years old); other risk factors include severity of pain (prodromal and acute), severity of rash, and ocular involvement.

Vesicles with crusting

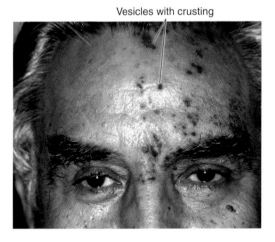

Figure 3-8 • Herpes zoster virus demonstrating unilateral V_1 dermatomal distribution (trigeminal ophthalmic branch).

- Cool saline or aluminum sulfate-calcium acetate (Domeboro) compresses bid to tid.
- Topical antibiotic ointment (erythromycin or bacitracin bid to tid) to affected skin.
- Systemic antiviral (acyclovir [Zovirax] 800 mg po 5 times/day for 7–10 days, or famciclovir [Famvir] 500 mg po or valacyclovir [Valtrex] 1 g po tid for 7 days). If immunocompromised, acyclovir 10–12 mg/kg/day IV, divided q8h for 10–14 days; resistant strains are treated with systemic vidarabine or foscarnet. Antiviral treatment within 72 hours of the rash decreases virus shedding, severity and duration of the rash, acute pain, and incidence of ocular involvement. Treatment with either famciclovir or valacyclovir is preferred to acyclovir because the former two medications reduce the incidence, duration, and severity of PHN.
- Rule out ocular involvement (see Chapters 5 and 6).
- Treatment of PHN consists of one or more of the following agents: tricyclic antidepressants (amitriptyline, doxepin, nortriptyline, or desipramine 25–100 mg po qd), gabapentin (Neurontin 600 mg po 2–6 times a day), pregabalin (Lyrica 300–600 mg po qd), opioids (oxycodone 10–30 mg po bid), topical analgesics (lidocaine 5% ointment, lidocaine-prilocaine cream, or lidoderm 5% patch q4-6h; capsaicin 0.025% [Zostrix] cream is poorly tolerated), and oral steroids (prednisone 60 mg po for 1 week, then 30 mg for 1 week, then 15 mg for 1 week); consider diphenhydramine (Benadryl 25–50 mg po qhs) for postherpetic itching. May rarely require nerve block or botulinum map injections.
- Vaccination in individuals ≥ 60 years old. Safety and efficacy demonstrated in the Shingles Prevention Study (SPS); vaccination reduces the incidence of herpes zoster by 51%, the incidence of PHN by 67%, and the severity and duration if shingles does occur; however, the efficacy of the vaccine decreases with increasing patient age.

Molluscum Contagiosum

DNA poxvirus infection, typically occurs in children and is spread by direct contact. Usually asymptomatic; appears as shiny dome-shaped waxy papules with central umbilication on the lid or lid margin; papules may appear anywhere on the body. May be associated with chronic follicular conjunctivitis, superficial pannus, and superficial punctate keratitis. Although disease is self-limited, resolution may take years; disseminated disease occurs in patients with acquired immunodeficiency syndrome (AIDS).

Figure 3-9 • Molluscum contagiosum demonstrating characteristic shiny, domed papule with central umbilication on the lower eyelid.

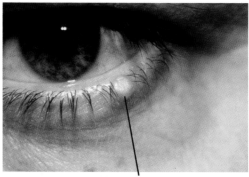

Molluscum papule

- Treatment is by curettage, cryotherapy, or cautery of one or more lesions with the intention of stimulating the immune system to eliminate satellite lesions. Suggested protocol includes excisional biopsy of one lesion with curettage of at least one additional lesion.

Demodicosis

Parasitic hair follicle infection with *Demodex folliculorum* or *D. brevis*; associated with blepharitis. Very common infestation but usually asymptomatic; may incite hordeolum formation. Examination of epilated hair follicles reveals sleeves of thin, semitransparent crusting at the base of the lashes.

- Lid scrubs may be effective: Commercial preparations are available; alternatively, a warm solution of baby shampoo and water (50:50 mixture) may be applied rigorously to the lids and lashes using cotton, a face cloth, or cotton-tipped applicator. Tea tree shampoo can also be considered.

Phthiriasis or Pediculosis

Infestation of eyelashes with lice (*Phthirus pubis*); usually sexually transmitted or from very close contact with an infected individual. Patients note itching and burning; signs include small, pearly, white nits (eggs) attached to lashes, adult lice, preauricular lymphadenopathy, blood-tinged lids and lashes, blepharoconjunctivitis, conjunctival follicles, and conjunctival injection.

Phthirus pubis lice

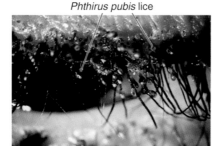

Phthirus pubis lice

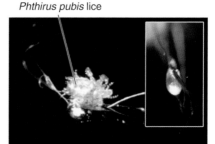

Figure 3-10 • Infestation of eyelashes with *Phthirus pubis*. Note the chronic skin changes at the base of the lashes.

Figure 3-11 • Close-up of eyelash with *Phthirus pubis*.

- Mechanical removal of lice and nits with fine forceps.
- Topical ointment (erythromycin or Lacrilube tid for 14 days) to suffocate lice.
- Physostigmine 0.25% ointment × 1, repeat in 1 week, or fluorescein 20% 1–2 drops to lid margins plus delousing creams and shampoo (not for ocular use): permethrin cream rinse 1% (Nix), lindane 1%, γ-benzene hexachloride (Kwell), or pyrethrins liquid with piperonyl butoxide (RID, A-200 Pyrinate liquid) (Warning: Kwell and RID not recommended for pregnant women and children.)
- Discard or thoroughly wash in hot cycle all bedding, linens, and clothing.
- Treat sexual partner.

Leprosy

Chronic infectious disease caused by *Mycobacterium leprae*, a pleomorphic, acid-fast bacillus. Of the four variants, tuberculoid and lepromatous leprosy can have eyelid involvement, including loss of eyelashes and eyebrows (madarosis), trichiasis, paralytic ectropion, lagophthalmos with exposure keratitis, and reduced blink rate; may develop corneal ulceration and perforation.

- Systemic multidrug treatment with dapsone (100 mg po qd) and rifampin (600 mg po qd); consider adding clofazimine (100 mg po qd).

- Reduce corneal exposure with temporary or permanent tarsorrhaphy.

Eyelid Inflammations

Chalazion or Hordeolum (Stye)

Definition

Chalazion

Obstruction and inflammation of meibomian gland with leakage of sebum into surrounding tissue and resultant lipogranuloma formation; often evolving from an internal hordeolum; associated with meibomitis and rosacea.

Hordeolum

Acute bacterial infection of sebaceous eyelid gland; most commonly meibomian gland (internal hordeolum) or gland of Zeis or Moll (external hordeolum); associated with *Staphylococcus aureus*.

Symptoms Painful, hot, swollen, red eyelid lump; chronic chalazia become nontender.

Signs Erythematous subcutaneous nodule, sometimes tender with visible pointing or drainage; usually solitary, but can be multiple or bilateral; occasionally, severe swelling prevents visualization or palpation of a discrete nodule; may have signs of blepharitis, meibomitis and rosacea; may develop super-infection with associated cellulitis.

Chalazion   Chalazion

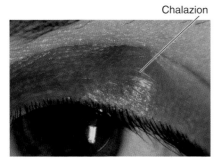

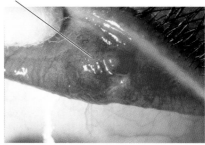

Figure 3-12 • Chalazion of the upper eyelid.

Figure 3-13 • Everted eyelid of the same patient as Figure 3-12, demonstrating the chalazion.

Differential Diagnosis Preseptal cellulitis, sebaceous cell carcinoma, pyogenic granuloma.

Evaluation
- Complete ophthalmic history and eye exam with attention to previous episodes, fever, facial skin, lids, meibomian gland orifices, eyelid eversion, lashes, motility, and cornea.

Management

- Warm compresses with gentle massage for 10 minutes qid.
- Topical antibiotic ointment (erythromycin or bacitracin bid to tid) in the inferior fornix if lesion is draining.
- Consider short course (1–2 weeks) of topical antibiotic-steroid ointment (Tobradex bid).
- Consider incision and curettage after 1 month if no improvement.
- Consider intralesional steroid injection (triamcinolone acetate 10 or 40 mg/mL; inject 0.5 mL with 30-gauge needle) for chalazia near lacrimal system or if only partially responsive to incision and curettage.
- Recurrent lesion must be evaluated by biopsy to rule out malignancy.
- Treat underlying meibomitis and rosacea.
- Multiple and recurrent chalazia may respond to oral antibiotic (doxycycline 50 mg po or minocycline 25 mg po bid). Tetracycline 250 mg is also effective but requires more frequent dosing and is associated with more frequent gastrointestinal side effects. These agents are not offered to women in their childbearing years or to children with deciduous dentition. Alternatively, erythromycin 250 mg po bid may be used.

Prognosis Good; may take weeks to months to resolve fully; recurrence is common (especially in blepharitis or acne rosacea); conservative treatment is recommended; surgical drainage through a posterior incision with curettage and excision of the lipogranulomatous material can lead to scarring and further episodes; steroid injection may produce hypopigmentation or local fat atrophy.

Contact Dermatitis

Definition Acute skin inflammation resulting from chemical or mechanical irritants, or from immunologic hypersensitivity to an allergic stimulus.

Symptoms Swelling, redness, itching, tearing, foreign body sensation, and ocular and eyelid discomfort.

Signs Erythematous, flaking, or crusting rash accompanied by edema; may have vesicular or weeping lesions; lichenified plaques suggest chronic exposure to irritant.

Figure 3-14 • Contact
dermatitis, demonstrating bilateral
erythematous, flaking rash.

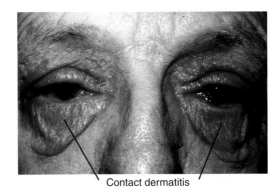

Contact dermatitis

Differential Diagnosis Herpes simplex, herpes zoster, preseptal cellulitis; chemical, ultraviolet, or thermal burns.

Evaluation
- Complete history with attention to exposure to irritants such as soaps, fragrances, cosmetics, hairspray, nail polish, jewelry, medications, poison ivy; and chemical, ultraviolet, or thermal exposure.
- Complete eye exam with attention to facial skin, lids, conjunctiva, and cornea.
- Consider dermatology consultation.

Management

- A stepwise approach is required given the wide range of severity that can occur in eyelid dermatitis. Periocular steroids should not be used for more than 2 weeks without ophthalmic supervision.
- Identify and remove inciting agent(s); may require allergic patch testing to determine causative allergens.
- Cold compresses.
- Topical antibiotic ointment (erythromycin or bacitracin bid) to crusted or weeping lesions.
- Consider mild steroid cream (<1% hydrocortisone cream bid to tid for 7–10 days) on eyelids; avoid lid margins and ocular exposure (for this reason, it is safer to use an ophthalmic preparation, e.g., fluorometholone [FML] ointment).
- Alternatively, ophthalmic steroid solution may be massaged onto affected eyelids bid.
- Tacrolimus 0.1% (Protopic), a nonsteroidal ointment, is very effective in the treatment of eyelid dermatitis and can be considered a first-line medication in advance of topical steroids.
- Oral antihistamine (diphenhydramine 25–50 mg po tid to qid) for severe or widespread lesions or excessive itching.

Continued

> ## Management—Cont'd
>
> - Consider short-term oral steroids (prednisone 40–80 mg po qd tapered over 10–14 days) for severe cases; check purified protein derivative (PPD) and controls, blood glucose, and chest radiographs before starting systemic steroids.
> - Add H_2-blocker (Zantac 150 mg po bid) or proton pump inhibitor when administering systemic steroids.

Prognosis Usually good; resolution occurs 1–2 weeks after removal of inciting agent; rebound can occur if steroids tapered too rapidly.

Blepharochalasis

Idiopathic, recurrent episodes of painless edema of the upper eyelids with or without redness and itching. Over time, repeated episodes may result in atrophy and laxity of the upper eyelid tissues, causing premature wrinkling of the skin, ptosis, deep superior sulci from fat atrophy, and lacrimal gland prolapse. Typically occurs in young females, first episode usually occurs before the age of 20. Inflammation may be treated acutely with topical steroid ointment; there is no treatment to prevent or shorten the episodes. Blepharoplasty may be helpful in addressing the long-term sequelae of multiple inflammatory episodes.

Madarosis

Definition Local or diffuse loss of eyelashes or eyebrows or both.

Etiology

Local

Chronic blepharitis, eyelid neoplasm (basal cell, squamous cell, or sebaceous cell carcinoma), burn, trauma, trichotillomania, eyelid infection (zoster, varicella, vaccinia, syphilis, tuberculosis, fungal).

Systemic

Endocrine (hypothyroidism, pituitary insufficiency), dermatologic (psoriasis, seborrheic dermatitis, alopecia syndromes, acne vulgaris, neurodermatitis, ichthyosis, impetigo, lichen planus), medications (topical epinephrine, gold, arsenic, barbiturates, PTU, quinine, chemotherapeutic agents), connective tissue disease (systemic lupus erythematosus), chronic malnutrition.

Symptoms Asymptomatic; may have redness, itching.

Signs Madarosis; may have lid or skin lesions.

Evaluation
- Complete ophthalmic history and eye exam with attention to facial skin, scalp, eyebrows, lids, and lashes. High suspicion for neoplasm, especially with focal areas of madarosis.
- Evaluation for underlying hormonal or nutritional deficits.
- Consider medical or dermatology consultation.

Figure 3-15 • Madarosis demonstrating an almost complete loss of eyelashes as well as some eyebrow loss.

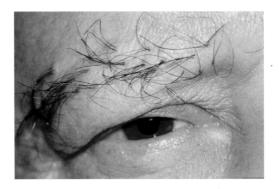

Management

- Treat underlying etiology.
- May require eyelid biopsy.
- Consider en bloc eyelash transplantation.

Prognosis Depends on underlying etiology.

Vitiligo and Poliosis

Total absence of melanin in hair follicles of the eyelashes or eyebrows (poliosis) and in skin (vitiligo), leading to focal patches of white hair or skin; associated with severe dermatitis, Vogt–Koyanagi–Harada syndrome, tuberous sclerosis, localized irradiation, sympathetic ophthalmia, and Waardenburg's syndrome (autosomal dominant, white forelock, congenital poliosis, nasal root abnormalities, synophrys [hypertrophy and fusion of the eyebrows], congenital deafness, iris heterochromia, and hypertelorism).

Figure 3-16 • Lower eyelid vitiligo and poliosis (white eyelashes) caused by total loss of melanin in a patient with Vogt–Koyanagi–Harada syndrome.

Poliosis

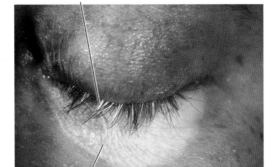

Vitiligo

- Treat underlying medical condition.

Acne Rosacea

Definition Chronic inflammatory disorder of the midline facial skin and eyelids.

Etiology Unknown; there is a genetic predilection and it is more common in certain ethnic backgrounds (e.g., Northern European ancestry); more common in women (2–3×). Rosacea may result from degenerative changes in perivascular collagen resulting in blood vessel dilation and leakage of inflammatory substances into the skin. It has also been suggested that the pathophysiology may include an inflammatory response to *D. folliculorum*. Facial flushing is associated with triggers such as alcohol, spicy foods, caffeine, extreme temperatures, and prolonged sunlight exposure.

Symptoms Facial flushing, tearing, dry eye, and foreign-body sensation.

Signs Acne, facial and eyelid telangiectasia, flushing most predominantly involving the nose and malar skin, persistent facial erythema, rhinophyma, blepharitis, recurrent chalazia/hordeola, conjunctivitis, keratitis, pannus, decreased tear break-up time, tear film debris and foam.

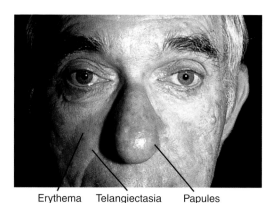

Erythema   Telangiectasia   Papules

Figure 3-17 • Acne rosacea demonstrating rhinophyma (bulbous nose) and midline facial erythema in the malar and brow regions.

Evaluation
- Complete ophthalmic history and eye exam with attention to facial skin, lids, tear film, conjunctiva, and cornea.

Management

DERMATOLOGIC MANIFESTATIONS

- Oral antibiotic (doxycycline 100 mg po or minocycline 50 mg po bid for 3 weeks, followed by qd for 3–4 months). Tetracycline 250 mg is also effective but requires more frequent dosing and is associated with more frequent gastrointestinal side effects. These agents are not offered to women in their childbearing years or to children with deciduous dentition. Alternatively, erythromycin 250 mg po bid then qd may be used.

Management—Cont'd

- Topical agents: metronidazole 0.75% (MetroGel, MetroCream) bid for 2–4 weeks; also, azeleic acid 20% (Azelex, Finevin), clindamycin 1% (Cleocin-T), or permethrin 5% (Elimite) cream.
- Consider topical tea tree oil.
- Avoidance of triggers of flushing.
- Telangiectasis can be treated with green tinted cosmetics or pulsed dye laser.
- Advanced rhinophyma can be treated with carbon dioxide laser, incisional surgery, or electrocauterization.

OPHTHALMIC MANIFESTATIONS

- Oral antibiotic (see above).
- Consider topical azithromycin (Azasite bid for 2 days, then qd for 2–4 weeks).
- Lid hygiene: daily application of hot compresses to the eyelids followed by massage and cleansing of the lid margins with commercial lid scrub pads, or face cloth or cotton-tipped applicator soaked in dilute baby shampoo or tea tree shampoo solution.
- Consider short course of topical antibiotic-steroid (see Blepharitis section) or compounded metronidazole 0.75% ointment for refractory cases.

Prognosis Clinical course is variable; depends on severity of disease and response to treatment.

Eyelid Malpositions

Ptosis

Definition Drooping of the upper eyelid(s).

Etiology

Aponeurotic (Involutional)

Disinsertion, central dehiscence, or attenuation of the levator aponeurosis causing lowering of the upper eyelid. Most common form of ptosis, often associated with advanced age, eye surgery, ocular trauma, pregnancy, chronic eyelid swelling, and blepharochalasis; good levator function.

Mechanical

Poor upper eyelid elevation due to mass effect of tumors, or to tethering of the eyelid by scarring (cicatricial ptosis); good levator function.

Myogenic

Inherent weakness of levator palpebrae superioris due to muscular disorders including chronic progressive external ophthalmoplegia, myotonic dystrophy, and oculopharyngeal dystrophy; extremely poor levator function.

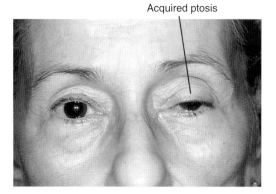

Acquired ptosis

Figure 3-18 • Significant acquired ptosis of the left eye. Most commonly caused by levator aponeurosis attenuation or dehiscence.

Neurogenic

Defects in innervation to cranial nerve III (oculomotor palsy) or sympathetic input to Müller's muscle (Horner's syndrome) or generalized dysfunction of neuromuscular junction such as myasthenia gravis; variable levator function depending on etiology.

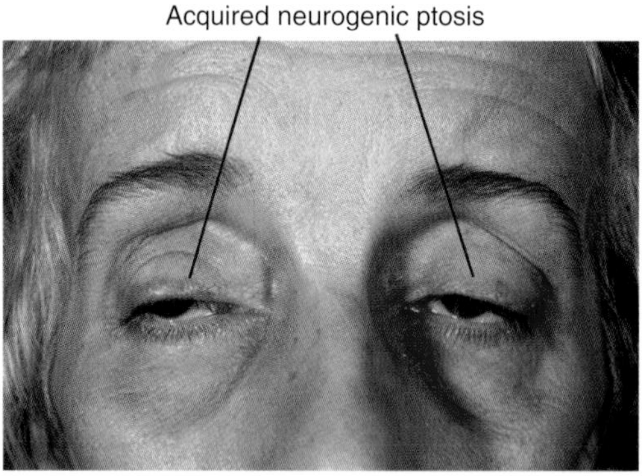

Acquired neurogenic ptosis

Figure 3-19 • Bilateral acquired ptosis due to myasthenia gravis.

Congenital

Poor levator function from birth; usually unilateral, nonhereditary, and myogenic with fibrosis and fat infiltration of levator muscle; rarely results from aponeurosis dehiscence (possibly birth trauma), in which case good levator function would be expected. Congenital Horner's syndrome (ptosis, miosis, anhidrosis, iris hypopigmentation) with poor Müller's muscle function from decreased sympathetic tone, or congenital neurogenic with Marcus Gunn jaw-winking syndrome from aberrant connections between cranial nerve V (innervating the pterygoid muscles) and the levator muscle.

Congenital ptosis

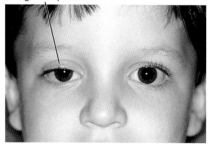

Poor levator function

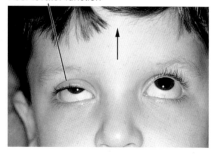

Figure 3-20 • Congenital ptosis of the right eye in a child.

Figure 3-21 • Same patient as Figure 3-20, demonstrating poor levator function with upgaze of the right eye. Note reduced levator excursion.

Symptoms Superior visual field defect, brow ache, loss of depth perception; may have decreased vision (congenital cases with deprivation amblyopia).

Signs Drooping of upper eyelid(s) with impaired elevation on upgaze, recruitment of brow muscles with brow furrows, higher lid crease and apparently smaller eye on ptotic side, abnormally high contralateral eyelid (Hering's law); in downgaze, affected lid may be higher than contralateral lid in congenital ptosis (lid lag) and lower in acquired cases; may have decreased visual acuity when visual axis obscured or head tilt with chin-up position when bilateral; other associated abnormalities in congenital ptosis include lagophthalmos, decreased superior rectus function, high astigmatism, anisometropia, strabismus, amblyopia, epicanthus, and blepharophimosis.

Differential Diagnosis Dermatochalasis (excess skin of upper eyelids, pseudoptosis), lid swelling, enophthalmos (e.g., orbital floor fracture), hypotropia, contralateral eyelid retraction causing asymmetry (e.g., thyroid-related ophthalmopathy), and small eye (phthisis bulbi, microphthalmia, anophthalmia).

Evaluation
- Complete ophthalmic history with attention to age of onset, previous surgeries or trauma, degree of functional impairment and time of day when worst, associated symptoms such as generalized fatigue, breathing problems, diplopia.
- Complete eye exam with attention to amblyopia in children, visual acuity, pupils, motility, Bell's phenomenon, lids, corneal sensation, and cornea.
- Eyelid measurements: margin reflex distance (MRD, distance between upper eyelid margin and corneal light reflex – normal is 4.5 mm), palpebral fissure height, upper lid crease height (high in aponeurotic), and levator function (LF; distance the upper lid margin travels between downgaze and upgaze – normal is greater than 11 mm; normal in aponeurotic, decreased in congenital).
- Consider neurologic evaluation with edrophonium chloride (Tensilon) test to rule out myasthenia gravis.

- Consider phenylephrine 2.5% to stimulate Müller's muscle and rule out Horner's syndrome; may also use topical cocaine 4–10% or hydroxyamphetamine 1% or both.
- Check visual field test with and without upper lids being held up by tape or finger (ptosis visual fields) to document visual impairment prior to surgery.
- External photos to document lid appearance prior to surgery.

Management

- Ptosis is treated with surgery:

  Good levator function: levator aponeurosis advancement, levator resection, muellerectomy, Fasanella-Servat tarsoconjunctival resection.

  Poor levator function (<6 mm): frontalis suspension with silicone rods, polytetrafluoroethylene sling, fascia lata, or frontalis flap. Maximal levator resection may be useful in some cases.

  Horner's syndrome or mild ptosis with good levator function: superior tarsal (Müller's muscle) resection.

- Surgery for aponeurotic ptosis is performed in an awake mildly sedated patient with intraoperative adjustment. Surgery for mechanical ptosis involves removal of any mechanical elements (i.e., excision of tumors or removal of tethering adhesions) followed by levator adjustment as needed. Surgery for congenital ptosis depends on the levator function: with normal levator function, a levator advancement works well but still has variability because many patients are children who require general anesthesia which prevents intraoperative fine-tuning, as the levator function approaches 6 mm the success of levator advancement decreases, and under 6 mm most surgeons will opt for a frontalis sling procedure.
- Ptosis is a difficult surgical challenge that often is confused with the simpler technique of blepharoplasty. Ptosis surgery should be performed by an experienced eyelid surgeon.
- Avoid surgery or undercorrect when poor Bell's reflex or decreased corneal sensation exists.
- Treat underlying medical condition.

Prognosis Excellent for aponeurotic and mechanical ptosis; fair to good for congenital ptosis, depending on the levator function; variable for myogenic and neurogenic ptosis.

Dermatochalasis

Laxity of the upper eyelid tissues resulting in redundancy of skin and subcutaneous tissue. Frequently associated with herniation of orbital fat through an attenuated orbital septum. May be associated with upper lid ptosis or pseudoptosis (mechanical effect of dermatochalasis). Profound dermatochalasis may result in superior visual field defect. Management is surgical with careful attention given preoperatively to coexisting conditions (e.g., ptosis). Lower lid dermatochalasis, on very rare occasion, may limit vision in downgaze due to extreme orbital fat herniation.

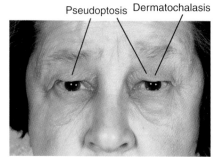

Pseudoptosis Dermatochalasis

Figure 3-22 • A patient with pseudoptosis from dermatochalasis.

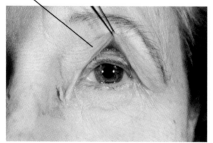

Dermatochalasis

Figure 3-23 • Dermatochalasis with redundant upper eyelid skin and subcutaneous tissue and herniated orbital fat. When the excess skin is retracted, the upper lid margin can be seen in the normal position.

Ectropion

Definition Eversion of the eyelid margin.

Etiology

Cicatricial

Due to burns (thermal or chemical), ocular trauma (surgical or mechanical), or chronic inflammation with anterior lamellar contraction.

Congenital

Due to vertical shortening of anterior lamella (skin and orbicularis oculi), rarely isolated, may be associated with blepharophimosis syndrome (blepharophimosis, ptosis, epicanthus inversus, and telecanthus).

Inflammatory

Due to chronic eyelid skin inflammation (atopic dermatitis, herpes zoster infections, rosacea).

Involutional

Due to horizontal lid laxity and tissue relaxation, followed by lid elongation, sagging, and conjunctival hypertrophy; usually involves lower eyelid; most frequent cause of ectropion in adults.

Mechanical

Due to lid edema, bulky lid tumors, orbital fat herniation, or lid-riding spectacles.

Paralytic

Usually follows cranial nerve VII (Bell's) palsy; can be temporary.

Symptoms Tearing, chronic eyelid or ocular irritation, or asymptomatic.

Signs Eversion of eyelid margin, conjunctival keratinization, injection and hypertrophy, superficial punctate keratitis, dermatitis (from chronic tearing and rubbing); may have corneal ulceration or scarring.

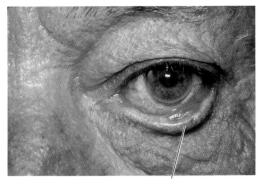

Figure 3-24 • Involutional ectropion of the left lower eyelid.

Ectropion

Evaluation
- Complete ophthalmic history with attention to history of eye surgery, trauma, burns, infections, or facial droop (Bell's palsy).
- Complete eye exam with attention to lids, orbicularis function, lateral canthal tendon laxity, herniated fat and scarring, conjunctiva, and cornea.

Management

- Treat ectropion-related corneal and conjunctival exposure with topical lubrication with preservative-free artificial tears (see Appendix) up to q1h and ointment (Refresh PM) qhs.

CICATRICIAL

- Four-step procedure: (1) cicatrix release and relaxation; (2) horizontal lid tightening with lateral tarsal strip; (3) anterior lamella lengthening with full-thickness skin graft or cheek lift; and (4) posterior lamellar spacer (with ear cartilage or other material).

CONGENITAL

- Mild ectropion often requires no treatment. Moderate or severe ectropion treated like cicatricial ectropion with horizontal lid tightening and full-thickness skin graft to vertically lengthen anterior lamella.

INFLAMMATORY

- Treat underlying dermatologic condition. Temporizing measures include taping temporal side of eyelid, using moisture chamber goggles, and topical lubrication with preservative-free artificial tears (see Appendix) up to q1h.

Management—Cont'd

INVOLUTIONAL

- Three procedures may be used individually or in combination: (1) medial spindle procedure for punctal ectropion; (2) horizontal lid shortening using lateral tarsal strip procedure, lateral lid wedge resection, or canthal tendon plication; and (3) lower lid retractor reinsertion.

MECHANICAL

- Relieve mechanical force causing ectropion (tumor or fat removal, eyeglass adjustment, etc.).

PARALYTIC

- Often resolves spontaneously within 6 months if due to Bell's palsy. Temporizing measures include taping temporal side of eyelid, suture tarsorrhaphy, using moisture chamber goggles, and topical lubrication with preservative-free artificial tears (see Appendix) up to q1h; rarely, if chronic, consider canthoplasty, lateral tarsorrhaphy, brow suspension, and horizontal lid tightening with or without middle lamellar buttress such as ear cartilage.

Prognosis Usually good with surgical treatment; cicatricial and inflammatory ectropion are prone to recurrence; paralytic ectropion may resolve spontaneously within 6 months after Bell's palsy.

Entropion

Definition Inversion of the eyelid margin; may affect either eyelid, although the lower lid is affected more frequently.

Etiology

Cicatricial

Due to posterior lamella (tarsus and conjunctiva) shortening with lid inversion and rubbing of lashes and lid margin on globe; associated with Stevens–Johnson syndrome, ocular cicatricial pemphigoid, trachoma, herpes zoster, eye surgery, ocular trauma, thermal or chemical burns, and chronic conjunctivitis from long-term topical glaucoma medications.

Congenital

Due to structural tarsal plate defects, shortened posterior lamellae, or eyelid retractor dysgenesis; horizontal tarsal kink is an unusual form of congenital entropion that usually affects the upper eyelid.

Involutional

Most common cause of entropion in older patients, usually affects lower lid; predisposing factors include horizontal lid laxity, overriding preseptal orbicularis, disinserted or atrophied lid retractors, and involutional enophthalmos.

Spastic

Due to ocular inflammation or irritation; often occurs following eye surgery in patients with early underlying involutional changes.

Symptoms Tearing, foreign body sensation, and red eye.

Signs Inturned eyelid margin, keratinized eyelid margins (cicatricial), horizontal lid laxity, overriding preseptal orbicularis, enophthalmos, symblepharon (cicatricial), conjunctival injection, superficial punctate keratitis; may have corneal ulceration or scarring.

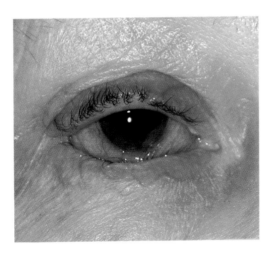

Figure 3-25 • Cicatricial entropion of the right lower eyelid.

Differential Diagnosis Trichiasis, distichiasis, blepharospasm.

Evaluation
- Complete ophthalmic history with attention to history of eye surgery, trauma, burns, or infections.
- Complete eye exam with attention to lids, lid tone (snapback test), lower lid margin (sagging), medial and lateral canthal tendons, inferior fornix (unusually deep), digital eversion test at the inferior border of tarsus to distinguish involutional from cicatricial entropion (involutional rotates, cicatricial does not).

Management

- If corneal involvement exists, topical antibiotic ointment (erythromycin or bacitracin bid to qid).

CICATRICIAL

- Excision of scar and consider anterior lamellar resection or recession for minimal involvement; tarsal fracture procedure for lower lid involvement; tarsal graft from preserved sclera, ear cartilage, or hard palate if the tarsus is badly damaged; may also require conjunctival and mucous membrane grafts in severe cases.

CONGENITAL

- Rarely improves and often requires surgical treatment to correct underlying anatomic defect.

INVOLUTIONAL

- Three procedures may be used individually or in combination: (1) temporizing measure with lid taping below lower lid, Quickert suture, or thermal cautery; (2) horizontal lid tightening with lateral tarsal strip procedure; and (3) lid retractor repair with full-thickness transverse blepharoplasty and eyelid margin rotation (Wies' procedure) or retractor reinsertion.

SPASTIC

- Break entropion–irritation cycle by taping inturned lid to evert margin, thermal cautery, or suture techniques to temporarily evert lid; often requires more definitive procedure as involutional changes progress (see above).

Prognosis　Good except for autoimmune or inflammatory-related cicatricial entropion.

Blepharospasm

Definition　Bilateral, uncontrolled, episodic contraction of the orbicularis oculi.

Essential Blepharospasm

Thought to be caused by a disorder of the basal ganglia; usually with gradual onset during the fifth to seventh decade; some association with other movement disorders, and high incidence of movement disorders among first-degree relatives.

Meige's Syndrome

Essential blepharospasm with facial grimacing; may have cog-wheeling in the neck and extremities.

Symptoms Uncontrollable blinking, squeezing, or twitching of eyelids or facial muscles.

Signs Spasms of orbicularis oculi or facial muscles; may prevent examiner from prying open lids during episodes; may be absent during sleep.

Differential Diagnosis Reflex blepharospasm (caused by eyelid irritation, dry eye, entropion, trichiasis, contact lens overuse, or meningeal irritation), hemifacial spasm, facial myokymia, Tourette's syndrome, tic douloureux (trigeminal neuralgia), Parkinson's disease, Huntington's disease, basal ganglia infarct.

Evaluation
- Complete ophthalmic history with attention to causes of ocular irritation, stress and caffeine use, and history of neurologic disorders.
- Complete eye exam with attention to cranial nerves, motility, and lids.
- Consider head magnetic resonance imaging (MRI) with attention to the posterior fossa for atypical history or presentation.

Management

- Injection of botulinum type A toxin (Botox) into the orbicularis muscle to weaken contractions; repeat injections are often required every 12 weeks as the therapeutic effect declines; transient ptosis and diplopia are uncommon side effects.
- Medical therapy with haloperidol, clonazepam, bromocriptine, or baclofen has limited success.

Prognosis Good with appropriate therapy; in most cases, repeat injections every few months are needed indefinitely.

Bell's Palsy

Definition Acutely acquired, isolated, peripheral facial paralysis of unknown cause involving the facial nerve (CN VII).

Etiology By definition, the etiology is unknown; neural inflammation has been identified by MRI and on autopsy; herpes virus is thought to play a role in most cases.

Symptoms Acute onset of unilateral facial paralysis over a period of 24 hours, often accompanied by headache and numbness; dry eye, foreign body sensation, tearing, drooling, dysarthria, and dysphagia. Long-term symptoms include oral-ocular synkinesis, gustatory lacrimation, decreased vision, corneal irritation.

Signs Unilateral facial paralysis including all divisions of cranial nerve VII. Chronic signs include brow ptosis, ipsilateral hypertonicity, lagophthalmos, exposure keratopathy with epiphora, ulceration, and scarring.

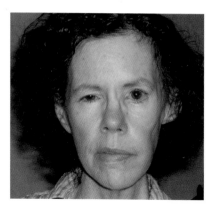

Figure 3-26 • Patient with left-sided Bell's palsy. Note hypertonicity on left side of face.

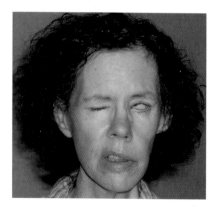

Figure 3-27 • Same patient as Figure 3-26 with left-sided Bell's palsy during attempted lid closure. Note the large lagophthalmos and good Bell's reflex of the left eye.

Table 3-1 House-Brackmann Facial Nerve Grading System

Grade	Description	Characteristics
I	Normal	Normal facial function
II	Mild dysfunction	Very slight weakness found on close inspection; good forehead function; complete and quick eyelid closure
III	Moderate dysfunction	Obvious but not disfiguring asymmetry; mild synkinesis; slight forehead movement; complete eyelid closure with effort
IV	Moderately severe dysfunction	Disfiguring asymmetry; no forehead movement; incomplete eyelid closure
V	Severe dysfunction	Barely perceptible facial movement; incomplete eyelid closure
VI	Total paralysis	No movement

Adapted from House JW, Brackmann DE: Facial nerve grading system, *Otolaryngol Head Neck Surg* 93:146, 1985.

Differential Diagnosis Tumor of parotid gland or facial nerve, trauma (temporal bone fracture), congenital facial nerve palsy, herpes zoster cephalicus, central nervous system (CNS) disease, postsurgical.

Evaluation
- Complete history with attention to date, time, and nature of onset, duration of symptoms, evidence of improvement within first 4 months.
- Complete eye exam with attention to cranial nerves, lids, orbicularis function, brow position, lower lid retraction, and cornea.

- Delayed onset with progression over more than 1 week requires MRI of facial nerve and CT of temporal bone.
- Additional cranial nerve involvement requires further brain stem investigation.

Management

- Initially, aggressive lubrication of ocular surface with viscous artificial tears (see Appendix) up to q1h and ointment qhs.
- Consider taping lid closed at night, some patients prefer Tegaderm dressing instead of tape.
- Consider gold weight implantation or temporary lateral tarsorrhaphy.
- Follow monthly for signs of improvement. Lack of improvement after 4 months is ominous and requires further investigation (MRI and CT scan).
- Consider antiviral (acyclovir) and antiinflammatory (prednisone) treatment.
- Chronic sequelae can be treated surgically (persistent paralysis) or with botulinum toxin (aberrant regeneration).
- There is no evidence to support the use of electrical facial stimulation, nor is there strong evidence supporting the efficacy of facial physical therapy.

Prognosis Typically excellent with most patients returning to nearly complete function (grade 2); 90% of function returns within 1 year, 99% within 2 years.

Floppy Eyelid Syndrome

Definition Chronic papillary conjunctivitis with lax tarsi, spontaneous eyelid eversion, and loss of eyelid–globe contact when lying prone.

Etiology Nocturnal lid eversion with rubbing of the tarsal conjunctiva against bedding.

Epidemiology Often occurs in obese men with obstructive sleep apnea.

Symptoms Chronically red and irritated eyes, particularly upon awakening; mild mucous discharge.

Signs Loose, rubbery eyelids (particularly upper lids), very easily everted, palpebral conjunctival papillae, conjunctival injection, superficial punctate keratitis.

Figure 3-28 • Floppy eyelid syndrome demonstrating extreme laxity of upper eyelid. Note upper eyelid papillary conjunctivitis due to nocturnal lid eversion.

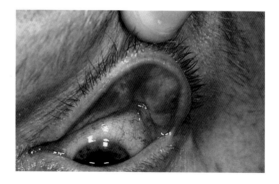

Differential Diagnosis Giant papillary conjunctivitis, adult inclusion conjunctivitis, superior limbic keratoconjunctivitis, vernal keratoconjunctivitis, atopic keratoconjunctivitis, medicamentosa.

Evaluation

- Complete ophthalmic history and eye exam with attention to lids, upper lid laxity, palpebral conjunctiva, and cornea.
- Formal sleep study to evaluate for obstructive sleep apnea.

Management

- Topical lubrication with preservative-free artificial tears (see Appendix) up to q1h.
- Topical antibiotic ointment (erythromycin or bacitracin bid to qid for 5–7 days) if cornea involved.
- Metal eye shield when sleeping.
- Consider surgical correction using eyelid wedge resection.
- Consider sleep study with otolaryngologist.

Prognosis Excellent.

Trichiasis

Definition Misdirected eyelashes.

Etiology Entropion, cicatricial eye disease, chronic eyelid inflammation, or idiopathic.

Symptoms Red eye, foreign body sensation, and tearing.

Signs Eyelashes directed toward and rubbing against the eye, conjunctival injection, superficial punctate keratitis; may have corneal scarring in chronic cases.

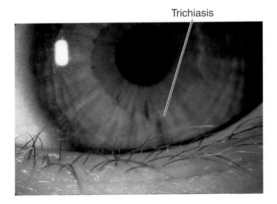

Trichiasis

Figure 3-29 • Trichiasis demonstrating posterior misdirection of eyelid lashes touching the corneal epithelium. Not to be confused with distichiasis (see Figure 3-32).

Differential Diagnosis   Distichiasis (ectopic eyelashes).

Evaluation
- Complete ophthalmic history and eye exam with attention to lids, lashes, conjunctiva, and cornea.

Management

- Topical lubrication with preservative-free artificial tears (see Appendix) up to q1h.
- Topical antibiotic ointment (erythromycin or bacitracin bid to qid for 5–7 days) if cornea involved.
- Mechanical epilation using fine forceps if only a few lashes are misdirected.
- For segmental trichiasis, consider cryotherapy using a double freeze–thaw technique, lashes then mechanically removed using fine forceps; complications include lid edema, eyelid notching, and skin depigmentation.
- Electroepilation for extensive or recurrent trichiasis; use limited application because of the potential of scarring adjacent follicles and eyelid tissue.
- Consider full-thickness wedge resection with primary closure for segmental trichiasis, or tarsal fracture (tarsotomy) or entropion repair (see Entropion section) for large areas of trichiasis; should be performed by an oculoplastic surgeon.
- Consider oral azithromycin (single dose) to reduce postsurgical recurrence of trachoma induced trichiasis.

Prognosis   Frequent recurrences with mechanical technique, usually good with permanent removal.

Congenital Eyelid Anomalies

Ankyloblepharon

Partial or complete eyelid fusion. Severe forms may be associated with craniofacial abnormalities. Prognosis usually good unless severe associated defects.

- Simple cases treated with incision of skin webs after clamping with hemostat for 10–15 seconds with reapproximation of skin and conjunctiva; severe cases may necessitate major surgical revision.

Blepharophimosis

Tight, foreshortened (vertically and horizontally) palpebral fissures with poor eyelid function and no levator fold. May be sporadic or part of congenital syndrome (autosomal dominant [AD]) with blepharophimosis, blepharoptosis, epicanthus inversus, and telecanthus. Prognosis depends on extent of syndrome and need for additional surgery. Mapped to chromosome 3q.

- Surgery usually is performed at 4–5 years of age to allow nasal bridge to develop fully.
- Congenital syndrome: consider staged oculoplastic repair with medial canthoplasty via Y–V plasty and transnasal wiring, followed by frontalis suspension for ptosis 3 to 4 months later, and finally full-thickness skin graft from periauricular or supraclavicular area.

Figure 3-30 • Blepharophimosis syndrome demonstrating small palpebral fissures, lack of upper lid folds, ptosis, epicanthus inversus, and telecanthus.

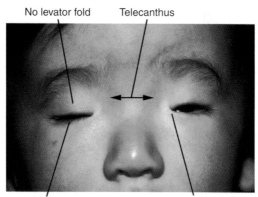

No levator fold   Telecanthus

Blepharophimosis   Epicanthus inversus

Coloboma

Small notch to full-thickness defect of the eyelid due to incomplete union of frontonasal or maxillary mesoderm at the eyelid margin, usually superonasal and unilateral. Inferolateral defects are often bilateral and associated with systemic anomalies such as mandibulofacial dysostosis (AD; Treacher Collins syndrome); corneal exposure and dryness may occur. Small defects (<25%) have good prognosis; prognosis of medium and larger defects depends on location and associated abnormalities. Associated with microphthalmos, iris coloboma, and anterior polar cataract.

Lid coloboma

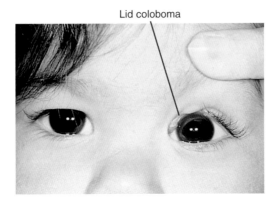

Figure 3-31 • Superonasal coloboma of left upper eyelid in a child.

- Topical lubrication with preservative-free artificial tears or ointments (see Appendix) up to q1h.
- Surgical repair (delay until preschool age): small defects (<25%) via pentagonal resection with direct layered closure, medium defects (25–50%) via Tenzel flap with or without lateral cantholysis, large defects (>50%) via myocutaneous flap or full-thickness lid rotation flap.
- Beware of lid-sharing procedures in children because occlusion amblyopia may result.

Cryptophthalmos

Congenital defects of the first, second, and third wave of neural crest migration leading to abnormal lid and anterior eye structure development, including partial or complete absence of eyebrow, palpebral fissure, eyelashes, and conjunctiva; may have hidden or buried eye with smooth skin stretching from brow to cheek; more posterior orbital structures are usually normal. Prognosis often poor due to underlying structural ocular defects.

- Treatment focuses on progressive expansion of the understimulated bony orbit to prevent midfacial hypoplasia; multiple surgeries or expanding conformers often are required with eyelid reconstruction.

Distichiasis

Ectopic eyelashes growing posterior to or out of the meibomian gland orifices. May be congenital or acquired (i.e., from chronic inflammation), sometimes hereditary. Lashes are usually shorter, softer, and finer than normal cilia, and may or may not contact the conjunctival and corneal surfaces; usually well tolerated. In congenital distichiasis, the embryonic pilosebaceous units inappropriately develop into hair follicles. Treat if corneal involvement exists, but with caution because treatment can be more damaging than disease.

- Topical lubrication with preservative-free artificial tears or ointments (see Appendix) or bandage contact lens in mild cases.
- Epilation, tarsal fracture surgery, electrolysis, cryotherapy, or laser thermal ablation in more severe cases.

Figure 3-32 • Distichiasis with lashes originating from meibomian gland orifice.

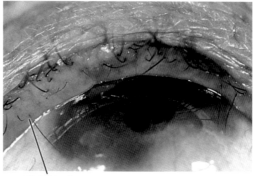

Distichiasis

Epiblepharon

Redundant skin and orbicularis muscle leading to inward rotation of the lower eyelid margins, turning lashes against the globe; usually resolves spontaneously. More common in Asians. Prognosis excellent even if surgery necessary.

- Conservative treatment in infants, because condition tends to resolve with facial maturation.
- Subciliary myocutaneous excision is extremely effective; care is taken to avoid overexcision with resultant ectropion.

Figure 3-33 • Epiblepharon of lower eyelid demonstrating upwardly directed lashes.

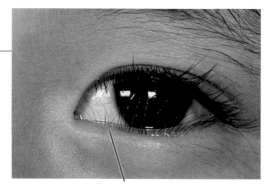

Epiblepharon

Epicanthus

Crescentic vertical skin folds in the medial canthal area overlying the medial canthal tendon; usually bilateral. Caused by immature facial bones or redundant skin and underlying tissue. May be most prominent superiorly (epicanthus tarsalis), inferiorly (epicanthus inversus), or equally distributed (epicanthus palpebralis). Epicanthus tarsalis is frequently associated with Asian eyelids, while epicanthus inversus is associated with blepharophimosis syndrome. Good prognosis.

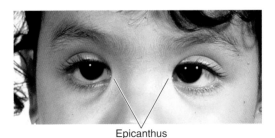

Figure 3-34 • Epicanthus demonstrating pseudostrabismus. Note vertical skin fold over medial canthal areas.

Epicanthus

- If due to facial bone immaturity, delay treatment.
- When treatment required (delay until preschool age), Z-plasty or Y-V plasty often effective; eyelid crease construction may be required.

Euryblepharon

Horizontal widening of the palpebral fissure, often temporally; usually involves the lower eyelid with an antimongoloid appearance due to inferior insertion of the lateral canthal tendon. Patients have a poor blink, poor lid closure, and lagophthalmos with exposure keratitis. Usually good prognosis.

- Topical lubrication with preservative-free artificial tears (see Appendix) in mild cases.
- If symptoms severe and corneal pathology exists, full-thickness eyelid resection with repositioning of lateral canthal tendon may be required. If necessary, vertical eyelid lengthening can be achieved with skin grafts.

Microblepharon

Rare, bilateral, vertical foreshortening of the eyelids, sometimes causing exposure and dry eye symptoms; may be related to cryptophthalmos. Usually stable with good prognosis if no exposure keratitis exists.

- Topical lubrication with preservative-free artificial tears (see Appendix) in mild cases.
- Pedicle rotation skin flaps from cheek or brow, eyelid-sharing procedures, or full-thickness skin grafts for severe exposure with a normal globe.
- Beware of lid-sharing procedures in children because occlusion amblyopia may result.

Telecanthus

Increased distance between medial canthi caused by long medial canthal tendons (in contrast to hypertelorism in which the distance between the medial walls of the orbits is increased). Most frequent ocular finding in fetal alcohol syndrome; also associated with Waardenburg's syndrome and blepharophimosis syndrome. Good prognosis.

- Transnasal wiring to shorten distance between medial canthi and remove excess medial canthal skin.

Figure 3-35 • Telecanthus. Note increased distance between medial canthi.

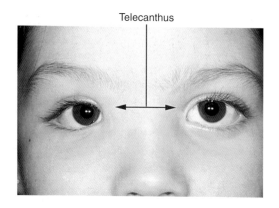

Telecanthus

Benign Eyelid Tumors

Pigmented Benign Eyelid Tumors

Acquired Nevus

Darkly pigmented lesion that contains modified melanocytes called nevocellular nevus cells. Classified according to location in skin: junctional (epidermis), compound (epidermis and dermis), or dermal (dermis); may contain hair. Malignant transformation rare, although the Halo nevus, a type of compound nevus, is associated with remote cutaneous malignant melanoma. The Spitz nevus, another type of compound nevus, may be confused histologically with malignant melanoma in children and young adults.

Figure 3-36 • Nevus of the upper eyelid along the lid margin.

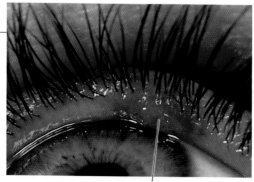

Eyelid nevus

- No treatment usually required.
- Consider excision for cosmesis, chronic irritation, or evidence of malignant transformation.

Ephelis (Freckle)

Focal regions of cutaneous melanocytic overactivity; cells slightly larger than normal. Found in sun-exposed areas; occurs in individuals with fair complexions. No malignant potential.

- No treatment recommended.

Oculodermal Melanocytosis (Nevus of Ota)

Unilateral, blue-gray, pigmented macule; usually in the distribution of the first and second division of cranial nerve V with ipsilateral melanocytosis of the sclera and uveal tract; 10% bilateral; melanosis of the ipsilateral orbit and leptomeninges may occur. Histologically, composed of dermal fusiform dendritic melanocytes. May be present at birth or during the first year of life. Increased risk of congenital glaucoma; risk of malignant transformation is very low; however, cutaneous and ocular melanoma can occur, especially in Caucasians.

- No treatment usually required.
- Periodic examinations to monitor for evidence of malignant transformation.

Seborrheic Keratosis

Waxy, pigmented, hyperkeratotic, plaquelike, crusty lesion; occurs in the elderly; histologically, composed of intradermal proliferation of basal epithelioid cells; irritation is frequent; no malignant potential.

- Shave excision or curettage for small lesions.
- Complete surgical excision for larger lesions.

Oculodermal melanocytosis

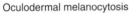
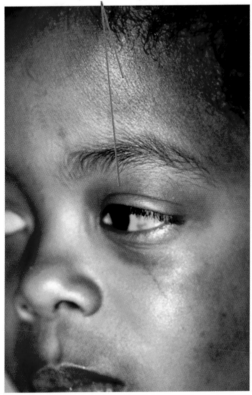

Figure 3-37 • Nevus of Ota of the left eye and orbit demonstrating unilateral, blue-gray, pigmented macule and pigmented sclera.

Figure 3-38 • Seborrheic keratosis on the eyelid.

Seborrheic keratosis

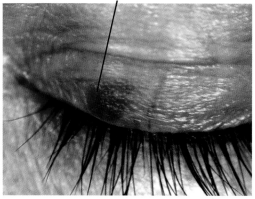

Squamous Papilloma

Most common benign eyelid growth; occurs in older adults. Benign hyperplasia of the squamous epithelium; may be sessile or pedunculated with color similar to that of skin; grows slowly and in groups. Etiology is unclear; viral papillomas are found in groups and more common in children, while the elderly usually develop individual or widely spaced papillomas that are not thought to be viral in origin. Histologically, papillomas display epithelial hyperkeratosis and acanthosis around a central vascular core.

Figure 3-39 • Squamous papilloma demonstrating abundant multiple lesions of the lower eyelid.

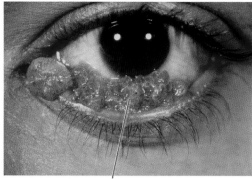
Squamous papilloma

• Complete surgical excision.

Verruca Vulgaris (Viral Papilloma)

Viral-related growth with potential for malignant transformation. Usually asymptomatic; appears as a pedunculated or sessile hyperemic mass on eyelid or tarsal conjunctiva with minimal surrounding inflammation. Associated with human papillomavirus (strains 6, 11, and 16). Frequently resolves spontaneously.

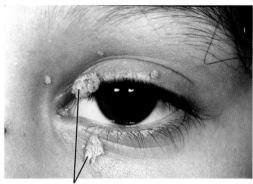

Figure 3-40 • Verruca vulgaris demonstrating multiple large and small lesions of the eyelids.

Verruca vulgaris

- Observation if small and no inflammation.
- Larger or multiple lesions may be entirely excised, scraped, cauterized, or treated with cryotherapy; satellite lesions are thought to respond to initial treatment of selected lesions.

Nonpigmented Benign Eyelid Tumors
Xanthelasma

Xanthomas of the eyelids that appear as flat or slightly elevated creamy yellow plaques; usually bilateral, involving the medial upper lids. Histologically composed of foamy histiocytes surrounded by localized inflammation. Occurs in older patients; most patients with xanthelasma are normolipidemic. Systemic diseases that demonstrate xanthomatosis include biliary cirrhosis, diabetes, pancreatitis, renal disease, and hypothyroidism. Xanthelasma is the least specific of the xanthomas (nodular, tendinous, eruptive, and plaques). Excellent prognosis, usually recur after excision.

Xanthelasma

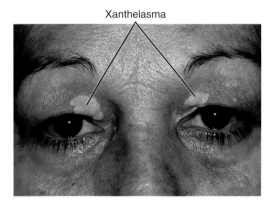

Figure 3-41 • Xanthelasma demonstrating characteristic yellow plaques on upper eyelids bilaterally.

- **Lab tests**: In extreme cases, serum cholesterol and triglycerides.
- Full-thickness excision with flaps or grafts, carbon dioxide laser treatment, or chemical cauterization with trichloroacetic acid as needed.

Moll's Gland Cyst (Hidrocystoma, Sudoriferous Cyst)

Benign cystic lesion resulting from abnormal proliferation of apocrine secretory gland (gland of Moll); also known as sudoriferous cyst or cystadenoma. Smooth, translucent, and several millimeters in size; usually slow growing and painless; frequently involves the eyelid, particularly the inner canthus in a peripunctal location. No predilection for race or gender but more common in adults than in children. Differential diagnosis includes cystic basal cell carcinoma and milia (pilosebaceous cysts). Recurrence after complete excision is rare, but incision alone to drain the fluid contained within the hidrocystoma typically results in recurrence.

- Marsupialization or complete excision.
- Peripunctal excision may require canalicular probing to avoid or detect canalicular injury.

Figure 3-42 • Moll's gland cyst (hidrocystoma) with smooth translucent appearance.

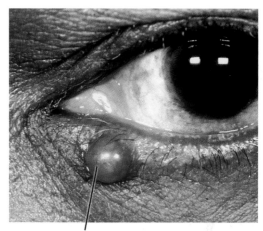

Moll's gland cyst

Epidermal Inclusion Cyst

Firm, freely mobile, subepithelial lesion (1–5 mm in diameter); cyst contains cheesy keratin material produced by cyst lining. Thought to arise from occluded surface epithelium or

Figure 3-43 • Epidermal inclusion cyst containing firm, cheesy keratin material.

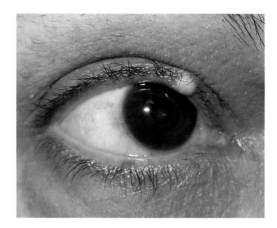

pilosebaceous follicles. Often has a central pore representing the remaining pilar duct, or occasionally a dark or even black center indicating oxidized keratin. Multiple epidermal inclusion cysts may be associated with Gardner's syndrome or Torre's syndrome.

• Complete surgical excision.

Inverted Follicular Keratosis

Small, solitary, benign lesion with a nodular or verrucous appearance. Occurs in older adults; male predilection. May arise over months and is thought to have a viral etiology. Histologically, lobular acanthosis of the epithelium with squamous and basal cell proliferation; represents a type of irritated seborrheic keratosis.

• Complete surgical excision.

Milia

Multiple, umbilicated, well-circumscribed, pinhead-sized, elevated, round, white nodules (1–3 mm in diameter). May arise spontaneously, or after trauma, radiation, herpes zoster ophthalmicus, or epidermolysis bullosa. Thought to represent retention follicular cysts caused by blockage of pilosebaceous units.

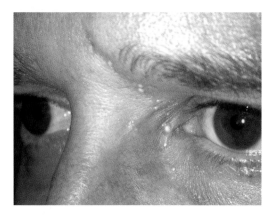

Figure 3-44 • Milia, appearing as small white lumps in the medial canthus.

• Complete surgical excision, electrolysis, or diathermy. Frequently treated with curettage using a 25–30-gauge needle.

Sebaceous (Pilar) Cyst

Yellow, elevated, smooth, subcutaneous tumor with central comedo plug caused by sebaceous or meibomian gland obstruction; occurs in the elderly. Less common than epithelial inclusion cysts; may be associated with chalazia.

• Complete surgical excision with inclusion of epithelial lining.

Figure 3-45 • Sebaceous cyst appearing as a smooth nodule in the upper eyelid.

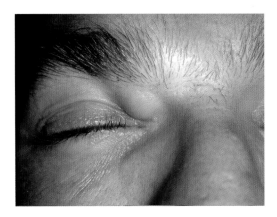

Pilomatrixoma (Calcifying Epithelioma of Malherbe)

Small (<3 cm), solitary, firm, nodular lesion consisting of cells that demonstrate features of hair cells; slow, progressive growth; usually flesh colored but may have a red or purple hue. Occur in the head and neck, often along the brow or lid. More common in Caucasians and slight female predilection. Differential diagnosis includes dermoid cyst, preseptal cellulitis, and cutaneous abscess. Histology reveals characteristic calcification. Recurrence after complete excision is rare.

• Biopsy or complete surgical excision.

Vascular Benign Eyelid Tumors

Capillary Hemangioma

Most common pediatric eyelid tumor, usually appears within 1 month of life with a bluish subcutaneous mass and normal overlying dermis, or as a superficial vascular lesion (sometimes erroneously called strawberry nevus) representing hamartomatous growth of capillary blood vessels. Rapid growth occurs in two phases with peaks at 3 and 8 months; spontaneous involution begins after 1 year and may proceed up to 10 years; slight female predilection.

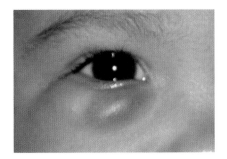

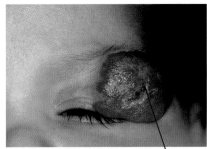

Capillary hemangioma

Figure 3-46 • Capillary hemangioma demonstrating lower-eyelid swelling with bluish doscoloration.

Figure 3-47 • Large capillary hemangioma of the left upper eyelid in an infant causing ptosis.

Possible amblyopia due to occlusion of the visual axis or induced astigmatism; myopia or strabismus may occur. Prognosis usually good if visual axis clear and no amblyopia.

- Routine follow-up visits to monitor for amblyopia and refractive error.

- Large lesions may be treated with intralesional steroid injection, systemic corticosteroids, or surgical excision. Interferon (Lupron) should be avoided due to spastic diplegia. Pulsed dye laser may be useful in treating the superficial component of some lesions.

Lymphangioma

Congenital malformation with a predilection for the head and neck. Around the eye, the orbit is more often involved. The eyelid can be involved, but is rarely involved in isolation (see Chapter 1).

Port Wine Stain (Nevus Flammeus)

Congenital venular malformation often confused with eyelid hemangioma. Always present at birth and follows dermatomal distribution. Typically lighter with a more purple hue than hemangioma; facial involvement may include any or multiple branches of the trigeminal nerve (CN V); does not blanch on palpation. Risk of glaucoma (from increased venous pressure) and the Sturge–Weber syndrome (facial port wine stain, choroidal "hemangioma", intracranial vascular anomalies [see Phakomatoses section in Chapter 10]) occurs primarily in patients with V_1 and V_2 involvement; risk of Sturge–Weber with isolated V_1 involvement is extremely small.

- Early examination for choroidal involvement and glaucoma is critical.
- Pulsed dye laser treatment is recommended as early as 1 month of life.
- Cranial nerve V2 involvement is an indication for MRI of the brain.

Malignant Eyelid Tumors

Basal Cell Carcinoma

Firm, pearly nodule or flatter, less well-defined lesion with central ulceration, telangiectasia, madarosis (lash loss), and inflammation. Associated with ultraviolet radiation exposure and fair skin. Most common (90%) malignant eyelid tumor; occurs in older adults with male predilection (2:1). Usually found on lower lid (67%) followed in frequency by upper lid (20%), medial canthus (10%), and lateral canthus (3%). Locally invasive, but rarely metastatic (usually occurs with canthal involvement). Two growth patterns:

Nodular

Most common; appears as small, painless, umbilicated nodule with sharp pearly borders and superficial telangiectasia that can be ulcerative ("rodent ulcer"); rarely pigmented; less invasive. Nests of cells with peripheral palisading on histopathologic examination.

Morpheaform or sclerosing

Appears as flat, indurated plaque that lacks distinct margins; often ulcerated; more invasive. Associated with nevoid basal cell carcinoma syndrome, linear unilateral basal cell nevus, and Bazex syndrome. Excellent prognosis with appropriate treatment, but 2–10% local recurrence; metastasis in 0.02–0.1%.

Figure 3-48 • Basal cell carcinoma of the lower eyelid demonstrating central ulceration with pearly, nodular border containing telangiectatic vessels.

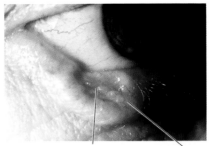

Central ulceration Basal cell carcinoma

Figure 3-49 • Basal cell carcinoma of the lower eyelid demonstrating central ulceration with scab and pearly, nodular borders.

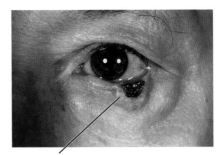

Basal cell carcinoma

- Protect against further sun damage.
- Complete surgical excision with margin controls (frozen sectioning); Mohs micrographic surgery sometimes useful in preserving critical eyelid tissue.
- Extremely advanced cases involving both upper and lower lids may benefit rarely from external beam irradiation.
- Canthal tumors require orbital CT scan to evaluate posterior (orbital) involvement. Radiation or cryotherapy should not be used in these lesions, because posterior portions of the tumor may go untreated.

Squamous Cell Carcinoma

Flat or slightly elevated, scaly, ulcerated, erythematous plaque, often arising from actinic keratosis (better prognosis), may also arise from Bowen's disease (in situ) and radiation dermatosis. Constitutes less than 5% of malignant eyelid tumors (although second most common it is 40–50 times less common than basal cell carcinoma). Usually found on lower lid with lid margin involvement. Risk factors include sun exposure, radiation injury, fair skin, or other irritative insults; male predilection. Potentially metastatic (low) and locally invasive (faster growth than basal cell carcinoma), regional lymph node spread from eyelids occurs in 13–24% of cases. Prognosis varies with tumor size, degree of differentiation, underlying etiology, and depth of tumor invasion.

- Protect against further sun damage.
- Incisional or excisional biopsy with wide surgical margins (wider than basal cell carcinoma).

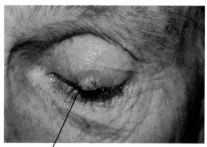

Figure 3-50 • Squamous cell carcinoma of the left upper eyelid, demonstrating erythematous lesion with central scaly plaque.

Squamous cell carcinoma

- Adjunctive radiation, cryotherapy, or chemotherapy, or a combination.
- Postseptal involvement typically requires orbital exenteration.

Actinic Keratosis

Most common precancerous skin lesion; 25% develop squamous cell carcinoma. Round, scaly, flat, or papillary keratotic growth with surrounding erythema; found in sun-exposed areas. Occurs in older adults with fair complexions. Histologically, cellular atypia with mitotic figures and hyperkeratosis; squamous carcinoma-in-situ.

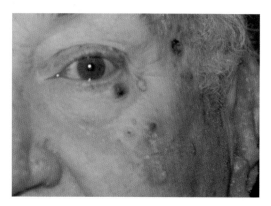

Figure 3-51 • Actinic keratosis of the molar region demonstrating flat, erythematous, scaly appearance. The pigmented lesions are seborrheic keratoses.

- Periocular lesions require incisional or excisional biopsy to rule out malignant lesions.
- Cryotherapy or additional surgery can be performed once diagnosis is confirmed.

Keratoacanthoma

Rapidly growing lesion usually found in sun-exposed areas with a central ulcerated, keratin-filled crater and hyperkeratotic margins; occurs in older adults. Lid or lash involvement may cause permanent damage; spontaneous resolution is common. A form of pseudoepitheliomatous hyperplasia; neither distinction is used any longer in some pathology laboratories, where these lesions are all classified as squamous carcinomas. May have viral origin; multiple keratoacanthomas occur in Ferguson–Smith syndrome.

Figure 3-52 • Keratoacanthoma of the right upper eyelid demonstrating keratin-filled crater with hyperkeratotic margins.

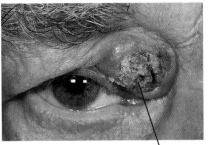

Keratoacanthoma

- Complete surgical excision is treatment of choice for single lesions.

Sebaceous Cell Carcinoma

Highly malignant, rare neoplasm of the sebaceous glands in the caruncle or lids; most common in fifth to seventh decades. May masquerade as chronic unilateral blepharitis (20–50% of patients) or recurrent chalazion; usually found on upper lid. Constitutes 1–15% of malignant eyelid tumors (approximately equal incidence to squamous carcinoma of the eyelid, and 40–50 times less common than basal cell carcinoma); female predilection. Sometimes related to previous radiotherapy. Pagetoid spread common (discontinuous areas of tumor spread through epithelium). Cardinal signs include madarosis, poliosis, and thick, red lid margin inflammation; tumor is typically yellow and hard; lymphadenopathy common. Poor prognosis when symptomatic for longer than 6 months (38% mortality vs. 14% for less than 6 months), size greater than 2 cm (60% mortality vs. 18% when <1 cm), upper and lower lid involvement (83% mortality), poor differentiation, and local vascular or lymphatic infiltration. Muir–Torre syndrome (multiple internal malignancies and external sebaceous tumors) is more common in sebaceous gland hyperplasia than sebaceous carcinoma.

Figure 3-53 • Sebaceous cell carcinoma with chronic lid changes of the left upper eyelid.

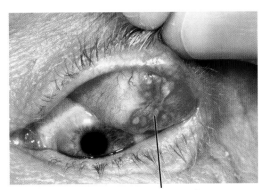

Sebaceous cell carcinoma

- Incisional full-thickness eyelid biopsy required to make the diagnosis. Prior to planning total resection in advanced cases extensive conjunctival map biopsies to evaluate extent of disease is recommended (since pagetoid spread with skip lesions is common). Map biopsies can be done as fresh frozen sections with oil-red-O (stains intracytoplasmic lipid droplets) or as permanent sections taken prior to planned resection. Mohs surgery is not beneficial because skip lesions are often present.

- Orbital exenteration required in advanced cases.
- Palliative radiation.

Malignant Melanoma

Tan, black, or gray nodule or plaque with irregular, notched borders; often rapidly growing with color changes. Most lethal primary skin tumor, but rare (<1% of eyelid malignancies); prognosis related to histology, depth of invasion, and tumor thickness. Acral lentiginous melanoma does not occur in the eyelids. Orderly growth with stage 1: localized disease without lymph node spread; stage 2: palpable regional lymph nodes (preauricular from upper lid, submandibular from lower lid); and stage 3: distant metastases; choroidal melanoma may reach lids via extrascleral extension into orbit. Fair prognosis for stage 1, poor for stages 2 and 3. Three histologic types:

Nodular Melanoma

Very rare on eyelid (10% of cases), aggressive, worst prognosis.

Superficial Spreading Melanoma

Most common (80% of cases), onset usually 20–60 years of age. Presents as flat, variegated, multicolored lesion that invades dermis, rapidly leading to raised nodule.

Lentigo Maligna Melanoma

Ten percent of cases, related to sun exposure, usually in the elderly. Appears as flat, tan-brown lesion with irregular borders that enlarges radially with black flecks; largest when identified, often due to underdiagnosis.

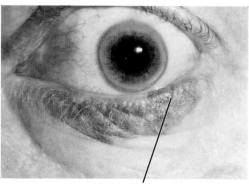

Figure 3-54 • Malignant melanoma of the lower eyelid.

Malignant melanoma

- Incisional or excisional biopsy or complete excision with or without wide margins (frozen sectioning is contraindicated); for lentigo maligna and superficial spreading this results in almost total cure.
- Orbital exenteration and neck dissection required in advanced cases.
- Dermatologic evaluation.

Merkel Cell Tumor

Rare, rapidly growing, solitary, violaceous, vascularized, occasionally ulcerated tumor of the amino precursor uptake and decarboxylation (APUD) system; usually found in sun-exposed areas. Onset in seventh decade; reported only in Caucasians. Potential for recurrence and lymphatic spread with lymph node enlargement. Generally poor prognosis due to early spread after local excision alone, 39% recur locally and 46% recur regionally; after adjuvant radiation therapy or node dissection, 26% recur locally and 22% regionally; 67% tumor mortality for locoregional spread.

Figure 3-55 • Merkel cell tumor of the right lower eyelid.

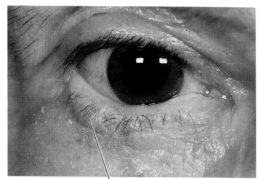

Merkel cell tumor

- Wide local excision and immunohistochemical stains for enkephalin, calcitonin, somatostatin, corticotropin, and neuron-specific enolase.
- Lymph node resection.
- Supplemental radiation therapy.

Metastatic Tumors

Metastatic eyelid lesions are very rare. Female predilection; occur in older adults. Primary sites include breast and lung (most common) carcinoma, cutaneous malignancies, gastrointestinal and genitourinary carcinomas, and lymphoma. Three patterns: (1) single nontender

Figure 3-56 • Metastatic lymphoma to left upper eyelid.

Lymphoma

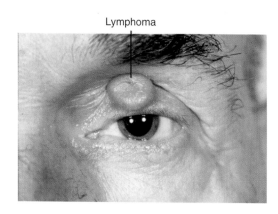

nodule, (2) painless diffuse induration, (3) ulcerating lesion of eyelid skin or conjunctiva. Evidence of primary tumor elsewhere, lymph node enlargement; usually poor prognosis but variable.

- Local excision, radiation, or observation.
- Systemic treatment for primary tumor.

Kaposi's Sarcoma

Soft tissue sarcoma usually associated with acquired immunodeficiency syndrome (AIDS), may also rarely occur in Africans and older men of Mediterranean descent; very malignant in immunocompromised patients. Appears as violaceous nodules on the eyelids that are nontender and progress over several months; may have associated distortion of the eyelid with entropion, edema, trichiasis, and corneal scarring.

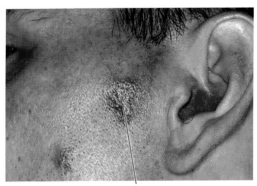

Figure 3-57 • Kaposi's sarcoma demonstrating characteristic purple nodule.

Kaposi's sarcoma

- Complete surgical excision.
- May require cryotherapy, radiotherapy, chemotherapy, immunotherapy, or a combination.

▌Systemic Diseases

Neurofibromatosis

Definition Neurofibromatosis (NF) is one of the classic phakomatoses and is an AD inherited disorder of the neuroectodermal system, affecting primarily neural crest-derived tissue (Schwann cells and melanocytes), manifesting with neural, cutaneous, and ocular hamartomas. The disorder displays highly variable expressivity. Two types:

NF-1 (Von Recklinghausen's disease)

Mapped to chromosome 17q with a prevalence of 1 in 3000; 50% of cases represent new mutations. Diagnosis requires two or more of the following criteria:

(1) Six or more café-au-lait spots 15 mm or larger in adults, 5 mm or larger in children.

(2) Two or more neurofibromas; or one plexiform neurofibroma.

(3) Axillary or inguinal freckling.

(4) Optic nerve or tract glioma.

(5) Two or more iris Lisch nodules.

(6) Characteristic osseous lesion (i.e., sphenoid dysplasia).

(7) First-degree relative with NF-1 by these criteria.

NF-2 (bilateral acoustic neurofibromatosis)

Mapped to chromosome 22q with a prevalence of 1 in 50,000. Diagnostic criteria include:

(1) Bilateral acoustic neuromas.

(2) First-degree relative with NF-2 and either a single acoustic neuroma or two of the following: glioma, neurilemoma, meningioma, neurofibroma, or a premature posterior subcapsular cataract.

Signs

NF-1

Café-au-lait spots, neurofibromas (fibroma molluscum), plexiform neurofibromas (bag of worms), intertriginous freckling, CNS and spinal cord gliomas, meningiomas, nerve root neurofibromas, intracranial calcifications, mild intellectual deficit, kyphoscoliosis and pseudoarthroses, gastrointestinal neurofibromas, pheochromocytoma, plus various other malignant tumors.

NF-1 ocular findings

Lisch nodules (iris melanocytic hamartomas), eyelid café-au-lait spots, neurofibromas, and plexiform neurofibroma; may have ipsilateral congenital glaucoma, proptosis secondary to tumors or bony defects, conjunctival neurofibromas, enlarged corneal nerves, diffuse uveal thickening, choroidal hamartomas, retinal astrocytic and combined hamartomas, optic nerve glioma.

S-shaped lid deformity

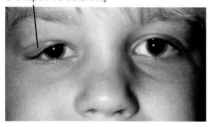

Eyelid neurofibroma

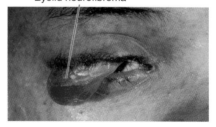

Figure 3-58 • Neurofibroma demonstrating characteristic S-shaped lid deformity of the right upper eyelid in a child with type 1 neurofibromatosis.

Figure 3-59 • Right eyelid neurofibroma in a patient with type 1 neurofibromatosis.

NF-2

Paucity of cutaneous lesions (few or small café-au-lait spots), bilateral acoustic neuromas, CNS and spinal cord gliomas, meningiomas, nerve root neurofibromas, intracranial calcifications, pheochromocytoma, plus various other malignant tumors.

NF-2 ocular findings

Premature posterior subcapsular cataracts (40%), combined retinal hamartomas, optic nerve meningioma, and glioma; no Lisch nodules.

Evaluation
- Complete ophthalmic history and eye exam with attention to family history (examine family members), color vision, pupils, lids, cornea, tonometry, iris, lens, ophthalmoscopy, visual field testing, general dermatologic evaluation (especially intertriginous regions), and neurologic screening.
- Brain and orbital MRI or CT scan.
- **Lab tests**: Complete blood count (CBC), electrolytes, and urine catecholamines (vanillylmandelic acid, metanephrine).
- Audiography for patients with NF-2.
- Intelligence testing.

Management

- Genetic counseling.
- Routine (every 6–12 months) eye exams to monitor for glaucoma, cataracts, and ocular malignancies.
- Surgical removal of eyelid fibromas possible, but recurrence rate is high.

Prognosis Increased morbidity if associated with CNS or other malignant neoplasm.

Sarcoidosis

Idiopathic multisystem disease, with abnormalities in cell-mediated and humoral immunity and granulomatous inflammation in many organs; commonly affects the lungs, skin, and eyes including the eyelid skin, lacrimal gland and sac, and nasolacrimal duct. May cause redness, pain, swelling of involved lids or lacrimal glands (usually bilateral), painless subcutaneous nodular masses of eyelids, ptosis, diplopia, severe cicatrizing conjunctival inflammation, conjunctival nodules, keratoconjunctivitis sicca, band keratopathy, granulomatous anterior or posterior uveitis, cataract, chorioretinitis, retinal periphlebitis or neovascularization, optic nerve disease, glaucoma, and orbital involvement. Variable prognosis depending on organs involved.

- Biopsy of conjunctival, lacrimal, or eyelid nodule (with stains to rule out acid-fast bacteria).
- **Lab tests**: Angiotensin converting enzyme (ACE), CBC, lysozyme, serum calcium, chest radiographs, and purified protein derivative (PPD) and controls; additional tests may be ordered by pulmonologist or internist and include chest CT and gallium scans.
- Sarcoid dacryoadenitis is treated with systemic corticosteroids. Tuberculosis must be ruled out prior to initiating therapy.
- Uveitis is treated with topical corticosteroids (see Chapter 6).
- Retinal consultation as indicated.
- Treatment of systemic disease (steroids and chemotherapy) by internist.

Amyloidosis

Definition Group of diseases (systemic or localized; primary or secondary) characterized by abnormal protein production and tissue deposition.

Etiology Nonfamilial and familial forms. Familial amyloidosis (autosomal dominant [AD]) is caused by substitution errors in coding of prealbumin. Associated with multiple myeloma.

Symptoms Asymptomatic; may notice eyelid discoloration, droopy eyelids, dryness, decreased vision, diplopia, floaters.

Signs

Systemic findings

Nonfamilial form

Polyarthralgias, pulmonary infiltrates, waxy, maculopapular skin lesions, renal failure, postural hypotension, congestive heart failure, and gastrointestinal bleeds.

Familial form

Autonomic dysfunction, peripheral neuropathies, and cardiomyopathy.

Ocular findings

Decreased visual acuity; may have flat or nodular purpuric lesions of the eyelids, lacrimal gland, caruncle, or conjunctiva (ruptured, fragile, amyloid-infiltrated blood vessels in abnormal tissue), or may occur without hemorrhage as elevated, yellowish, waxy eyelid papules; ptosis, proptosis, ophthalmoplegia, dry eye, corneal deposits, iris stromal infiltrates, vitreous opacities, retinal vascular occlusions, cotton-wool spots, retinal neovascularization, and compressive optic neuropathy.

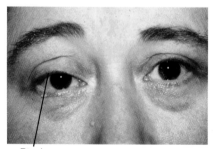

Ptosis

Figure 3-60 • Amyloidosis of the right upper eyelid causing ptosis.

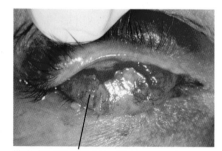

Nodular amyloid deposition

Figure 3-61 • Same patient as Figure 3-60, demonstrating thickened everted eyelid with plaquelike appearance.

Evaluation
* Complete ophthalmic history and eye exam with attention to motility, lids, conjunctiva, cornea, iris, anterior vitreous, and ophthalmoscopy.

- **Lab tests:** Complete blood count (CBC), serum and urine protein electrophoresis, serum total protein, albumin and globulin, liver function tests, blood urea nitrogen (BUN) and creatinine, erythrocyte sedimentation rate (ESR), ANA, RF, VDRL, FTA-ABS, urinalysis, PPD and controls, chest radiographs, electrocardiogram (ECG), bone scan.
- Diagnosis made by biopsy (birefringence and dichroism with Congo red stain, metachromasia with crystal violet, and fluorescence with thioflavine-T).
- Medical consultation.

Management

- Surgical excision/debulking, radiotherapy where feasible.
- Consider pars plana vitrectomy for vitreous opacities affecting vision.
- Underlying systemic disease should be treated by an internist.

Prognosis Variable depending on systemic involvement; very poor when associated with multiple myeloma.

Canaliculitis

Definition Inflammation of the canaliculus (duct between the punctum and lacrimal sac), often resulting in recurrent conjunctivitis.

Etiology *Actinomyces israelii* (Streptothrix), a filamentous anaerobic (or facultative anaerobic) gram-positive rod, is the most common cause; other organisms include *Candida albicans, Aspergillus, Nocardia asteroides*, and herpes simplex or zoster virus; more common in middle-aged women; usually insidious onset.

Symptoms Medial eyelid tenderness, tearing, and redness.

Signs Erythema and swelling of punctum and adjacent tissue ("pouting punctum"), follicular conjunctivitis around medial canthus, expression of discharge from punctum,

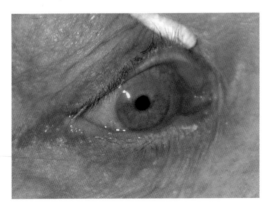

Figure 3-62 • Canaliculitis, demonstrating swollen, erythematous, pouting upper punctum with discharge.

concretions in canaliculus, grating sensation on lacrimal duct probing, dilated canaliculus on dacryocystography.

Differential Diagnosis Conjunctivitis, dacryocystitis, nasal lacrimal duct obstruction, and carunculitis.

Evaluation
- Complete ophthalmic history with attention to history of recurrent conjunctivitis and tearing.
- Complete eye exam with attention to lids, lacrimal system, expression of discharge from punctum, and conjunctiva.
- Compression medial to the punctum observing for discharge.
- **Lab tests**: Culture and Gram stain (*Actinomyces* branching filaments and sulfur granules on Gram stain).
- Probing and possible irrigation to determine patency of canalicular system.
- Consider dacryocystography to confirm a dilated canaliculus, concretions, or normal out-flow function in the lower excretory system.

Management

- Warm compresses to canalicular region bid to qid.
- Marsupialization of the involved canaliculus.
- *Actinomyces israelii*: canalicular irrigation with antibiotic solution (penicillin G 100,000 U/mL) and systemic antibiotic (penicillin V 500 mg po qid for 7 days).
- *Candida albicans*: systemic antifungal (fluconazole 600 mg po qd for 7–10 days).
- *Aspergillus*: topical antifungal (amphotericin B 0.15% tid) and systemic antifungal (itraconazole 200 mg po bid for 7–10 days).
- *Nocardia asteroides*: topical antibiotic (sulfacetamide tid) and systemic antibiotic (trimethoprim-sulfamethoxazole [Bactrim] one double-strength tablet po qd for 7–10 days).
- Herpes simplex or zoster virus: topical antiviral (trifluridine 0.1% 5 times/day for 2 weeks); if stenosis present may need silicone intubation.
- Consider curettage or canaliculotomy of the lateral horizontal canaliculus for recalcitrant cases.

Prognosis Often good; depends on infecting organism.

Dacryocystitis

Definition Acute or chronic infection of the lacrimal sac, often with overlying cellulitis.

Etiology *Streptococcus pneumoniae*, *Staphylococcus* species, and *Pseudomonas* species; *Haemophilus influenzae* in children is less common now that they receive *H. influenzae* vaccination.

Associated with conditions that cause lacrimal sac tear stasis and predispose to infection, including strictures, long and narrow nasolacrimal ducts, lacrimal sac diverticulum, trauma, dacryoliths, congenital or acquired nasolacrimal duct obstruction, and inflammatory sinus and nasal problems.

Symptoms Pain, swelling, and redness over nasal portion of lower eyelid with tearing and crusting; may have fever.

Signs Edema and erythema below the medial canthal tendon with lacrimal sac swelling; tenderness on palpation of the lacrimal sac, expression of discharge from the punctum; may have fistula formation or lacrimal sac cyst.

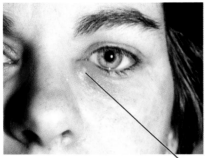

Dacryocystitis

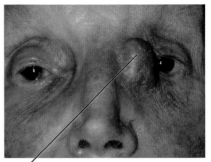

Dacryocystitis

Figure 3-63 • Dacryocystitis demonstrating erythema and swelling of lacrimal sac of the left eye.

Figure 3-64 • Dacryocystitis with massive medial canthal swelling.

Differential Diagnosis Ethmoid sinusitis, preseptal or orbital cellulitis, lacrimal sac neoplasm, dacryocystocele (infants) and encephalocele (infants, blue mass above medial canthal tendon), and facial abscess.

Evaluation
- Complete ophthalmic history with attention to history of tearing (absence of tearing calls diagnosis into question) and previous history of sinus or upper respiratory infection.
- Complete eye exam with attention to lids, lacrimal system, expression of discharge from punctum, digital massage of lacrimal sac, motility, exophthalmometry, and conjunctiva.
- **Lab tests**: Culture and Gram stain any punctal discharge (chocolate agar in children).
- Do not probe nasolacrimal duct during acute infection.
- Orbital CT scan for limited motility, proptosis, sinus disease, or atypical cases not responding to antibiotic therapy.

Management

- Warm compresses tid.

ACUTE

- Systemic antibiotic (amoxicillin-clavulanate [Augmentin] 500 mg po tid for 10 days or amoxicillin-sulbactam [Unasyn] 15–30 mg IV q6h); if penicillin-allergic, use trimethoprim-sulfamethoxazole ([Bactrim] one double-strength tablet po bid for 10 days).
- Topical antibiotic (erythromycin ointment bid) if conjunctivitis exists.
- Percutaneous aspirate lacrimal sac contents with 18-gauge needle for culture and Gram stain.
- If pointing abscess, consider incision and drainage of lacrimal sac.
- Consider dacryocystorhinostomy once infection has resolved.

CHRONIC

- Cultures to determine antibiotic therapy (see above).
- Dacryocystorhinostomy required to relieve obstruction after infection resolved. Occasionally responds to lacrimal probing with intubation.

Prognosis Good; usually responds to therapy, but surgery almost always required; if untreated, sequelae include mucocele formation, recurrent lacrimal sac abscess, orbital cellulitis, and infectious keratitis.

Nasolacrimal Duct Obstruction

Definition Obstruction of the nasolacrimal duct.

Etiology

Congenital

Most frequently due to an imperforate membrane over the valve of Hasner at the nasal end of the duct; occurs clinically in 2–4% of full-term infants at 1–2 weeks of age; bilateral in one-third of cases. Spontaneous opening frequently occurs 1–2 months after birth; may be complicated by acute dacryocystitis.

Acquired

Due to chronic sinus disease, involutional stenosis, dacryocystitis, or nasoorbital trauma; uncommonly caused by obstruction from neoplasm such as nasal/sinus or lacrimal sac/duct tumors. Involutional stenosis is the most common cause in older individuals; female predilection (2:1); may be associated with granulomatous diseases such as Wegener's granulomatosis and sarcoidosis; increased risk of dacryocystitis.

Symptoms Tearing, discharge, crusting, recurrent conjunctivitis.

Signs Watery eyes, eyelash crusting and debris, mucus reflux from punctum with compression over the lacrimal sac, medial lower eyelid erythema.

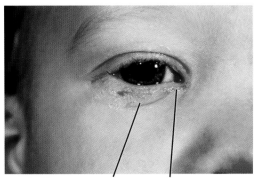

Figure 3-65 • Nasolacrimal duct obstruction with tearing, crusting of eyelids, and lower lid erythema.

Erythema   Crusting

Differential Diagnosis

Congenital tearing

Congenital glaucoma, trichiasis, conjunctivitis, nasal lacrimal duct anomalies (punctal atresia), dacryocystocele, corneal abrasion, corneal trauma from forceps delivery, ocular surface foreign body.

Acquired tearing

Conjunctivitis, trichiasis, entropion, ectropion, corneal abnormalities, dry eye syndrome, blepharitis, punctal stenosis, canalicular stenosis.

Evaluation
- Complete ophthalmic history and eye exam with attention to lids, lashes, expression of discharge from punctum, conjunctiva, cornea (diameter, breaks in Descemet's membrane, staining with fluorescein), and tonometry.
- Dye disappearance test with fluorescein, particularly helpful in infants.
- Jones I test: fluorescein is instilled in conjunctival cul-de-sac; a cotton-tipped applicator is used to attempt fluorescein retrieval via the external naris. Positive test result indicates functional blockage.
- Jones II test: nasolacrimal irrigation with saline following positive Jones I test; fluorescein retrieval is attempted once again. Positive test result indicates anatomic blockage.
- Nasolacrimal irrigation: 23-gauge cannula mounted on 3-cc to 5-cc syringe is inserted into canaliculus, and irrigation is attempted. Retrograde flow through opposite canaliculus and punctum indicates nasolacrimal blockage. Reflux through same punctum indicates canalicular obstruction. Successful irrigation into nose and throat eliminates anatomic blockage but does not rule out functional blockage.
- Consider orbital and sinus CT scan for atypical demographics or presentation.
- Consider nasal endoscopy especially before surgical intervention.

Management

- Treat dacryocystitis if present.

CONGENITAL

- Crigler massage bid to qid (parent places index finger over infant's canaliculi [medial corner of eyelid] and makes several slow downward strokes).
- Nasolacrimal duct probing at 13 months if no spontaneous resolution, sooner if infection or discharge occurs, probing may be repeated.
- Consider balloon dacryoplasty with silicone intubation of the nasolacrimal duct if initial probing does not resolve the tearing.

ACQUIRED

- Treat partial nasolacrimal duct obstruction with topical antibiotic-steroid (neomycin-polymyxin-dexamethasone [Maxitrol] qid).
- Consider silicone intubation of the nasolacrimal duct or dacryoplasty for persistent partial obstruction.
- Complete nasolacrimal duct obstruction with patent canaliculi and functional lacrimal pump requires dacryocystorhinostomy (anastomosis between lacrimal sac and nasal cavity through a bony ostium).

Prognosis Excellent for congenital; often good for acquired, depends on cause of obstruction.

Dacryoadenitis

Definition Inflammation of the lacrimal gland.

Etiology Usually of idiopathic, noninfectious origin, viral, bacterial, or rarely parasitic etiology.

Acute

Most commonly due to infection (*Staphylococcus* species, mumps, Epstein–Barr virus, herpes zoster, or *Neisseria gonorrhoeae*); palpebral lobe affected more frequently than orbital lobe; most cases associated with systemic infection; typically occurs in children and young adults.

Chronic

More common than acute form; usually due to inflammatory disorders including idiopathic orbital inflammation, sarcoidosis, thyroid-related ophthalmopathy, Sjögren's syndrome, and benign lymphoepithelial lesions; also with syphilis and tuberculosis.

Symptoms

Acute

Temporal upper eyelid redness, swelling, and pain with tearing and discharge.

Chronic

Temporal upper eyelid swelling; occasional redness and discomfort.

Signs

Acute

Edema, tenderness, and erythema of upper eyelid with S-shaped deformity, enlarged and erythematous lacrimal gland (palpebral lobe), preauricular lymphadenopathy, and fever; may have inferonasal globe displacement and proptosis if orbital lobe involved.

Chronic

Tenderness in superotemporal area of upper eyelid, globe displacement, restricted ocular motility, and enlarged lacrimal gland.

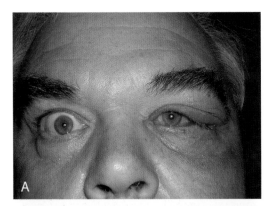

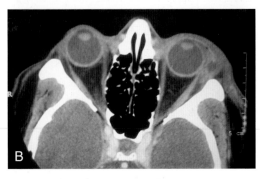

Figure 3-66 • Dacryoadenitis, demonstrating erythema and edema of the left upper eyelid laterally and conjunctival injection (A), and lacrimal gland enlargement on CT scan (B).

Differential Diagnosis Malignant lacrimal gland neoplasm, preseptal or orbital cellulitis, viral conjunctivitis, chalazion, dermoid tumor, lacrimal gland cyst (dacryops).

Evaluation

Acute

- Complete ophthalmic history and eye exam with attention to constitutional signs, palpation of parotid glands, lymph nodes, and upper lid, examination of palpebral lacrimal lobe (lift upper lid) for enlargement, globe retropulsion, exophthalmometry, and motility.
- **Lab tests**: culture and Gram stain of discharge, CBC with differential; consider blood cultures for suspected systemic involvement.
- Orbital CT scan for proptosis, motility restriction, or suspected mass.

Chronic

- Complete ophthalmic history and eye exam with attention to constitutional signs, palpation of parotid glands, lymph nodes, and upper lid; examination of palpebral lacrimal lobe (lift upper lid) for enlargement, globe retropulsion, exophthalmometry, motility, and signs of previous anterior or posterior uveitis.
- **Lab tests**: Chest radiographs, CBC with differential, ACE, lysosyme, VDRL, FTA-ABS, PPD and controls.
- Orbital CT scan.
- Consider chest CT scan or gallium scan.
- Consider lacrimal gland biopsy if diagnosis uncertain or malignancy suspected.

Management

ACUTE

- Mumps or Epstein–Barr virus: warm compresses bid to tid.
- Herpes simplex or zoster virus: systemic antiviral (acyclovir [Zovirax] 800 mg po 5 times/day for 10 days or famciclovir [Famvir] 500 mg po tid for 7 days); in immunocompromised patients use acyclovir 10–12 mg/kg/day IV divided into 3 doses for 7–10 days.
- *Staphylococcus* and *Streptococcus* species: systemic antibiotic (amoxicillin-clavulanate [Augmentin] 500 mg po q8h); in severe cases ampicillin-sulbactam [Unasyn] 1.5–3 g IV q6h.
- *Neisseria gonorrhoeae*: systemic antibiotic (ceftriaxone 1 g IV × 1); warm compresses and incision and drainage if suppurative.
- *Mycobacterium* species: surgical excision and systemic treatment with isoniazid (300 mg po qd) and rifampin (600 mg po qd) for 6–9 months, follow liver function tests for toxicity; consider adding pyrazinamide (25–35 mg/kg po qd) for first 2 months.
- *Treponema pallidum*: systemic antibiotic (penicillin G 24 million U/day IV for 10 days).

CHRONIC

- Treat underlying inflammatory disorder.
- Treat infections (rare) as above.

Prognosis Depends on etiology; most infections respond well to treatment.

Lacrimal Gland Tumors

Approximately 50% of all lacrimal gland masses are inflammatory; the other 50% are neoplasms. Of these, 50% are of epithelial origin while 50% are primarily lymphoproliferative (see Chapter 1). Of all epithelial tumors, 50% are pleomorphic adenomas (benign mixed tumors), and 50% are malignant. Lacrimal gland lesions appear in the superotemporal quadrant of the orbit. Patients often have inferior and medial globe displacement, limitation of ocular movements, lid edema and erythema, and a palpable mass under the superotemporal orbital rim. Conditions that may present in a similar fashion include dermoids, sarcoidosis, idiopathic orbital inflammation, and dacryops.

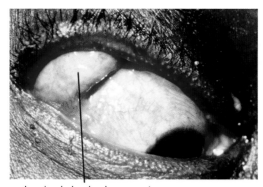

Lacrimal gland enlargement

Figure 3-67 • Lacrimal gland enlargement due to reactive lymphoid hyperplasia.

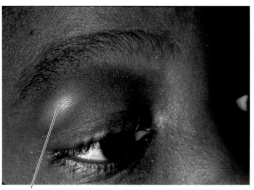

Lacrimal gland tumor

Figure 3-68 • Lacrimal gland tumor of the right orbit.

Benign Mixed Cell Tumor (Pleomorphic Adenoma)

Most common epithelial tumor of the lacrimal gland, usually appearing insidiously in the fourth and fifth decade, often with inferior and medial displacement of the globe. A firm, circumscribed mass can be palpated under the superior temporal orbital rim, often with bony remodeling (not osteolytic) on radiographic images. Histologically, these tumors contain a pseudocapsule, a double row of epithelial cells forming lumens, and stroma containing spindle-shaped cells with mucinous, osteoid, or cartilaginous metaplasia. Complete resection is critical in order to avoid malignant degeneration. Excellent prognosis if tumor is excised completely.

- Orbital CT scan: Well-circumscribed mass with lacrimal gland fossa enlargement.
- Fine-needle aspiration biopsy of the lacrimal gland may be useful in some cases.
- En bloc excision via a lateral orbitotomy; rupture of pseudocapsule may lead to recurrence and malignant transformation. Incisional biopsy should be avoided.

Malignant Mixed Cell Tumor (Pleomorphic Adenocarcinoma)

Occurs in the elderly with pain and rapid progression; contains the same epithelial and mesenchymal features of pleomorphic adenoma, but with malignant components; associated with longstanding or incompletely excised pleomorphic adenomas. Treatment and prognosis are similar to adenoid cystic carcinoma (see below).

Adenoid Cystic Carcinoma (Cylindroma)

Most common malignant tumor of the lacrimal gland, rapid onset with infiltrative capacity; associated with pain due to perineural invasion; bony erosion and proptosis common; CT scan shows a poorly defined mass with adjacent bony destruction. Histologically, the tumor is composed of densely staining, small cells that grow in nests, tubules, or a Swiss cheese (cribriform) pattern; the basaloid pattern carries the worst prognosis. Five-year survival rate is 47%, and at 15 years is only 22%; major cause of death is intracranial extension due to perineural spread.

- Orbital CT scan: Irregular mass with or without adjacent bony erosion
- En bloc resection with wide margins including orbital rim at a minimum. Orbital exenteration with adjunctive chemotherapy and irradiation may be required, and must be discussed with each patient on a case-by-case basis.

Trauma 131
Telangiectasia 135
Microaneurysm 136
Dry Eye Disease 136
Inflammation 141
Conjunctivitis 144
Degenerations 153
Ocular Cicatricial Pemphigoid 156
Stevens–Johnson Syndrome 157
Tumors 158
Episcleritis 168
Scleritis 169
Scleral Discoloration 171

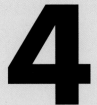

4

Conjunctiva and Sclera

Trauma

Foreign Body

Exogenous material on, under, or embedded within the conjunctiva or sclera; commonly dirt, glass, metal, or cilia. Patients usually note foreign body sensation and redness; may have corneal staining, particularly linear vertical scratches due to blinking with a foreign body trapped on the upper tarsal surface. Good prognosis.

- Remove foreign body; evert lids to check tarsal conjunctiva.
- Topical broad spectrum antibiotic (polymyxin B sulfate-trimethoprim [Polytrim] drops or bacitracin ointment qid).

Laceration

Partial-thickness or full-thickness cut in conjunctiva with or without partial-thickness cut in the sclera; very important to rule out open globe (see below); good prognosis.

- Seidel test for suspected open globe (see below).
- Topical broad spectrum antibiotic (gatifloxacin [Zymar] or moxifloxacin [Vigamox] qid).
- Conjunctival and partial-thickness scleral lacerations rarely require surgical repair.

Open Globe

Full-thickness defect in eye wall (cornea or sclera), commonly from penetrating or blunt trauma; the latter usually causes rupture at the limbus, just posterior to the rectus muscle insertions, or at previous surgical incision sites; double penetrating injuries are called perforations; an open globe may also be due to corneal or scleral melting. Associated signs include lid and orbital trauma, corneal abrasion or laceration, wound dehiscence, positive

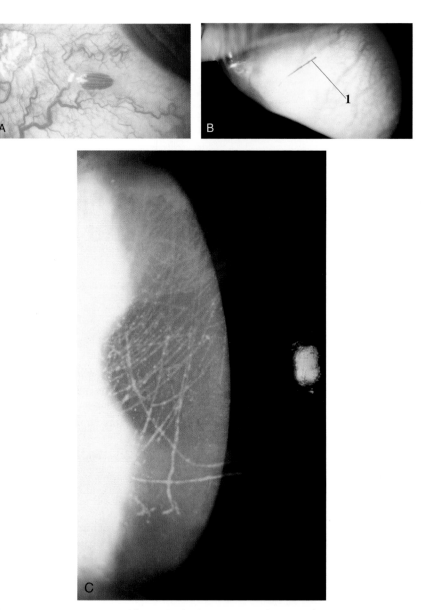

Figure 4-1 • (A) Conjunctival foreign body, demonstrating a fragment of corn husk embedded in the conjunctiva. (B) Conjunctival foreign body, demonstrating a grasshopper leg embedded in the conjunctiva. (C) Same patient as in (B), demonstrating multiple vertical corneal abrasions from a grasshopper leg in the superior tarsal conjunctiva. Such a pattern of linear abrasions suggests a foreign body under the upper eyelid, and therefore the examiner should always evert the eyelid to inspect for this.

Figure 4-2 • Conjunctival laceration with gaping edges.

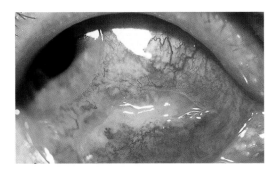

Seidel test (see Laceration section in Chapter 5), low intraocular pressure, flat or shallow anterior chamber, anterior chamber cells and flare, hyphema, peaked pupil, iris transillumination defect, sphincter tears, angle recession, iridodialysis, cyclodialysis, iridodonesis, phacodonesis, dislocated lens, cataract, vitreous and retinal hemorrhage, commotio retinae, retinal tear, retinal detachment, choroidal rupture, intraocular foreign body or gas bubbles, and extruded intraocular contents. Guarded prognosis.

Figure 4-3 • Full-thickness corneoscleral limbal laceration with wound gape. Note discontinuity of slit-beam as it crosses the wound edge (arrowhead).

Slit-beam   Laceration

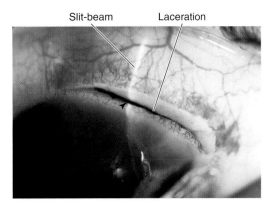

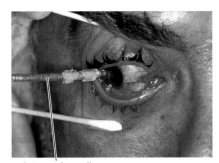

Intraocular nail

Figure 4-4 • Penetrating injury with foreign body (nail) protruding from globe.

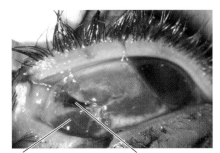

Bullous conjunctival   Uveal prolapse
hemorrhage

Figure 4-5 • Open globe. There is a temporal full-thickness scleral laceration with uveal prolapse. Also note the extensive subconjunctival hemorrhage and upper and lower eyelid lacerations.

OPHTHALMIC EMERGENCY

- Admit for surgical exploration and repair; protect eye with metal eye shield; minimize ocular manipulations; examine globe only enough to verify the diagnosis of an open globe; remainder of examination and exploration should be performed in the operating room. Postoperatively, start antibiotics and steroids.
- Consider B-scan ultrasonography if unable to visualize the fundus.
- Consider orbital computed tomography (CT) scan or orbital radiographs to rule out intraocular foreign body; magnetic resonance imaging (MRI) is *contraindicated* if foreign body is metallic.
- Subconjunctival antibiotics and steroids:

  Vancomycin (25 mg).

  Ceftazidime (50–100 mg) or gentamicin (20 mg).

  Dexamethasone (12–24 mg).
- Topical fortified antibiotics (alternate every 30 minutes):

  Vancomycin (25–50 mg/mL q1h).

  Ceftazidime (50 mg/mL q1h).
- Topical steroid (prednisolone acetate 1% q1–2h initially) and cycloplegic (scopolamine 0.25% or atropine 1% tid).
- Systemic intravenous antibiotics for marked inflammation or severe cases:

  Vancomycin (1 g IV q12h).

  Ceftazidime (1 g IV q12h).
- Small corneal lacerations (<2 mm) that are self-sealing or intermittently Seidel positive may be treated with a bandage contact lens, topical broad spectrum antibiotic (gatifloxacin [Zymar] or moxifloxacin [Vigamox] q2h to q6h), cycloplegic (cyclopentolate 1% bid), and an aqueous suppressant (timolol maleate [Timoptic] 0.5% or brimonidine [Alphagan-P] 0.15% bid); observe daily for 5–7 days; consider suturing laceration if wound has not sealed after 1 week.

Subconjunctival Hemorrhage

Diffuse or focal area of blood under the conjunctiva. Appears bright red, otherwise asymptomatic. May be idiopathic, associated with trauma, sneezing, coughing, straining, emesis, aspirin or anticoagulant use, or hypertension, or due to an abnormal conjunctival vessel. Excellent prognosis.

- Reassurance if no other ocular findings.
- Consider blood pressure measurement if recurrent.
- Medical or hematology consultation for recurrent, idiopathic, subconjunctival hemorrhages, or other evidence of systemic bleeding (ecchymoses, epistaxis, gastrointestinal bleeding, hematuria, etc.).

Figure 4-6 • Subconjunctival hemorrhage demonstrating bright red blood under the conjunctiva. As the hemorrhage resorbs, the edges may spread, become feathery, and turn yellowish (arrowhead).

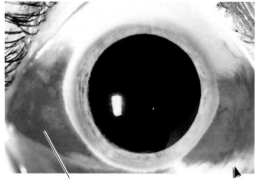

Subconjunctival hemorrhage

Telangiectasia

Definition Abnormal, dilated conjunctival capillary formation.

Symptoms Asymptomatic red spot on eye; patient may have epistaxis and gastrointestinal bleeding depending on etiology.

Signs Telangiectasia of conjunctival vessels, subconjunctival hemorrhage.

Figure 4-7 • Conjunctival telangiectasia appearing as dotlike, corkscrew, irregular vessels near the limbus.

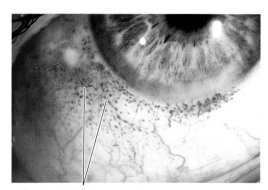

Conjunctival telangiectasia

Differential Diagnosis Idiopathic, Osler–Weber–Rendu syndrome, ataxia-telangiectasia, Fabry's disease, Sturge–Weber syndrome.

Evaluation

• Complete ophthalmic history and eye exam with attention to conjunctiva, cornea, lens, and ophthalmoscopy.

• Consider CT scan for multisystem disorders.

• Medical consultation to rule out systemic disease.

Management

- No treatment recommended.

Prognosis Usually benign; may bleed; depends on etiology.

Microaneurysm

Definition Focal dilation of conjunctival vessel.

Symptoms Asymptomatic; may notice red spot on eye.

Signs Microaneurysm; may have associated retinal findings.

Differential Diagnosis Diabetes mellitus, hypertension, sickle cell anemia (Paton's sign), arteriosclerosis, carotid occlusion, fucosidosis, polycythemia vera.

Evaluation
- Complete ophthalmic history and eye exam with attention to conjunctiva and ophthalmoscopy.
- Check blood pressure.
- **Lab tests**: Fasting blood glucose (diabetes mellitus), sickle cell prep, hemoglobin electro-phoresis (sickle cell).
- Medical consultation.

Management

- No treatment recommended.
- Treat underlying medical condition.

Prognosis Usually benign.

Dry Eye Disease (Dry Eye Syndrome, Keratoconjunctivitis Sicca)

Definition Sporadic or chronic ocular irritation with visual disturbance due to a tear film and ocular surface abnormality.

Etiology Any condition that causes a deficiency or imbalance in the aqueous, lipid, or mucin components of the tear film. Dry eye can be classified by mechanism (decreased tear production or increased tear evaporation), category (lid margin disease (i.e., blepharitis, mei-bomitis), no lid margin disease, altered tear distribution/clearance), or severity (Table 4-1).

It is usually multifactorial with an inflammatory component; tear hyperosmolarity and tear film instability create a cycle of ocular surface inflammation, damage, and symptoms.

Aqueous-deficient dry eye

Characterized by abnormal lacrimal gland function causing decreased tear production.

Sjögren syndrome

Dry eye, dry mouth, and arthritis with autoantibodies (to Ro (SSA) and/or La (SSB) antigens) and no connective tissue disease (primary, >95% female) or with connective tissue disease, including rheumatoid arthritis and collagen vascular diseases (secondary).

Non-Sjögren

Hypofunction of the lacrimal gland due to other causes:

Primary lacrimal gland deficiencies Age-related (historically labeled KCS), congenital alacrima, familial dysautonomia (Riley Day syndrome).

Secondary lacrimal gland deficiencies Lacrimal gland infiltration, lymphoma, sarcoidosis, amyloidosis, AIDS, graft-versus-host disease, lacrimal gland ablation or denervation.

Obstruction of the lacrimal ducts Cicatrizing conjunctivitis (Stevens–Johnson syndrome, ocular cicatricial pemphigoid, trachoma, chemical burns, radiation).

Neurosecretory block Sensory (corneal surgery, contact lens wear, diabetes, neurotrophic keratopathy), motor (cranial nerve VII damage, systemic medications (β-blockers, antimuscarinics, antidepressants, diuretics)).

Evaporative dry eye

Characterized by normal lacrimal gland function but increased tear evaporation.

Intrinsic causes

Meibomian gland dysfunction (MGD) Primary, secondary, simple, or cicatricial (see posterior blepharitis and acne rosacea in Chapter 3).

Lid/globe abnormalities Conditions that result in a malposition, lagophthalmos, or proptosis with exposure of the ocular surface (see Exposure Keratopathy in Chapter 5).

Reduced blink rate Reading/computer work (decreases blink rate by up to 60%), Parkinson's disease.

Medications Systemic retinoids (Accutane).

Extrinsic causes

Vitamin A deficiency Malnutrition or malabsorption causes conjunctival xerosis and night blindness (nyctalopia) with progressive retinal degeneration; major cause of blindness worldwide.

Topical drugs Anesthetics, preservatives (BAK – benzalkonium chloride).

Contact lens wear Approximately 50% of contact lens wearers have dry eye symptoms.

Ocular surface disease Cicatrizing conjunctivitis (see above), allergic conjunctivitis.

Epidemiology Dry eye disease is estimated to affect 5–30% of the population ≥ 50 years old and is more common in women. Associated factors include age, hormone levels (menopause, androgen deficiency), environmental conditions (low humidity, wind, heat, air-conditioning, pollutants, irritants, allergens), and smoking.

Symptoms Irritation, dryness, burning, stinging, grittiness, foreign body sensation, tearing, red eye, discharge, blurred or fluctuating vision, photophobia, contact lens intolerance, increased blinking; symptoms are variable and exacerbated by wind, smoke, and activities that reduce the blink rate (i.e., reading and computer work).

Signs Conjunctival injection, decreased tear break-up time (<10 seconds), decreased tear meniscus height (<1–1mm), excess tear film debris, corneal filaments, dry corneal surface, irregular and dull corneal light reflex, corneal and/or conjunctival staining with lissamine green, rose Bengal, and fluorescein (typically in the interpalpebral space or on the inferior cornea); may have Bitot's spot (white, foamy patch of keratinized bulbar conjunctiva [pathognomonic for vitamin A deficiency]), conjunctivochalasis (loosened bulbar conjunctiva resting on lid margin); severe cases can cause corneal ulceration, descemetocele, or perforation. May also have signs of an underlying condition (i.e., rosacea, blepharitis, lid abnormality).

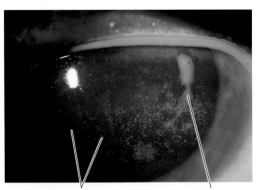

Fluorescein staining of SPK   Filament

Figure 4-8 • Keratoconjunctivitis sicca demonstrating superficial punctate keratitis (SPK) and filaments stained with fluorescein dye.

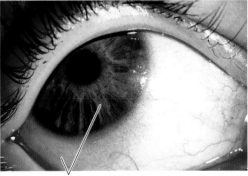

Rose bengal staining

Figure 4-9 • Dry eye due to vitamin A deficiency, demonstrating diffuse staining of cornea, inferior limbus, and interpalpebral conjunctiva with rose bengal.

Figure 4-10 • Dry eye demonstrating lissamine green staining of the interpalpebral conjunctiva.

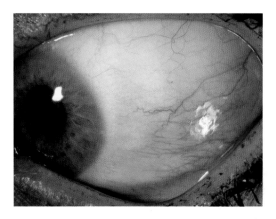

Differential Diagnosis See above; also allergic conjunctivitis, medicamentosa, contact lens overwear, trichiasis.

Evaluation

- Complete history with attention to severity, duration, exacerbating factors, prior treatment, contact lens wear, previous eye/eyelid surgery, systemic diseases and medications. Consider using a questionnaire such as the Ocular Surface Disease Index (OSDI), Dry Eye Questionnaire (DEQ), National Eye Institute Visual Function Questionnaire (NEI VFQ-25), or McMonnies questionnaire.

- Complete eye exam with attention to lids, tear film (break-up time and height of meniscus), conjunctiva, and cornea (staining with lissamine green or rose Bengal [dead and degenerated epithelial cells], and/or fluorescein [only dead epithelial cells]).

- Schirmer's test: Two tests exist, but they are usually not performed as originally described. One is done without and one is done with topical anesthesia. The inferior fornix is dried with a cotton-tipped applicator, and a strip of standardized filter paper (Whatman #41, 5-mm width) is placed in each lower lid at the junction of the lateral and middle thirds. After 5 minutes, the strips are removed and the amount of wetting is measured. Normal results are 15 mm or greater without anesthesia (basal + reflex tearing), and 10 mm or greater with topical anesthesia (basal tearing). Schirmer's test often produces variable results so its usefulness may be limited.

- Alternatively, consider phenol red thread test: Similar to the Schirmer's test but uses a special cotton thread that changes color as tears are absorbed for 30 seconds; less irritating and may be more reproducible.

- **Lab tests**: Consider tear lactoferrin and lysozyme (decreased), tear osmolarity (>316 mOsm/L), and impression cytology (detects reduced goblet cell density and squamous metaplasia; rarely used clinically).

- Consider corneal topography (computerized videokeratography): Irregular or broken mires with resulting abnormal topography and blank areas due to poor quality tear film and dry spots. Surface regularity index (SRI) value correlates with severity of dry eye.

- Electroretinogram (reduced), electro-oculogram (abnormal), and dark adaptation (prolonged) in vitamin A deficiency.

- Consider medical consultation for systemic diseases.

Management

- Reduce/eliminate associated factors.
- The mainstay of therapy is topical lubrication with artificial tears (see Appendix) up to q1h and gel or ointment qhs. Preservative-free tear formulations should be used if the frequency of administration is greater than qid.
- Additional treatment is performed in a stepwise fashion and includes: hydroxypropyl methylcellulose (Lacrisert), topical cyclosporine 0.05% (Restasis) bid for at least 3 months, short course (1–2 weeks) of topical steroid (Lotemax, Alrex, Pred Mild, or FML) bid to qid, punctal occlusion (with plugs or cautery), nutritional supplements (i.e., oral flaxseed/fish oils [omega-3 fatty acids]), bandage contact lens, moisture chamber goggles, lid taping at bedtime, and tarsorrhaphy for more severe cases. Recommendations of the 2007 Dry Eye Workshop (DEWS) are based on severity (1–4) of symptoms (discomfort, fatigue, visual disturbance) and signs (lid, tear film, conjunctiva, cornea) (see Table 4-1).
- Consider acetylcysteine 10% (Mucomyst) qd to qid for mucus strands or filaments.
- Consider autologous serum drops in severe cases.
- Consider oral cholinergic agonists (pilocarpine, cevimeline) to increase tear production, especially in patients with Sjögren syndrome.
- Treat underlying condition:
  - **Acne rosacea/blepharitis:** see Chapter 3
  - **Vitamin A deficiency:** Vitamin A replacement (vitamin A 15,000 IU po qd)
  - **Lid malposition:** Consider surgical repair.

Table 4-1 Dry Eye Severity and Treatment (DEWS recommendations)

Severity Level	Signs and Symptoms	Treatment (Additive)
1	Mild symptoms Mild conjunctival signs No staining	Education, modify/eliminate associated factors, lubrication (artificial tears, gels, ointments), nutritional supplements, lid hygiene
2	Moderate symptoms Tear film and visual signs Conjunctival staining Mild corneal staining	Topical steroids, cyclosporine, secretogogues, punctal plug, tetracyclines, moisture chamber goggles
3	Severe symptoms Marked corneal staining Filamentary keratitis	Permanent punctal occlusion, bandage contact lenses, autologous serum drops
4	Extremely severe symptoms Severe corneal staining Corneal erosions Conjunctival scarring	Systemic anti-inflammatory agents, acetylcysteine, surgery (i.e., lid, tarsorrhaphy; mucus membrane, salivary gland, amniotic membrane transplantation)

Prognosis Depends on underlying condition; severe cases may be difficult to manage.

Inflammation

Definition

Chemosis

Edema of conjunctiva; may be mild with boggy appearance or massive with tense ballooning.

Figure 4-11 • Chemosis with extensive ballooning of conjunctiva and prolapse over lower lid nasally. Temporally, the edges of the elevated conjunctiva are delineated by the light reflexes from the tear film.

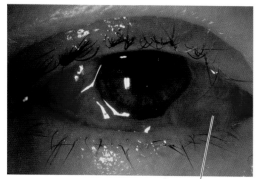

Chemosis

Follicles

Small, translucent, avascular mounds of plasma cells and lymphocytes found in epidemic keratoconjunctivitis (EKC), herpes simplex virus, chlamydia, molluscum, or drug reactions.

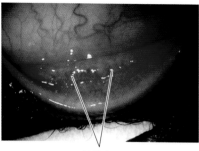

Follicles

Figure 4-12 • Follicular conjunctivitis demonstrating inferior palpebral follicles with the typical gelatinous bump appearance.

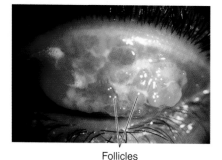

Follicles

Figure 4-13 • Large, gelatinous, tarsal follicles in a patient with acute trachoma.

Granuloma

Collection of giant multinucleated cells found in chronic inflammation from sarcoid, foreign body, or chalazion.

Hyperemia

Redness and injection of conjunctiva.

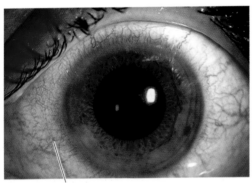

Figure 4-14 • Hyperemia. The dilated conjunctival vessels produce a diffuse redness (injection).

Conjunctival hyperemia

Membranes

A true membrane is a firmly adherent, fibrinous exudate that bleeds and scars when removed; found in bacterial conjunctivitis (*Streptococcus* species, *Neisseria gonorrhoeae*, *Corynebacterium diphtheriae*), Stevens–Johnson syndrome, and burns. A pseudomembrane is a loosely attached, avascular, fibrinous exudate found in EKC and mild allergic or bacterial conjunctivitis.

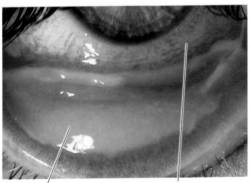

Figure 4-15 • Pseudomembrane evident as a thick yellow coating in a patient with epidemic keratoconjunctivitis.

Pseudomembrane   Conjunctival injection

Papillae

Vascular reaction consisting of fibrovascular mounds with central vascular tuft; nonspecific finding in any conjunctival irritation or conjunctivitis; can be large ("cobblestones" or giant papillae).

Figure 4-16 • Large papillae in a patient with vernal keratoconjunctivitis. The central vascular cores are clearly visible as dots within the papillae.

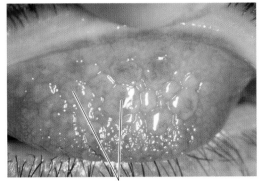

Papillae

Phlyctenule

Focal, nodular, vascularized infiltrate of polymorphonuclear leukocytes and lymphocytes with central necrosis due to hypersensitivity to *Staphylococcus* species, *Mycobacterium* species, *Candida* species, *Coccidioides*, *Chlamydia*, or nematodes; located on the bulbar conjunctiva or at the limbus; can march across the cornea, causing vascularization and scarring behind the leading edge.

Figure 4-17 • Phlyctenule creeping across the cornea is demonstrated by the white infiltrate with trailing neovascularization.

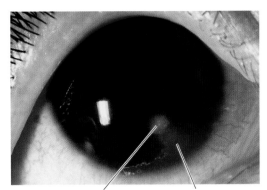

Phlyctenule   Neovascularization

Symptoms Red eye, swelling, itching, foreign body sensation; may have discharge, photophobia, and tearing.

Signs See above; depends on type of inflammation.

Differential Diagnosis Any irritation of conjunctiva (allergic, infectious, autoimmune, chemical, foreign body, idiopathic).

Evaluation
- Complete ophthalmic history and eye exam with attention to preauricular lymphadenopathy, everting lids, conjunctiva, cornea, and characteristics of discharge if present.
- **Lab tests**: Cultures and smears of conjunctiva, cornea, and discharge for infectious causes.

Management

- Treatment depends on etiology; usually supportive.
- Topical vasoconstrictor, nonsteroidal antiinflammatory drug (NSAID), antihistamine, mast cell stabilizer, or mast cell stabilizer and antihistamine combination (see Table 4-2); severe cases may require topical steroid (prednisolone acetate 1% qid) or topical antibiotic (bacitracin-polymixin B sulfate [Polysporin] drops or erythromycin ointment qid or both).
- Membranes and pseudomembranes may require debridement.
- Discontinue offending agent if due to allergic reaction.

Prognosis Depends on etiology; most are benign and self-limited (see Conjunctivitis section).

Conjunctivitis

Definition Infectious or noninfectious inflammation of the conjunctiva classified as acute (shorter than 4-weeks' duration) or chronic (longer than 4-weeks' duration).

Acute Conjunctivitis

Infectious

Gonococcal

Hyperacute presentation with severe purulent discharge, chemosis, papillary reaction, preauricular lymphadenopathy, and lid swelling. *N. gonorrhoeae* can invade intact corneal epithelium and cause infectious keratitis (see Chapter 5).

Nongonococcal Bacterial

Seventy percent due to Gram-positive organisms, 30% due to Gram-negative organisms; usually caused by *Staphylococcus aureus*, *Streptococcus pneumoniae*, *Haemophilus* species, or *Moraxella catarrhalis*. Spectrum of clinical presentations ranging from mild (signs include minimal lid edema, scant purulent discharge) to moderate (significant conjunctival injection, membranes); usually no preauricular lymphadenopathy or corneal involvement.

Figure 4-18 • Bacterial conjunctivitis with mucopurulent discharge adherent to the upper tarsal conjunctiva.

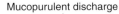
Mucopurulent discharge

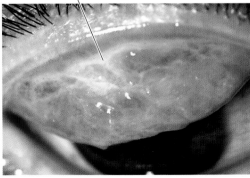

Adenoviral

Most common cause of viral conjunctivitis ("pink eye"); signs include lid edema, serous discharge, pseudomembranes; may have preauricular lymphadenopathy and corneal subepithelial infiltrates. Transmitted by contact and contagious for 12–14 days; 51 serotypes, 1/3 associated with eye infection:

Epidemic keratoconjunctivitis (EKC) Caused by types 8, 19, and 37.

Pharyngoconjunctival fever Caused by types 3, 4, 5, and 7.

Nonspecific follicular conjunctivitis Caused by types 1–11 and 19.

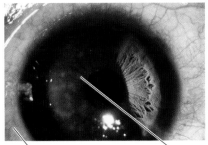

Conjunctival injection   Subepithelial infiltrates

Figure 4-19 • Adenoviral conjunctivitis due to epidemic keratoconjunctivitis with characteristic subepithelial infiltrates.

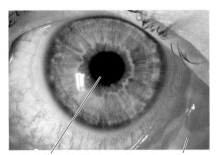

Subepithelial infiltrates   Pseudomembrane

Figure 4-20 • Adenoviral conjunctivitis due to epidemic keratoconjunctivitis demonstrating small, white, punctate subepithelial infiltrates in the central cornea and a yellow pseudomembrane in the inferior fornix.

Herpes Simplex Virus

Primary disease in children causes lid vesicles; may also have fever, preauricular lymphadenopathy, and an upper respiratory infection.

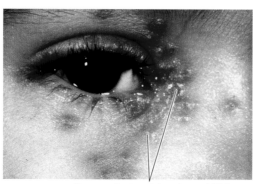

Figure 4-21 • Herpes simplex viral conjunctivitis with characteristic lid vesicles.

Seropurulent vesicles due to HSV

Herpes Zoster Virus

Herpes zoster ophthalmicus can cause conjunctival injection, hemorrhages, vesicles, papillary or follicular reaction, membrane or pseudomembrane; may develop ulceration, scarring, and symblepharon; may have other ocular complications (see Chapters 3 and 5).

Pediculosis

Results from contact with pubic lice (sexually transmitted); may be unilateral or bilateral (see Chapter 3).

Allergic

Seasonal

Most common (50% of allergic conjunctivitis); occurs in individuals of all ages; associated with hay fever, airborne allergens (i.e., pollen).

Atopic Keratoconjunctivitis

Rare (3% of allergic conjunctivitis); occurs in adults; not seasonal; associated with atopy (rhinitis, asthma, dermatitis). Similar features as vernal keratoconjunctivitis but papillae usually smaller and conjunctiva has milky edema; also thickened and erythematous lids, corneal neovascularization, cataracts (10%), and keratoconus.

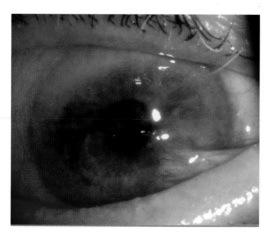

Figure 4-22 • Atopic keratoconjunctivitis demonstrating corneal vascularization and scarring with symblepharon.

Vernal Keratoconjunctivitis

Very rare (<1% of allergic conjunctivitis); occurs in children; seasonal (warm months); male predilection; lasts 5–10 years, then resolves. Associated with family history of atopy; signs include intense itching, ropy discharge, giant papillae (cobblestones), Horner–Trantas dots (collections of eosinophils at limbus), shield ulcer, and keratitis (50%). Histologically, more than two eosinophils per high-power field is pathognomonic.

Figure 4-23 • Vernal keratoconjunctivitis demonstrating "cobblestones" (giant papillae).

Giant papillae (cobblestones)

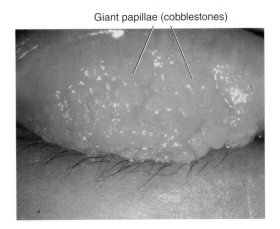

Figure 4-24 • Horner–Trantas dot appears as an elevated white bump at the limbus.

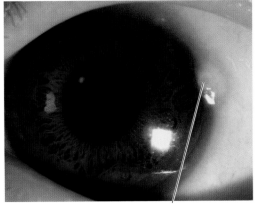

Horner–Trantas dot

Toxic

Follicular reaction due to eye drops (especially neomycin, aminoglycoside antibiotics, antiviral medications, atropine, miotic agents, brimonidine [Alphagan], apraclonidine [Iopidine], epinephrine, and preservatives including contact lens solutions [i.e., thimerosal]).

Chronic Conjunctivitis

Infectious

Chlamydial

Trachoma Leading cause of blindness worldwide; caused by serotypes A–C. Signs include follicles, Herbert's pits (scarred limbal follicles), superior pannus, superficial punctate keratitis, upper tarsal scarring (Arlt's line).

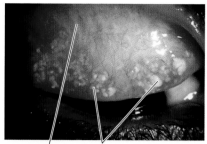

Arlt's line   Concretions

Figure 4-25 • Trachoma demonstrating linear pattern of upper tarsal scarring. Also note the abundant concretions that appear as yellow granular aggregates.

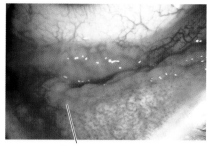

Follicles

Figure 4-26 • Chlamydial conjunctivitis with follicles in the inferior fornix.

Inclusion conjunctivitis Caused by serotypes D–K. Signs include chronic, follicular conjunctivitis, subepithelial infiltrates, and no membrane; associated with urethritis in 5%.

Lymphogranuloma venereum Caused by serotype L. Associated with Parinaud's oculoglandular syndrome (see below), conjunctival granulomas, and interstitial keratitis.

Molluscum Contagiosum

Usually appears with one or more, umbilicated, shiny papules on the eyelid. Associated with follicular conjunctivitis; with multiple lesions, consider human immunodeficiency virus (HIV) (see Chapter 3).

Allergic

Perennial

Occurs in individuals of all ages. Associated with animal dander, dust mites.

Giant Papillary Conjunctivitis

Occurs in contact lens wearers (>95% of giant papillary conjunctivitis cases); also secondary to prosthesis, foreign body, or exposed suture. Signs include itching, ropy discharge, blurry vision, and pain/irritation with contact lens wear.

Figure 4-27 • Giant papillary conjunctivitis demonstrating large papillae in upper tarsal conjunctiva.

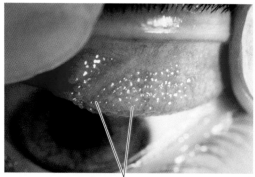

Giant papillary conjunctivitis

Toxic

Follicular reaction due to eye drops or contact lens solutions (see above).

Other

Superior Limbic Keratoconjunctivitis

Occurs in middle-aged females; 50% have thyroid disease; usually bilateral and asymmetric; may be secondary to contact lens use (see Chapter 5). Signs include boggy edema, redundancy and injection of superior conjunctiva, superficial punctate keratitis, filaments, and no discharge; symptoms are worse than signs.

Figure 4-28 • Superior limbic keratoconjunctivitis demonstrating the typical staining of the central superior conjunctiva with rose bengal dye.

Rose bengal staining

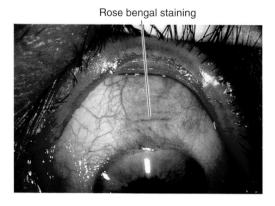

Kawasaki's Disease

Mucocutaneous lymph node syndrome of unknown etiology; occurs in children under 5 years old; more common in Japanese. Diagnosis based on 5 of 6 criteria: (1) fever (=5 days), (2) bilateral conjunctivitis, (3) oral mucosal changes (erythema, fissures, "strawberry tongue"), (4) rash, (5) cervical lymphadenopathy, and (6) peripheral extremity changes (edema, erythema, desquamation). Associated with polyarteritis especially of coronary arteries; may be fatal (1–2%).

Ligneous

Rare, idiopathic, bilateral, membranous conjunctivitis; occurs in children. A thick, white, woody infiltrate and plaque develops on the upper tarsal conjunctiva.

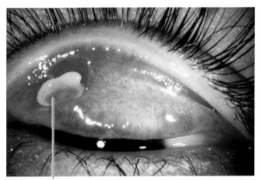

Ligneous plaque

Figure 4-29 • Ligneous conjunctivitis demonstrating thick, yellow-white plaque on superior tarsal conjunctiva.

Parinaud's Oculoglandular Syndrome

Unilateral conjunctivitis with conjunctival granulomas and preauricular/submandibular lymphadenopathy; may have fever, malaise, and rash. Due to cat-scratch fever, tularemia, sporotrichosis, tuberculosis, syphilis, lymphogranuloma venereum, Epstein–Barr virus, mumps, fungi, malignancy, or sarcoidosis.

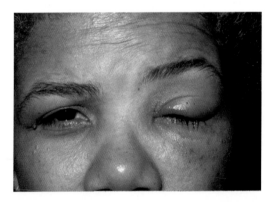

Figure 4-30 • Parinaud's oculoglandular syndrome. There is marked eyelid swelling and erythema in this patient with an affected left eye.

Ophthalmia Neonatorum

Occurs in newborns; may be toxic (silver nitrate) or infectious (bacteria [especially *N. gonorrhoeae*], herpes simplex virus, chlamydia [may have otitis and pneumonitis]).

Figure 4-31 • Hyperacute gonorrheal conjunctivitis demonstrating conjunctival injection and purulent discharge in a newborn.

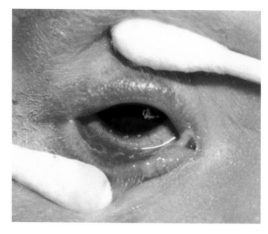

Symptoms Red eye, swelling, itching, burning, foreign body sensation, tearing, discharge, crusting of lashes; may have photophobia and decreased vision.

Signs Normal or decreased visual acuity, lid edema, conjunctival injection, chemosis, papillae, follicles, membranes, petechial hemorrhages, concretions, discharge; may have preauricular lymphadenopathy, tarsal conjunctival filament, subepithelial corneal infiltrates, punctate corneal staining, corneal ulcers, and cataract.

Differential Diagnosis See above; also blepharitis (may present as "recurrent conjunctivitis"), medicamentosa (toxic reaction commonly associated with preservatives [i.e., benzalkonium chloride (BAK)] in medications, as well as antiviral medications, antibiotics, miotic agents, dipivefrin [Propine], apraclonidine [Iopidine], and atropine), dacryocystitis, nasolacrimal duct obstruction.

Evaluation
- Complete ophthalmic history and eye exam with attention to preauricular lymphadenopathy, everting lids, characteristics of discharge, conjunctiva, cornea, and anterior chamber.
- **Lab tests**: Consider cultures and smears of conjunctiva and cornea (mandatory for suspected bacterial cases). Consider RPS Adeno Detector test (for suspected viral cases).
- Consider pediatric consultation.

Management

- Treatment depends on etiology; usually supportive with medications, compresses, and debridement of membranes for symptomatic relief.

BACTERIAL
- Topical broad spectrum antibiotic (gatifloxacin [Zymar] qid, moxifloxacin [Vigamox] tid, or azithromycin [Azasite] bid/qd).
- May require systemic antibiotics especially in children.
- Remove discharge with irrigation and membranes with sterile cotton-tipped applicator.

Continued

Management—Cont'd

VIRAL

- Topical lubrication with artificial tears (see Appendix) and topical vasoconstrictor, NSAID, antihistamine, mast cell stabilizer, or mast cell stabilizer and antihistamine combination (see Table 4-2).
- Topical antibiotic (polymyxin B sulfate-trimethoprim [Polytrim] drops qid, erythromycin or bacitracin ointment qid to tid) for corneal epithelial defects.
- Topical steroid (fluorometholone alcohol 0.1% [FML] qid) for subepithelial infiltrates in EKC.
- Topical antiviral (trifluridine [Viroptic] 5 times/day) for herpes simplex.
- Topical antibiotic (polymyxin B sulfate-trimethoprim [Polytrim] drops qid, erythromycin or bacitracin ointment tid) for herpes zoster; consider topical steroid (prednisolone acetate 1% qid) if severe.

OTHER INFECTIONS

- *N. gonorrhoeae, chlamydia,* and Parinaud's oculoglandular syndrome (e.g., cat-scratch disease, tularemia, syphilis, tuberculosis, etc.) require systemic antibiotics based on causative organism.

ALLERGIC

- Identify and avoid/eliminate inciting agent(s); may require allergic patch testing to determine causative allergens.
- Topical vasoconstrictor, NSAID, antihistamine, mast cell stabilizer, or mast cell stabilizer and antihistamine combination (see Table 4-2).
- Consider mild topical steroid especially for severe allergic keratoconjunctivitis; start with fluorometholone alcohol 0.1% (FML) qid or loteprednol etabonate 0.2% (Alrex) qid, change to prednisolone 1% qid to q1h in severe cases. Solution (phosphate [Inflamase Mild, AK-Pred]) works better than suspension (acetate [Pred Mild, Econopred]).
- Consider systemic antihistamine (diphenhydramine [Benadryl] 25–50 mg po q6h prn).

GIANT PAPILLARY CONJUNCTIVITIS

- Clean, change, or discontinue use of contact lenses; change to preservative free contact lens cleaning solution (see Chapter 5).

SUPERIOR LIMBIC KERATOCONJUNCTIVITIS

- Silver nitrate solution, bandage contact lens, conjunctival cautery, or conjunctival recession and resection.
- Steroids do not help.
- Cromolyn sodium 4% [Crolom] qid or olopatadine hydrochloride 0.1% [Patanol] bid may be useful (see Chapter 5).

Management—Cont'd

ATOPIC AND VERNAL KERATOCONJUNCTIVITIS

- Consider topical cyclosporine (1–2%) qid.
- Consider supratarsal steroid injection (0.25–0.50 ml dexamethasone or triamcinolone acetate [Kenalog]).

KAWASAKI'S DISEASE

- Pediatric consultation and hospital admission.
- Systemic steroids are contraindicated.

LIGNEOUS

- May respond to topical steroids, mucolytics, or cyclosporine.

Table 4-2 Topical Medications Available for Management of Allergic Conjunctivitis

Mechanism	Trade Name	Pharmacologic Name	Dosage
Antihistamine	Emadine	Emadastine 0.05%	qid
	Livostin	Levocabastine 0.05%	qid
Mast cell stabilizer	Alamast	Pemirolast 0.1%	qid
	Alocril	Nedocromil 2%	bid
	Alomide	Lodoxamide 0.1%	qid
	Crolom	Cromolyn sodium 4%	qid
Mast cell stabilizer and antihistamine combination	Optivar	Azelastine 0.05%	bid
	Patanol, Pataday	Olopatadine 0.1%, 0.2%	bid, qd
	Elestat	Epinastine hydrochloride 0.05%	bid
	Zaditor, Alaway	Ketotifen fumarate 0.025%	bid
Nonsteroidal antiinflammatory	Acular	Ketorolac tromethamine 0.5%	qid
Steroidal anti-inflammatory	Alrex	Loteprednol etabonate 0.2%	up to qid
Vasoconstrictor	Naphcon-A	Naphazoline 0.025% and pheniramine 0.3%	up to qid
	Vasocon-A	Naphazoline 0.05% and antazoline 0.5%	up to qid

Prognosis Usually good; subepithelial infiltrates in adenoviral conjunctivitis cause variable decreased vision for months.

Degenerations

Definition Secondary degenerative changes of the conjunctiva.

Amyloidosis

Yellow-white or salmon-colored, avascular deposits; may be due to primary (localized) or secondary (systemic) amyloidosis.

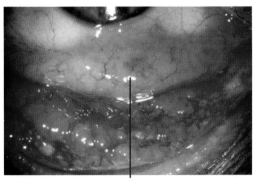

Figure 4-32 • Yellowish avascular deposits in inferior conjunctiva from amyloidosis.

Conjunctival amyloidosis

Concretions

Yellow-white inclusion cysts filled with keratin and epithelial debris in fornix or palpebral conjunctiva; associated with aging and chronic conjunctivitis; can erode through overlying conjunctiva causing foreign body sensation (see Figure 4-25).

Pinguecula

Yellow-white, subepithelial lesion of abnormal collagen at the medial or temporal limbus; due to actinic changes; elastotic degeneration seen histologically; may become inflamed (pingueculitis); may calcify over time.

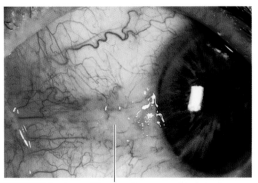

Figure 4-33 • Pinguecula appears as a yellow-white elevated mass near the medial limbus.

Pinguecula

Pterygium

Triangular fibrovascular tissue in interpalpebral space involving cornea; often preceded by pinguecula; destroys Bowman's membrane; may have iron line at leading edge (Stocker's line); induces astigmatism and may cause decreased vision.

Figure 4-34 • Large nasal and smaller temporal pterygia. Note the typical triangular, wedge-shaped configuration, and also the white corneal scarring at the leading edges.

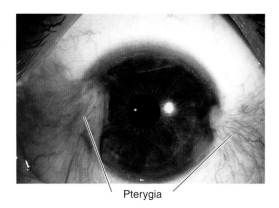

Pterygia

Symptoms Asymptomatic; may have red eye, foreign body sensation, decreased vision; may notice bump or growth; may have contact lens intolerance.

Signs See above.

Differential Diagnosis Cyst, squamous cell carcinoma, conjunctival intraepithelial neoplasia, episcleritis, scleritis, phlyctenule.

Evaluation
• Complete ophthalmic history and eye exam with attention to conjunctiva and cornea.

Management

• Often no treatment necessary.
• Topical lubrication with artificial tears (see Appendix) up to q1h.
• Consider limited use of vasoconstrictor (naphazoline [Naphcon] qid) for inflamed pinguecula or pterygium.
• Consider short course (1–2 weeks) of topical steroid (FML) bid to qid for pingueculitis.
• Surgical excision of pterygium for chronic inflammation, cosmesis, contact lens intolerance, or involvement of visual axis.
• Concretions are easily unroofed and removed with a 27–30-gauge 1/2 inch needle if symptomatic.

Prognosis Good; about one-third of pterygia recur after simple excision, recurrences are reduced by conjunctival autograft, β-irradiation, thiotepa, or mitomycin C.

Ocular Cicatricial Pemphigoid

Definition Systemic vesiculobullous disease of mucous membranes resulting in bilateral, chronic, cicatrizing conjunctivitis; other mucous membranes frequently involved, including oral (up to 90%), esophageal, tracheal, and genital; skin involved in up to 30% of cases.

Etiology Usually idiopathic (probably autoimmune mechanism) or drug induced (may occur with epinephrine, timolol, pilocarpine, echothiophate iodide [Phospholine Iodide], or idoxuridine).

Epidemiology Incidence of 1 in 20,000; usually occurs in females (2:1) over 60 years old; associated with HLA-DR4, DQw3.

Symptoms Red eye, dryness, foreign body sensation, tearing, decreased vision; may have dysphagia or difficulty breathing.

Signs Normal or decreased visual acuity, conjunctival injection and scarring, dry eye, symblepharon (fusion or attachment of eyelid to bulbar conjunctiva), ankyloblepharon (fusion or attachment of upper and lower eyelids), foreshortened fornices, trichiasis, entropion, keratitis, corneal ulcer, scarring, and vascularization, conjunctival and corneal keratinization, and oral lesions; corneal perforation and endophthalmitis can occur.

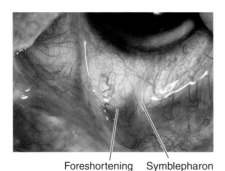

Foreshortening   Symblepharon

Figure 4-35 • Ocular cicatricial pemphigoid demonstrating symblepharon and foreshortening of the inferior fornix.

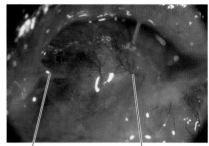

Symblepharon   Neovascularization

Figure 4-36 • Ocular cicatricial pemphigoid demonstrating advanced stage with corneal vascularization and symblepharon.

Differential Diagnosis Stevens–Johnson syndrome, chemical burn, squamous cell carcinoma, scleroderma, infectious or allergic conjunctivitis, trachoma, sarcoidosis, ocular rosacea, radiation, linear immunoglobulin A dermatosis, practolol-induced conjunctivitis.

Evaluation
- Complete ophthalmic history and eye exam with attention to lids, conjunctiva, and cornea.
- Conjunctival biopsy (immunoglobulin and complement deposition in basement membrane).

Management

- Topical lubrication with preservative-free artificial tears (see Appendix) up to q1h and ointment (Refresh PM) qhs.
- Topical antibiotic (polymyxin B sulfate-trimethoprim [Polytrim] drops qid or erythromycin ointment tid) for corneal epithelial defects.
- Consider punctal occlusion, tarsorrhaphy.
- Often requires treatment with systemic steroids or immunosuppressive agents (dapsone [contraindicated in patients with glucose 6-phosphate dehydrogenase deficiency], cyclophosphamide); should be performed by a cornea or uveitis specialist.
- Consider surgery for entropion, trichiasis, symblepharon, ankyloblepharon, or corneal scarring; may require mucous membrane grafting; keratoprosthesis in advanced cases.

Prognosis Poor; chronic progressive disease with remissions and exacerbations, surgery often initiates exacerbations.

Stevens–Johnson Syndrome (Erythema Multiforme Major)

Definition Acute, usually self-limited (up to 6 weeks), cutaneous, bullous disease with mucosal ulceration resulting in acute membranous conjunctivitis.

Etiology Usually drug-induced (may occur with sulfonamides, penicillin, aspirin, barbiturates, isoniazid, or phenytoin [Dilantin]) or infectious (herpes simplex virus, *Mycoplasma* species, adenovirus, *Streptococcus* species).

Symptoms Fever, upper respiratory infection, headache, malaise, skin eruption, decreased vision, pain, red eye, swelling, and oral mucosal ulceration.

Signs Fever, skin eruption (target lesions), mucous membrane ulceration and crusting, decreased visual acuity, conjunctival injection, discharge, membranes, dry eye, symblepharon (fusion or attachment of eyelid to bulbar conjunctiva), trichiasis, keratitis, corneal ulcer, scarring, vascularization, and keratinization.

Differential Diagnosis Ocular cicatricial pemphigoid, chemical burn, squamous cell carcinoma, scleroderma, infectious or allergic conjunctivitis, trachoma, sarcoidosis, ocular rosacea, radiation.

Evaluation
- Complete ophthalmic history and eye exam with attention to systemic mucous membranes, lids, conjunctiva, and cornea.
- Medical consultation.

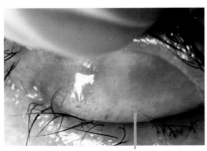

Tarsal scarring

Figure 4-37 • Stevens–Johnson syndrome demonstrating tarsal scarring.

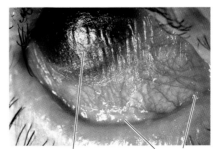

Corneal keratinization   Symblepharon

Figure 4-38 • • Stevens–Johnson syndrome demonstrating keratinization of the ocular surface with a dry, wrinkled appearance. Note the resulting irregular, diffuse corneal reflex.

Management

- Supportive, topical lubrication with preservative-free artificial tears (see Appendix) up to q1h and ointment (Refresh PM) qhs.
- Topical antibiotic (polymyxin B sulfate-trimethoprim [Polytrim] drops qid or erythromycin ointment tid) for corneal epithelial defects.
- Consider topical steroid (prednisolone acetate 1% up to q2h) depending on severity of inflammation.
- Consider steroids (prednisone 60–100 mg po qd) in very severe cases; check purified protein derivative (PPD) and controls, blood glucose, and chest radiographs before starting systemic steroids.
- Add H_2-blocker (ranitidine [Zantac] 150 mg po bid) or proton pump inhibitor when administering systemic steroids.
- May require punctal occlusion, tarsorrhaphy for more severe cases.
- Consider surgery for trichiasis, symblepharon, or corneal scarring.

Prognosis Fair; not progressive (in contrast to ocular cicatricial pemphigoid), recurrences are rare, but up to 30% mortality.

Tumors

Congenital

Hamartoma

Derived from abnormal rest of cells, composed of tissues normally found at same location (e.g., telangiectasia, lymphangioma).

Choristoma

Derived from abnormal rest of cells, composed of tissues not normally found at that location.

Dermoid

White-yellow, solid, round, elevated nodule, often with visible hairs on surface and lipid deposition anterior to its corneal edge; composed of dense connective tissue with pilosebaceous units and stratified squamous epithelium; usually located at inferotemporal limbus; may be part of Goldenhar's syndrome with dermoids, preauricular skin tags, and vertebral anomalies (see Chapter 5).

Dermolipoma

Similar appearance to dermoid but composed of adipose tissue with keratinized surface; usually located superotemporally extending into orbit.

Epibulbar osseous choristoma

Solitary, white nodule composed of compact bone that develops from episclera; freely moveable; usually located superotemporally.

Epithelial

Cysts

Fluid-filled cavity within the conjunctiva, defined by its lining (ductal or inclusion). Often due to trauma or inflammation, can be congenital.

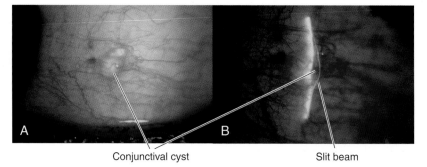

Conjunctival cyst   Slit beam

Figure 4-39 • Conjunctival inclusion cyst appears as a clear elevation over which the slit beam bends.

- No treatment necessary.
- Consider excision; must remove inner lining to prevent recurrence.

Papilloma

Red, gelatinous lesions composed of proliferative epithelium with fibrovascular cores; may be pedunculated or sessile, solitary or multiple. Often associated with human papillomavirus.

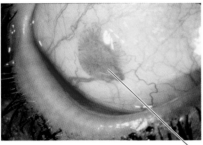

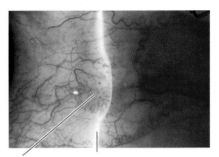

Papilloma

Papilloma   Slit-beam

Figure 4-40 • Papilloma demonstrating the typical elevated appearance with central vascular fronds.

Figure 4-41 • Squamous papilloma with elevated, gelatinous appearance.

- May resolve spontaneously.
- Consider excision with or without cryotherapy, topical interferon alpha-2b, or topical mitomycin C.
- Consider oral cimetidine or carbon dioxide laser treatment for recalcitrant cases.

Conjunctival Intraepithelial Neoplasia

White, gelatinous, conjunctival dysplasia confined to the epithelium; usually begins at limbus and is a precursor of squamous cell carcinoma.

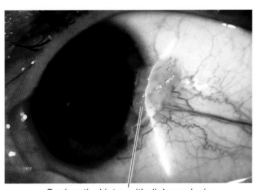

Figure 4-42 • Conjunctival intraepithelial neoplasia demonstrating pink, nodular, gelatinous, vascularized appearance at the limbus.

Conjunctival intraepithelial neoplasia

- Excisional biopsy; consider topical 5-fluorouracil or mitomycin C.

Squamous Cell Carcinoma

Interpalpebral, exophytic, gelatinous, papillary appearance with loops of abnormal vessels; may have superficial invasion and extend onto cornea. Most common conjunctival malignancy in the US; more common in elderly, Caucasian (90%) and males (81%); associated with ultraviolet radiation, human papillomavirus, and heavy smoking; suspect AIDS in patients <50 years of age. Intraocular invasion (2–8%), orbital invasion (12–16%), and metastasis are rare; recurrence after excision is <10%; mortality rate of up to 8%.

Figure 4-43 • Squamous cell carcinoma with gelatinous growth and abnormal vascular loops.

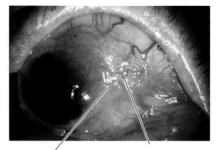

Squamous cell carcinoma   Vascular loops

- MRI to rule out orbital involvement if suspected.
- Excisional biopsy with episclerectomy, corneal epitheliectomy with 100% alcohol, and cryotherapy to bed of lesion; should be performed by a cornea or tumor specialist.
- Consider topical 5-fluorouracil or mitomycin C, especially for recurrence.
- Exenteration with adjunctive radiation therapy for orbital involvement.
- Medical consultation and systemic workup.

Melanocytic

Nevus

Mobile, discrete, elevated, variably pigmented lesion that contains cysts; may be junctional, subepithelial, or compound. May enlarge during puberty; rarely becomes malignant.

- Observation; consider serial photographs and clinical examination for any growth that would be suspicious for malignant melanoma.

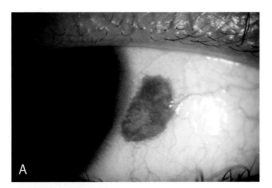

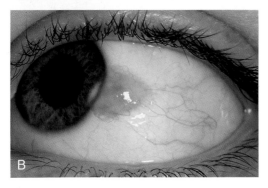

Figure 4-44 • Elevated (A) pigmented and (B) non-pigmented conjunctival nevus.

Ocular Melanocytosis

Unilateral, increased uveal, scleral, and episcleral pigmentation appearing as blue-gray patches. More common in Caucasians.

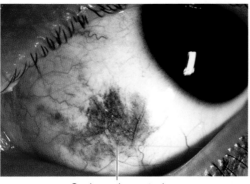

Ocular melanocytosis

Figure 4-45 • Ocular melanocytosis demonstrating blue-gray, patchy pigmentation.

• No treatment necessary.

Oculodermal Melanocytosis (Nevus of Ota)

Increased uveal, scleral, episcleral, and periorbital skin pigmentation; more common in Asians and African Americans; increased risk of congenital glaucoma; uveal melanoma may rarely develop in Caucasians (see Chapter 10).

Figure 4-46 • Oculodermal melanocytosis (nevus of Ota) of the left eye. Note the prominent scleral pigmentation; the periorbital skin changes are difficult to see in this photo.

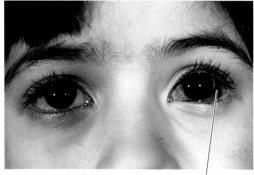

Oculodermal melanocytosis (nevus of Ota)

• Periodic examinations to monitor for evidence of malignant transformation.

Primary Acquired Melanosis

Mobile, patchy, diffuse, flat, brown lesions without cysts; indistinct margins, may grow and involve the cornea. Occurs in middle-aged Caucasian adults; accounts for 11% of conjunctival tumors and 21% of pigmented lesions. Histologically may have atypia; 13% with severe atypia progress to malignant melanoma.

Figure 4-47 • Primary acquired melanosis demonstrating mottled, brown, patchy pigmentation.

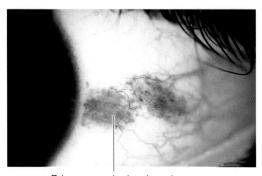

Primary acquired melanosis

• Excisional biopsy with cryotherapy.
• Consider topical interferon alpha-2b or mitomycin C for recurrence.

Secondary Acquired Melanosis

Hyperpigmentation due to racial variations, actinic stimulation, radiation, pregnancy, Addison's disease, or inflammation; usually perilimbal.

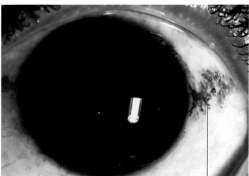

Figure 4-48 • Secondary acquired melanosis (racial pigmentation) demonstrating typical perilimbal, brown, homogeneous pigmentation.

Secondary acquired melanosis

* No treatment necessary.

Malignant Melanoma

Nodular, pigmented lesion containing vessels, but no cysts; may arise from primary acquired melanosis (50–75%), nevus (20%), or de novo (25%). Mainly occurs in middle-aged Caucasian adults. 25% risk of metastasis; 25–45% mortality.

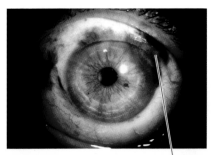

Malignant melanoma

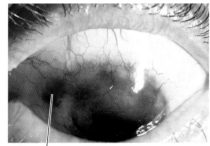

Malignant melanoma

Figure 4-49 • Malignant melanoma with nodular, pigmented, vascular lesion at the limbus.

Figure 4-50 • Malignant melanoma demonstrating irregular pigmented growth at limbus and onto cornea with vascularization.

* Consider ultrasound biomicroscopy (UBM) to rule out extrascleral extension of ciliary body melanoma.
* Excisional biopsy using "no touch" technique with episclerectomy, corneal epitheliectomy with 100% alcohol, and cryotherapy; consider topical mitomycin C; should be performed by a cornea or tumor specialist.
* May require exenteration, but does not improve prognosis.
* Medical consultation and systemic workup.

Stromal

Cavernous Hemangioma

Red patch on conjunctiva; may bleed and be associated with other ocular hemangiomas or systemic disease.

Figure 4-51 • Cavernous hemangioma demonstrating red patch of dilated blood vessels in the inferior fornix.

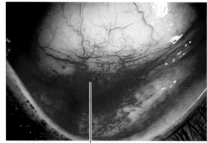
Cavernous hemangioma

- No treatment necessary.

Juvenile Xanthogranuloma

Yellow-orange nodules composed of vascularized, lipid-containing histiocytes; can also involve iris and skin; often regresses spontaneously.

- No treatment necessary.

Kaposi's Sarcoma

Single or multiple, flat or elevated, deep red to purple plaques (malignant granulation tissue); may cause recurrent subconjunctival hemorrhage; may involve orbit; also found on skin. Occurs in immunocompromised individuals, especially HIV-positive patients.

Figure 4-52 • Kaposi's sarcoma demonstrating beefy, red, large, nodular mass in the inferior fornix.

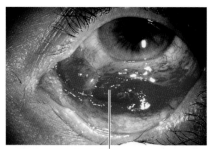
Kaposi's sarcoma

- Consider excision, cryotherapy, chemotherapy, or radiation therapy; should be performed by a cornea or tumor specialist.
- Medical consultation and systemic workup.

Lymphangiectasis

Cluster of elevated clear cysts that represent dilated lymphatics; may have areas of hemorrhage.

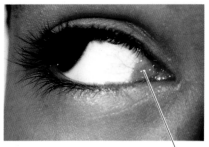

Lymphangiectasis

Figure 4-53 • Lymphangiectasis demonstrating cluster of cysts medially near the caruncle.

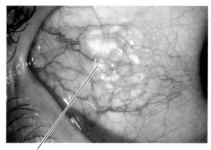

Lymphangiectasis

Figure 4-54 • Lymphangiectasis with clear cysts.

• Consider excision.

Lymphoid

Single or multiple, smooth, flat, salmon-colored patches. Usually occurs in middle-aged adults. Spectrum of disease from benign reactive lymphoid hyperplasia to malignant lymphoma (non-Hodgkin's; less aggressive MALT [mucosa associated lymphoid tissue] or more malignant non-MALT); may involve orbit, may develop systemic lymphoma (see Chapter 1).

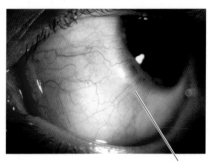

Lymphoid tumor

Figure 4-55 • Malignant lymphoma with salmon-colored lesion.

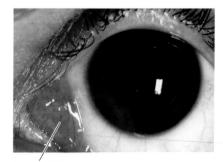

Lymphoid tumor

Figure 4-56 • Lymphoid tumor demonstrating typical salmon-patch appearance.

Figure 4-57 • Lymphoma involving the entire conjunctiva.

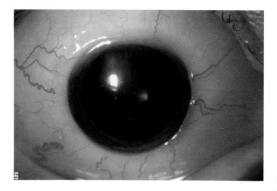

- Tissue biopsy with immunohistochemical studies on fresh specimens required for diagnosis; should be performed by a cornea or tumor specialist.
- External beam radiation for lesion limited to conjunctiva.
- May require systemic chemotherapy.
- Medical and oncology consultations and systemic workup.

Pyogenic Granuloma

Red, fleshy, polypoid mass at the site of chronic inflammation; often follows surgical or accidental trauma. Misnomer, because it is neither pyogenic nor a granuloma, but rather granulation tissue.

Figure 4-58 • Pyogenic granuloma appearing as a large, fleshy, vascular, pedunculated growth.

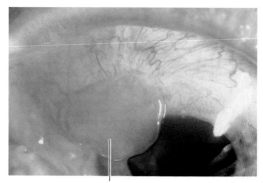

Pyogenic granuloma

- Topical steroid.
- Consider excision.

Caruncle

Tumors that affect the conjunctiva may also occur in the caruncle, including (in order of frequency): papilloma, nevus, inclusion cyst, malignant melanoma, also sebaceous cell carcinoma, and oncocytoma (oxyphilic adenoma; fleshy, yellow-tan cystic mass from transformation of epithelial cells of accessory lacrimal glands; slowly progressive).

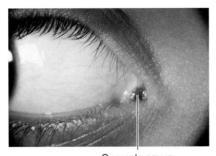

Caruncle nevus

Figure 4-59 • Nevus of the caruncle appearing as a brown pigmented spot.

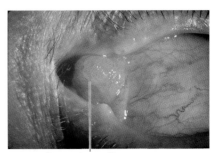

Caruncle papilloma

Figure 4-60 • Papilloma of the caruncle appearing as a large, vascular, pedunculated mass.

- Consider excisional biopsy.
- Medical consultation and systemic workup for malignant lesions.

Episcleritis

Definition Sectoral (70%) or diffuse (30%) inflammation of episclera.

Epidemiology Eighty percent simple; 20% nodular; 33% bilateral.

Etiology Idiopathic, tuberculosis, syphilis, herpes zoster, rheumatoid arthritis, other collagen vascular diseases.

Symptoms Red eye; may have mild pain.

Signs Subconjunctival and conjunctival injection, usually sectoral; may have chemosis, episcleral nodules, anterior chamber cells and flare.

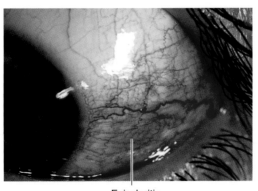

Figure 4-61 • Episcleritis demonstrating characteristic sectoral injection.

Episcleritis

Differential Diagnosis Scleritis, iritis, pingueculitis, myositis, phlyctenule, staphylococcal marginal keratitis, superior limbic keratoconjunctivitis.

Evaluation
- Complete ophthalmic history and eye exam with attention to pattern of conjunctival and scleral injection and blanching with topical phenylephrine (scleritis is painful, has violaceous hue, and does not blanch with topical vasoconstrictor [phenylephrine 2.5%]), cornea, and anterior chamber.
- Consider scleritis workup (see below) in recurrent or bilateral cases.

Management

- Consider limited use of vasoconstrictor (naphazoline [Naphcon] qid) for mild cases.
- May require topical steroid (fluorometholone acetate [Flarex] qid) or oral NSAID (indomethacin 50 mg po qd to bid) for severe cases.

Prognosis Good; usually self-limited; may be recurrent in 67% of cases.

Scleritis

Definition Inflammation of sclera, can be anterior (98%) or posterior (2%) (see Chapter 10).

Epidemiology Anterior form may be diffuse (40%), nodular (44%), or necrotizing (14%) with or without (scleromalacia perforans) inflammation; more than 50% are bilateral; associated systemic disease in 50% of cases.

Etiology Collagen vascular disease in 30% of cases (most commonly rheumatoid arthritis, ankylosing spondylitis, systemic lupus erythematosus, polyarteritis nodosa, Wegener's granulomatosis, and relapsing polychondritis); also herpes zoster, syphilis, tuberculosis, leprosy, gout, porphyria, postsurgical, and idiopathic.

Symptoms Pain, photophobia, swelling, red eye, decreased vision (except scleromalacia).

Signs Normal or decreased visual acuity, subconjunctival and conjunctival injection with violaceous hue, chemosis, scleral edema, scleral nodule(s), globe tenderness to palpation; may have anterior chamber cells and flare (30%), corneal infiltrate or thinning, scleral thinning (30%); posterior type may have chorioretinal folds, focal serous retinal detachments, vitritis, and optic disc edema (see Figures 10-168 and 10-169).

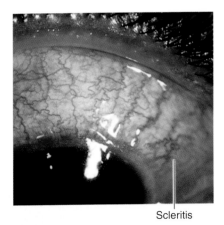

Scleritis

Figure 4-62 • Diffuse anterior scleritis demonstrating characteristic deep red, violaceous hue.

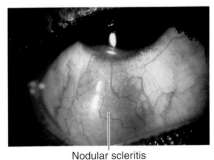

Nodular scleritis

Figure 4-63 • Nodular anterior scleritis. Note the elevated nodule within the deep, red, sectoral injection.

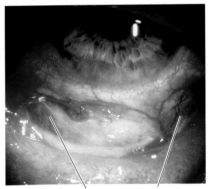

Necrotizing scleritis

Figure 4-64 • Necrotizing scleritis demonstrating thinning of sclera superiorly with increased visibility of the underlying blue uvea.

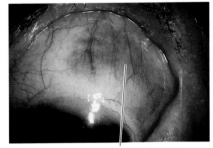

Scleromalacia perforans

Figure 4-65 • Scleromalacia perforans demonstrating characteristic blue appearance due to visible uvea underneath thin sclera.

Differential Diagnosis Episcleritis, iritis, phlyctenule, retrobulbar mass, myositis, scleral ectasia, and staphyloma.

Evaluation

- Complete ophthalmic history and eye exam with attention to pattern of conjunctival and scleral injection and failure of area to blanch with topical vasoconstrictor (phenylephrine 2.5%), cornea, anterior chamber, and ophthalmoscopy.
- **Lab tests**: Complete blood count (CBC), rheumatoid factor (RF), antinuclear antibody (ANA), antineutrophil cytoplasmic antibody (ANCA), Venereal Disease Research Laboratory (VDRL) test, fluorescent treponemal antibody absorption (FTA-ABS) test, PPD and controls, and chest radiographs.
- **B-scan ultrasonography:** Thickened sclera and "T-sign" in posterior scleritis (see Figure 10-170).
- Medical consultation.

Management

- Depending on severity, consider using one or a combination of the following:
  - Systemic NSAID (indomethacin 50 mg po bid to tid, Dolobid 500 mg po qd to bid, Celebrex 200 mg po bid).
  - Oral steroids (prednisone 60–100 mg po qd); check PPD and controls, blood glucose, and chest radiographs before starting systemic steroids. Note: topical steroids and NSAIDs are ineffective.
  - Add H_2-blocker (ranitidine [Zantac] 150 mg po bid) or proton pump inhibitor when administering systemic NSAIDs or steroids.
  - Immunosuppressive agents (see Anterior Uveitis section in Chapter 6) in severe cases; should be administered by a uveitis specialist.
- Sub-Tenon's steroid injection is contraindicated.
- May require surgery (patch graft) for globe perforation.

Prognosis Depends on etiology; poor for necrotizing form, which may perforate; scleromalacia perforans rarely perforates; recurrences common.

Scleral Discoloration

Definition

Alkaptonuria (Ochronosis)

Recessive inborn error of metabolism (accumulation of homogentisic acid) causing brown pigment deposits in eyes, ears, nose, joints, and heart; triangular patches in interpalpebral space near limbus, pigmentation of tarsus and lids.

Ectasia (Staphyloma)

Congenital, focal area of scleral thinning usually near limbus; underlying uvea is visible and may bulge through defect; perforation is uncommon.

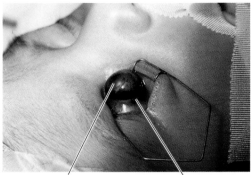

Figure 4-66 • Scleral and corneal staphylomas with bulging blue appearance.

Corneal staphyloma   Scleral staphyloma

Osteogenesis Imperfecta

Congenital disorder of collagen; sclera is thin and appears blue due to underlying uvea (also found in Ehlers–Danlos syndrome). If patient develops scleral icterus, then the sclera may appear green.

Scleral Icterus

Yellow sclera due to hyperbilirubinemia.

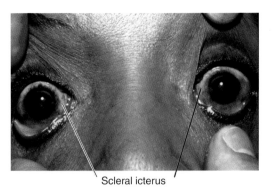

Figure 4-67 • Scleral icterus in patient with jaundice.

Scleral icterus

Senile Scleral Plaque

Blue-gray discoloration of sclera located near horizontal rectus muscle insertions due to hyalinization; occurs in elderly patients.

Figure 4-68 • Senile scleral plaque demonstrating discoloration of sclera near horizontal rectus muscle insertions due to hyalinization.

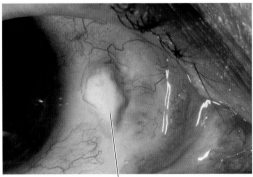

Senile scleral plaque

Symptoms Asymptomatic; may notice scleral discoloration.

Signs Focal or diffuse discoloration of sclera in one or both eyes.

Differential Diagnosis See above; also foreign body, melanoma, mascara, intrascleral nerve loop, adrenochrome deposits (epinephrine), scleromalacia perforans.

Evaluation
- Complete ophthalmic history and eye exam with attention to conjunctiva, sclera, and ophthalmoscopy.
- B-scan ultrasonography and gonioscopy to rule out suspected extension of uveal melanoma.
- Medical consultation for systemic diseases.

Management

- No treatment recommended.
- Treat underlying disorder.

Prognosis Good; discoloration itself is benign.

Trauma	175
Peripheral Ulcerative Keratitis	180
Contact Lens-Related Problems	183
Miscellaneous	189
Corneal Edema	193
Graft Rejection or Failure	194
Infectious Keratitis	196
Interstitial Keratitis	203
Pannus	205
Degenerations	206
Ectasias	211
Congenital Anomalies	214
Dystrophies	218
Metabolic Diseases	225
Deposits	226
Enlarged Corneal Nerves	230
Tumors	231

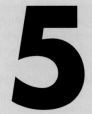

Cornea

Trauma

Abrasion

Corneal epithelial defect usually due to trauma. Patients note pain, foreign body sensation, photophobia, tearing, and red eye. May have normal or decreased visual acuity, conjunctival injection, and an epithelial defect that stains with fluorescein.

- Topical antibiotic drop (polymyxin B sulfate-trimethoprim [Polytrim], moxifloxacin [Vigamox], or tobramycin [Tobrex] qid) or ointment (polymyxin B sulfate-bacitracin [Polysporin] qid).

- Consider topical nonsteroidal antiinflammatory drugs (NSAID) (ketorolac tromethamine [Acular], nepafenac [Nevanac], bromfenac [Xibrom], or diclofenac sodium [Voltaren] tid for 48–72 hours) for pain.

Figure 5-1 • Central corneal abrasion demonstrating fluorescein staining with white light.

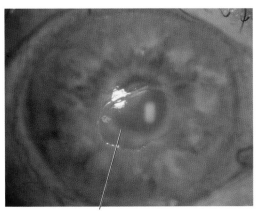

Corneal abrasion with fluorescein staining

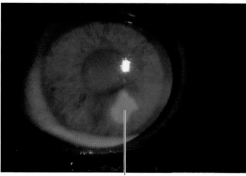

Figure 5-2 • Corneal abrasion demonstrating fluorescein staining with blue light.

Corneal abrasion

- Consider topical cycloplegic (cyclopentolate 1% bid) for pain and photophobia.
- Pressure patch or bandage contact lens if area larger than 10 mm². (Note: do not patch if patient is contact lens wearer, there is corneal infiltrate, or injury caused by plant material, because these scenarios represent high risk for infectious keratitis if patched; no patching necessary if area of abrasion is <10 mm².)

Birth Trauma

Vertical or oblique breaks in Descemet's membrane due to forceps injury at birth. Results in acute corneal edema, scars in Descemet's membrane; associated with astigmatism and amblyopia; may develop corneal decompensation and bullous keratopathy in later life.

- No treatment necessary.
- Consider Descemet's stripping automated endothelial keratoplasty (DSAEK) or penetrating keratoplasty for corneal decompensation.

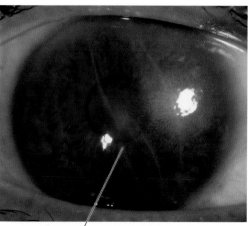

Figure 5-3 • Birth trauma demonstrating vertical scars in the cornea and hazy edema.

Breaks in Descemet's membrane

Figure 5-4 • Same patient as Figure 5-3 demonstrating the corneal scars as seen with sclerotic scatter of the slit-beam light.

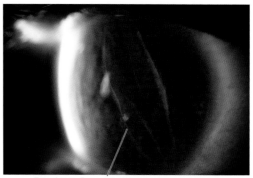

Breaks in Descemet's membrane

Burn

Corneal tissue destruction (epithelium and stroma) due to chemical (acid or base) or thermal (e.g., welding, intense sunlight, tanning lamp) injury; alkali causes most severe injury (penetrates and disrupts lipid membranes) and may cause perforation. Patients note pain, foreign body sensation, photophobia, tearing, and red eye. May have normal or decreased visual acuity, conjunctival injection, ciliary injection, epithelial defects that stain with fluorescein, and scleral or limbal blanching due to ischemia in severe chemical burns. Prognosis variable, worst for severe alkali burns.

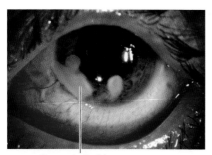

Corneal alkali burn

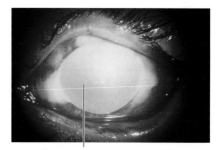

Corneal alkali burn

Figure 5-5 • Alkali burn demonstrating corneal burns and conjunctival injection on the day of the accident.

Figure 5-6 • Complete corneal tissue destruction 7 days after alkali burn.

OPHTHALMIC EMERGENCY

- Immediate copious irrigation with sterile water, saline, or Ringer's solution.
- Measure pH before and after irrigation, continue irrigation until pH is neutralized.
- Remove any chemical particulate matter from surface of eye and evert lids to sweep fornices with sterile cotton swab.

Continued

OPHTHALMIC EMERGENCY—Cont'd

- Topical lubrication with preservative-free artificial tears (see Appendix) up to q1h and ointment (Refresh PM) qhs.
- Topical broad spectrum antibiotic (gatifloxacin [Zymar] or moxifloxacin [Vigamox] qid).
- Topical cycloplegic (cyclopentolate 1%, scopolamine 0.25%, or atropine 1% bid to qid depending on severity).
- For more severe damage, consider topical steroids (prednisolone acetate 1% up to q2h then taper; only use during first week, then if steroids are still necessary, change to medroxyprogesterone [Provera 1%]), topical citrate (10% qid), or sodium ascorbate (10% qid and 2 g po qid), collagenase inhibitor (acetylcysteine [Mucomyst] up to q4h).
- Consider oral doxycycline 100 mg po bid (collagenase inhibitor).
- May require treatment of increased intraocular pressure (see Chapter 11).
- In severe cases, surgery may be required including symblepharon lysis, conjunctival and mucous membrane transplantation, and tarsorrhaphy; consider amniotic membrane or Prokera (Biotissue) for extensive limbal ischemia. Later, consider penetrating keratoplasty or keratoprosthesis.

Foreign Body

Foreign material on or in cornea; usually metal, glass, or organic material; may have associated rust ring if metallic. Patients note pain, foreign body sensation, photophobia, tearing, and red eye; may be asymptomatic if deep and chronic. May have normal or decreased visual acuity, conjunctival injection, ciliary injection, foreign body, rust ring, epithelial defect that stains with fluorescein, corneal edema, anterior chamber cells and flare. Good prognosis unless rust ring or scarring involves visual axis.

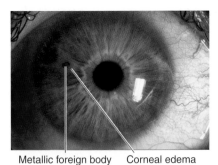

Metallic foreign body   Corneal edema

Figure 5-7 • Metallic foreign body appears as brown spot on cornea.

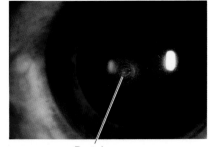

Rust ring

Figure 5-8 • Rust ring from iron foreign body in central cornea.

- Remove foreign material with needle tip or foreign body removal instruments unless it is deep, nonpenetrating, unexposed, and inert material (may be observed).
- Remove rust ring with Alger brush or automated burr.

- Seidel test if deep foreign body to rule out open globe (see below).
- Topical antibiotic (polymyxin B sulfate-trimethoprim [Polytrim], moxifloxacin [Vigamox], or tobramycin [Tobrex] qid).
- Consider topical cycloplegic (cyclopentolate 1% bid) for pain.
- Pressure patch or bandage contact lens as needed (same indications as for corneal abrasion; see above).

Laceration

Partial or full-thickness cut in cornea (see Open Globe section in Chapter 4) due to trauma. Patients note pain, foreign body sensation, photophobia, tearing, and red eye. May have normal or decreased visual acuity, conjunctival injection, ciliary injection, intraocular foreign body, positive Seidel test, corneal edema, breaks or scars in Descemet's membrane, anterior chamber cells and flare, low intraocular pressure. Potentially good prognosis unless laceration crosses visual axis.

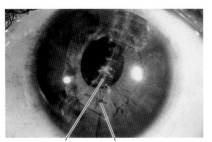

Corneal laceration   Nylon sutures

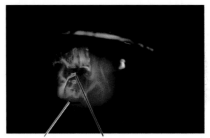

Nylon sutures   Positive Seidel test

Figure 5-9 • Large corneal laceration through visual axis. Note the linear scar from the wound and around the multiple, interrupted, nylon sutures of various lengths used to repair the laceration.

Figure 5-10 • Corneal laceration demonstrating positive Seidel test (bright stream of fluorescein around the central suture).

- **Seidel test (to rule out open globe):** Concentrated fluorescein is used to cover the suspected leakage site by placing a drop of sterile 2% fluorescein in the eye or wetting a sterile fluorescein strip and painting the area of the wound. Slit-lamp examination is then performed looking for a stream of diluted fluorescein emanating from the wound. This will appear as a fluorescent yellow area on a dark blue background with the cobalt blue light, or a light yellow-green area on a dark orange background with the white light.
- Partial thickness lacerations require topical broad spectrum antibiotic (gatifloxacin [Zymar] or moxifloxacin [Vigamox] qid) and cycloplegic (cyclopentolate 1% or scopolamine 0.25% tid).
- Daily follow-up until wound has healed.
- Pressure patch or bandage contact lens as needed for self-sealing or small wounds; if wound gape exists, consider surgical repair.
- Full-thickness lacerations usually require surgical repair (see Open Globe section in Chapter 4).

- Consider orbital radiographs or computed tomography (CT) scan to rule out intraocular foreign body when full-thickness laceration exists; magnetic resonance imaging (MRI) is *contraindicated* if foreign body is metallic.

Recurrent Erosion

Recurrent bouts of pain, foreign body sensation, photophobia, tearing, red eye, and spontaneous corneal epithelial defect usually upon awakening. Associated with anterior basement membrane dystrophy in 50% of cases, or previous traumatic corneal abrasion (usually from fingernail, paper, plant, or brush); also occurs in Meesman's, Reis–Bücklers, lattice, granular, Fuchs', and posterior polymorphous dystrophies.

- Same treatment as for corneal abrasion until reepithelialization occurs, then add hypertonic saline ointment (Adsorbonac or Muro 128 5% qhs for 3 months).
- Topical lubrication with preservative-free artificial tears (see Appendix) up to q1h or Muro 128 drops.
- Consider debridement (manual or with 20% alcohol for 30–40 seconds), diamond burr polishing, bandage contact lens, anterior stromal puncture/reinforcement, Nd:YAG laser reinforcement, superficial keratectomy, or phototherapeutic keratectomy (PTK) for multiple recurrences.
- Consider doxycycline 50 mg po bid for 2 months (matrix metalloproteinase-9 inhibitor) and topical steroid tid for 2–3 weeks (experimental).

Peripheral Ulcerative Keratitis

Definition   Progressive stromal ulceration and thinning of the peripheral cornea with an overlying epithelial defect associated with inflammation.

Etiology   Due to noninfectious systemic or local diseases as well as systemic or local infections.

Marginal Keratolysis

Acute peripheral ulcerative keratitis (PUK) due to an autoimmune or collagen vascular disease (rheumatoid arthritis, systemic lupus erythematosus, polyarteritis nodosa, relapsing polychondritis, and Wegener's granulomatosis).

Mooren's Ulcer

Idiopathic. Two types:

Type I

More common (75%), benign, and unilateral; occurs in older patients; responds to conservative management.

Type II

Progressive and bilateral; occurs in younger patients; more common in African American males; may be associated with coexistent parasitemia.

Staphylococcal Marginal Keratitis

Immune response (hypersensitivity) to *Staphylococcus aureus*; associated with staphylococcal blepharitis, rosacea, phlyctenule, and vascularization.

Symptoms Pain, tearing, photophobia, red eye, and decreased vision; may be asymptomatic.

Signs Normal or decreased visual acuity, conjunctival injection, ciliary injection, corneal thinning, corneal edema, anterior chamber cells and flare, hypopyon; may have corneal infiltrate; may perforate.

Marginal Keratolysis

Acute ulceration with rapid progression, usually in one sector; corneal epithelium absent; melting resolves after healing of overlying epithelium; may have associated scleritis.

Figure 5-11 • Marginal keratolysis due to Wegener's granulomatosis demonstrating peripheral corneal ulceration for 360°.

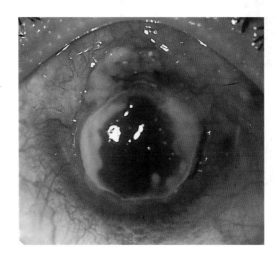

Mooren's Ulcer

Thinning and ulceration that spreads circumferentially and then centrally with undermining of the leading edge; may develop neovascularization.

Figure 5-12 • Mooren's ulcer demonstrating circumferential thinning and ulceration of almost the entire peripheral cornea. The leading edge of the ulcer can be seen as the thin, white, irregular line above the midsection of the iris from the 2 o'clock to 8 o'clock positions (counterclockwise) and then extending to the peripheral cornea. Neovascularization is most evident extending from the limbus at the 8 o'clock position. The inset demonstrates undermining of the ulcer's leading edge seen with a fine slit-beam.

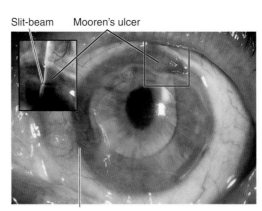

Slit-beam   Mooren's ulcer

Neovascularization

Staphylococcal Marginal Keratitis

Ulceration and white infiltrate(s) 1–2 mm from the limbus with an intervening clear zone; often stains with fluorescein; may progress to a ring ulcer or become superinfected.

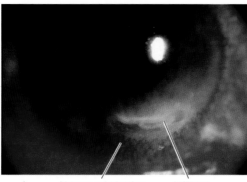

Figure 5-13 • Staphylococcal marginal keratitis demonstrating circumlimbal location of ulceration and infiltrate with intervening clear zone.

Neovascularization   Infiltrate

Differential Diagnosis Infectious ulcer, sterile ulcer (diagnosis of exclusion), Terrien's marginal degeneration, pellucid marginal degeneration.

Evaluation

- Complete ophthalmic history and eye exam with attention to lids, keratometry, cornea, fluorescein staining, anterior chamber, and ophthalmoscopy.
- Consider corneal topography (computerized videokeratography).
- **Lab tests**: Complete blood count (CBC), erythrocyte sedimentation rate (ESR), rheumatoid factor (RF), antinuclear antibody, antineutrophil cytoplasmic antibody (ANCA), blood urea nitrogen (BUN), creatinine, urinalysis (UA); consider hepatitis C antigen (Mooren's ulcer). Consider cultures or smears to rule out infectious etiology.
- Medical or rheumatology consultation for systemic disorders or when treatment with immunosuppressive medications is anticipated.

Management

- Topical lubrication with preservative-free artificial tears (see Appendix) up to q1h and ointment (Refresh PM) qhs.
- Consider topical cycloplegic (cyclopentolate 1% bid) for pain.
- Topical antibiotic (polymyxin B sulfate-trimethoprim [Polytrim] or tobramycin [Tobrex] qid) if epithelial defect exists.
- Consider topical collagenase inhibitor (acetylcysteine [Mucomyst] qd to qid).
- Consider oral doxycycline (50–100 mg po qd).
- Treat underlying medical condition; usually requires oral immunosuppressive agents.

Management—Cont'd

- Consider oral steroids (prednisone 60–100 mg po qd) for significant, progressive thinning; check purified protein derivative (PPD) and controls, blood glucose, and chest radiographs before starting systemic steroids. Topical steroids are controversial for PUK associated with an autoimmune disease.
- Add H_2-blocker (ranitidine [Zantac] 150 mg po bid) or proton pump inhibitor when administering systemic steroids.
- Lid hygiene with warm compresses and lid scrubs for blepharitis.
- Topical steroid (prednisolone acetate 1% or fluorometholone qid, adjust and taper as necessary) and topical antibiotic (polymyxin B sulfate-trimethoprim [Polytrim], moxifloxacin [Vigamox], or tobramycin [Tobrex] qid) for staph marginal keratitis.
- May require lamellar keratectomy with conjunctival resection, tectonic or penetrating keratoplasty if significant thinning exists; should be managed by a cornea or uveitis specialist.
- Consider protective eye wear to prevent perforation.

Prognosis Depends on etiology; poor for marginal keratolysis and Mooren's ulcer.

Contact Lens-Related Problems

Definition A variety of abnormalities induced by contact lenses. Several types of lenses exist, broadly divided into rigid and soft lenses. They are used primarily to correct refractive errors (myopia, hyperopia, astigmatism, and presbyopia), but also can serve as a therapeutic bandage lens for unhealthy corneal surfaces or even for cosmetic use (to apparently change iris color or create a pseudopupil).

Rigid Lenses

Hard

Polymethylmethacrylate (PMMA) lenses impermeable to oxygen; blinking allows tear film to enter the space beneath the lens providing nutrition to the cornea. Used for daily wear with good visual results but can lead to corneal edema and visual blur due to corneal hypoxia.

Figure 5-14 • Hard contact lens. The edge of the lens (arrowheads) as well as the central optical portion (line) are visible.

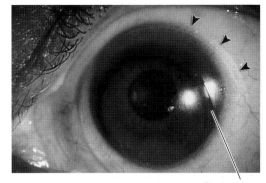

Contact lens

Gas-permeable

Rigid lenses composed of cellulose acetate butyrate, silicone acrylate, or silicone combined with polymethylmethacrylate; high oxygen permeability allows for greater comfort and improved corneal nutrition. Used for daily wear; lens of choice for patients with keratoconus and high astigmatism. Hardest contact lens to adjust to but lowest rate of contact lens related keratitis. Also available as specialized and hybrid lenses (i.e., SynergEyes, Boston [scleral] ocular surface prosthesis).

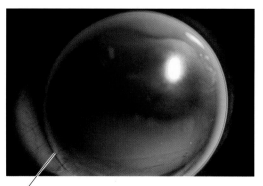

Figure 5-15 • Rigid gas-permeable contact lens demonstrating fluorescein staining pattern.

Contact lens

Soft Lenses

Daily wear

Hydrogel lenses (hydroxymethyl methacrylate); more comfortable and flexible than rigid lenses; conform to corneal surface, therefore poorly correct large degrees of astigmatism; length of time of wear depends on oxygen permeability and water content.

Extended wear

Disposable lenses discarded after extended wear from 1 week to 30 days; higher risk (10–15×) of infectious keratitis with overnight wear (occurs in approximately 1:500).

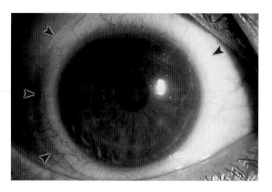

Figure 5-16 • Soft contact lens. Note the edge of the lens overlying the sclera (arrowheads).

Symptoms Foreign body sensation, decreased vision, red eye, tearing, itching, burning, pain, lens awareness, and reduced contact lens wear time.

Signs and Management

Corneal Abrasion

Corneal fluorescein staining due to epithelial defect; contact lens-related etiologies include foreign bodies under lens, damaged lens, poor lens fit, corneal hypoxia, poor lens insertion or removal technique (see Trauma: Corneal Abrasion section above).

- Treat as for traumatic corneal abrasion except do not patch any size abrasion.

Corneal Hypoxia

Acute

Conjunctival injection and epithelial defect (polymethylmethacrylate [PMMA] contact lens).

- Suspend contact lens use.
- Topical antibiotic ointment (polymyxin B sulfate-bacitracin [Polysporin] tid for 3 days).
- When acute hypoxia has resolved, refit with higher Dk/L (oxygen transmissibility) contact lens.

Chronic

Punctate staining, corneal epithelial microcysts, stromal edema, and corneal neovascularization.

- Suspend contact lens use or decrease contact lens wear time.
- Refit with higher Dk/L contact lens.

Contact Lens-Related Dendritic Keratitis

Conjunctivitis, pseudodendritic lesions.

- Suspend contact lens use.

Contact Lens Solution Hypersensitivity or Toxicity

Conjunctival injection, diffuse corneal punctate staining or erosion; occurs with solutions that contain preservatives (e.g., thimerosal).

- Suspend contact lens use.
- Identify and discontinue toxic source; thoroughly clean, rinse, and disinfect contact lenses; reinstruct patient in proper contact lens care or change system of care; replace soft contact lenses or polish rigid contact lens.
- Topical antibiotic ointment (erythromycin or bacitracin tid for 3 days); do not patch.

Corneal Neovascularization

Superficial or deep vascular ingrowth due to chronic hypoxia. Superior corneal pannus 1–2 mm in soft contact lens wearers is common and benign; larger than 2 mm is serious; deep vessels may cause stromal hemorrhage, lipid deposits, and scarring.

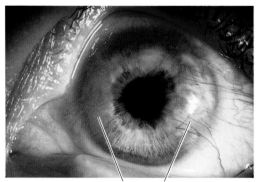

Figure 5-17 • Contact lens-induced corneal neovascularization and scarring.

Corneal neovascularization

- If neovascularization larger than 2 mm, suspend contact lens use and refit with higher Dk/L contact lens.
- Consider topical steroid (prednisolone acetate 1% qid) to cause regression.
- Consider argon laser photocoagulation of large or deep vessels to prevent stromal hemorrhage or rebleed.

Corneal Warpage

Change in corneal shape (regular and irregular astigmatism) not associated with corneal edema; related to lens material (hard > rigid gas-permeable contact lens [RGP] > soft), fit, and length of time of wear. Usually asymptomatic, but some patients may notice poorer vision with glasses or contact lens intolerance; may have loss of best spectacle-corrected visual acuity or change in refraction (especially axis of astigmatism); hallmark is abnormal corneal topography (computerized videokeratography), which shows irregular astigmatism and may mimic keratoconus (pseudokeratoconus).

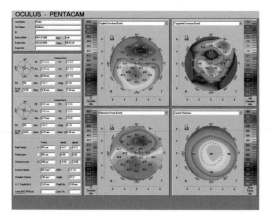

Figure 5-18 • Pentacam image demonstrating corneal topography and thickness maps of patient with contact lens induced corneal warpage. Note the irregular astigmatism in the top maps with inferior steepening similar to keratoconus. The lower right map shows normal corneal thickness without thinning inferiorly.

- Suspend contact lens use.
- Periodic evaluations with refraction and corneal topography until stabilization occurs.

Damaged Contact Lens

Pain with lens insertion and prompt relief with removal; look for chips in rigid lenses and fissures or tears in soft lenses.

- Replace defective contact lens.

Deposits on Contact Lens

Significant contact lens deposits (film or bumps), conjunctival injection, corneal erosion, excess contact lens movement, giant papillary conjunctivitis; old contact lens.

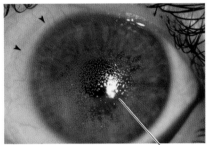

Deposits on contact lens

Figure 5-19 • Calcium phosphate deposits on soft contact lens.

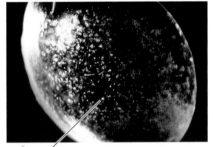

Deposits on contact lens

Figure 5-20 • Lipid deposits on contact lens.

- Reinstruct patient in proper contact lens care; institute regular enzyme cleaning (soft contact lens or RGP), frequent replacement schedule, or use of disposable contact lenses; polish rigid contact lens.

Giant Papillary Conjunctivitis

Due to contact lens protein deposits, conjunctival contact lens-related mechanical irritation, or soft contact lens material sensitivity reaction. Signs include large upper lid tarsal conjunctival papillae (>0.33 mm), ropy mucous discharge, contact lens coating, and possible contact lens decentration secondary to papillae; also caused by exposed suture or ocular prosthesis (see Giant Papillary Conjunctivitis in Chapter 4).

- **Mild:** Replace contact lenses and reinstruct patient in proper contact lens care; decrease contact lens wear time; increase frequency of enzyme cleanings; change to frequent or disposable contact lenses, or change lens material from soft contact lens to RGP; topical lodoxamide tromethamine 0.1% (Alomide qid) or cromolyn sodium 4% (Crolom qid).
- **Severe:** Suspend contact lens use; short course of topical steroid (prednisolone acetate 1% or fluorometholone qid).

Infectious Keratitis

Pain, red eye, infiltrate with epithelial defect, and anterior chamber cells and flare. All contact lens-related corneal infiltrates should be treated as an infection, suspect Pseudomonas or Acanthamoeba. Occurs more often in extended wear and soft contact lens wearers (see Infectious Keratitis section below); fungal infections are more common in warmer climates.

- Suspend contact lens use.
- **Lab tests**: Cultures of cornea, contact lenses, solutions, and contact lens cases.
- Topical broad spectrum antibiotic (fluoroquinolone [Vigamox, Iquix, or Zymar] or a fortified antibiotic q1h); be alert for Pseudomonas and Acanthamoeba.
- Never patch an infiltrate or epithelial defect in a contact lens wearer.

Sterile Corneal Infiltrates

Small (1 mm), peripheral, often multifocal, white, nummular, corneal lesions; corneal epithelium usually intact; diagnosis of exclusion.

- Suspend contact lens use.
- Use preservative-free solutions.
- Must treat as an infection (see above).

Poor Fit (Loose)

Upper eyelid irritation, limbal injection, excess contact lens movement with blinking, poor contact lens centration, lens edge bubbles, lens edge stand-off, variable keratometry mires with blinking, and lower portion of retinoscopy reflex darker and faster.

- Increase sagittal vault; choose steeper base curve or larger diameter contact lens.

Poor Fit (Tight)

Injection or indentation around limbus, minimal contact lens movement with blinking, blurred retinoscopic reflex, corneal edema, and distorted keratometry mires that clear with blinking.

- Decrease sagittal vault; choose flatter base curve or smaller diameter contact lens.

Superior Limbic Keratoconjunctivitis

Due to contact lens hypersensitivity reaction or poor contact lens fit. Signs include upper tarsal micropapillae, superior limbal injection, fluorescein staining of superior bulbar conjunctiva, and 12 o'clock micropannus (see Superior Limbic Keratoconjunctivitis in Chapter 4).

- Suspend contact lens use; replace or clean contact lenses; use preservative-free contact lens solutions (no thimerosal).
- For persistent cases, consider topical steroid (prednisolone acetate 1% or fluorometholone qid) or silver nitrate 0.5–1.0% solution.

Superficial Punctate Keratitis

Punctate fluorescein staining of corneal surface due to poor lens fit, dry eye, or contact lens solution reaction (see Superficial Punctate Keratitis section below).

- Suspend contact lens use.
- Topical lubrication with artificial tears (see Appendix) up to q1h.
- Consider topical broad spectrum antibiotic (polymyxin B sulfate-trimethoprim [Polytrim], moxifloxacin [Vigamox], or tobramycin [Tobrex] qid) if severe.
- Refit contact lens.
- Consider punctal plugs for dry eyes.

Evaluation
- Complete ophthalmic history with attention to contact lens wear and care habits.
- Complete eye exam with attention to contact lens fit, contact lens surface, everting upper lids, conjunctiva, keratometry, and cornea.
- Consider corneal topography (computerized videokeratography).
- Consider dry eye evaluation: tear meniscus, tear break-up time, lissamine green or rose bengal staining, and Schirmer's testing (see Chapter 4).
- **Lab tests**: Cultures or smears of cornea, contact lens, contact lens case, and contact lens solutions if infiltrate exists to rule out infection.

Prognosis Usually good except for severe or central corneal infections.

Miscellaneous

Definitions

Delle

Area of corneal thinning secondary to corneal drying from an adjacent area of tissue elevation. Appears as a focal excavation with overlying pooling of fluorescein dye; usually occurs near pterygium or filtering bleb.

Figure 5-21 • Delle appears as a depression or thinning of the cornea nasally.

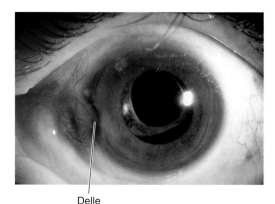

Delle

Exposure Keratopathy

Drying of the cornea with subsequent epithelial breakdown; due to neurotrophic (cranial nerve V palsy, cerebrovascular accident, aneurysm, multiple sclerosis, tumor, herpes simplex, herpes zoster), neuroparalytic (cranial nerve VII palsy), lid malposition, nocturnal lagophthalmos, or any cause of proptosis with lagophthalmos; sequelae include filamentary keratitis, corneal ulceration and scarring.

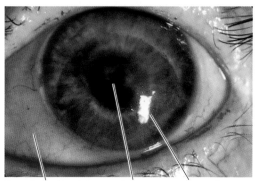

Figure 5-22 • Exposure keratopathy with interpalpebral rose bengal staining, a neurotrophic ulcer in the central cornea, and an irregular light reflex on the cornea.

Rose bengal staining   Ulcer   Irregular reflex

Filamentary Keratitis

Strands of mucus and desquamated epithelial cells adherent to corneal epithelium due to many conditions including any cause of dry eye, patching, recurrent erosion, bullous keratopathy, superior limbic keratoconjunctivitis, herpes simplex, medicamentosa, or ptosis; blinking causes pain as filaments pull on intact epithelium.

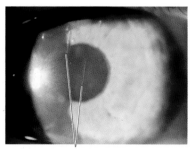

Corneal filament

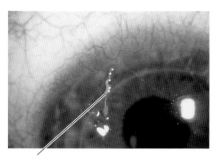

Corneal filament

Figure 5-23 • Filamentary keratitis demonstrating filaments, which appear as thin vertical strands adherent to the cornea.

Figure 5-24 • Corneal filament visible as an opaque strand attached to the superior cornea.

Keratic Precipitates

Fine, medium, or large deposits of inflammatory cells on the corneal endothelium due to a prior episode of inflammation. Usually round white spots, but can be translucent or pigmented; may have mutton fat (in granulomatous uveitis) or stellate (in Fuchs' heterochromic iridocyclitis) appearance; often melt or disappear or become pigmented with time.

Figure 5-25 • White, mutton fat, granulomatous, keratic precipitates on the central and inferior corneal endothelium in a patient with toxoplasmosis.

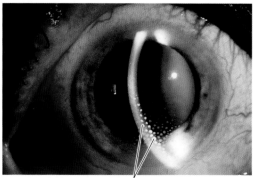

Keratic precipitates

Superficial Punctate Keratitis

Nonspecific, pinpoint, epithelial defects; punctate staining with fluorescein. Associated with blepharitis, any cause of dry eye, trauma, foreign body, trichiasis, ultraviolet or chemical burn, medicamentosa, contact lens-related, exposure, and conjunctivitis.

Figure 5-26 • Superficial punctate keratitis demonstrating diffuse epithelial staining of the central cornea with fluorescein.

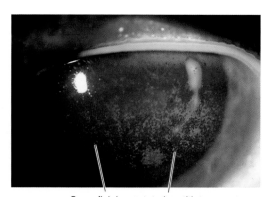

Superficial punctate keratitis

Thygeson's Superficial Punctate Keratitis

Bilateral, recurrent, gray-white, slightly elevated epithelial lesions (similar to early subepithelial infiltrates in adenoviral keratoconjunctivitis) in a white and quiet eye; minimal or no staining with fluorescein. Unknown etiology, possibly viral; usually occurs in second to third decade.

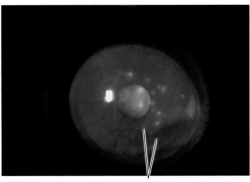

Figure 5-27 • Thygeson's superficial punctate keratitis demonstrating multiple, white, stellate, corneal opacities with cobalt blue light.

Thygeson's superficial punctate keratitis

Symptoms Asymptomatic; may have dryness, foreign body sensation, discharge, tearing, photophobia, red eye, and decreased vision.

Signs Normal or decreased visual acuity; may have lagophthalmos, conjunctival injection, decreased corneal sensation, corneal staining, superficial punctate keratitis (inferiorly or in a central band in exposure keratopathy), filaments (stain with fluorescein), subepithelial infiltrates, keratic precipitates, anterior chamber cells, and flare.

Differential Diagnosis See above.

Evaluation
• Complete ophthalmic history and eye exam with attention to lids, conjunctiva, cornea, anterior chamber, and cranial nerve testing.

Management

• Topical lubrication with preservative-free artificial tears (see Appendix) up to q1h and ointment (Refresh PM) qhs.

• Topical antibiotic ointment (erythromycin, Polysporin, or bacitracin tid) for moderate superficial punctate keratitis and exposure keratitis; consider cycloplegic (cyclopentolate 1% or scopolamine 0.25% bid) and pressure patch (except in contact lens wearer) if severe.

• Consider punctal occlusion, lid taping at bedtime, moisture chamber goggles, bandage contact lens, or tarsorrhaphy for moderate-to-severe dry eye symptoms and exposure keratopathy.

• Clean, change, or discontinue contact lens use.

• Debridement of filaments with sterile cotton-tipped applicator; consider collagenase inhibitor (acetylcysteine 10% [Mucomyst] qd to qid) or bandage contact lens for prolonged episodes of filamentary keratitis.

• Topical mild steroid (fluorometholone qid for 1–2 weeks then taper slowly) for Thygeson's superficial punctate keratitis.

• Consider bandage contact lens for comfort.

Prognosis Usually good.

Corneal Edema

Definition Focal or diffuse hydration and swelling of the corneal stroma (stromal edema due to endothelial dysfunction) or epithelium (intercellular or microcystic edema due to increased intraocular pressure or epithelial hypoxia).

Etiology Inflammation, infection, Fuchs' dystrophy, posterior polymorphous dystrophy, congenital hereditary endothelial dystrophy, hydrops (keratoconus or pellucid marginal degeneration), acute angle-closure glaucoma, congenital glaucoma, previous ocular surgery (aphakic or pseudophakic bullous keratopathy or graft failure), contact lens overwear, hypotony, trauma, postoperative, iridocorneal endothelial syndrome, Brown–McLean syndrome (peripheral edema in aphakic patients possibly from endothelial contact with floppy iris), anterior segment ischemia.

Symptoms Asymptomatic; may have photophobia, foreign body sensation, tearing, pain, halos around lights, decreased vision.

Signs Normal or decreased visual acuity, poor corneal light reflex, thickened cornea, epithelial microcysts and bullae, nonhealing epithelial defects, superficial punctate keratitis, stromal haze, Descemet's folds, guttata, anterior chamber cells and flare, decreased or increased intraocular pressure, iridocorneal touch, aphakia, pseudophakia, vitreous in anterior chamber.

Figure 5-28 • Pseudophakic bullous keratopathy demonstrating corneal edema with central corneal folds, hazy stroma, and distorted light reflex.

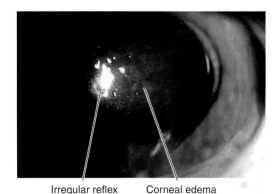

Irregular reflex   Corneal edema

Differential Diagnosis Interstitial keratitis, corneal scar, Salzmann's nodular degeneration, crocodile shagreen, band keratopathy, anterior basement membrane dystrophy, Meesman dystrophy.

Evaluation
- Complete ophthalmic history and eye exam with attention to visual acuity, cornea, tonometry, anterior chamber, gonioscopy, and iris.
- Check pachymetry
- Consider specular or confocal microscopy.

Management

- Symptomatic relief with hypertonic saline ointment (Adsorbonac or Muro 128 5% tid); consider topical steroid (prednisolone acetate 1% up to qid) and cycloplegic (scopolamine 0.25% bid to qid).
- Topical broad spectrum antibiotic (polymyxin B sulfate-trimethoprim [Polytrim], moxifloxacin [Vigamox], or tobramycin [Tobrex] qid) for epithelial defects; consider bandage contact lens or tarsorrhaphy for persistent epithelial defects.
- Treat underlying cause (e.g., penetrating keratoplasty or DSAEK for aphakic or pseudophakic bullous keratopathy, Fuchs' dystrophy, and congenital hereditary endothelial dystrophy; intraocular pressure control and iridotomy for angle-closure glaucoma; observation and symptomatic relief for acute hydrops and birth trauma).

Prognosis Depends on etiology.

Graft Rejection or Failure

Definition

Graft Rejection

Allograft rejection is an immune response that may occur early or late after corneal transplant surgery. Epithelial rejection is rare but occurs early, stromal rejection may appear with subepithelial infiltrates, and endothelial rejection usually does not occur before 2 weeks after transplantation.

Graft Failure

Corneal edema and opacification due to primary donor failure (graft does not clear within 6 weeks after surgery), allograft rejection, recurrence of disease, glaucoma, or neovascularization.

Symptoms Pain, photophobia, red eye, and decreased vision.

Signs Decreased visual acuity, conjunctival injection, ciliary injection, corneal edema, vascularization, subepithelial infiltrates, epithelial rejection line, endothelial rejection line (Khodadoust line), keratic precipitates, anterior chamber cells and flare; may have increased intraocular pressure.

Differential Diagnosis Endophthalmitis, herpes simplex virus (HSV) keratitis, adenoviral keratoconjunctivitis, anterior uveitis, anterior segment ischemia.

Evaluation

- Complete ophthalmic history and eye exam with attention to visual acuity, conjunctiva, cornea, suture integrity, tonometry, and anterior chamber.
- Consider pachymetry.

Figure 5-29 • Clear corneal graft with running and interrupted sutures. The edge of the graft is visible as a faint white scar between the suture bites.

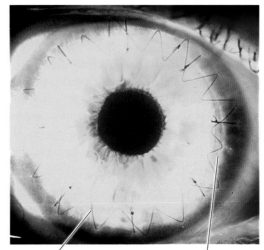

Running suture   Graft interface

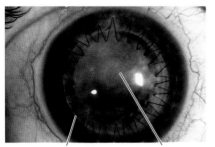

Running suture   Graft failure

Figure 5-30 • Graft failure with opaque central cornea. Note the running suture and the edge of the graft (white line under suture).

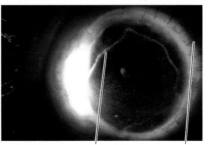

Rejection line   Sutures

Figure 5-31 • Graft failure with rejection line and keratic precipitates.

Management

- Topical steroid (prednisolone acetate 1% up to q1h initially, taper slowly) and cycloplegic (cyclopentolate 1% or scopolamine 0.25% tid).

- Consider oral steroids (prednisone 60–80 mg po qd initially, then taper rapidly over 5–7 days) or sub-Tenon's steroid injection (triamcinolone acetonide 40 mg/mL); check PPD and controls, blood glucose, and chest radiographs before starting systemic steroids.

- Add H_2-blocker (ranitidine [Zantac] 150 mg po bid) or proton pump inhibitor when administering systemic steroids.

Continued

Management—Cont'd

- Topical cyclosporine is controversial.
- Treat recurrent HSV keratitis if this is the inciting event with systemic antiviral (acyclovir 400 mg po tid for 10–21 days, then bid for 12–18 months).
- May require treatment of increased intraocular pressure (see Chapter 11).

Prognosis Thirty percent of patients have rejection episodes within 1 year after surgery. Often good if treated early and aggressively; poorer for a penetrating keratoplasty secondary to prior graft failure, HSV keratitis, acute corneal ulcer, chemical burn, and eyes with other ocular disease (dry eye disease, exposure keratopathy, ocular cicatricial pemphigoid, Stevens–Johnson syndrome, uveitis, and glaucoma); better for a penetrating keratoplasty secondary to corneal edema (aphakic or pseudophakic bullous keratopathy, Fuchs' dystrophy), keratoconus, corneal scar or opacity, and dystrophy.

Infectious Keratitis (Corneal Ulcer)

Definition Destruction of corneal tissue (epithelium and stroma) due to inflammation from an infectious organism. Risk factors include contact lens wear, trauma, dry eye, exposure keratopathy, bullous keratopathy, neurotrophic cornea, and lid abnormalities.

Etiology

Bacterial

Most common infectious source; usually due to *Pseudomonas aeruginosa, Staphylococcus aureus, Staphylococcus epidermidis, Streptococcus pneumoniae, Haemophilus influenzae, Moraxella catarrhalis*; beware of *Neisseria* species, *Corynebacterium diphtheriae, Haemophilus aegyptius*, and *Listeria* because they can penetrate intact epithelium. *Streptococcus viridans* causes crystalline keratopathy (central branching cracked glass appearance without epithelial defect; associated with chronic topical steroid use).

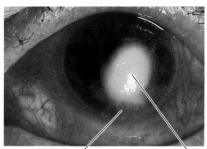

Neovascularization   Corneal ulcer

Figure 5-32 • Bacterial keratitis demonstrating large, central, *Streptococcus pneumoniae* corneal ulcer. Note the dense, white, corneal infiltrate and the extreme conjunctival injection.

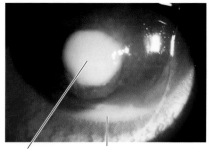

Corneal ulcer   Hypopyon

Figure 5-33 • Bacterial keratitis demonstrating *Pseudomonas aeruginosa* corneal ulcer with surrounding corneal edema and hypopyon.

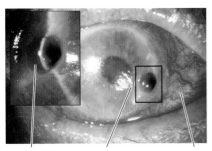

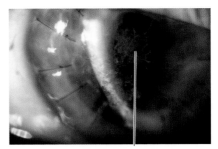

Iris plug   Corneal ulcer   Conjunctival injection

Crystalline keratopathy

Figure 5-34 • Perforated corneal ulcer. The cornea is opaque, scarred, and vascularized, and there is a paracentral perforation with iris plugging the wound. Inset shows slit-beam over iris plugging perforated wound.

Figure 5-35 • Crystalline keratopathy due to *Streptococcus viridans* demonstrating white branching opacities.

Fungal

Usually *Aspergillus, Candida,* or *Fusarium* species. Often have satellite infiltrates, feathery edges, endothelial plaques; can penetrate Descemet's membrane. Associated with trauma, especially involving vegetable matter.

Figure 5-36 • Fungal keratitis demonstrating a central corneal infiltrate with feathery borders, severe conjunctival injection, and a small hypopyon.

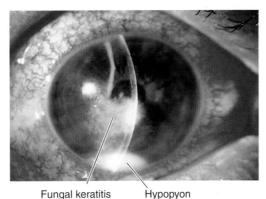

Fungal keratitis   Hypopyon

Parasitic

Acanthamoeba

Resembles HSV epithelial keratitis early, perineural and ring infiltrates later; usually occurs in contact lens wearers who use nonsterile water or have poor contact lens cleaning habits. Patients usually have pain out of proportion to signs.

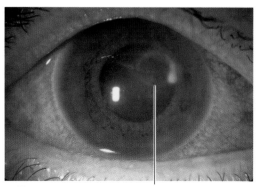

Figure 5-37 • *Acanthamoeba* keratitis demonstrating the characteristic ring infiltrate.

Acanthamoeba ring infiltrate

Microsporidia

Causes diffuse epithelial keratitis with small, white, intraepithelial infiltrates (organisms); occurs in patients with acquired immunodeficiency syndrome (AIDS).

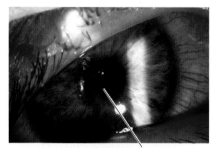

Microsporidia keratitis

Figure 5-38 • *Microsporidia* keratitis demonstrating diffuse, whitish epithelial keratitis.

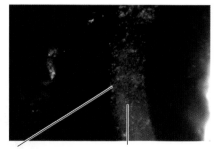

Microsporidia keratitis   Intraepithelial infiltrate

Figure 5-39 • Same patient as Figure 5-38 demonstrating the intraepithelial infiltrates of *Microsporidia* keratitis.

Viral

Herpes simplex virus

Recurrent HSV is the most common cause of central infectious keratitis. Associated with sun exposure, fever, stress, menses, trauma, illness, and immunosuppression. Recurrence rate = 25% during first year, 50% during second year. Various types of HSV keratitis exist:

Epithelial Keratitis Can appear as a superficial punctate keratitis, dendrite (ulcerated, classically with terminal bulbs), or geographic ulcer; associated with scarring and decreased corneal sensation (neurotrophic cornea).

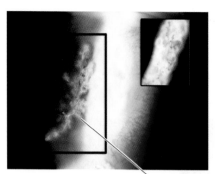

Herpes simplex virus dendrite

Figure 5-40 • Herpes simplex epithelial keratitis demonstrating dendrite with terminal bulbs. Inset shows staining of dendrite with rose bengal.

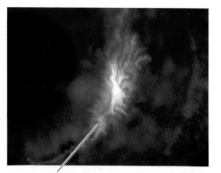

Herpes simplex virus dendrite

Figure 5-41 • Same patient as Figure 5-40 demonstrating staining of herpes simplex virus dendrite with fluorescein.

Disciform Keratitis Self-limited (2–6 months), cell-mediated, immune reaction with focal disc-like area of stromal edema, folds, fine keratic precipitates, and scarring.

Figure 5-42 • Herpes simplex disciform keratitis demonstrating central round area of hazy edema.

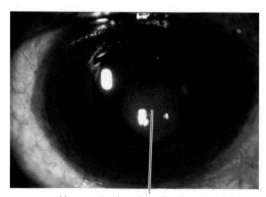

Herpes simplex virus disciform keratitis

Necrotizing Interstitial Keratitis Antigen-antibody-complement mediated immune reaction with dense stromal inflammation, ulceration, and severe iritis.
Endotheliitis Keratouveitis with corneal edema, keratic precipitates, increased intraocular pressure, anterior chamber cells and flare.

Metaherpetic or Trophic Ulcer Noninfectious, nonhealing epithelial defect with heaped-up gray edges due to HSV basement membrane disease with possible neurotrophic component.

Herpes zoster virus

Ocular involvement and complications of herpes zoster ophthalmicus (HZO; see Chapter 3) are due to infection, inflammation, immune response, and scarring; may be acute, chronic, or recurrent, and can be sight threatening. In addition to keratitis (65%), there may be lid changes, conjunctivitis, episcleritis, scleritis, uveitis, retinitis, optic neuritis, vasculitis (iris atrophy, orbital apex syndrome), and cranial nerve (III, IV, or IV) palsies; patients may also develop glaucoma and cataracts. Various types of HSV keratitis exist:

Epithelial Keratitis Can appear as a superficial punctate keratitis (early) or pseudodendrites (early or late; coarser, heaped-up epithelial plaques without terminal bulbs); virus may persist on corneal surface for 1 month.

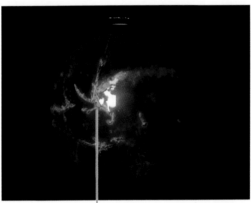

Figure 5-43 • Herpes zoster ophthalmicus demonstrating fluorescein staining of coarse pseudodendrites with heaped-up epithelium and no terminal bulbs.

Herpes zoster virus pseudodendrite

Stromal Keratitis Can be anterior stromal infiltrates or disciform or peripheral edema (late) that may become chronic and cause vascularization, scarring, ulceration, and lipid keratopathy.

Endotheliitis Viral infection or immune response that causes a keratouveitis with focal stromal edema, keratic precipitates, anterior chamber cells and flare; chronic corneal edema occurs with extensive endothelial damage.

Mucus Plaque Keratopathy Mucus plaques months or years later; vary in size, shape, and location daily; associated with decreased corneal sensation, stromal keratitis, anterior segment inflammation, increased intraocular pressure, and cataracts.

Interstitial Keratitis Corneal vascularization and scarring (see Interstitial Keratitis section below).

Neurotrophic Keratopathy Decreased corneal sensation due to nerve damage; often improves spontaneously, but if not poor blink response and tear dysfunction can cause epithelial breakdown with infections, ulceration, and perforation.

Exposure Keratopathy Due to lid scarring, lagophthalmos, and neurotrophic cornea; may develop severe dry eye with ulceration and scarring (see Exposure Keratopathy section above).

Symptoms Pain, discharge, tearing, photophobia, red eye, decreased vision; may notice white spot on cornea.

Signs Normal or decreased visual acuity, conjunctival injection, ciliary injection, white corneal infiltrate with overlying epithelial defect that stains with fluorescein, satellite lesions (fungal), corneal edema, Descemet's folds, dendrite (HSV), pseudodendrite (HZV), cutaneous herpes vesicles, perineural and ring infiltrates *(Acanthamoeba)*, corneal thinning, descemetocele, anterior chamber cells and flare, hypopyon, mucopurulent discharge; may have scleritis, increased intraocular pressure, iris atrophy, cataracts, retinitis, optic neuritis, or cranial nerve palsy.

Differential Diagnosis Sterile ulcer, shield ulcer (vernal keratoconjunctivitis), staphylococcal marginal keratitis, epidemic keratoconjunctivitis subepithelial infiltrates, ocular rosacea, marginal keratolysis, Mooren's ulcer, Terrien's marginal degeneration, corneal abrasion, recurrent erosion, stromal scar, Thygeson's superficial punctate keratitis, anesthetic abuse (nonhealing epithelial defect usually with ragged edges and "sick"-appearing surrounding epithelium with or without haze or an infiltrate), tyrosinemia (pseudodendrite).

Evaluation

- Complete ophthalmic history with attention to trauma and contact lens use and care regimen.
- Complete eye exam with attention to visual acuity, lids, sclera, cornea (sensation, size and depth of ulcer, character of infiltrate, fluorescein and rose bengal staining, amount of thinning), tonometry, and anterior chamber.
- **Lab tests**: Scrape corneal ulcer with sterile spatula or blade and smear on microbiology slides; send for routine cultures (bacteria), Sabouraud's media (fungi), chocolate agar (*H. influenzae, Neisseria gonorrhoeae*), Gram stain (bacteria), Giemsa stain (fungi, *Acanthamoeba*); consider calcofluor white (*Acanthamoeba*) and acid fast (*Mycobacteria*) if these entities are suspected.
- Consider biopsy for progressive disease, culture-negative ulcer, or deep abscess (usually fungal, *Acanthamoeba*, crystalline keratopathy).
- Consider confocal microscopy to identify fungal hyphae and *Acanthamoeba* cysts.

Management

- Suspend contact lens use.
- May require treatment of increased intraocular pressure (see Chapter 11), especially HZV.
- Never patch a corneal ulcer.
- Ulcers require daily follow-up initially, and severe ones require hospital admission.
- If organism is in doubt, treat as a bacterial ulcer until culture results return.
- Consider autologous serum drops, punctal occlusion, bandage contact lens, or surgery (temporary or permanent tarsorrhaphy, amniotic membrane graft, partial or complete conjunctival flap) to heal persistent epithelial defects due to exposure or neurotrophic keratopathy.
- May require cyanoacrylate glue and contact lens to seal a small perforation (≤1.5 mm) or patch graft for a larger perforation.
- May eventually require PTK, lamellar or penetrating keratoplasty for central scarring; consider keratoprosthesis for failed grafts in HZV.

Continued

Management—Cont'd

BACTERIAL

- **Small ulcers (<2 mm)**: topical broad spectrum antibiotic (gatifloxacin [Zymar], levofloxacin [Iquix], or moxifloxacin [Vigamox] q1h initially, then taper slowly).
- **Larger ulcers**: topical broad spectrum fortified antibiotics (tobramycin 13.6 mg/mL and cefazolin 50 mg/mL or vancomycin 50 mg/mL [in patients allergic to penicillin and cephalosporin] alternating q1h [which means taking a drop every 30 minutes] for 24–72 hours, then taper slowly); consider subconjunctival antibiotic injections in noncompliant patients.
- Adjust antibiotics based on culture and Gram stain results.
- Topical cycloplegic (scopolamine 0.25% or atropine 1% bid to qid).
- Topical steroid (prednisolone acetate 1% dosed at lower frequency than topical antibiotics) should be avoided until improvement is noted (usually after 48–72 hours).
- Systemic antibiotics for corneal perforation or scleral involvement.

FUNGAL

- Topical antifungal (natamycin 50 mg/mL q1h, amphotericin B 1.0–2.5 mg/mL q1h, miconazole 10 mg/mL q1h, or voriconazole 1% for 24–72 hours, then taper slowly).
- For severe infection, add systemic antifungal (ketoconazole 200–400 mg po qd or amphotericin B 1 mg/kg IV over 6 hours).
- Topical cycloplegic (scopolamine 0.25% or atropine 1% bid to qid).
- Topical steroids are *contraindicated*.

PARASITIC

- *Acanthamoeba*: topical agents (combination of propamidine isethionate [Brolene] 0.1% or hexamidine 0.1%, and miconazole 1% or clotrimazole 1%, and polyhexamethylene biguanide [Baquacil] 0.02% or chlorhexidine 0.02%, q1h for 1 week, then taper very slowly over 2–3 months), topical broad spectrum antibiotic (neomycin or paromomycin q2h), and oral antifungal (ketoconazole 200 mg or itraconazole 100 mg po bid).
- Topical steroids are controversial, consider for severe necrotizing keratitis (prednisolone phosphate 1% qid).
- Topical cycloplegic (scopolamine 0.25% or atropine 1% bid to qid).
- Consider repeated epithelial debridement to reduce antigen load and improve penetration of medication.
- *Microsporidia*: topical fumagillin up to q2h initially, then taper slowly.

VIRAL

- **HSV Epithelial Keratitis**: topical antiviral (trifluridine [Viroptic] 9 times/day for 5–7 days, then 5 times/day for another 1–2 weeks or vidarabine monohydrate [Vira-A] 5 times/day for 10–14 days); alternatively, consider oral antiviral (acyclovir [Zovirax]

Management—Cont'd

400 mg po tid, or famciclovir [Famvir] 250 mg po or valacyclovir [Valtrex] 500 mg po bid for 14–21 days), débride dendrite.

- **HSV Disciform Keratitis or Endotheliitis**: topical steroid (prednisolone phosphate 0.12–1.0% qd to qid depending on severity of inflammation, adjust and then taper slowly over months depending on response); consider cycloplegic (scopolamine 0.25% bid to qid); add topical antiviral (trifluridine [Viroptic] qid) if epithelium is involved or prophylactically when using steroid doses greater than prednisolone phosphate 0.12% bid (alternatively, can use acyclovir 400 mg po bid).

- **HSV Metaherpetic or Trophic Ulcer**: topical lubrication with preservative-free artificial tears (see Appendix) up to q1h and ointment (Refresh PM) qhs; topical broad spectrum antibiotic (gatifloxacin [Zymar], moxifloxacin [Vigamox], polymyxin B sulfate-trimethoprim [Polytrim], or tobramycin [Tobrex] qid), bandage contact lens; mild topical steroid (fluorometholone qd to bid) if stromal inflammation exists.

- Long-term suppressive therapy with acyclovir ([Zovirax] 400 mg po bid) for 1 year with 6-month additional follow-up reduces the incidence of recurrent keratitis by almost 50% (Herpetic Eye Disease Study conclusion). Alternatively, may use famciclovir ([Famvir] 250 mg po qd) or valacyclovir ([Valtrex] 500 mg po qd).

- **HZV**: systemic antiviral (acyclovir [Zovirax] 800 mg po 5 times a day for 7–10 days, or famciclovir [Famvir] 500 mg po or valacyclovir [Valtrex] 1 g po tid for 7 days) for acute HZO should be started within 72 hours of the rash; topical antibiotic ointment (erythromycin or bacitracin tid) for conjunctival or corneal epithelial involvement; topical steroid (prednisolone acetate 1% qid to q4h, then taper slowly over months) and cycloplegic (scopolamine 0.25% bid to qid) for stromal keratitis or iritis, some patients may require low dose topical steroid indefinitely to prevent recurrence. May require treatment of increased intraocular pressure (see Chapter 11; do not use miotic agents or prostaglandin analogues), eyelid abnormalities (see Chapter 3), or postherpetic neuralgia (see Chapter 3).

- **HZV Mucus Plaque Keratitis**: debridement of plaques, topical steroid and collagenase inhibitor (acetylcysteine 10% [Mucomyst] qd to qid); consider topical or systemic antiviral.

Prognosis Depends on organism, size, location, and response to treatment; sequelae may range from a small corneal scar without alteration of vision to corneal perforation requiring emergent grafting. Poor for fungal, *Acanthamoeba*, and chronic herpes zoster keratitis; herpes simplex and *Acanthamoeba* commonly recur in corneal graft. Neurotrophic corneas are at risk for melts and perforation.

Interstitial Keratitis

Definition Diffuse or sectoral vascularization and scarring of the corneal stroma due to nonnecrotizing inflammation and edema; may be acute or chronic.

Etiology Most commonly congenital syphilis (90% of cases), tuberculosis, and herpes simplex; also herpes zoster, leprosy, onchocerciasis, mumps, lymphogranuloma venereum, sarcoidosis, and Cogan's syndrome (triad of interstitial keratitis, vertigo, and deafness).

Symptoms

Acute

Decreased vision, pain, photophobia, red eye.

Chronic

Usually asymptomatic.

Signs Normal or decreased visual acuity.

Acute

Conjunctival injection, salmon patch (stromal vascularization), stromal edema, anterior chamber cells and flare, keratic precipitates.

Chronic

Deep corneal haze, scarring, thinning, vascularization, ghost vessels; may have other stigmata of congenital syphilis (optic nerve atrophy, salt-and-pepper fundus, deafness, notched teeth, saddle nose, sabre shins).

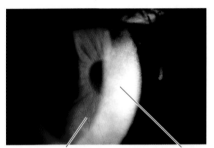

Figure 5-44 • Interstitial keratitis demonstrating diffuse stromal scarring of the central cornea and extensive corneal neovascularization.

Stromal neovascularization Central scarring

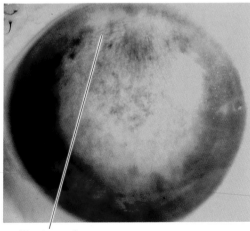

Figure 5-45 • Interstitial keratitis demonstrating ghost vessels that appear as clear, linear, branching lines within the dense, white, corneal scarring.

Ghost vessels

Evaluation

- Complete ophthalmic history and eye exam with attention to lids, conjunctiva, cornea, anterior chamber, and ophthalmoscopy.
- **Lab tests**: Venereal Disease Research Laboratory (VDRL) test, fluorescent treponemal antibody absorption (FTA-ABS) test, PPD and controls, and chest radiographs; consider angiotensin converting enzyme (ACE).
- Consider medical and otolaryngology (Cogan's syndrome) consultation.

Management

ACUTE

- Topical steroid (prednisolone acetate 1% qid to q4h, then taper) and cycloplegic (scopolamine 0.25% bid to qid).

CHRONIC

- Treat underlying etiology (e.g., syphilis, tuberculosis).
- May require lamellar or penetrating keratoplasty if vision is affected by corneal scarring.
- Early oral steroids in Cogan's syndrome may prevent permanent hearing loss.

Prognosis Good; corneal opacity is nonprogressive.

Pannus

Definition Superficial vascularization and scarring of the peripheral cornea due to inflammation; histologically, fibrovascular tissue between epithelium and Bowman's layer. Two types:

Inflammatory

Bowman's layer destruction, with inflammatory cells.

Degenerative

Bowman's layer intact, with areas of calcification.

Etiology Trachoma, contact lens-related neovascularization, vernal keratoconjunctivitis, superior limbic keratoconjunctivitis, atopic keratoconjunctivitis, staphylococcal blepharitis, Terrien's marginal degeneration, ocular rosacea, herpes simplex, chemical injury, ocular cicatricial pemphigoid, Stevens–Johnson syndrome, aniridia, or idiopathic.

Symptoms Asymptomatic; may have decreased vision if visual axis is involved.

Signs Corneal vascularization and opacification past the normal peripheral vascular arcade; micropannus (1–2 mm), gross pannus (>2 mm).

Neovascularization   Pannus

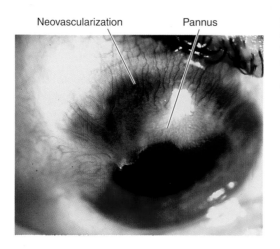

Figure 5-46 • Large pannus demonstrating scarring and vascularization of the superior cornea in a patient with a chemical burn.

Differential Diagnosis Arcus senilis, staphylococcal marginal keratitis, phlyctenulosis, Salzmann's nodular degeneration.

Evaluation
• Complete ophthalmic history and eye exam with attention to everting lids, conjunctiva, and cornea.

Management

• Treat underlying etiology.

Prognosis Good; may progress.

Degenerations

Definition Acquired lesions secondary to aging or previous corneal insult.

Arcus Senilis

Bilateral, white ring in peripheral cornea; occurs in elderly individuals due to lipid deposition at level of Bowman's and Descemet's membranes; clear zone exists between arcus and limbus. Check lipid profile if patient is under 40 years old; unilateral is due to contralateral carotid occlusive disease; arcus juvenilis is the congenital form.

Figure 5-47 • Arcus senilis evident as a peripheral white ring in the inferior cornea.

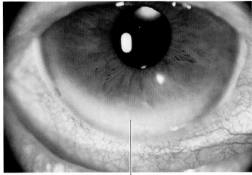

Arcus senilis

Band Keratopathy

Interpalpebral, subepithelial, patchy calcific changes in Bowman's membrane; Swiss cheese pattern; due to chronic ocular inflammation (edema, uveitis, glaucoma, interstitial keratitis, phthisis, dry eye syndrome), hypercalcemia, gout, mercury vapors, or hereditary.

Figure 5-48 • Band keratopathy demonstrating characteristic Swiss cheese pattern of central corneal opacification.

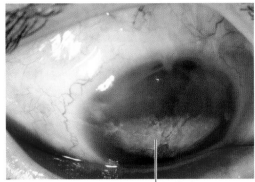

Band keratopathy

Crocodile Shagreen

Bilateral, gray-white opacification at the level of Bowman's layer (anterior) or the deep stroma (posterior); mosaic or cracked ice pattern.

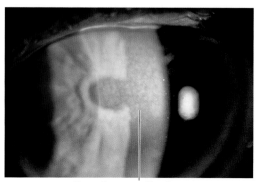

Figure 5-49 • Posterior crocodile shagreen with hazy, cracked ice appearance.

Posterior crocodile shagreen

Furrow Degeneration

Corneal thinning in the clear zone between arcus senilis and the limbus (more apparent than real); perforation is rare; nonprogressive.

Lipid Keratopathy

Yellow-white, subepithelial and stromal infiltrate with feathery edges due to lipid deposition from chronic inflammation and vascularization.

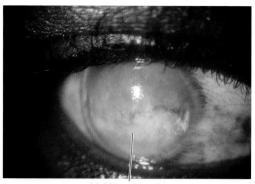

Figure 5-50 • Lipid keratopathy demonstrating dense white corneal infiltration.

Lipid keratopathy

Spheroidal Degeneration (Actinic Degeneration, Labrador Keratopathy, Climatic Droplet Keratopathy, Bietti's Nodular Dystrophy)

Bilateral, elevated, interpalpebral, yellow, stromal droplets due to sun exposure. Male predilection; associated with band keratopathy.

Salzmann's Nodular Degeneration

Elevated, usually midperipheral, smooth, opaque, blue-white, subepithelial, hyaline nodules due to chronic keratitis. Female predilection.

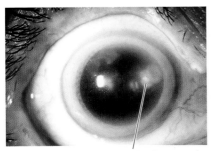

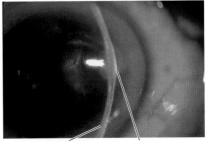

Salzmann's nodular degeneration

Slit-beam   Elevation of nodule

Figure 5-51 • Salzmann's nodular degeneration with several white, elevated, nummular opacities.

Figure 5-52 • Same patient as Figure 5-51, demonstrating elevation of nodule with fine slit-beam.

Terrien's Marginal Degeneration

Noninflammatory, slowly progressive, peripheral thinning of cornea with pannus; starts superiorly and spreads circumferentially; epithelium intact. Slight male predilection. Causes progressive against-the-rule astigmatism; rarely perforates.

Figure 5-53 • Terrien's marginal degeneration with superior thinning (note how slit-beam bends downward) bounded by white scarring.

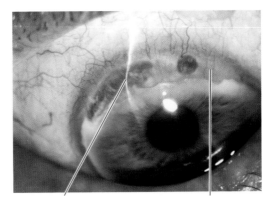

Peripheral thinning   Pannus

White Limbal Girdle of Vogt

Bilateral, white, needle-like opacities in interpalpebral peripheral cornea; occurs in elderly patients. Two types:

Type I

Calcific (lucid interval at limbus).

Type II

Elastotic (no lucid interval).

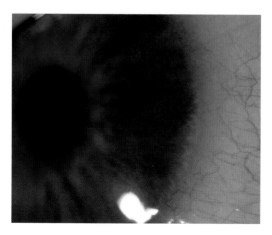

Figure 5-54 • White limbal girdle of Vogt appears as short, white, linear corneal opacities at the limbus.

Symptoms Asymptomatic; may have tearing, photophobia, decreased vision, and foreign body sensation.

Signs Normal or decreased visual acuity, corneal opacity.

Differential Diagnosis See above, corneal dystrophy, metabolic disease, corneal deposits.

Evaluation
- Complete ophthalmic history and eye exam with attention to cornea.
- Consider corneal topography (computerized videokeratography) for Terrien's marginal degeneration.

Management

- No treatment usually recommended.
- Consider 3% topical sodium ethylenediaminetetraacetic acid (EDTA) chelation, superficial keratectomy, or PTK for band keratopathy.
- Consider lamellar or penetrating keratoplasty for lipid keratopathy.
- Salzmann's nodules are often easily removed with superficial keratectomy; may also be treated with PTK.
- Correct astigmatism in Terrien's marginal degeneration with glasses or RGP contact lens; may rarely require tectonic or penetrating keratoplasty.

Prognosis Good, most are benign incidental findings; poor for band and lipid keratopathy, because these are progressive conditions secondary to chronic processes.

Ectasias

Definition

Keratoconus

Bilateral, asymmetric, cone-shaped deformity of the cornea due to progressive central or paracentral corneal thinning. Patients develop irregular astigmatism, corneal striae, superficial scarring from breaks in Bowman's membrane, acute painful stromal edema from breaks in Descemet's membrane (hydrops). Usually sporadic, but may have positive family history (10% of cases); occurs in up to 0.6% of the population (1:2000) and has been reported in up to 10% of individuals in contact lens or refractive surgery clinics; associated with atopy and vernal keratoconjunctivitis (eye rubbing), Down's syndrome, Marfan's syndrome, and contact lens wear (hard lenses).

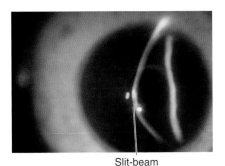

Slit-beam

Figure 5-55 • Keratoconus demonstrating central "nipple" cone as seen with a fine slit-beam. Note the central scarring at the apex of the cone.

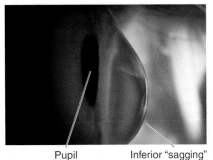

Pupil   Inferior "sagging"

Figure 5-56 • Keratoconus demonstrating inferior "sagging" cone as viewed from the side. Note that the apex of the cone is below the center of the pupil.

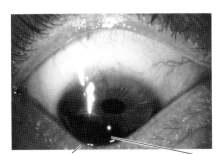

Munson's sign   Keratoconus

Figure 5-57 • Munson's sign in a patient with keratoconus demonstrating protrusion of the lower eyelid with downgaze.

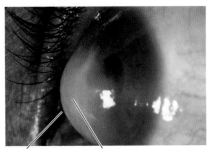

Keratoconus   Hydrops

Figure 5-58 • Hydrops in a patient with keratoconus demonstrating hazy, white, central edema.

Keratoglobus

Rare, globular deformity of the cornea due to diffuse thinning that is maximal at the base of the protrusion. Sporadic; associated with Ehlers–Danlos syndrome.

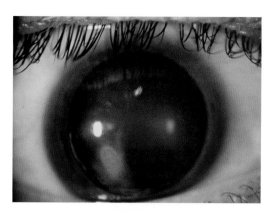

Figure 5-59 • Keratoglobus demonstrating globular corneal deformity with inferior scarring.

Pellucid Marginal Degeneration

Bilateral, inferior, peripheral corneal thinning (2 mm from limbus) with protrusion above thinned area. Patients develop irregular against-the-rule astigmatism; no scarring, cone, or striae occurs.

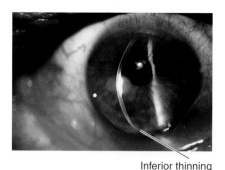

Inferior thinning

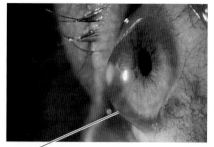

Inferior thinning

Figure 5-60 • Pellucid marginal degeneration demonstrating inferior thinning. Note how thin the slit-beam becomes at the inferior cornea.

Figure 5-61 • Side view of same patient as Figure 5-60 demonstrating protrusion of cornea.

Symptoms Decreased vision; may have sudden loss of vision, pain, photophobia, tearing, and red eye in hydrops.

Signs Decreased visual acuity, abnormally shaped cornea, astigmatism, steep keratometry with irregular mires, abnormal corneal topography. In keratoconus may have central thinning, scarring, Fleischer ring (epithelial iron deposition around base of cone, best seen with blue light),

Vogt's striae (deep, stromal, vertical stress lines at apex of cone), Munson's sign (protrusion of lower lid with downgaze), and Rizzuti's sign (triangle of light on iris from penlight beam focused by cone). In keratoconus and pellucid marginal degeneration may have hydrops (opaque edematous cornea, ciliary injection, and anterior chamber cells and flare).

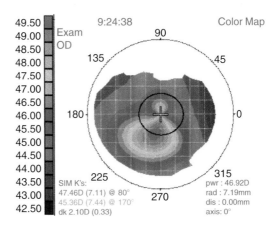

Figure 5-62 • Corneal topography of keratoconus demonstrating characteristic pattern of inferior steepening.

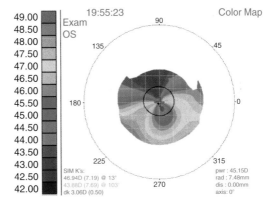

Figure 5-63 • Corneal topography of pellucid marginal degeneration demonstrating irregular astigmatism with characteristic claw or lazy-C shape appearance of corneal steepening.

Differential Diagnosis See above; Terrien's marginal degeneration, contact lens-induced corneal warpage (pseudokeratoconus), corneal topography artifact.

Evaluation

• Complete ophthalmic history and eye exam with attention to cornea, keratometry, retinoscopy reflex, and anterior chamber.

• Corneal topography (computerized videokeratography, CVK): Characteristic pattern of irregular astigmatism (central or inferior steepening in KC, and similar pattern or asymmetric skewed bow-tie pattern in form fruste or KC suspects; inferior claw or lazy-C pattern of steepening in PMD). Three specific CVK parameters have classically been used to aid in the diagnosis of KC (central corneal power > 47.2 D, difference in corneal power between fellow eyes > 0.92 D, and I-S value (difference between average inferior and superior corneal powers 3 mm from the center of the cornea) >1.4 D). Many CVK instruments have built-in software to identify early and subclinical ectasias, and elevation maps may provide increased sensitivity.

Management

- Correct refractive errors with glasses or RGP contact lenses.
- Instrastromal corneal ring segments (Intacs, see Chapter 12) or cross-linking corneal collagen with riboflavin (C3-R: apply topical riboflavin and activate with UV light for 30 minutes to increase the amount of collagen cross-linking in the cornea) may help stabilize the cornea and improve vision in keratoconus.
- Consider lamellar or penetrating keratoplasty when acuity declines or if patient is intolerant of contact lenses.
- Supportive treatment for acute hydrops with hypertonic saline ointment (Adsorbonac or Muro 128 5% qid); add topical broad spectrum antibiotic (polymyxin B sulfate-trimethoprim [Polytrim], moxifloxacin [Vigamox], or tobramycin [Tobrex] qid) for epithelial defect; consider topical steroid (prednisolone acetate 1% qid) and cycloplegic (cyclopentolate 1% tid) for severe pain.
- Corneal refractive surgery is contraindicated in these unstable corneas.

Prognosis Good; penetrating keratoplasty has high success rate for keratoconus and keratoglobus.

Congenital Anomalies

Definition Variety of developmental corneal abnormalities.

Cornea Plana (Autosomal Dominant or Autosomal Recessive)

Flat cornea (curvature often as low as 20–30 diopters); corneal curvature equal to scleral curvature is pathognomonic; associated with sclerocornea and microcornea; increased incidence of angle-closure glaucoma. Mapped to chromosome 12q.

Dermoid

Choristoma (normal tissue in abnormal location) composed of dense connective tissue with pilosebaceous units and stratified squamous epithelium; usually located at inferotemporal limbus, can involve entire cornea. May cause astigmatism and amblyopia; may be associated with preauricular skin tags and vertebral anomalies (Goldenhar's syndrome).

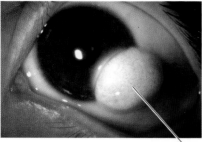

Limbal dermoid

Figure 5-64 • Limbal dermoid at inferotemporal limbus.

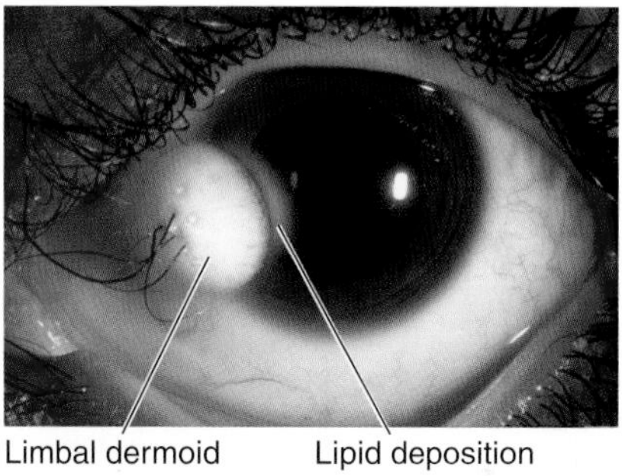

Limbal dermoid   Lipid deposition

Figure 5-65 • Limbal dermoid with central hairs and lipid deposition along the corneal edge.

Haab's Striae

Horizontal breaks in Descemet's membrane due to increased intraocular pressure in children with congenital glaucoma.

Figure 5-66 • Haab's striae appear as clear parallel lines in the cornea.

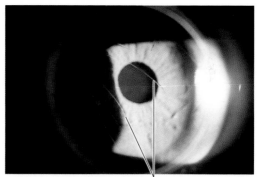

Haab's striae

Megalocornea (X-Linked)

Enlarged cornea (horizontal diameter ≥13 mm); male predilection (90%). Usually isolated, nonprogressive, and bilateral; associated with weak zonules and lens subluxation.

Figure 5-67 • Megalocornea demonstrating abnormally large diameter of both corneas.

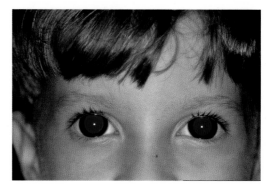

Microcornea (Autosomal Dominant and Recessive)

Small cornea (diameter <10 mm); increased incidence of hyperopia and angle-closure glaucoma.

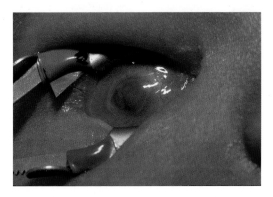

Figure 5-68 • Microcornea demonstrating abnormally small diameter of the right cornea.

Posterior Keratoconus

Focal, central indentation of the posterior cornea with intact endothelium and Descemet's membrane; no change in anterior corneal surface. Rare, usually unilateral, and nonprogressive; female predilection.

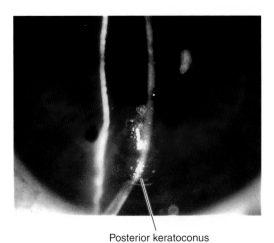

Figure 5-69 • Posterior keratoconus demonstrating focal Descemet's defect with posterior corneal indentation and scarring.

Posterior keratoconus

Sclerocornea

Scleralized peripheral or entire cornea; nonprogressive. 50% sporadic, 50% hereditary (autosomal recessive (AR) more severe); 90% bilateral; 80% associated with cornea plana.

Figure 5-70 • Sclerocornea demonstrating peripheral opacification due to scleralized cornea.

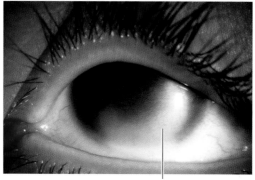

Sclerocornea

Symptoms Asymptomatic; may have decreased vision.

Signs Normal or decreased visual acuity, abnormal corneal size or shape, corneal opacity, edema, or scarring; may have other anterior segment abnormalities (angle, iris, or lens) and increased intraocular pressure.

Differential Diagnosis
- **Small cornea:** microphthalmos, nanophthalmos.
- **Large cornea:** congenital glaucoma (buphthalmos).
- **Cloudy cornea:** interstitial keratitis, birth trauma, metabolic disease, Peter's anomaly, edema, dystrophy, rubella, staphyloma.
- **Posterior keratoconus:** internal ulcer of von Hippel (excavation of the posterior cornea with scarring due to focal absence of endothelium and Descemet's membrane), Peter's anomaly.

Evaluation
- Complete ophthalmic history and eye exam with attention to refraction, cornea, keratometry, tonometry, gonioscopy, iris, lens, and ophthalmoscopy.
- May require examination under anesthesia.

Management

- Correct any refractive error.
- May require patching or occlusion therapy for amblyopia (see Chapter 12), treatment of increased intraocular pressure (see Congenital Glaucoma section in Chapter 11), or even penetrating keratoplasty in severe cases.
- Consider surgical excision of dermoid.

Prognosis Depends on etiology.

Dystrophies

Definition Primary, hereditary, corneal diseases; usually bilateral, symmetric, central, and progressive with early onset.

Anterior (Epithelial and Bowman's Membrane)

Anterior Basement Membrane Dystrophy (Epithelial Basement Membrane Dystrophy, Map-Dot-Fingerprint Dystrophy, Cogan's Microcystic Dystrophy) (Autosomal Dominant)

Most common anterior corneal dystrophy. Abnormal epithelial adhesion causes intraepithelial and subepithelial basement membrane reduplication with intraepithelial microcysts (dots) and subepithelial ridges and lines (map-like and fingerprint-like). 10% of patients with anterior basement membrane dystrophy (ABMD) develop recurrent erosions, whereas 50% of patients with recurrent erosions have ABMD; may develop scarring and decreased vision (due to irregular astigmatism) starting after age 30 years. Slight female predilection.

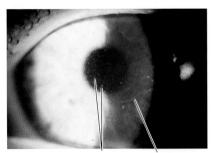

Intraepithelial   Subepithelial
microcysts   ridges

Figure 5-71 • Anterior basement membrane dystrophy demonstrating central dots and lines.

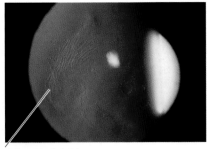

Subepithelial ridges

Figure 5-72 • Anterior basement membrane dystrophy demonstrating dots and lines as viewed with retroillumination.

Gelatinous Droplike Dystrophy (Autosomal Recessive)

Subepithelial, central, mulberry-like, protuberant opacity. Composed of amyloid; lack Bowman's membrane; rare. Decreased vision, photophobia, and tearing occur in first decade.

Meesman Dystrophy (Autosomal Dominant)

Intraepithelial microcystic blebs concentrated in the interpalpebral zone extending to the limbus; surrounded by clear epithelium. Blebs contain periodic acid-Schiff (PAS)-positive material ("peculiar substance") and appear as numerous dots with retroillumination. Rare; recurrent erosions common; retain good vision.

Figure 5-73 • Meesman dystrophy demonstrating dotlike blebs as viewed with retroillumination.

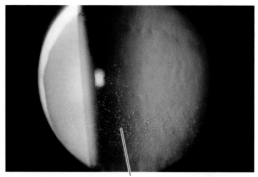

Intraepithelial microcystic blebs

Reis-Bückler Dystrophy (Honeycomb Dystrophy, Thiel-Behnke Dystrophy) (Autosomal Dominant)

Progressive subepithelial opacification and scarring of Bowman's membrane with honeycomb appearance. Recurrent erosions early, usually in the first or second decade; often recurs after penetrating keratoplasty. Mapped to chromosome 5q (BIGH3 gene).

Figure 5-74 • Reis–Bückler dystrophy demonstrating central honeycomb pattern of opacification.

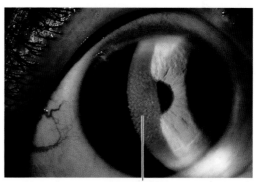

Subepithelial honeycomb opacification

Stromal

Avellino Dystrophy (Autosomal Dominant)

Combination of granular and lattice dystrophies (see below) with discrete granular appearing opacities; intervening stroma contains lattice-like branching lines and dots (not clear like in granular dystrophy). Composed of a combination of hyaline and amyloid that stains with Congo red and Masson's trichrome, respectively. Mapped to chromosome 5q (BIGH3 gene).

Central Cloudy Dystrophy of François (Autosomal Dominant)

Small, indistinct, cloudy gray areas in central posterior stroma with intervening clear cracks (like crocodile shagreen, but does not extend to periphery). Nonprogressive; usually asymptomatic.

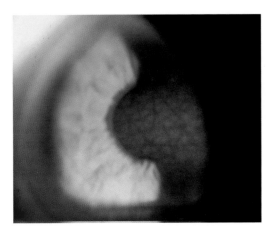

Figure 5-75 • Central cloudy dystrophy demonstrating cracked ice appearance of central cornea with clear periphery.

Schnyder's Central Crystalline Dystrophy (Autosomal Dominant)

Central, yellow-white ring of fine, needle-like, polychromatic crystals with stromal haze; also have dense arcus and limbal girdle. Composed of cholesterol and neutral fats that stain with oil-red-O. Very rare and nonprogressive; associated with hyperlipidemia, genu valgum, and xanthelasma; usually asymptomatic. Mapped to chromosome 1p36.

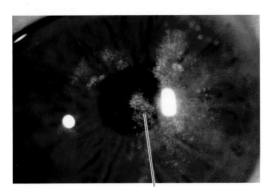

Figure 5-76 • Schnyder's central crystalline dystrophy demonstrating crystalline deposits and stromal haze.

Central crystalline dystrophy

Congenital Hereditary Stromal Dystrophy (Autosomal Dominant)

Superficial, central, feathery, diffuse opacity; alternating layers of abnormal collagen lamellae. Nonprogressive; associated with amblyopia, esotropia, and nystagmus.

François-Neetans Fleck (Mouchetée) Dystrophy (Autosomal Dominant)

Subtle, gray-white, dandruff-like specks that extend to the limbus. Composed of abnormal glycosaminoglycans that stain with Alcian blue. Can be unilateral and asymmetric; nonprogressive and usually asymptomatic.

Figure 5-77 • Fleck dystrophy demonstrating tiny, white, stromal opacities.

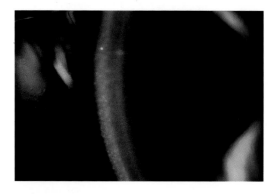

Granular Dystrophy (Autosomal Dominant)

Most common stromal dystrophy. Central, discrete, white, breadcrumb or snowflake-like opacities; intervening stroma usually clear, but may become hazy late; corneal periphery spared. Composed of hyaline that stains with Masson's trichrome. Recurrent erosions rare; decreased vision late. Mapped to chromosome 5q (BIGH3 gene).

Figure 5-78 • Granular dystrophy demonstrating abundant central opacities.

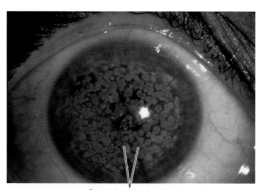

Granular dystrophy

Lattice Dystrophy (Autosomal Dominant)

Refractile branching lines, white dots, and central haze; intervening stroma becomes cloudy, with ground glass appearance. Composed of amyloid that stains with Congo red. Recurrent erosions common, decreased vision in third decade; often recurs after penetrating keratoplasty. Mapped to chromosome 5q (BIGH3 gene).

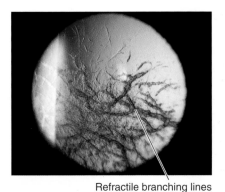

Figure 5-79 • Lattice dystrophy demonstrating branching lines, dots, and central haze as viewed with retroillumination.

Refractile branching lines

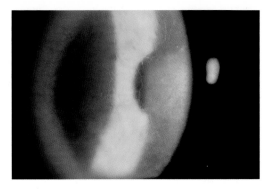

Figure 5-80 • Lattice dystrophy demonstrating branching lines.

Macular Dystrophy (Autosomal Recessive)

Diffuse haze with focal, irregular, gray-white spots that have a sugar-frosted appearance; extends to limbus. Composed of abnormal glycosaminoglycans that stain with Alcian blue. Rare; recurrent erosions occasionally; decreased vision early. Mapped to chromosome 16q22 (CHST6 gene).

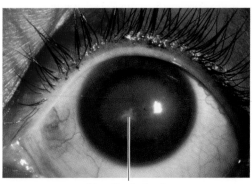

Figure 5-81 • Macular dystrophy demonstrating diffuse central haze with focal area of white spots.

Macular dystrophy

Pre-Descemet's Dystrophy (Deep Filiform Dystrophy) (Autosomal Dominant)

Fine, gray, posterior opacities; various morphologies. Composed of lipid. Onset in fourth to seventh decade; usually asymptomatic. Four types: pre-Descemet's, polymorphic stromal, cornea farinata, and pre-Descemet's associated with ichthyosis and pseudoxanthoma elasticum.

Posterior (Endothelial)

Congenital Hereditary Endothelial Dystrophy (Autosomal Recessive > Autosomal Dominant)

Opacified, edematous corneas at birth due to endothelial dysfunction; rare. Mapped to chromosome 20p. Two types:

Type 1

More common, autosomal recessive, nonprogressive; no pain or tearing.

Type II

Autosomal dominant, delayed onset (age 1–2 years old), progressive; pain and tearing; may require penetrating keratoplasty.

Figure 5-82 • Congenital hereditary endothelial dystrophy demonstrating bilateral corneal edema and opacification.

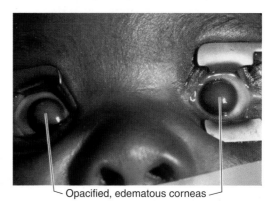

Opacified, edematous corneas

Fuchs' Endothelial Dystrophy (Autosomal Dominant)

Cornea guttata (thickened Descemet's membrane with PAS-positive excrescences [orange peel appearance]) and endothelial dysfunction. Decreased endothelial cell density, increased

Figure 5-83 • Fuchs' endothelial dystrophy demonstrating endothelial pigment, guttata and endothelial scarring. Inset demonstrates guttata and corneal edema when viewed with fine slit-beam.

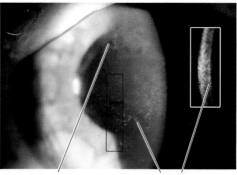

Endothelial scarring   Guttata

pleomorphism, and increased polymegathism; endothelial pigment; early stromal edema, late epithelial edema, bullae, and fibrosis. Female predilection; may have decreased vision (worse in the morning), pain with ruptured bullae, and subepithelial scarring.

Posterior Polymorphous Dystrophy (Autosomal Dominant)

Asymmetric patches of grouped vesicles, scalloped bands, and geographic, gray, hazy areas; epithelial-like endothelium (loss of contact inhibition with proliferation and growth over angle and iris). May develop stromal edema, iris and pupil changes similar to those in iridocorneal endothelial syndrome (see Chapter 7), broad peripheral anterior synechiae, and glaucoma; usually asymptomatic. Mapped to chromosome 20q.

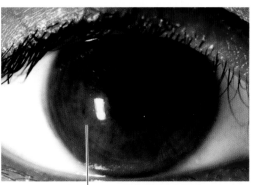

Figure 5-84 • Posterior polymorphous dystrophy demonstrating diffuse, hazy, endothelial opacities.

Posterior polymorphous dystrophy

Symptoms Asymptomatic; may have pain, foreign body sensation, tearing, photophobia, decreased vision.

Signs Normal or decreased visual acuity, corneal opacities; may have corneal edema or scarring.

Differential Diagnosis See above, corneal degeneration, corneal deposits, metabolic diseases, interstitial keratitis.

Evaluation
- Complete ophthalmic history and eye exam with attention to refraction, cornea, tonometry, gonioscopy, iris, and ophthalmoscopy.
- B-scan ultrasonography if unable to visualize the fundus.

Management

- No treatment recommended if asymptomatic.
- May require treatment of recurrent erosions (see Trauma: Recurrent Erosion section).
- May require superficial keratectomy, phototherapeutic keratectomy, lamellar keratoplasty, or penetrating keratoplasty for central scarring.
- Consider DSAEK for edema in Fuchs' dystrophy or congenital hereditary endothelial dystrophy.
- May require treatment of increased intraocular pressure (see Chapter 11) for posterior polymorphous dystrophy.

- Consider pachymetry and specular microscopy for Fuchs' dystrophy.
- **Lab tests**: Lipid profile for Schnyder's central crystalline dystrophy.

Prognosis Usually good; may recur in graft (Reis-Bückler > macular > granular > lattice); may develop glaucoma (posterior polymorphous).

Metabolic Diseases

Definition Hereditary (autosomal recessive) enzymatic deficiencies that result in accumulation of substances in various tissues as well as bilateral corneal opacities.

Etiology Mucopolysaccharidoses, mucolipidoses, sphingolipidoses, gangliosidosis type 1; corneal clouding does not occur in Hunter's or Sanfilippo's syndromes.

Symptoms Decreased vision.

Signs Decreased visual acuity and corneal stromal opacification; may have nystagmus, cataracts, retinal pigment epithelial changes, macular cherry red spot, optic nerve atrophy, and other systemic abnormalities.

Table 5-1 Ocular Involvement of the Metabolic Diseases

Disease	Conjunctiva	Cornea	Retina	Optic nerve
Mucopolysaccharidoses (autosomal recessive)				
MPS I-H (Hurler)	–	+	+	+
MPS I-S (Scheie)	–	+	+	+
MPS II (Hunter; X-linked recessive)	–	–	+	+
MPS III (Sanfilippo)	–	–	+	+
MPS IV (Morquio)	–	+	–	+
MPS VI (Maroteaux-Lamy)	–	+	–	+
MPS VII (Sly)	–	+	–	–
Lipidoses (autosomal recessive)				
GM2 gangliosidosis type I (Tay-Sachs)	–	–	+	+
GM2 gangliosidosis type II (Sandhoff)	–	–	+	+
Fabry's disease (X-linked recessive)	+	+	+	+
Niemann-Pick disease	–	–	+	+

MPS=Mucopolysaccharidosis.

Differential Diagnosis See above; congenital glaucoma, birth trauma, congenital hereditary endothelial dystrophy, Peter's anomaly, sclerocornea, dermoid, interstitial keratitis, corneal ulcer, rubella, staphyloma.

Evaluation
- Complete ophthalmic history and eye exam with attention to cornea, tonometry, lens, and ophthalmoscopy.

- May require examination under anesthesia.
- Pediatric consultation.

Management

- Treat underlying disease.
- May require penetrating keratoplasty.

Prognosis Poor.

Deposits

Definition Pigment or crystal deposition at various levels of the cornea.

Calcium

Yellow-white deposits in Bowman's membrane (see Degenerations: Band Keratopathy section).

Copper

Chalcosis

Green-yellow pigmentation of Descemet's membrane and iris; causes sunflower cataract. Occurs with intraocular foreign body composed of less than 85% copper; pure copper causes suppurative endophthalmitis.

Wilson's disease

Ninety-five percent have Kayser–Fleischer ring at Descemet's membrane (brown-yellow-green peripheral pigmentation that starts inferiorly, no clear interval at limbus); best identified by gonioscopy.

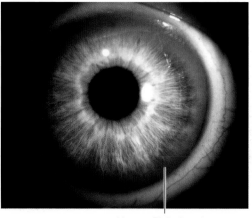

Figure 5-85 • Copper deposition in a patient with Wilson's disease, demonstrating peripheral, brown, Kayser–Fleischer ring.

Kayser-Fleischer ring

Cysteine (Cystinosis)

Stromal, polychromatic crystals.

Drugs

Epinephrine

Black, conjunctival and corneal adrenochrome deposits.

Ciprofloxacin

White precipitate over epithelial defect of corneal ulcer; dose related (i.e., topical drops every 1–2 hours).

Figure 5-86 • Drug deposition demonstrating chalky, white, ciprofloxacin (Ciloxan) precipitates in the bed of a corneal ulcer.

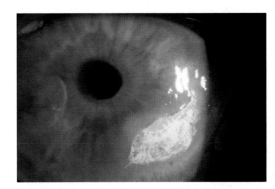

Gold (chrysiasis)

Deposits in conjunctival and stromal periphery; dose related.

Mercury

Preservative in drops causes orange-brown band in Bowman's membrane.

Silver (argyrosis)

Conjunctival and deep stromal deposits.

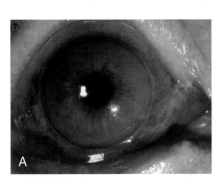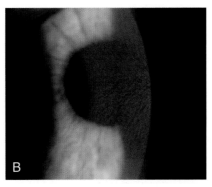

Figure 5-87 • Argyrosis demonstrating gray discoloration of (A) conjunctiva, caruncle, puncta, and (B) cornea due to silver deposits.

Thorazine or stelazine

Brown, stromal deposits; also anterior subcapsular lens deposits.

Immunoglobulin (Multiple Myeloma)

Stromal deposits (also occur in Waldenström's macroglobulinemia and benign monoclonal gammopathy).

Iron

Blood staining

Stromal deposits, from hyphema.

Ferry line

Epithelial deposits, under filtering bleb.

Fleischer ring

Epithelial deposits, at base of cone in keratoconus.

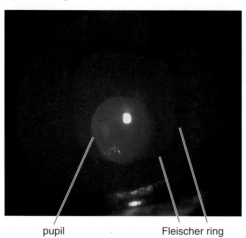

Figure 5-88 • Fleischer ring is often more evident when viewed with blue light.

pupil   Fleischer ring

Hudson-Stahli line

Epithelial deposits, across inferior one third of cornea.

Siderosis

Stromal deposits, from intraocular metallic foreign body.

Stocker line

Epithelial deposits, at head of pterygium.

Lipid or Cholesterol (Dyslipoproteinemias)

Hyperlipoproteinemia

Arcus in types 2, 3, and 4.

Fish-eye disease

Diffuse corneal clouding, denser in periphery.

Lecithin-cholesterol acyltransferase deficiency

Dense arcus and diffuse, fine, gray, stromal dots.

Tangier's disease (familial high-density lipoprotein deficiency)

Diffuse or focal, small, deep, stromal opacities.

Melanin
Krukenberg spindle

Endothelial deposits, central vertical distribution in pigment dispersion syndrome.

Scattered endothelial pigment

Ingested by abnormal endothelial cells (Fuchs' dystrophy).

Tyrosine (Tyrosinemia) Type II

Epithelial and subepithelial pseudodendritic opacities; may ulcerate and cause vascularization and scarring.

Urate (Gout)

Epithelial, subepithelial, and stromal, fine, yellow crystals; may form brown, band keratopathy with ulceration and vascularization.

Verticillata (Vortex Keratopathy)

Brown, epithelial, whorl pattern involving inferior and paracentral cornea; occurs in Fabry's disease (X-linked recessive) including carriers (women); also due to amiodarone, chloroquine, indomethacin, chlorpromazine, or tamoxifen deposits.

Figure 5-89 • Cornea verticillata demonstrating golden brown deposits in a whorl pattern in the inferior central cornea of a Fabry's disease carrier.

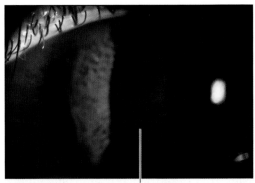

Cornea verticillata

Symptoms Asymptomatic; may have photophobia and, rarely, decreased vision.

Signs Normal or decreased visual acuity, corneal deposits; may have iris heterochromia (siderosis and chalcosis), cataract (Wilson's disease, intraocular metallic foreign body, tyrosinemia), corneal ulcer (tyrosinemia, gout).

Differential Diagnosis See above; dieffenbachia plant sap, ichthyosis (may have fine, white, deep, stromal opacities), hyperbilirubinemia.

Evaluation

• Complete ophthalmic history and eye exam with attention to conjunctiva, cornea, anterior chamber, iris, and lens.

• Electroretinogram (ERG) for intraocular metallic foreign body.

• Medical consultation for systemic diseases.

Management

• Treat underlying disease.

• Remove offending agent.

• May require surgical removal of intraocular metallic foreign body.

Prognosis Good except for siderosis, chalcosis, Wilson's disease, and multiple myeloma.

Enlarged Corneal Nerves

Definition Prominent, enlarged corneal nerves.

Etiology Multiple endocrine neoplasia type IIb (MEN-IIb), leprosy, Fuchs' dystrophy, amyloidosis, keratoconus, ichthyosis, Refsum's syndrome, neurofibromatosis, congenital glaucoma, trauma, posterior polymorphous dystrophy, and idiopathic.

Symptoms Asymptomatic.

Signs Prominent, white, branching, lines in the cornea.

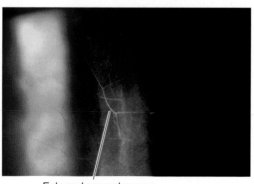

Enlarged corneal nerves

Figure 5-90 • Enlarged corneal nerves appear as prominent, white, branching lines.

Differential Diagnosis See above; lattice dystrophy.

Evaluation
- Complete ophthalmic history and eye exam with attention to cornea, tonometry, lens, and ophthalmoscopy.
- Medical consultation for systemic diseases.

Management

- No treatment recommended.
- Treat underlying medical disorder.

Prognosis Enlarged nerves are benign; underlying etiology may have poor prognosis (i.e., MEN-IIb).

Tumors

Definition Corneal intraepithelial neoplasia (CIN) or squamous cell carcinoma involving the cornea; usually arises from conjunctiva near limbus (see Chapter 4).

Epidemiology Usually unilateral; more common in elderly, Caucasian males; associated with ultraviolet radiation, human papillomavirus, and heavy smoking; suspect AIDS in patients <50 years of age.

Symptoms Asymptomatic; may have foreign body sensation, red eye, decreased vision, or notice growth (white spot) on cornea.

Signs Gelatinous, thickened, white, nodular or smooth, limbal or corneal mass with loops of abnormal vessels.

Figure 5-91 • Corneal intraepithelial neoplasia demonstrating thickened, white, gelatinous lesion at limbus with vascularization.

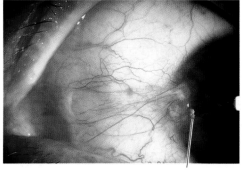

Corneal intraepithelial neoplasia

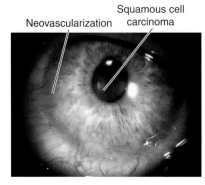

Figure 5-92 images:
Neovascularization
Squamous cell carcinoma

Figure 5-93 images:
Squamous cell carcinoma

Figure 5-92 • Squamous cell carcinoma of the cornea.

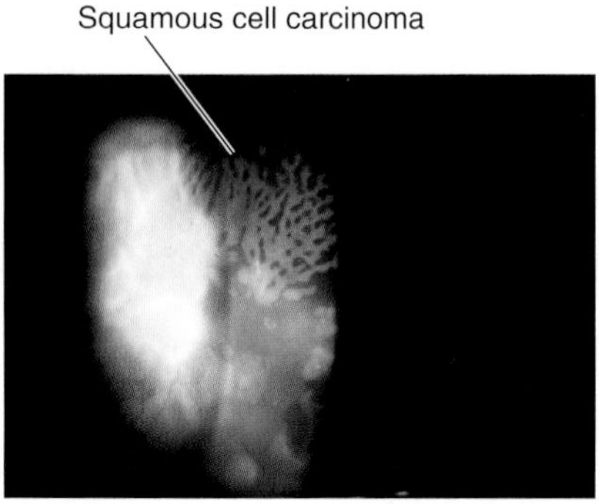

Figure 5-93 • Same patient as Figure 5-92 demonstrating a close-up of the white gelatinous lesion.

Differential Diagnosis Pinguecula, pterygium, pannus, dermoid, Bitot's spot, papilloma, pyogenic granuloma, pseudoepitheliomatous hyperplasia ([PEH] benign, rapid, conjunctival proliferation onto cornea), hereditary benign intraepithelial dyskeratosis ([HBID] elevated white-gray interpalpebral conjunctival plaques with abnormal vessels; may involve cornea and affect vision; oral mucosa also affected; occurs in American Indians from North Carolina; AD, mapped to chromosome 4q35).

Evaluation

- Complete ophthalmic history and eye exam with attention to conjunctiva and cornea.
- MRI to rule out orbital involvement if suspected.
- Medical consultation and systemic workup.

Management

- Excisional biopsy with episclerectomy, corneal epitheliectomy with 100% alcohol, and cryotherapy to bed of lesion; should be performed by a cornea or tumor specialist.
- Consider topical 5-fluorouracil or mitomycin C, especially for recurrence.
- Exenteration with adjunctive radiation therapy for orbital involvement.

Prognosis Depends on extent and ability to completely excise. Intraocular spread, orbital invasion, and metastasis are rare; recurrence after excision is <10%; mortality rate of up to 8%.

Primary Angle-Closure Glaucoma 233
Secondary Angle-Closure Glaucoma 236
Hypotony 238
Hyphema 240
Cells and Flare 241
Hypopyon 243
Endophthalmitis 244
Anterior Uveitis 248
Uveitis-Glaucoma-Hyphema Syndrome 255

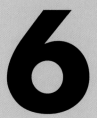

Anterior Chamber

Primary Angle-Closure Glaucoma

Definition Glaucoma due to obstruction of the trabecular meshwork by peripheral iris; classified as acute, subacute (intermittent), or chronic.

Etiology/Mechanism

Pupillary Block

Most common. Lens-iris apposition interferes with aqueous flow and causes the iris to bow forward and occlude the trabecular meshwork.

Plateau Iris Syndrome (Without Pupillary Block)

Peripheral iris occludes the angle in patients with an atypical iris configuration (anteriorly positioned peripheral iris with steep insertion due to anteriorly rotated ciliary processes) (see Chapter 7).

Epidemiology Approximately 5% of the general population over 60 years old have occludable angles, 0.5% of these develop angle-closure. Usually bilateral (develops in 50% of untreated fellow eyes within 5 years); higher incidence in Asians and Eskimos; female predilection (4:1). Associated with hyperopia, nanophthalmos, anterior chamber depth less than 2.5 mm, thicker lens, and lens subluxation.

Symptoms

Acute Angle-Closure

Pain, red eye, photophobia, decreased or blurred vision, halos around lights, headache, nausea, emesis.

Subacute Angle-Closure

May be asymptomatic or have symptoms of acute form but less severe; episodes evolve over the course of days or weeks and resolve spontaneously.

Chronic Angle-Closure

Asymptomatic; may have decreased vision or constricted visual fields in late stages.

Signs

Acute Angle-Closure

Decreased visual acuity, increased intraocular pressure, ciliary injection, corneal edema, anterior chamber cells and flare, shallow anterior chamber, narrow angles on gonioscopy, mid-dilated nonreactive pupil, iris bombé; may have signs of previous attacks including sector iris atrophy, anterior subcapsular lens opacities (glaukomflecken; due to lens epithelial cell ischemia and necrosis from high intraocular pressure), dilated irregular pupil, and peripheral anterior synechiae (PAS).

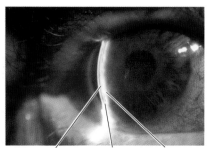

Posterior cornea   Slit-beam   Iris surface

Figure 6-1 • Primary angle-closure glaucoma with very shallow anterior chamber and iridocorneal touch (no space between slit-beam view of cornea and iris).

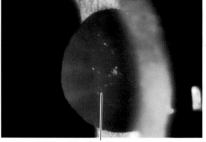

Glaukomflecken

Figure 6-2 • Glaukomflecken appear as dotlike anterior subcapsular lens opacities.

Subacute and Chronic Angle-Closure

Narrow angles; may have increased intraocular pressure, PAS, sector iris atrophy, glaukomflecken, optic nerve cupping, nerve fiber layer defects, and visual field defects.

Evaluation
- Complete ophthalmic history and eye exam with attention to pupils, cornea, tonometry, anterior chamber, indentation gonioscopy (Zeiss lens), iris, lens, and ophthalmoscopy.
- Check visual fields.
- Consider provocative testing (prone test, dark room test, prone dark room test, and pharmacologic dilation; intraocular pressure increase of >8 mmHg is considered positive).

Management

ACUTE ANGLE-CLOSURE

- Topical β-blocker (timolol [Timoptic] 0.5% q 15 minutes × 2, then bid), α-agonist (apraclonidine [Iopidine] 1% q 15 minutes × 2), and topical steroid (prednisolone acetate 1% q 15 minutes × 4, then q1h).

- Topical miotic (pilocarpine 1–2% × 1 initially, then qid if effective; usually not effective if intraocular pressure >40 mmHg due to iris sphincter ischemia; in 20% of patients pilocarpine will exacerbate the situation due to forward displacement of the lens-iris diaphragm); can also consider topical α-antagonist (thymoxamine 0.5% q 15 minutes for 2–3 hours).

- Systemic acetazolamide (Diamox 500 mg po STAT, then bid) and hyperosmotic (isosorbide up to 2 g/kg po of 45% solution).

- **Laser peripheral iridotomy (LPI) with or without iridoplasty:** Definitive treatment after acute attack is broken medically; may require application of topical glycerin (Ophthalgan) to clear corneal edema for adequate visualization of iris.

  - *Procedure parameters:* a contact lens is used to stabilize the eye, better focus the beam, and place laser spots peripherally; patency of the iridotomy is confirmed by visualization of the lens capsule (often a rush of aqueous fluid through the hole is seen) not by the appearance of a red reflex.

  - *Argon laser (depends on iris pigmentation):*

    Dark brown: 0.02–0.05-second duration, 50 μ spot size, 600–1000 mW power; then 0.1 second and 400–600 mW through pigment epithelium.

    Medium brown: 0.1–0.2-second duration, 50 μ spot size, 600–1000 mW power.

    Blue: 0.05-second duration, 500 μ spot size, 200–500 mW power contraction burns; then 0.1-second duration, 50μ spot size, 600–1000 mW power through stroma and 400–600 mW through pigment epithelium.

  - *Nd:YAG laser:* 4–10 mJ power.

- Prophylactic laser peripheral iridotomy in fellow eye with narrow angle to prevent an acute attack in the future.

- If unable to perform laser peripheral iridotomy, consider surgical iridectomy.

- Consider goniosynechiolysis for recent peripheral anterior synechiae (<12 months).

- Plateau iris syndrome may require long-term miotic therapy and peripheral iridectomy to reduce risk of pupillary block; consider **argon laser iridoplasty or gonioplasty**.

  - *Procedure parameters:* 0.2–0.5-second duration, 200–500 μ spot size, 200–400 mW power, approximately 10 spot applications per quadrant, spots are placed on the iris as peripheral as possible and the power setting is adjusted until movement of the iris is observed.

SUBACUTE AND CHRONIC ANGLE-CLOSURE

- Laser peripheral iridotomy even without evidence of pupillary block.

- Treatment of increased intraocular pressure (see Primary Open Angle Glaucoma section in Chapter 11); may require trabeculectomy or glaucoma drainage implant to lower pressure adequately.

Prognosis Good if prompt treatment is initiated for acute attack; poorer for chronic cases but depends on extent of optic nerve damage and subsequent intraocular pressure control.

Secondary Angle-Closure Glaucoma

Definition Acute or chronic angle-closure glaucoma caused by a variety of ocular disorders.

Etiology/Mechanism

With Pupillary Block

Lens-induced (phacomorphic, dislocated lens, microspherophakia), seclusio pupillae, aphakic or pseudophakic pupillary block, silicone oil, nanophthalmos.

Without Pupillary Block

Posterior "Pushing" Mechanism

Mechanical or anterior displacement of the lens-iris diaphragm.
- Anterior rotation of ciliary body due to:
  - Inflammation (scleritis, uveitis, panretinal photocoagulation).
  - Congestion (scleral buckling, nanophthalmos).
  - Choroidal effusion (hypotony, uveal effusion, medication [Topamax]).
  - Suprachoroidal hemorrhage.
- Aqueous misdirection (malignant glaucoma).
- Pressure from posterior segment (tumor, expanding gas, exudative retinal detachment).
- Persistent hyperplastic primary vitreous.
- Retinopathy of prematurity.

Anterior "Pulling" Mechanism

Adherence of iris to the trabecular meshwork or membranes over the trabecular meshwork.
- Epithelial (downgrowth or ingrowth).
- Endothelial (iridocorneal endothelial syndrome, posterior polymorphous dystrophy).
- Neovascular (neovascular glaucoma; see Chapter 7).
- Postinflammatory peripheral anterior synechiae.
- Adhesion from trauma.

Symptoms

Acute Angle-Closure

Pain, red eye, photophobia, decreased or blurred vision, halos around lights, headache, nausea, emesis.

Chronic Angle-Closure

Asymptomatic; may have decreased vision or constricted visual fields in late stages.

Signs

Acute Angle-Closure

Decre ased visual acuity, increased intraocular pressure, ciliary injection, corneal edema, anterior chamber cells and flare, shallow anterior chamber, narrow angles on gonioscopy, mid-dilated nonreactive pupil, iris bombé; signs of underlying etiology.

Figure 6-3 • Secondary angle-closure due to pseudophakic pupillary block. The intact anterior vitreous face (visible with pigment) is blocking the pupil and superior iridectomy. The slit-beam shows the peripheral iris bowing forward, obstructing the angle and bulging around the anterior chamber intraocular lens.

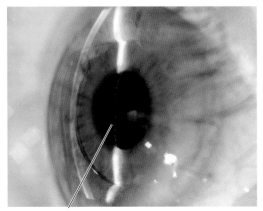

Anterior vitreous face

Chronic Angle-Closure

Narrow angles, increased intraocular pressure, PAS, signs of underlying etiology; may have sector iris atrophy, glaukomflecken, optic nerve cupping, nerve fiber layer defects, and visual field defects.

Evaluation
- Complete ophthalmic history and eye exam with attention to pupils, cornea, tonometry, anterior chamber, indentation gonioscopy, iris, lens, and ophthalmoscopy.
- Check visual fields.

Management

- Treat underlying etiology.
- Laser peripheral iridotomy for pupillary block.
- Topical cycloplegic (scopolamine 0.25% qid or atropine 1% bid) for malignant glaucoma, microspherophakia, after scleral buckle or after panretinal photocoagulation (do not use miotic agents).

Continued

Management—Cont'd

- May require pars plana vitrectomy and lens extraction in refractory cases of malignant glaucoma or Nd:YAG laser disruption of the anterior hyaloid face in patient with pseudophakia and aphakia.
- Topical cycloplegic (scopolamine 0.25% qid), steroid (prednisolone acetate 1% qid), and panretinal photocoagulation for neovascular glaucoma.
- Cataract extraction may be necessary in some cases of lens-induced angle-closure glaucoma.
- Treatment of increased intraocular pressure (see Primary Open Angle Glaucoma section in Chapter 11); may require trabeculectomy or glaucoma drainage implant to lower pressure adequately.

Prognosis Poorer than primary angle-closure because usually due to chronic process; depends on etiology, extent of optic nerve damage, and subsequent intraocular pressure control.

Hypotony

Definition Low intraocular pressure (≤5 mmHg).

Etiology

Increased Outflow (Excessive Drainage of Aqueous or Vitreous Fluid)

Trauma (cyclodialysis), surgery (wound leak, bleb overfiltration), choroidal effusion, retinal detachment.

Decreased Production (Ciliary Body Shutdown)

Inflammation (uveitis), medication (ciliary body toxicity: 5-fluorouracil, mitomycin-C, cidofovir, mannitol, anesthetic agents [fentanyl, succinylcholine, propofol, sevoflurane]), systemic disorder (bilateral hypotony: dehydration, ketoacidosis, uremia), cyclitic membrane, anterior proliferative vitreoretinopathy, ocular ischemic syndrome, phthisis.

Symptoms Asymptomatic; may have pain and decreased vision.

Signs Normal or decreased visual acuity, low intraocular pressure, functional and structural changes usually occur; may have refractive (hyperopic) shift, corneal folds and edema, positive Seidel test, filtering bleb, anterior chamber cells and flare, shallow anterior chamber, cyclodialysis cleft, cataract, cyclitic membrane, choroidal effusion, chorioretinal folds (hypotony maculopathy), cystoid macular edema, retinal detachment, proliferative vitreoretinopathy, optic disc edema, phthisis (end-stage; see Chapter 1).

Figure 6-4 • Hypotony maculopathy with choroidal folds after trabeculectomy surgery.

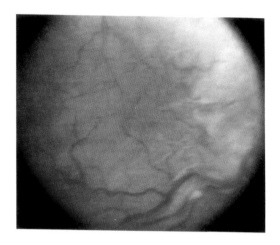

Evaluation

- Complete ophthalmic history with attention to trauma, surgery, medications, and systemic conditions.
- Complete eye exam with attention to cornea, tonometry, anterior chamber, gonioscopy, and ophthalmoscopy.
- Seidel test (see Trauma: Laceration section in Chapter 5) to rule out open globe or wound leak in traumatic or postsurgical cases.
- B-scan ultrasonography to evaluate choroidal effusion, retinal detachment, and intraocular foreign body if unable to visualize the fundus.
- Consider ultrasound biomicroscopy (UBM) to identify cyclitic membrane, cyclodialysis cleft, and ciliary body detachment (≥ 2 clock hours).
- Consider fluorescein angiogram or OCT to identify choroidal folds.

Management

- Treat underlying etiology.
- Topical cycloplegic (cyclopentolate 1%, scopolamine 0.25%, atropine 1% bid to tid).
- Topical antibiotic for wound leak (gatifloxacin [Zymar] or moxifloxacin [Vigamox] qid).
- Bandage contact lens or pressure patch may work for small wound leaks.
- May require drainage of choroidal effusion or surgical repair of wound leak, retinal detachment, or ciliary body detachment.
- Consider Simmons' shell or anterior chamber injection of viscoelastic or gas for bleb overfiltration.
- Steroids (topical, sub-Tenon's, intravitreal, or oral), especially in cases due to uveitis.
- Consider topical ibopamine 2%.

Prognosis   Depends on etiology and duration.

Hyphema

Definition Blood in the anterior chamber. Hyphema forms a layer of blood, whereas a microhyphema cannot be visualized with the naked eye (can only see red blood cells floating in the anterior chamber on slit-lamp examination).

Etiology Usually traumatic (60% also have angle recession); may be spontaneous when associated with neovascularization of the iris or angle, iris lesions, or a malpositioned or loose intraocular lens (IOL).

Symptoms Decreased vision; may have pain, photophobia, red eye.

Signs Normal or decreased visual acuity, red blood cells in the anterior chamber (layer or clot); may have subconjunctival hemorrhage, increased intraocular pressure, rubeosis, iris sphincter tears, unusually deep anterior chamber, angle recession, iridodonesis, iridodialysis, cyclodialysis, and other signs of ocular trauma; may have iris lesion or pseudophacodonesis of IOL implant.

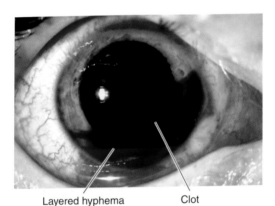

Figure 6-5 • Hyphema demonstrating layered blood inferiorly and suspended red blood cells and clot.

Layered hyphema　　　　Clot

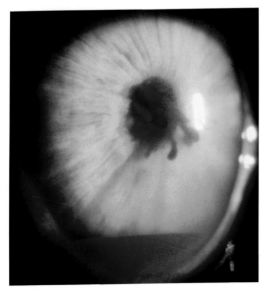

Figure 6-6 • Hyphema with active bleeding from the pupil margin.

Differential Diagnosis Trauma, uveitis-glaucoma-hyphema (UGH) syndrome, juvenile xanthogranuloma, leukemia, child abuse, postoperative, Fuchs' heterochromic iridocyclitis, rubeosis irides.

Evaluation

- Complete ophthalmic history and eye exam with attention to cornea, tonometry, anterior chamber, iris, and ophthalmoscopy; wait 2–4 weeks to perform gonioscopy and scleral depression in traumatic cases.
- B-scan ultrasonography to rule out open globe if unable to visualize the fundus.
- Consider UBM to evaluate angle structures.
- **Lab tests**: Sickle cell prep and hemoglobin electrophoresis to rule out sickle cell disease.

Management

- Topical steroid (prednisolone acetate 1% up to q1h initially, then taper over 3–4 weeks as hyphema and inflammation resolve).
- Topical cycloplegic (scopolamine 0.25% or atropine 1% bid to tid).
- Consider aminocaproic acid ([Amicar] 50–100 mg/kg q4h).
- May require treatment of increased intraocular pressure (see Primary Open Angle Glaucoma section in Chapter 11; do not use carbonic anhydrase inhibitors in patients with sickle cell disease; do not use miotic agents or prostaglandin analogues).
- Instruct patient to avoid aspirin-containing products, sleep with head of bed elevated at 30° angle, protect eye with metal shield at all times, and remain at bed rest.
- Daily examination for first 5 days (when risk of recurrent bleed is highest) then slowly space out visits.
- May require anterior chamber washout for corneal blood staining, uncontrolled elevated intraocular pressure, persistent clot, rebleed (8-ball hyphema).
- IOL removal or exchange for UGH syndrome.

- **Prognosis** Good in traumatic cases if intraocular pressure is controlled and there is no rebleed; may be at risk for angle recession glaucoma in the future.

Cells and Flare

Definition Cells and increased protein (flare) in the anterior chamber due to breakdown of the blood–aqueous barrier by inflammation.

Cells

Appear as small particles floating in the aqueous; usually white blood cells, sometimes red blood cells (microhyphema) or pigment cells (from iris after dilation and in pigment dispersion syndrome). If severe, cells settle inferiorly in anterior chamber and form layer (hypopyon, hyphema, or pseudohypopyon).

Flare

Appears as hazy or cloudy aqueous; severe fibrinous exudate produces a jelly-like plasmoid aqueous appearance with strands of fibrin (4+ flare).

Etiology Exudation from blood vessels due to anterior segment inflammation; usually uveitis, trauma, postoperative, scleritis, and keratitis.

Symptoms Variable pain, photophobia, tearing, red eye, decreased vision; may be asymptomatic.

Signs Normal or decreased visual acuity, ciliary injection, miosis, anterior chamber cells and flare (best seen when viewed with a short narrow slit-lamp beam directed at an angle through the pupil producing an effect similar to shining a flashlight through a dark room; cells demonstrate brownian motion and flare looks like smoke in the light beam; graded on a 1 to 4 scale [i.e., 1+ = 1–10 cells; 2+ = 11–20 cells; 3+ = 21–50 cells; 4+ = >50 cells]); may have scleritis, keratic precipitates, keratitis, iris nodules, posterior synechiae, increased or decreased intraocular pressure, hypopyon, hyphema, pseudohypopyon, cataract, vitritis, vitreous hemorrhage, or retinal or choroidal lesions.

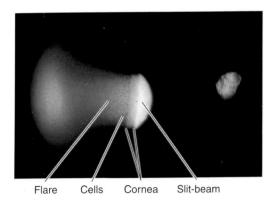

Flare   Cells   Cornea   Slit-beam

Figure 6-7 • Grade 4+ anterior chamber cells and flare visible with fine slit-beam between the cornea and iris.

Differential Diagnosis See above.

Evaluation
- Complete ophthalmic history and eye exam with attention to sclera, cornea, tonometry, anterior chamber, gonioscopy, iris, lens, and ophthalmoscopy.
- Consider uveitis workup (see Anterior Uveitis section).

Management

- Treat underlying etiology.
- Topical steroid (prednisolone acetate 1% up to q1h initially, then taper slowly) and cycloplegic (cyclopentolate 1%, scopolamine 0.25%, or atropine 1% bid to tid).
- Consider sub-Tenon's steroid injection (triamcinolone acetonide 40 mg/mL), oral steroids (prednisone 60–100 mg po qd), or cytotoxic agents for severe inflammation after ruling out infectious etiologies (see Anterior Uveitis section).
- May require treatment of increased intraocular pressure (see Primary Open Angle Glaucoma section in Chapter 11; do not use miotic agents or prostaglandin analogues).

Prognosis Depends on etiology.

Hypopyon

Definition Layer of white blood cells in the anterior chamber.

Etiology Usually due to inflammation (uveitis, especially HLA-B27 associated and Behçet's disease) or infection (corneal ulcer, endophthalmitis).

Symptoms Pain, red eye, and decreased vision.

Signs Normal or decreased visual acuity, conjunctival injection, hypopyon, and anterior chamber cells and flare; may have scleritis, corneal infiltrate, keratic precipitates, iris nodules, cataract, vitritis, or retinal or choroidal lesions.

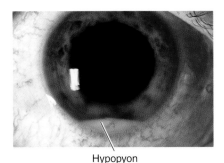
Hypopyon

Figure 6-8 • Hypopyon demonstrating layered white blood cells inferiorly.

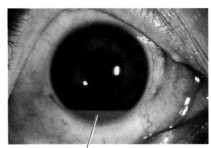
Pseudohypopyon

Figure 6-9 • Pseudohypopyon composed of khaki-colored ghost cells layered inferiorly.

Differential Diagnosis Pseudohypopyon (layer of other cells in the anterior chamber including pigment cells, ghost cells, tumor cells, or macrophages).

Evaluation

- Complete ophthalmic history and eye exam with attention to sclera, cornea, tonometry, anterior chamber, iris, lens, and ophthalmoscopy.
- B-scan ultrasonography if unable to visualize the fundus.
- **Lab tests**: Cultures and smears for infectious keratitis (see Chapter 5) or endophthalmitis (see Endophthalmitis section).
- Consider uveitis workup (see Anterior Uveitis section).

Management

- Treat underlying etiology.
- Antimicrobial medications if infectious (see Infectious Keratitis in Chapter 5 and Endophthalmitis sections below).
- Topical steroid (prednisolone acetate 1% up to q1–2h initially) and cycloplegic (cyclopentolate 1%, scopolamine 0.25%, or atropine 1% bid to tid).
- Monitor treatment response by hypopyon resorption.
- Rarely requires surgery, except in cases of endophthalmitis.

Prognosis Depends on etiology and treatment response.

Endophthalmitis

Definition Intraocular infection; may be acute, subacute, or chronic; localized or involving anterior and posterior segments.

Etiology

Postoperative (70%)

Acute postoperative (<6 weeks after surgery)

Ninety-four percent Gram-positive bacteria including coagulase-negative staphylococci (70%), *Staphylococcus aureus* (10%), *Streptococcus* species (11%); only 6% Gram-negative organisms.

Delayed postoperative (>6 weeks after surgery)

Propionibacterium acnes, coagulase-negative staphylococci, and fungi (*Candida* species).

Conjunctival filtering bleb associated

Streptococcus species (47%), coagulase-negative staphylococci (22%), *Haemophilus influenzae* (16%).

Posttraumatic (20%)

Bacillus (*B. cereus*) species (24%), *Staphylococcus* species (39%), and Gram-negative organisms (7%).

Endogenous (2–15%)

Rare, usually fungal (*Candida* species); bacterial endogenous is usually due to *Staphylococcus aureus* and Gram-negative bacteria. Occurs in debilitated, septicemic, or immunocompromised patients, especially after surgical procedures.

Epidemiology Incidence following cataract surgery is less than 0.1%; risk factors include loss of vitreous, disrupted posterior capsule, poor wound closure, and prolonged surgery. Incidence following penetrating trauma is 4–13%, may be as high as 30% after injuries in rural settings; risk factors include retained intraocular foreign body, delayed surgery (>24 hours), rural setting (soil contamination), disrupted crystalline lens.

Symptoms Pain, photophobia, discharge, red eye, decreased vision; may be asymptomatic or have chronic uveitis appearance in delayed onset and endogenous cases.

Signs Decreased visual acuity (usually severe; only 14% of patients in the Endophthalmitis Vitrectomy Study (EVS) had better than 5/200 vision), lid edema, proptosis, conjunctival injection, chemosis, wound abscess, corneal edema, keratic precipitates, anterior chamber cells and flare, hypopyon, vitritis, poor red reflex; may have positive Seidel test and other signs of an open globe (see Chapter 4).

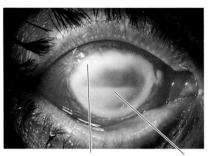

Corneal infiltrate   Hypopyon

Figure 6-10 • Endophthalmitis with large hypopyon (almost 50% of anterior chamber height). There is severe inflammation with 4+ conjunctival injection and a white ring corneal infiltrate at the limbus.

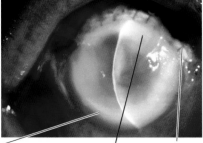

Hypopyon   Ring infiltrate   Sutures

Figure 6-11 • *Staphylococcus* endophthalmitis with ring infiltrate. There is marked corneal edema and the corneal sutures across the surgical wound are visible at the superior limbus.

Differential Diagnosis Uveitis, sterile inflammation (usually from prolonged intraoperative manipulations, especially involving vitreous; retained lens material; rebound inflammation after sudden decrease in postoperative steroids; or toxic anterior segment syndrome (TASS; acute postoperative anterior chamber reaction and corneal edema due to contaminants from surgical instruments, intraocular solutions, or IOL implant)), intraocular foreign body, intraocular tumor, sympathetic ophthalmia, anterior segment ischemia (from carotid artery disease [ocular ischemic syndrome] or following muscle surgery [usually on three or more rectus muscles in same eye at the same surgery]).

Evaluation

- Complete ophthalmic history with attention to surgery and trauma.
- Complete eye exam with attention to visual acuity, conjunctiva, sclera, cornea, tonometry, anterior chamber, vitreous cells, red reflex, and ophthalmoscopy.
- Seidel test (see Trauma: Laceration section in Chapter 5) to rule out wound leak or open globe in postsurgical or traumatic cases.
- B-scan ultrasonography if unable to visualize the fundus.
- **Lab tests**: STAT evaluation of intraocular fluid cultures and smears; conjunctival and nasal swabs can also be collected for culture but have low yield.
- Medical consultation for endogenous endophthalmitis.

Management

OPHTHALMIC EMERGENCY

Acute Postoperative Endophthalmitis

- If vision is better than light perception (>LP), then anterior chamber and vitreous tap to collect specimens for culture, and intravitreal antibiotics (see below).
- If vision is LP only, then anterior chamber tap, pars plana vitrectomy, and intravitreal antibiotics (EVS conclusion); should be performed by a vitreoretinal specialist.
- Intravitreal antibiotics ± steroid:

  Vancomycin (1 mg/0.1 mL)

  Ceftazidime (2.25 mg/0.1 mL) or amikacin (0.4 mg/0.1 mL)

  Dexamethasone (0.4 mg/0.1 mL; controversial, because intravitreal steroids were not evaluated in the EVS).

- Subconjunctival antibiotics ± steroid, which only included cataract surgery and secondary IOL cases:

  Vancomycin (25 mg)

  Ceftazidime (100 mg) or gentamicin (20 mg)

  Dexamethasone (12–24 mg).

- Topical broad spectrum fortified antibiotics (alternate every 30 minutes):

  Vancomycin (50 mg/mL q1h)

  Ceftazidime (50 mg/mL q1h).

- Topical steroid (prednisolone acetate 1% q1–2h initially) and cycloplegic (atropine 1% tid or scopolamine 0.25% qid).
- Systemic intravenous antibiotics for marked inflammation, severe cases, or rapid onset (controversial, because EVS found no benefit with systemic antibiotics):

  Vancomycin (1 g IV q12h).

  Ceftazidime (1 g IV q12h).

Management—Cont'd

Delayed, Filtering Bleb Associated, Posttraumatic, and Endogenous

- EVS guidelines do not apply and treatment should be based on the clinical situation.

- Intravitreal antibiotics or steroids similar to acute postoperative guidelines (see above); amphotericin B (0.005 mg/0.1 mL) if endogenous fungal or delayed onset with presumed fungal etiology.

- Subconjunctival antibiotics or steroids similar to acute postoperative guidelines (see above).

- Topical broad spectrum fortified antibiotics similar to acute postoperative guidelines (see above); amphotericin B (1.0–2.5 mg/mL q1h) or natamycin (50 mg/mL q1h) if fungal.

- Topical steroid (prednisolone acetate 1% q1–2h initially) and cycloplegic (atropine 1% tid).

- Systemic intravenous antibiotics for marked inflammation similar to acute postoperative guidelines (see above); amphotericin B (0.25–1.0 mg/kg IV divided equally q6h) if disseminated fungal disease exists.

- Delayed postoperative endophthalmitis may require partial or total capsulectomy, pars plana vitrectomy, or IOL removal or exchange.

- Consider repeat tap (or pars plana vitrectomy) and intravitreal injections if clinical worsening after 48–72 hours.

- Adjust antibiotics based on culture results.

- **Vitreous tap and injection:** This procedure is performed under controlled aseptic conditions with sterile gloves and sterile field (or equivalent). The eye is anesthetized with either sterile cotton swabs soaked in 2% lidocaine, or a subconjunctival injection of 2% lidocaine in the quadrant of the procedure; some patients may require a peribulbar or even retrobulbar block. The eye and lids are prepped with providone iodine, chlorhexidine, or betadine, and a sterile wire lid speculum is placed. A 27-gauge needle on a 1 ml syringe is used to enter the anterior chamber at the limbus, avoiding the iris, and approximately 0.1 ml of aqueous humor and hypopyon is withdrawn. The appropriate distance posterior to the limbus for the vitreous tap and injection sites is measured with sterile calipers (3 mm for pseudophakic patients or 4 mm for phakic patients or use the hub of a 1 ml syringe). Then a 27-gauge needle on a 1 ml syringe is used to enter the posterior chamber at the preplaced mark so that the needle is in the midvitreous cavity, and approximately 0.1 ml of vitreous is withdrawn. Intravitreal injections with a 30-gauge needle attached to the syringes containing the antibiotics are immediately performed, and the injection sites are covered with a sterile cotton-tipped applicator to avoid vitreous exit. Subconjunctival injections should then be performed in the anesthetized quadrant. The aqueous and vitreous samples are immediately plated or sent to the microbiology lab for appropriate smears and cultures. Following the intravitreal injections, patients should be evaluated for possible increased intraocular pressure; this consists of ophthalmoscopy of the optic nerve head for ocular perfusion (if the view is clear) or tonometry.

Prognosis Depends on etiology, duration, and organism; usually poor, especially for traumatic cases.

Anterior Uveitis (Iritis, Iridocyclitis)

Definition Inflammation of the anterior uvea (iris [iritis] and ciliary body [cyclitis]) with exudation of white blood cells and protein into the anterior chamber secondary to breakdown of the blood–aqueous barrier and increased vascular permeability from a variety of disorders. Minimal spill-over into the retrolental space can be present. Classified by pathology (nongranulomatous [lymphocyte and plasma cell infiltrates] or granulomatous [epithelioid and giant cell infiltrates]), location (keratouveitis, sclerouveitis, anterior uveitis, intermediate uveitis, posterior uveitis, endophthalmitis, panuveitis), course (acute, chronic, recurrent), or etiology.

Etiology Most commonly idiopathic or autoimmune, but it is critical to rule out other causes such as infection, malignancy, medication, and trauma.

Infectious Anterior Uveitis

Herpes Simplex and Herpes Zoster Ophthalmicus

Acute or chronic, recurrent iritis, especially herpes zoster ophthalmicus (HZO); often with keratic precipitates underlying areas of dendritic or stromal keratitis; elevated intraocular pressure common; may have sector iris atrophy, corneal scarring, and decreased corneal sensation.

Lyme Disease

Patients have classic cutaneous erythema chronicum migrans at the site of a tick bite; due to *Borrelia burgdorferi* transmitted by *Ixodes dammini* or *I. pacificus* tick; 1–3 months later can develop neurologic involvement including encephalitis and meningitis. In addition to iritis, may also have conjunctivitis, keratitis, vitritis, and optic neuritis; may develop chronic skin changes, chronic arthritis, and cardiac manifestations.

Syphilis

Chronic or recurrent granulomatous anterior uveitis can be an ocular manifestation of acquired secondary syphilis; may also have interstitial keratitis, vitritis, chorioretinitis, papillitis, and mucocutaneous manifestations (see Chapters 5 and 10). This infection must be ruled out in every patient with persistent granulomatous iritis, because systemic antibiotics are necessary to prevent significant morbidity.

Tuberculosis

Chronic granulomatous iritis, may also have conjunctival nodules, phlyctenules, interstitial keratitis, scleritis, vitritis, and choroiditis (see Chapter 10). It is rarely caused by direct ocular infection of *Mycobacterium tuberculosis* and most of the time is an immune response directed toward the organism. Patients with a chronic granulomatous iritis who are immunocompromised or come from endemic areas should be evaluated for tuberculosis.

Noninfectious Anterior Uveitis

Nongranulomatous

Idiopathic (acute)

Most common cause of anterior uveitis (50%).

HLA-B27 associated (acute)

Recurrent iritis may affect one eye at a time. Accounts for up to 47% of anterior uveitis without an associated systemic condition; often male and tend to develop iritis at a younger age; distinct entity from the idiopathic form. Twenty-five percent have a seronegative spondyloarthropathy.

Seronegative spondyloarthropathies (acute)

Group of conditions sharing common features that include: radiographic sacroiliitis (with or without spondylitis), asymmetric peripheral arthritis without rheumatoid nodules, negative rheumatoid factor (RF) and antinuclear antibody (ANA), HLA-B27 association, variable mucocutaneous lesions, and anterior uveitis.

Ankylosing Spondylitis Thirty percent develop anterior uveitis, recurrent in 40%, also episcleritis and scleritis. Patients develop lower back pain and stiffness after inactivity; also associated with aortitis and pulmonary apical fibrosis; arthritis less severe in women, but eye disease can still be severe. Sacroiliac radiographs often show sclerosis and narrowing of joint spaces; untreated patients will progress to debilitating spinal fusion; 90% have positive HLA-B27 test results.

Reiter's Syndrome Triad of nonspecific urethritis, polyarthritis (80%), and mucopurulent, papillary conjunctivitis with iritis; arthritis starts within 30 days of infection; also associated with keratoderma blennorrhagicum, circinate balanitis, plantar fasciitis, Achilles tendonitis, sacroiliitis, palate or tongue ulcers, nail pitting, prostatitis, and cystitis. Occurs in males age 15–40 years old (90%); may be triggered by diarrhea or infectious organism (*Chlamydia, Ureaplasma, Yersinia, Shigella, Salmonella*); 85–95% have positive HLA-B27 test results.

Inflammatory Bowel Disease In contrast to the unilateral iritis associated with ankylosing spondylitis and Reiter's syndrome, the iritis associated with inflammatory bowel disease is usually bilateral and has a posterior component; may also develop dry eyes, conjunctivitis, episcleritis, scleritis, orbital cellulitis, and optic neuritis. Rare in Crohn's disease (2.4%), 5–10% in ulcerative colitis; associated with sacroiliitis, erythema nodosum, pyoderma gangrenosum, hepatitis, and sclerosing cholangitis; 60% of patients with sacroiliitis have positive HLA-B27 test results.

Psoriatic Arthritis Twenty percent develop iritis; also conjunctivitis and dry eyes. Patients have "sausage" digits from terminal phalangeal joint arthritic involvement, subungual hyperkeratosis, erythematous rash, nail pitting, and onycholysis; associated with sacroiliitis; iritis rarely occurs when psoriasis appears without arthritis; associated with HLA-B27.

Whipple's Disease Rare systemic disorder associated with *Tropheryma whippelii* infection, characterized by chronic diarrhea (due to malabsorption), joint inflammation, central nervous system manifestations, and anterior uveitis; associated with sacroiliitis, spondylitis, and HLA-B27.

Behçet's disease (acute)

Triad of recurrent hypopyon iritis, aphthous stomatitis, and genital ulcers; also develop arthritis, thromboembolism, and central nervous system problems; iritis is usually bilateral with posterior involvement, the hallmark is retinal vasculitis (see Chapter 10). More common in Asians and Middle Easterners; associated with HLA-B5 (subtypes Bw51 and B52) and HLA-B12.

Glaucomatocyclitic crisis (Posner-Schlossman syndrome) (acute)

Unilateral, mild, recurrent iritis with markedly elevated intraocular pressure, corneal edema, fine keratic precipitates, and a mid-dilated pupil; no synechiae; self-limited episodes (hours to days); associated with HLA-Bw54.

Kawasaki's disease (acute)

Exanthematous disease with bilateral conjunctivitis and anterior uveitis in children (see Chapter 4); may be fatal.

Drugs (acute)

Certain systemic medications may cause anterior uveitis, specifically rifabutin and cidofovir.

Interstitial nephritis (acute)

Usually bilateral, anterior uveitis that occurs more frequently in children, may have posterior involvement; female predilection. Patients have fever, malaise, arthralgias; urinalysis shows white blood cells without infection. May be due to allergic reaction to a nonsteroidal antiinflammatory or antibiotic; can progress to renal failure if not treated with oral steroids.

Other autoimmune disease (acute and chronic)

Systemic lupus erythematosus, relapsing polychondritis, and Wegener's granulomatosis.

Juvenile rheumatoid arthritis (acute and chronic)

Most common cause of uveitis in children, typically bilateral, anterior uveitis with minimal redness and pain. Type I is pauciarticular (90%), rheumatoid factor (RF) negative, antinuclear antibody (ANA) positive, female predilection (4:1), no sacroiliitis, and earlier onset (by age 4 years); type II is pauciarticular, RF negative, ANA negative, HLA-B27 positive, male predilection, sacroiliitis common, and later onset (by age 8 years); both have a chronic course with poor prognosis. Another subset is childhood spondyloarthropathy, which causes an acute, unilateral, self-limited, anterior uveitis; usually in males, older than 12 years, and HLA-B27 positive. Iritis is rare in polyarticular RF-negative JRA and Still's disease.

Fuchs' heterochromic iridocyclitis (chronic)

Accounts for 2% of anterior uveitis. Usually unilateral (90%), low-grade iritis with small, white, stellate keratic precipitates, fine vascularization of the angle, diffuse iris atrophy, and no synechiae; predilection for blue-eyed patients; iris of affected eye may be lighter; associated with glaucoma (15%) and cataracts (70%). Good prognosis; poor response to topical steroids (therefore, not indicated).

Figure 6-12 • Fuchs'
heterochromic iridocyclitis with fine,
white, stellate keratic precipitates.

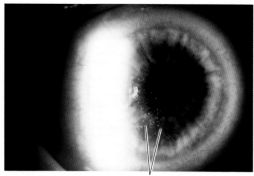

Keratic precipitates

Postoperative or trauma (acute or chronic)

Ocular injury including surgery produces variable anterior chamber inflammation, and must be distinguished from: exacerbation of preexisting uveitis, TASS, retained lens fragments, UGH syndrome, endophthalmitis, and sympathetic ophthalmia.

Granulomatous

Autoimmune

Sarcoidosis (see Chapter 10), Vogt–Koyanagi–Harada syndrome (see Chapter 10), sympathetic ophthalmia (see Chapter 10), Wegener's granulomatosis, multiple sclerosis, and lens-induced (phacoanaphylactic endophthalmitis; an immune-mediated [type 3] hypersensitivity reaction to lens particles after trauma or surgery causing a zonal granulomatous reaction after a latent period).

HLA Associations (Located on Chromosome 6)

A11   Sympathetic ophthalmia.

A29   Bird-shot retinochoroidopathy.

B5   Behçet's disease (also B12).

B7   Presumed ocular histoplasmosis syndrome, serpiginous choroidopathy, ankylosing spondylitis.

B8   Sjögren's syndrome.

B12   Ocular cicatricial pemphigoid.

B27   Ankylosing spondylitis (88%), Reiter's syndrome (85–95%), inflammatory bowel disease (60%), psoriatic arthritis (also B17).

Bw54 Posner-Schlossman syndrome.

DR4   Vogt-Koyanagi-Harada syndrome, ocular cicatricial pemphigoid.

Symptoms Pain, photophobia, tearing, red eye; may have decreased vision.

Signs Normal or decreased visual acuity, ciliary injection, miosis, anterior chamber cells and flare; may have fine (nongranulomatous) or mutton fat (granulomatous) keratic precipitates, keratitis, iris nodules (Koeppe, Busacca, Berlin; see Figures 7-40 and 7-41), increased or decreased intraocular pressure, peripheral anterior synechiae, posterior synechiae, hypopyon (especially HLA-B27 associated and Behçet's disease), cataract, vitritis, retinal or choroidal lesions, cystoid macular edema.

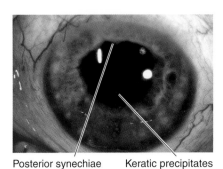

Posterior synechiae   Keratic precipitates

Figure 6-13 • Granulomatous uveitis demonstrating keratic precipitates and posterior synechiae.

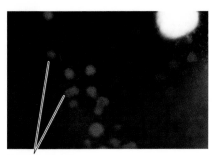

Keratic precipitates

Figure 6-14 • Close-up of granulomatous keratic precipitates.

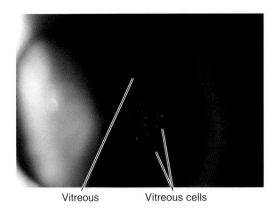

Vitreous   Vitreous cells

Figure 6-15 • Anterior vitreous cells are visible with fine slit-beam behind the lens. The cells are seen here as small white specks among vitreous strands.

Differential Diagnosis Masquerade syndromes: retinal detachment, retinoblastoma, malignant melanoma, leukemia, large cell lymphoma (reticulum cell sarcoma), juvenile xanthogranuloma, intraocular foreign body, anterior segment ischemia, ocular ischemic syndrome, and spill-over syndromes from any posterior uveitis (most commonly toxoplasmosis) (see Chapter 10).

Evaluation
• Complete ophthalmic history and eye exam with attention to corneal sensation, character of keratic precipitates, tonometry, anterior chamber, iris, vitreous cells, and ophthalmoscopy.
• Unilateral, nongranulomatous iritis is often idiopathic and treated without an extensive workup.

- If uveitis is recurrent, bilateral, granulomatous, or involving the posterior segment, consider workup as clinical examination and history dictate.

- **Lab tests**: Basic testing recommended for nongranulomatous anterior uveitis with a negative history, review of systems, and medical examination: complete blood count (CBC), erythrocyte sedimentation rate (ESR), Venereal Disease Research Laboratory (VDRL) test, fluorescent treponemal antibody absorption (FTA-ABS) test or microhemagglutination for treponema pallidum (MHA-TP) (syphilis), HLA-B27.

- **Other lab tests that should be ordered according to history and/or evidence of granulomatous inflammation:** ANA, RF (juvenile rheumatoid arthritis), serum lysozyme, angiotensin converting enzyme (ACE) (sarcoidosis), purified protein derivative (PPD) and controls (tuberculosis), herpes simplex and herpes zoster titers, enzyme-linked immunosorbent assay (ELISA) for Lyme immunoglobulin M and immunoglobulin G, human immunodeficiency virus (HIV) antibody test, chest radiographs (sarcoidosis, tuberculosis), chest CT scan (sarcoidosis), sacroiliac radiographs (ankylosing spondylitis), knee radiographs (juvenile rheumatoid arthritis, Reiter's syndrome), gallium scan (sarcoidosis), urinalysis (interstitial nephritis), and urethral cultures (Reiter's syndrome).

- **Special diagnostic lab tests**: HLA typing, antineutrophil cytoplasmic antibodies (ANCA) (Wegener's granulomatosis, polyarteritis nodosa), Raji cell and C1q binding assays for circulating immune complexes (systemic lupus erythematosus, systemic vasculitides), complement proteins: C3, C4, total complement (systemic lupus erythematosus, cryoglobulinemia, glomerulonephritis), soluble interleukin-2 receptor.

- Medical or rheumatology consultation.

Management

- Topical steroid (prednisolone acetate 1% up to q1h initially, then taper very slowly over weeks to months depending on etiology and response). Patients who are steroid responsive should still be treated with prednisolone acetate 1% initially and the intraocular pressure treated with ocular hypotensive agents, then consider switching to a steroid with less IOP-elevating potential (i.e., Lotemax, Alrex, Vexol, Pred Mild, FML). Some patients with HZO uveitis may require indefinite topical steroid treatment to prevent recurrence.

- Topical cycloplegic (scopolamine 0.25%, homatropine 2%, or atropine 1% bid to tid).

- May require treatment of increased intraocular pressure, especially glaucomatocyclitic crisis (see Primary Open Angle Glaucoma section in Chapter 11; do not use miotic agents or prostaglandin analogues).

- Systemic antibiotics for Lyme disease, tuberculosis, syphilis, Whipple's disease, and toxoplasmosis (see Chapter 10).

- Topical antiviral (trifluridine [Viroptic] 9 times/day) for herpes simplex infections with concomitant corneal epithelial involvement.

- Systemic antiviral (acyclovir [Zovirax] 800 mg 5 times/day for 7–10 days or famciclovir [Famvir] 500 mg po or valacyclovir [Valtrex] 1 g po tid for 7 days) for acute herpes zoster infection (see Chapter 3).

Continued

Management—Cont'd

- Consider oral steroids (prednisone 60–100 mg po qd for 1 week, then taper according to response) or orbital steroid injection (triamcinolone acetonide 40 mg/ml peribulbar q 2 weeks prn) for severe cases; check purified protein derivative (PPD) and controls, blood glucose, and chest radiographs before starting systemic steroids.

- Add H_2-blocker (ranitidine [Zantac] 150 mg po bid) or proton pump inhibitor when administering systemic steroids.

- Consider sub-Tenon's steroid injection (triamcinolone acetonide 40 mg/ml) or intravitreal steroid injection (triamcinolone acetonide 4 mg/0.1 ml) for resistant cases with associated cystoid macular edema. Biodegradable and nonerodable sustained release steroid implants may also be an option. Use with caution because of possible steroid response.

- If the uveitis becomes steroid dependent, does not respond or becomes refractory to steroids, or is vision threatening, then consider alternate agents:

  NSAIDs: diclofenac (Voltaren) 75 mg po bid or diflunisal (Dolobid) 250 mg po bid. Other nonselective NSAIDs that can be used as a second line of therapy include indomethacin (Indocin SR) 75 mg po bid or naproxen (Naprosyn) 250 mg po bid. In patients with a known history of gastritis or peptic ulceration, the use of COX-2 selective inhibitors should be considered (celecoxib (Celebrex) 100 mg po bid).

  Immunosuppressive chemotherapy: should be managed by a uveitis specialist or in coordination with a medical specialist familiar with these agents; indications include Behçet's disease, sympathetic ophthalmia, Vogt–Koyanagi–Harada syndrome, serpiginous choroidopathy, rheumatoid necrotizing scleritis or peripheral ulcerative keratitis, Wegener's granulomatosis, polyarteritis nodosa, relapsing polychondritis, juvenile rheumatoid arthritis, or sarcoidosis unresponsive to conventional therapy. Methotrexate is most commonly used first.

    Antimetabolites: azathioprine 1–3 mg/kg/day, methotrexate 0.15 mg/kg/day, mycophenolate mofetil (CellCept) 1–2 g po qd ("off-label" use for autoimmune ocular inflammatory diseases).

    Inhibitors of leukocyte signaling: cyclosporine 2.5–5.0 mg/kg/day, tacrolimus (Prograf) 0.1–0.15 mg/kg/day.

    Alkylating agents: cyclophosphamide 1–3 mg/kg/day, chlorambucil 0.1 mg/kg/day.

    Biologic agents: TNF-alpha inhibitors (infliximab [Remicade], etanercept [Enbrel], adalimumab [Humira]).

    Other agents: dapsone 25–50 mg bid or tid, colchicine 0.6 mg po bid for Behçet's disease is controversial.

- Lens extraction for phacoanaphylactic endophthalmitis.

Prognosis Depends on etiology; usually good if inflammation controlled. Poor if sequelae of chronic inflammation exist including cataract, glaucoma, posterior synechiae, band keratopathy, iris atrophy, cystoid macular edema, retinal detachment, retinal vasculitis, optic neuritis, neovascularization, hypotony, phthisis.

Uveitis-Glaucoma-Hyphema Syndrome

Definition Triad of findings in patients with closed-loop and rigid anterior chamber, iris-supported, or loose sulcus IOLs secondary to trauma to angle structures, iris, or ciliary body.

Symptoms Pain, photophobia, red eye, and decreased vision; may have constricted visual fields in late stages.

Signs Decreased visual acuity, increased intraocular pressure, anterior chamber cells and flare, hyphema, IOL implant; may have corneal edema, optic nerve cupping, retinal nerve fiber layer defects, and visual field defects.

Differential Diagnosis Neovascular glaucoma, trauma.

Evaluation
- Complete ophthalmic history and eye exam with attention to cornea, tonometry, anterior chamber, gonioscopy, iris, and ophthalmoscopy.
- Check visual fields.

Management

- Treatment of increased intraocular pressure (see Primary Open Angle Glaucoma section in Chapter 11; do not use miotic agents or prostaglandin analogues).
- Topical steroid (prednisolone acetate 1% up to q1h then taper slowly over weeks to months) and cycloplegic (scopolamine 0.25% tid or atropine 1% bid).
- Usually requires surgery for IOL removal or exchange; may require glaucoma surgery.

Prognosis Variable; depends on duration and extent of ocular damage; visual loss is permanent.

Trauma 257
Corectopia 261
Seclusio Pupillae 262
Peripheral Anterior Synechiae 263
Rubeosis Iridis 264
Neovascular Glaucoma 265
Pigment Dispersion Syndrome 266
Pigmentary Glaucoma 268
Iris Heterochromia 269
Anisocoria 271
Adie's Tonic Pupil 272
Argyll Robertson Pupil 274
Horner's Syndrome 275
Relative Afferent Pupillary Defect 277
Leukocoria 279
Congenital Anomalies 280
Mesodermal Dysgenesis Syndromes 282
Iridocorneal Endothelial Syndromes 285
Tumors 287

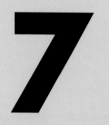

Iris and Pupils

Trauma

Definition

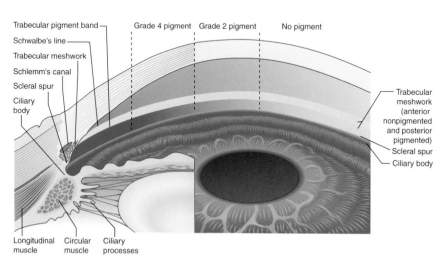

Figure 7-1 • Composite drawing of the microscopic and gonioscopic anatomy (reproduced with permission from Becker B, Shaffer RN: Diagnosis and Therapy of the Glaucomas. St. Louis, CV Mosby Co, 1965).

Angle Recession

Tear in ciliary body between longitudinal and circular muscle fibers. Appears as broad blue-gray band (ciliary body) on gonioscopy; associated with hyphema at time of injury. If more than two-thirds of the angle is involved, 10% develop glaucoma from scarring of angle structures.

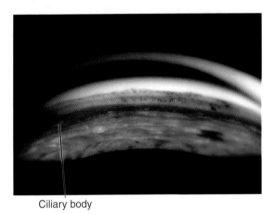

Figure 7-2 • Gonioscopic view of angle recession demonstrating deepened angle and blue-gray face of the ciliary body.

Ciliary body

Cyclodialysis

Disinsertion of ciliary body from scleral spur. Appears as broad white band (sclera) on gonioscopy; associated with hyphema at time of injury; may develop hypotony.

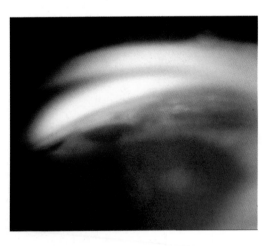

Figure 7-3 • Gonioscopic view of cyclodialysis demonstrating deepened angle and white face of the scleral spur.

Iridodialysis

Disinsertion of iris root from ciliary body. Appears as peripheral iris hole; associated with hyphema at time of injury.

Figure 7-4 • Iridodialysis. The iris is disinserted for approximately 90 degrees (from the 3 o'clock to 6 o'clock position).

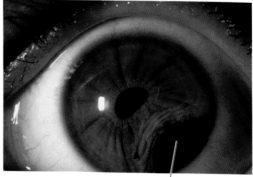

Iridodialysis

Sphincter Tears

Small radial iris tears at pupillary margin. May be associated with hyphema at time of injury; may result in permanent pupil dilation (traumatic mydriasis) and anisocoria.

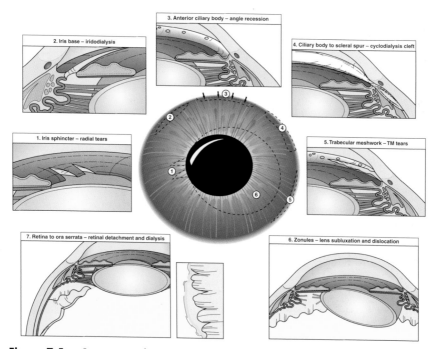

Figure 7-5 • Seven areas of traumatic ocular tears (shown in yellow) with the resultant findings. (Adapted from Campbell DG: Traumatic glaucoma. In Singleton BJ, Hersh PS, Kenyon KR [eds]: Eye Trauma, St. Louis, Mosby, 1991).

Symptoms Pain, photophobia, red eye; may have decreased vision, monocular diplopia or polyopia.

Signs Normal or decreased visual acuity, conjunctival injection, subconjunctival hemorrhage, anterior chamber cells and flare, hyphema, unusually deep anterior chamber, iris tears, abnormal pupil, angle tears, iridodonesis, increased or decreased intraocular pressure; may have other signs of ocular trauma including lid or orbital trauma, dislocated lens, phacodonesis, cataract, vitreous hemorrhage, commotio retinae, retinal tear or detachment, choroidal rupture, or traumatic optic neuropathy; may have signs of glaucoma with increased intraocular pressure, optic nerve cupping, nerve fiber layer defects, and visual field defects.

Differential Diagnosis See above, distinguish by careful gonioscopy; also, surgical iridectomy or iridotomy, iris coloboma, essential iris atrophy, Reiger's anomaly.

Evaluation
- Complete ophthalmic history and eye exam with attention to cornea, tonometry, iris, lens, and ophthalmoscopy.
- Check the angle with gonioscopy and rule out retinal tears or detachment with scleral depression if the globe is intact and there is no hyphema.
- B-scan ultrasonography if unable to visualize the fundus.
- Consider ultrasound biomicroscopy to evaluate angle structures and localize the injury.
- Rule out open globe and intraocular foreign body (see Chapter 4).

Management

- May require treatment of increased intraocular pressure (see Primary Open Angle Glaucoma section in Chapter 11).
- Treat other traumatic injuries as indicated.

ANGLE RECESSION
- Observe patients for angle-recession glaucoma.

CYCLODIALYSIS
- Consider surgical or laser reattachment for persistent hypotony.

IRIDODIALYSIS
- Consider cosmetic contact lens or surgical repair for disabling glare or diplopia/polyopia.

SPHINCTER TEARS
- No treatment required; consider cosmetic contact lens or surgical repair of dilated nonreactive pupil.

Prognosis Depends on amount of damage; poor when associated with angle recession glaucoma or chronic hypotony.

Corectopia

Definition Displaced, ectopic, or irregular pupil.

Etiology Mesodermal dysgenesis syndromes, iridocorneal endothelial (ICE) syndromes, chronic uveitis, trauma, postoperative, ectopia lentis et pupillae (corectopia associated with lens subluxation).

Symptoms Asymptomatic; may have glare or decreased vision.

Signs Normal or decreased visual acuity; distorted, malpositioned pupil.

Figure 7-6 • Corectopia demonstrating inferiorly displaced pupil.

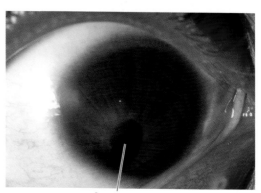

Corectopia

Evaluation
- Complete ophthalmic history and eye exam with attention to cornea, tonometry, anterior chamber, iris, and lens.
- Rule out open globe (peaked pupil after trauma, see Chapter 4).

Management

- No treatment recommended.
- May require treatment of iritis (see Chapter 6) or increased intraocular pressure (see Primary Open Angle Glaucoma section in Chapter 11).

Prognosis Depends on etiology and degree of malposition (distance from visual axis). Usually benign if mild, isolated, and non-progressive (i.e., postoperative). However, if associated with other findings or progressive, visual loss can occur.

Seclusio Pupillae

Definition Posterior synechiae (iris adhesions to the lens) at the pupillary border for 360°.

Etiology Inflammation (anterior uveitis, see Chapter 6).

Symptoms Asymptomatic; may have pain, red eye, and decreased vision.

Signs Normal or decreased visual acuity, posterior synechiae, poor or irregular pupil dilation, increased intraocular pressure, acute or chronic signs of iritis, including anterior chamber cells and flare, keratic precipitates, iris atrophy, iris nodules, cataract, and cystoid macular edema.

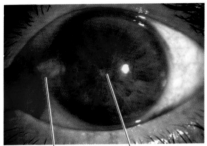

Pterygium   Seclusio pupillae

Figure 7-7 • Seclusio pupillae. The iris is completely bound down to the underlying cataractous lens visible as a white spot through the small pupil.

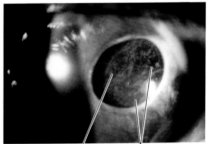

Occlusio pupillae   Neovascularization

Figure 7-8 • Occlusio pupillae with thin, white, fibrotic membrane and neovascularization covering the pupil.

Differential Diagnosis Occlusio pupillae (fibrotic membrane across the pupil), persistent pupillary membrane.

Evaluation
- Complete ophthalmic history and eye exam with attention to cornea, tonometry, anterior chamber, gonioscopy, iris, and ophthalmoscopy.
- Consider anterior uveitis workup (see Chapter 6).

Management

- Treat active uveitis and angle-closure glaucoma (see Chapter 6) if present.
- Consider laser iridotomy to prevent angle-closure glaucoma.

Prognosis Depends on etiology; poor if glaucoma has developed.

Peripheral Anterior Synechiae

Definition Peripheral iris adhesions to the cornea or angle structures; extensive PAS can cause increased intraocular pressure and angle-closure glaucoma.

Etiology Peripheral iridocorneal apposition due to previous pupillary block, flat or shallow anterior chamber, or inflammation.

Symptoms Asymptomatic; may have symptoms of angle-closure glaucoma (see Chapter 6).

Signs Iris adhesions to Schwalbe's line and cornea; may have signs of angle-closure glaucoma with increased intraocular pressure, optic nerve cupping, nerve fiber layer defects, and visual field defects.

Figure 7-9 • Peripheral anterior synechiae demonstrating a broad band of iris occluding the angle structures (area between arrowheads) as viewed with gonioscopy; also note that this patient has rubeosis with fine neovascularization.

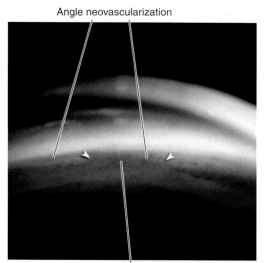

Angle neovascularization

Peripheral anterior synechiae

Differential Diagnosis Iris processes (mesodermal dysgenesis syndromes [see below]).

Evaluation
- Complete ophthalmic history and eye exam with attention to cornea, tonometry, anterior chamber, gonioscopy, iris, and ophthalmoscopy.
- Check visual fields in patients with elevated intraocular pressure or optic nerve cupping to rule out glaucoma.

Management

- May require treatment of increased intraocular pressure (see Primary Open Angle Glaucoma section in Chapter 11) or angle-closure glaucoma (see Chapter 6).
- Consider goniosynechiolysis for recent PAS (<12 months).

Prognosis Usually good; depends on extent of synechial angle closure and intraocular pressure control.

Rubeosis Iridis

Definition Neovascularization of the iris and angle.

Etiology Ocular ischemia; most commonly occurs with proliferative diabetic retinopathy, central retinal vein occlusion, and carotid occlusive disease; also associated with anterior segment ischemia, chronic retinal detachment, tumors, sickle cell retinopathy, chronic inflammation, and other rarer causes.

Symptoms Can be asymptomatic if no angle involvement; angle involvement may lead to neovascular glaucoma (see below) with decreased vision or other symptoms of angle-closure glaucoma (see Chapter 6).

Signs Normal or decreased visual acuity, abnormal blood vessels on iris and angle, particularly at pupillary margin and around iridectomies; may have spontaneous hyphema, or retinal lesions; may have signs of angle-closure glaucoma with increased intraocular pressure, optic nerve cupping, nerve fiber layer defects, and visual field defects.

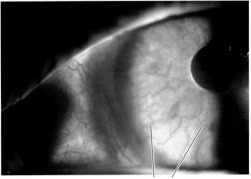

Rubeosis iridis

Figure 7-10 • Rubeosis iridis demonstrating florid neovascularization of the iris with large branching vessels.

Differential Diagnosis See above.

Evaluation
- Complete ophthalmic history and eye exam with attention to tonometry, gonioscopy, iris, and ophthalmoscopy.
- Check visual fields in patients with elevated intraocular pressure or optic nerve cupping to rule out glaucoma.
- Consider fluorescein angiogram to narrow differential diagnosis and determine cause of ocular ischemia if not apparent on direct examination.
- Consider medical consultation for systemic diseases including duplex and Doppler scans of carotid arteries to rule out carotid occlusive disease.

Management

- Topical steroid (prednisolone acetate 1% qid) and cycloplegic (atropine 1% bid) for inflammation.
- Usually requires laser photocoagulation for retinal ischemia if the cornea is clear; if the cornea is cloudy may require peripheral cryotherapy.
- Observe for neovascular glaucoma by monitoring intraocular pressure.
- May require treatment of increased intraocular pressure (see Primary Open Angle Glaucoma section in Chapter 11) and neovascular glaucoma (see below).

Prognosis
Poor; the rubeotic vessels may regress with appropriate therapy, but most causes of neovascularization are chronic progressive diseases.

Neovascular Glaucoma

Definition A form of secondary angle-closure glaucoma in which neovascularization of the iris and angle causes occlusion of the trabecular meshwork.

Etiology Any cause of rubeosis iridis (see above).

Symptoms Decreased vision and symptoms of angle-closure glaucoma (see Chapter 6).

Signs Decreased visual acuity; abnormal blood vessels on iris and angle, particularly at pupillary margin and around iridectomies; increased intraocular pressure, optic nerve cupping, nerve fiber layer defects, and visual field defects; may have corneal edema, spontaneous hyphema, or retinal lesions.

Differential Diagnosis As for rubeosis iridis (see above), and other forms of secondary angle-closure glaucoma (see Chapter 6).

Evaluation
- Complete ophthalmic history and eye exam with attention to cornea, tonometry, anterior chamber, gonioscopy, iris, and ophthalmoscopy.
- Check visual fields.
- Consider fluorescein angiogram to narrow differential diagnosis and determine cause of ocular ischemia if not apparent on direct examination.
- Consider medical consultation for systemic diseases, including duplex and Doppler scans of carotid arteries to rule out carotid occlusive disease.

Management

- Topical steroid (prednisolone acetate 1% qid) and cycloplegic (atropine 1% bid) for inflammation.
- Choice and order of topical glaucoma medications depend on many factors, including patient's age, intraocular pressure level and control, and amount and progression of optic nerve cupping and visual field defects. Treatment options are presented in the Primary Open-Angle Glaucoma section (see Chapter 11); more resistant to treatment than primary open-angle glaucoma.
- Usually requires laser photocoagulation for retinal ischemia if the cornea is clear; if the cornea is cloudy may require peripheral cryotherapy.
- Neovascular glaucoma with elevated intraocular pressure despite maximal medical therapy may require glaucoma filtering surgery, a glaucoma drainage implant, or a cyclodestructive procedure.

Prognosis Poor; the rubeotic vessels may regress with appropriate therapy, but most causes of neovascularization are chronic progressive diseases.

Pigment Dispersion Syndrome

Definition Liberation of pigment from the iris with subsequent accumulation on anterior segment structures.

Etiology Chafing of posterior iris surface on zonules produces pigment dispersion.

Epidemiology More common in 20- to 50-year-old Caucasian men and in patients with myopia; affected women are usually older; associated with lattice degeneration in 20% of cases and retinal detachment in up to 5% of cases; 25–50% develop pigmentary glaucoma. Mapped to chromosome 7q35–q36 (GLC1F gene).

Symptoms Asymptomatic; exercise or pupil dilation can cause pigment release with acute elevation of intraocular pressure and symptoms including halos around lights and blurred vision.

Signs Radial, midperipheral, iris transillumination defects, pigment on corneal endothelium (Krukenberg spindle), posterior bowing of midperipheral iris, dark pigment band overlying trabecular meshwork, pigment in iris furrows and on anterior lens capsule; may have signs of glaucoma with increased intraocular pressure, optic nerve cupping, nerve fiber layer defects, and visual field defects (see below); may have pigmented anterior chamber cells, especially following pupil dilation.

Differential Diagnosis Uveitis, albinism, pseudoexfoliation syndrome, iris atrophy.

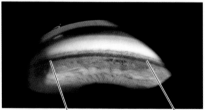

Pigment on TM   Pigment deposition

Figure 7-11 • Pigment dispersion syndrome demonstrating pigment deposition on the trabecular meshwork that appears as a dark brown band when viewed with gonioscopy.

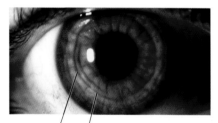

Pigment deposition

Figure 7-12 • Pigment dispersion syndrome demonstrating pigment deposition in concentric rings on the iris surface.

Figure 7-13 • Pigment dispersion syndrome demonstrating radial, midperipheral, slit-like iris transillumination defects for 360°.

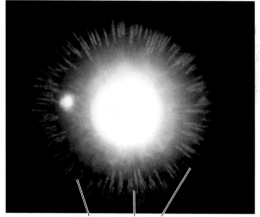

Transillumination defects

Evaluation

- Complete ophthalmic history and eye exam with attention to cornea, tonometry, anterior chamber, gonioscopy, the pattern of iris transillumination, lens, and ophthalmoscopy.
- Check visual fields in patients with elevated intraocular pressure or optic nerve cupping to rule out glaucoma.

Management

- Observe for pigmentary glaucoma by monitoring intraocular pressure.
- May require treatment of increased intraocular pressure (see Primary Open Angle Glaucoma section in Chapter 11) and pigmentary glaucoma (see below).

Prognosis Usually good; poorer if pigmentary glaucoma develops.

Pigmentary Glaucoma

Definition A form of secondary open-angle glaucoma caused by pigment liberated from the posterior iris surface (i.e., a sequela of uncontrolled increased intraocular pressure in pigment dispersion syndrome).

Epidemiology Develops in 25% to 50% of patients with pigment dispersion syndrome; same associations as in pigment dispersion syndrome (see above). Mapped to chromosome 7q35–q36 (GLC1F gene).

Mechanism Obstruction of the trabecular meshwork by dispersed pigment and pigment-laden macrophages.

Symptoms Asymptomatic; may have decreased vision or constricted visual fields in late stages; exercise or pupil dilation can cause pigment release with acute elevation of intraocular pressure and symptoms including halos around lights and blurred vision.

Signs Normal or decreased visual acuity, large fluctuations in intraocular pressure (especially with exercise); similar ocular signs as in pigment dispersion syndrome (see above), optic nerve cupping, nerve fiber layer defects, and visual field defects.

Differential Diagnosis Primary open-angle glaucoma, other forms of secondary open-angle glaucoma.

Evaluation
- Complete ophthalmic history and eye exam with attention to cornea, tonometry, anterior chamber, gonioscopy, iris, lens, and ophthalmoscopy.
- Check visual fields.
- Stereo optic nerve photos are useful for comparison at subsequent evaluations.

Management

- Choice and order of topical glaucoma medications depend on many factors, including patient's age, intraocular pressure level and control, and amount and progression of optic nerve cupping and visual field defects. Treatment options are presented in the Primary Open-Angle Glaucoma section (see Chapter 11).
- Consider initial treatment with pilocarpine 1–4% qid to minimize iris contact with lens zonules.
- Laser trabeculoplasty is effective, but action may be short lived.
- If posterior bowing of the iris exists, then consider laser peripheral iridotomy to alter iris configuration and minimize pigment liberation.
- May require glaucoma filtering surgery if medical treatment fails.

Prognosis Poorer than primary open-angle glaucoma.

Iris Heterochromia

Definition

Heterochromia Iridis

Unilateral; single iris with two colors (iris bicolor).

Figure 7-14 • Heterochromia iridis. The iris is bicolored.

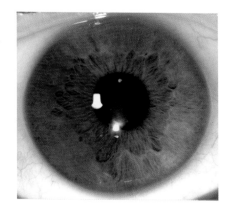

Heterochromia Iridum

Bilateral; irises are different colors (e.g., one blue, one brown).

Figure 7-15 • Heterochromia iridum. The patient's right iris is blue and the left iris is hazel.

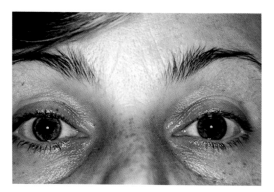

Etiology

Congenital

Hypochromic (involved eye lighter)

Congenital Horner's syndrome, Waardenburg's syndrome, Hirschsprung's disease, Perry-Romberg hemifacial atrophy.

Hyperchromic (involved eye darker)

Ocular or oculodermal melanocytosis, iris pigment epithelium hamartoma.

Acquired

Hypochromic

Acquired Horner's syndrome, juvenile xanthogranuloma, metastatic carcinoma, Fuchs' heterochromic iridocyclitis, stromal atrophy (glaucoma or inflammation).

Hyperchromic

Siderosis, hemosiderosis, chalcosis, medication (topical prostaglandin analogues for glaucoma), iris nevus or melanoma, iridocorneal endothelial syndrome, iris neovascularization.

Symptoms Usually asymptomatic; depends on etiology.

Signs Iris heterochromia; blepharoptosis, miosis, and anhidrosis in Horner's syndrome; white forelock, premature graying, leucism (cutaneous hypopigmentation), facial anomalies, dystopia canthorum, and deafness in Waardenburg's syndrome; skin, scleral, and choroidal pigmentation in ocular or oculodermal melanocytosis; anterior chamber cells and flare, keratic precipitates, and increased intraocular pressure in uveitis, siderosis, and chalcosis; may have intraocular foreign body (siderosis, chalcosis), old hemorrhage (hemosiderosis), or tumor.

Differential Diagnosis See above.

Evaluation
- Complete ophthalmic history and eye exam with attention to cornea, tonometry, anterior chamber, gonioscopy, iris, and ophthalmoscopy.
- Consider B-scan ultrasonography if unable to visualize the fundus.
- Consider orbital computed tomography (CT) scan or radiographs to rule out intraocular foreign bodies.
- Consider electroretinogram (ERG) to evaluate retinal function in siderosis, hemosiderosis, and chalcosis.
- Consider medical consultation.

Management

- Most forms do not require treatment.
- May require treatment of active uveitis (see Chapter 6), increased intraocular pressure (see Primary Open Angle Glaucoma section in Chapter 11), or malignancy (see Tumor section).
- Intraocular foreign body may require surgical removal.

Prognosis Depends on etiology.

Anisocoria

Definition Inequality in the size of the pupils.

Etiology

Greater Anisocoria in Dark (Abnormal Pupil is Smaller)

Horner's syndrome, Argyll Robertson pupil, iritis, pharmacologic (miotic agent, narcotic, insecticide).

Greater Anisocoria in Light (Abnormal Pupil is Larger)

Adie's tonic pupil, cranial nerve III palsy, Hutchinson's pupil (uncal herniation with cranial nerve III entrapment in a comatose patient), pharmacologic (mydriatic, cycloplegic, cocaine, hallucinogen), iris damage (traumatic, ischemic, or surgical).

Anisocoria Equal in Light and Dark

Physiologic (difference in pupil size ≤ 1 mm, and proportion of pupil areas is constant in all lighting).

Epidemiology Up to 20% of population has physiologic anisocoria; may fluctuate, be intermittent, and even reverse.

Symptoms Asymptomatic; may have glare, pain, photophobia, diplopia, or blurred vision, depending on etiology.

Signs Involved pupil may be larger or smaller, round or irregular, reactive or nonreactive; may constrict to accommodation but not to light (light-near dissociation; found in Adie's tonic pupil and Argyll Robertson pupil); may have ptosis and limitation of extraocular movements (cranial nerve III palsy); may have other signs depending on etiology.

Figure 7-16 • Anisocoria demonstrating larger pupil of the right eye.

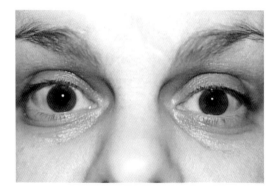

Evaluation

- Complete ophthalmic history and eye exam with attention to pupils (size in light and dark, pupil response to light and near), lids, motility, and iris.
- Gonioscopy and tonometry in traumatic cases to assess associated angle structure damage.
- **Greater anisocoria in dark (abnormal pupil is smaller)**: Pharmacologic pupil testing (*Note:* testing must be performed before cornea has been manipulated; i.e., before any drops, applanation, or other tests have been performed; otherwise the test may be invalid):

  (1) Topical cocaine 4–10% in each eye: after 40 minutes equal dilation = simple anisocoria; increased asymmetry = Horner's syndrome (see below).

  (2) Topical hydroxyamphetamine 1% (Paredrine): equal dilation = central or preganglionic Horner's syndrome; asymmetric dilation = postganglionic Horner's syndrome.

  Note: tests cannot be performed on the same day or will be invalid.
- **Greater anisocoria in light (abnormal pupil is larger)**: Pharmacologic pupil testing:

  (1) Topical pilocarpine 0.1% or methacholine 2.5%: constricts = Adie's tonic pupil (see below); no constriction = go to #2.

  (2) Topical pilocarpine 1%: constricts = cranial nerve III palsy; no constriction = pharmacologic dilation.
- **Lab tests:** Venereal Disease Research Laboratory (VDRL) test and fluorescent treponemal antibody absorption (FTA-ABS) test for syphilis (Argyll Robertson pupil).
- Lumbar puncture for VDRL, FTA-ABS, total protein, and cell counts to rule out neurosyphilis (Argyll Robertson pupil).
- Consider head, neck, or chest CT scan or magnetic resonance imaging (MRI) to rule out masses and vascular anomalies (Horner's syndrome, cranial nerve III palsy).
- May require medical consultation.

Management

- May require treatment of underlying etiology.
- Consider iris repair in traumatic cases.

Prognosis Often benign; depends on etiology.

Adie's Tonic Pupil

Definition Idiopathic, benign form of internal ophthalmoplegia.

Etiology Denervation hypersensitivity due to a lesion in the ciliary ganglion or short posterior ciliary nerves with receptor upregulation.

Epidemiology Usually occurs in 20–40-year-old women (90%); 80% unilateral (may become bilateral over time).

Symptoms Asymptomatic; may have blurred near vision and photophobia.

Signs In the acute stage, anisocoria greater in light than dark, dilated pupil with poor light response, segmental palsy with vermiform (worm-like) movements, slow or tonic near response (constriction and redilation), poor accommodation, light-near dissociation; 70% have decreased deep tendon reflexes (Adie's syndrome). In the chronic stage, the pupil often becomes small and poorly reactive. Similar pupillary findings may be associated with systemic autonomic dysfunction (Riley-Day Syndrome).

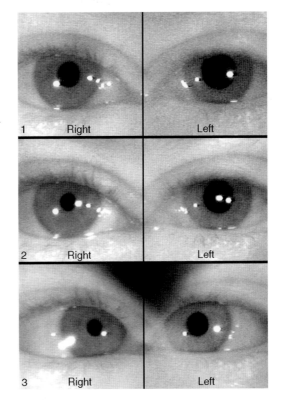

Figure 7-17 • Adie's pupil with light-near dislocation. (1) Anisocoria is evident in room light. (2) In bright light the normal right pupil constricts, but the left pupil responds poorly. (3) On near testing, the affected pupil responds better than to light.

Differential Diagnosis Iris ischemia or trauma, pupil-involving partial cranial nerve III palsy (almost always has oculomotor signs), botulism, and any cause of light-near dissociation (unilateral total afferent visual loss, Argyll Robertson pupil, dorsal midbrain syndrome, aberrant regeneration of cranial nerve III, diabetes mellitus, amyloidosis, sarcoidosis).

Evaluation
- Complete ophthalmic history, neurologic exam, and eye exam with attention to pupils (size in light and dark, pupil response to light and near), iris, and deep tendon reflexes.
- Pharmacologic testing with topical pilocarpine 0.1% or methacholine 2.5% (see Anisocoria section): Adie's tonic pupil constricts (normal does not) due to cholinergic supersensitivity; false-positive test result may occur in cranial nerve III palsy. (If recent onset, no response to dilute pilocarpine may be seen.)

Management

- No treatment recommended.

Prognosis Good; accommodative paresis is usually temporary (months).

Argyll Robertson Pupil

Definition Small, irregular pupil that reacts briskly to near (accommodation), but not to light; usually bilateral and asymmetric.

Etiology Associated with tertiary syphilis; thought to be due to damage to central pupillary pathways from the retina to the Edinger–Westphal nucleus in the midbrain.

Symptoms Asymptomatic.

Signs Miotic, irregular pupils, light-near dissociation (no reaction to light but normal near response (accommodation)), poor dilation; may have anisocoria (usually greater in dark than light), may have stigmata of congenital syphilis (e.g., Hutchinson's triad, fundus changes, skeletal deformities).

Differential Diagnosis Argyll Robertson-like pupils occur in diabetes mellitus (particulary after panretinal photocoagulation due to damage to the long ciliary nerves), alcoholism, multiple sclerosis, sarcoidosis.

Evaluation
- Complete ophthalmic history, neurologic exam, and eye exam with attention to pupils, iris, and ophthalmoscopy.
- **Lab tests**: VDRL, FTA-ABS.
- Lumbar puncture for VDRL, FTA-ABS, total protein, and cell counts to rule out neurosyphilis.
- Medical consultation.

Management

- If neurosyphilis present, treat with systemic penicillin G (2.4 million U IV q4h for 10–14 days, then 2.4 million U IM q week for 3 weeks), or tetracycline for penicillin-allergic patients.
- Follow serum VDRL to monitor treatment efficacy.

Prognosis Pupil abnormality itself is benign; poor for untreated tertiary syphilis.

Horner's Syndrome

Definition Group of findings that occurs in oculosympathetic paresis. Sympathetic damage may occur anywhere along the three-neuron pathway:

Central (first-order neuron)

Hypothalamus to ciliospinal center of Budge (C8–T2).

Preganglionic (second-order neuron)

Spinal cord to superior cervical ganglion.

Postganglionic (third-order neuron)

Along carotid artery to cranial nerve V and VI to orbit and finally to iris dilator muscle.

Etiology Failure of sympathetic nervous system to dilate affected pupil and to stimulate Müller's muscle in the upper eyelid and smooth muscle fibers of the lower eyelid.

Central

Cerebrovascular accident, neck trauma, tumor, demyelinating disease (rarely causes isolated Horner's syndrome).

Preganglionic

Pancoast's tumor, mediastinal mass, cervical rib, neck trauma, abscess, thyroid tumor, after thyroid or neck surgery.

Postganglionic

Neck lesion, head trauma, migraine, cavernous sinus lesion, carotid dissection, carotid-cavernous fistula, internal carotid artery aneurysm, nasopharyngeal carcinoma, vascular disease, infections (complicated otitis media). Congenital Horner's syndrome is usually due to birth trauma (brachial plexus injury during delivery).

Symptoms Asymptomatic; may have droopy eyelid, blurred vision, pain (especially with vascular postganglionic etiologies), and other symptoms depending on site and cause of lesion (central usually has other neurologic deficits). Initially, ipsilateral nasal stuffiness may occur.

Signs Triad of mild (1–2 mm) ptosis, miosis, and anhidrosis (anhidrosis usually indicates preganglionic lesion), anisocoria greater in dark than light (abnormal pupil is smaller and dilates poorly in the dark), upside-down ptosis (lower lid elevation), decreased intraocular pressure (1–2 mmHg lower in the involved eye), in congenital cases heterochromia iridum (iris on involved side is lighter). Initially, ipsilateral conjunctival hyperemia; may have cranial nerve VI palsy (localizes the lesion to the cavernous sinus).

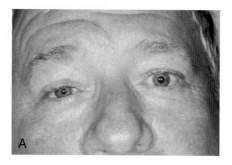

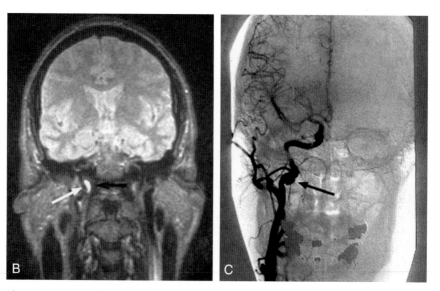

Figure 7-18 • (A) Patient with acute right Horner syndrome illustrating miosis and ptosis of the right eye. The dissection of the internal carotid artery is shown on (B) the magnetic resonance imaging scan and (C) angiogram (arrows).

Evaluation

- Complete ophthalmic history, neurologic exam, and eye exam, with attention to lids, motility, pupils, and iris.
- Pharmacologic pupil testing (*Note:* testing must be performed before cornea has been manipulated; i.e., before any drops, applanation, or other tests have been performed; otherwise the test result will be invalid):
  - (1) Topical cocaine 4–10% (place 2 drops in each eye, remeasure pupil after 30 minutes): determines presence of Horner's syndrome (normal pupil dilates; pupil does not dilate as well in patient with Horner's syndrome).
  - (2) Topical hydroxyamphetamine 1% (Paredrine): distinguishes between preganglionic (first-order and second-order neurons) and postganglionic (third-order neuron) lesions (pupil in patient with central or preganglionic Horner's syndrome dilates equal to normal pupil; pupil in postganglionic Horner's syndrome does not dilate as well); this test does not determine whether a preganglionic lesion affects the first-order or second-order neuron.

  Note: tests cannot be performed on the same day or will be invalid.
- In an infant with Horner's syndrome, consider evaluation for neuroblastoma with an MRI of the sympathetic chain from the hypothalamus down to the upper thoracic area and back up the neck to the cavernous sinus and orbit. If positive, additional workup includes, checking urine for vanillylmandelic acid and homovanillic acid and further imaging of the abdomen.
- Patients with a central or pre-ganglionic Horner's syndrome may have neck pain, shoulder pain, or abnormal taste in the mouth or other neurological signs, and should have an MRI of the sympathetic chain.
- Smokers should have a chest radiograph to rule out Pancoast's tumor.

Management

- Treat underlying etiology.
- Consider ptosis repair.

Prognosis Depends on etiology; postganglionic lesions are usually benign; most isolated Horner's syndrome without other findings are benign; preganglionic and central lesions are usually more serious.

Relative Afferent Pupillary Defect (Marcus Gunn Pupil)

Definition During the swinging flashlight test (see below), pupillary dilation of the affected eye when the light is on it due to the relatively lower amount of light perceived by the affected eye compared to the contralateral eye. In other words, the pupil of the affected eye constricts more from the consensual response when the light is on the contralateral eye than from the response from direct light.

Etiology Asymmetric optic nerve disease or widespread retinal damage. Most common causes include any optic neuropathy, optic neuritis, central retinal vein or artery occlusion, and retinal detachment. A mild relative afferent pupillary defect (RAPD) may rarely occur with a dense ocular media opacity, including vitreous hemorrhage and cataract (occasionally, a cataract may cause a contralateral RAPD because of light scatter to more retinal area); a very small RAPD may occur with amblyopia; optic tract lesions can cause a contralateral RAPD (due to more nasal crossing fibers in the chiasm).

Symptoms Decreased vision, dyschromatopsia, diminished sense of brightness.

Signs RAPD, decreased visual acuity, color vision, and contrast sensitivity; red desaturation; visual field defect; may have swollen or pale optic nerve, or retinal findings. A "reverse" RAPD can be detected even in an eye that is non-reactive because the contralateral eye will constrict more from response to direct light than from the consensual response when the light is on the affected eye.

NORMAL   DEFECT

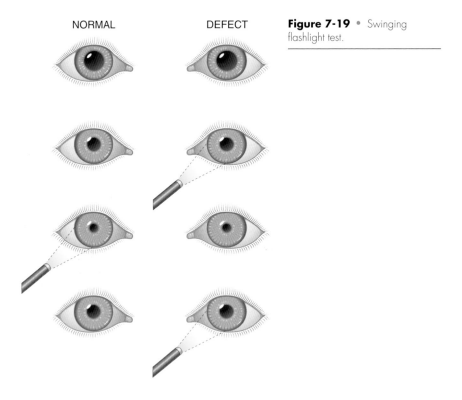

Figure 7-19 • Swinging flashlight test.

Differential Diagnosis Hippus (benign, rhythmic, variation in pupil size; more common in younger individuals).

Evaluation
• Complete ophthalmic history and eye exam with attention to visual acuity, color vision, pupils, iris, and ophthalmoscopy.

- **Swinging flashlight test:** Bright light is shined into one eye and then rapidly into the other in an alternating fashion; positive test result is when the pupil that the light is shined into dilates instead of constricts. When the pupil of the involved eye is nonreactive or nonfunctional, observe the fellow, normal eye for a "reverse" RAPD (dilation when light is on nonreactive eye, constriction when light is shined on reactive eye).
- Grading system with neutral density filters or 1+ to 4+ scale.

Management

- Treat underlying etiology.

Prognosis Depends on etiology.

Leukocoria

Definition Variety of disorders that cause the pupil to appear white; usually noted in infancy or early childhood.

Symptoms Decreased vision; may notice white pupil, eye turn, or abnormal size of eye.

Signs Leukocoria, decreased visual acuity; may have RAPD, nystagmus, strabismus, buphthalmos, microphthalmos, anterior chamber cells and flare, increased intraocular pressure, cataract, vitritis, retinal detachment, tumor, or other retinal findings; may have systemic findings.

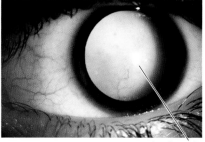
Leukocoria

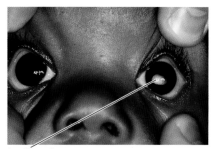
Leukocoria

Figure 7-20 • Leukocoria in a patient with toxocariasis. The large white reflex in the dilated pupil represents the retina; a retinal vessel is visible.

Figure 7-21 • Leukocoria due to retinoblastoma in the left eye. The white pupil in the left eye is strikingly evident in comparison with the normal (black) pupil of the fellow eye.

Differential Diagnosis Cataract, retinoblastoma, retinopathy of prematurity, persistent hyperplastic primary vitreous, Coats' disease, toxocariasis, toxoplasmosis, retinal/choroidal/optic nerve coloboma, myelinated nerve fibers, Norrie's disease, retinal dysplasia, cyclitic membrane, retinal detachment, incontinentia pigmenti, retinoschisis, and medulloepithelioma.

Evaluation

- Complete ophthalmic history and eye exam with attention to retinoscopy, pupils, tonometry, anterior chamber, lens, vitreous cells, and ophthalmoscopy.
- B-scan ultrasonography to evaluate retrolenticular area, vitreous, and retina if unable to visualize the fundus.
- Consider orbital radiograph, and head and orbital CT scans or MRI to rule out foreign body.
- Pediatric consultation.

Management

- Treat underlying etiology.

Prognosis Usually poor in the pediatric population; good with surgery if due to a mature white cataract in an adult.

Congenital Anomalies

Aniridia

Absence of the iris, except for a small, hypoplastic remnant or stump. Patients also have photophobia, nystagmus, glare, decreased visual acuity, amblyopia, and strabismus; associated with glaucoma in 28–50%, lens opacities in 50–85%, ectopia lentis, corneal pannus, and foveal hypoplasia. Occurs in 1:100,000 births; mapped to chromosome 11p. Three forms:

AN 1 (Autosomal Dominant)

Eighty-five percent of cases; only ocular findings.

AN 2

Thirteen percent of cases; includes Miller's syndrome with both aniridia and Wilms' tumor, and WAGR (Wilms' tumor, aniridia, genitourinary abnormalities, and mental retardation). Sporadic, but mapped to chromosome 11p (PAX6 gene).

AN 3 (Autosomal Recessive)

Two percent of cases; associated with mental retardation and cerebellar ataxia (Gillespie's syndrome); do not develop Wilms' tumor.

- May require treatment of increased intraocular pressure (see Primary Open Angle Glaucoma section in Chapter 11).
- May require cyclocryotherapy or glaucoma filtering surgery if medical treatment fails.
- Lensectomy if visually significant cataract develops; consider use of artificial iris segments.
- Consider painted contact lens to decrease photophobia or glare.

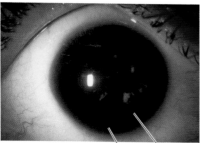

Aniridia Lens equator

Figure 7-22 • Aniridia with entire cataractous lens visible. The inferior edge of the lens is visible.

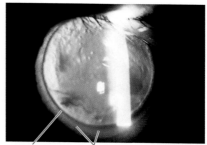

Lens equator   Zonules

Figure 7-23 • Aniridia with the lens equator and zonules visible on retroillumination.

Coloboma

Iris sector defect due to incomplete closure of the embryonic fissure. Usually located inferiorly; may have other colobomata (lid, lens, retina, choroid, optic nerve); associated with multiple genetic syndromes, including trisomy 22 (cat-eye syndrome), trisomy 18, trisomy 13, and chromosome 18 deletion.

Figure 7-24 • Coloboma of inferior iris.

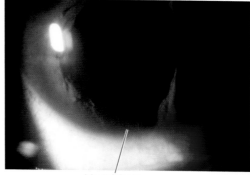

Iris coloboma

Persistent Pupillary Membrane

Benign, embryonic, mesodermal remnants (tunica vasculosa lentis) that appear as thin iris strands bridging the pupil. Most common ocular congenital anomaly; occurs in up to 80% of dark eyes and 35% of light eyes. Two types:

Type 1

Attached only to the iris.

Type 2

Iridolenticular adhesions.

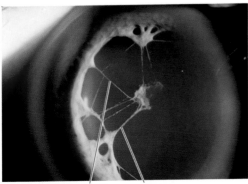

Figure 7-25 • Persistent pupillary membrane type 2 demonstrating multiple iris strands adhering to the anterior lens surface.

Type 2 persistent pupillary membrane

- No treatment required.
- If iris strands cross visual axis and are affecting vision, consider Nd:YAG (neodymium: yttrium-aluminum-garnet) laser treatment.

Plateau Iris (Configuration or Syndrome)

Atypical iris configuration (flat contour with steep insertion due to anteriorly rotated ciliary processes; anterior chamber is deep centrally and s-----hallow peripherally). Familial, more common in young, myopic women; 5–8% develop angle-closure glaucoma (plateau iris syndrome) (see Chapter 6).

- May require treatment of increased intraocular pressure (see Primary Open Angle Glaucoma section in Chapter 11).
- Consider miotic agents (pilocarpine 1% qid) or iridoplasty.

Mesodermal Dysgenesis Syndromes

Definition Group of bilateral, congenital, hereditary disorders involving anterior segment structures. Originally thought to be due to faulty cleavage of angle structures and, therefore, termed *angle cleavage syndromes*.

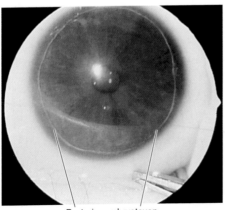

Figure 7-26 • Posterior embryotoxon can be clearly seen as a white ring in the peripheral cornea.

Posterior embryotoxon

Axenfeld's Anomaly

Posterior embryotoxon (anteriorly displaced Schwalbe's line that appears as a prominent, white, corneal line anterior to the limbus; occurs in 15% of normal individuals) and prominent iris processes; associated with secondary glaucoma in 50% of patients. Mapped to chromosome 4q25 (PITX2 gene), 6p25 (FOXC1 gene), 13q14 (RIEG2 gene).

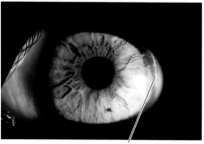

Posterior embryotoxon

Figure 7-27 • Axenfeld's anomaly with abnormal iris (extensive stromal atrophy) and posterior embryotoxon.

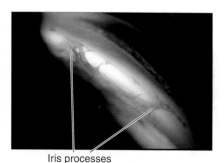

Iris processes

Figure 7-28 • Gonioscopic view of Axenfeld's anomaly demonstrating iris adhesions to the cornea.

Alagille's Syndrome

Axenfeld's anomaly and pigmentary retinopathy, corectopia, esotropia, and systemic abnormalities, including absent deep tendon reflexes, abnormal facies, pulmonic valvar stenosis, peripheral arterial stenosis, and skeletal abnormalities. Abnormal electroretinogram and electro-oculogram. Mapped to chromosome 20p12 (mutation in the JAG1 gene, a NOTCH receptor ligand).

Rieger's Anomaly

Axenfeld's anomaly and iris hypoplasia with holes; associated with secondary glaucoma in 50% of patients. Mapped to chromosome 4q25 (PITX2 gene), 6p25 (FOXC1 gene), 13q14 (RIEG2 gene).

Rieger's Syndrome

Combination of Rieger's anomaly with mental retardation and systemic abnormalities, including dental, craniofacial, genitourinary, and skeletal problems. Mapped to chromosome 4q25 (PITX2 gene), 6p25 (FOXC1 gene), 13q14 (RIEG2 gene).

Figure 7-29 • Dental abnormalities in patient with Rieger's syndrome.

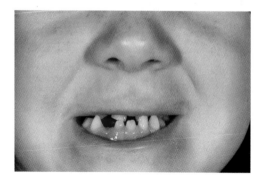

Peters' Anomaly

Corneal leukoma (white opacity due to central defect in Descemet's membrane and absence of endothelium) and iris adhesions with or without cataract. Usually sporadic; 80% bilateral; associated with secondary glaucoma in 50% of patients, congenital cardiac defects, cleft lip or palate, craniofacial dysplasia, and skeletal abnormalities. Mapped to chromosome 11p (PAX6 gene).

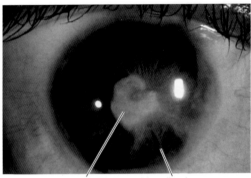

Figure 7-30 • Peters' anomaly demonstrating central, white, corneal opacity (leukoma).

Corneal leukoma   Iris adhesions

Symptoms Asymptomatic; may have decreased vision or iris abnormalities or a white spot on eye.

Signs Normal or decreased visual acuity, iris and cornea lesions (see above); may have systemic abnormalities and signs of glaucoma, including increased intraocular pressure, optic nerve cupping, and visual field defects.

Differential Diagnosis Iridocorneal endothelial syndromes, posterior polymorphous dystrophy, aniridia, coloboma, ectopia lentis et pupillae, iridodialysis, iridoschisis, trauma, corneal ulcer, hydrops.

Evaluation
- Complete ophthalmic history and eye exam with attention to cornea, tonometry, anterior chamber, gonioscopy, iris, lens, and ophthalmoscopy.
- Check visual fields in patients with elevated intraocular pressure or optic nerve cupping to rule out glaucoma.
- B-scan ultrasonography in Peters' anomaly if unable to visualize the fundus.

Management

- Often no treatment necessary.
- May require treatment of increased intraocular pressure (see Primary Open Angle Glaucoma section in Chapter 11).
- May require penetrating keratoplasty, cataract extraction, and treatment of amblyopia for Peter's anomaly.

Prognosis Poor for Peters' anomaly or when associated with glaucoma; otherwise fair.

Iridocorneal Endothelial Syndromes

Definition Unilateral, nonhereditary, slowly progressive abnormality of the corneal endothelium causing a spectrum of diseases with features including corneal edema, iris distortion, and secondary angle-closure glaucoma.

Essential Iris Atrophy (Progressive Iris Atrophy)

Iris atrophy with holes and corectopia, ectropion uveae, and focal stromal effacement.

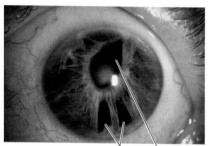

Iris atrophy   Corectopia

Figure 7-31 • Essential iris atrophy demonstrating iris atrophy and corectopia.

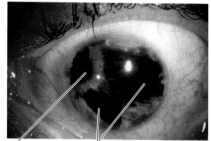

Corectopia   Iris atrophy

Figure 7-32 • Advanced essential iris atrophy demonstrating marked pupil displacement nasally and extreme atrophy with frank iris holes.

Chandler's Syndrome

Variant of essential iris atrophy with mild or no iris changes, corneal edema common, intraocular pressure may not be elevated.

Figure 7-33 • Chandler's syndrome with mild corectopia and moderate iris atrophy.

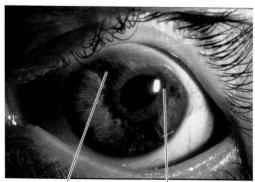

Iris atrophy   Corectopia

Iris Nevus (Cogan-Reese) Syndrome

Pigmented iris nodules, flattening of iris stroma, pupil abnormalities, and ectropion uveae.

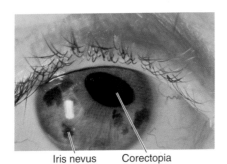

Iris nevus   Corectopia

Figure 7-34 • Iris nevus (Cogan–Reese) syndrome demonstrating iris nevi, iris atrophy, and corectopia.

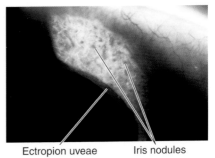

Ectropion uveae   Iris nodules

Figure 7-35 • Iris nevus (Cogan–Reese) syndrome with small, pigmented iris nodules and ectropion uveae.

Mechanism Altered, abnormal corneal endothelium proliferates across the angle and onto the iris, forming a membrane that obstructs the trabecular meshwork, distorts the iris, and may form nodules by contracting around the iris stroma.

Epidemiology Mostly young or middle-aged women; increased risk of secondary angle-closure glaucoma.

Symptoms Asymptomatic; may have decreased vision, glare, monocular diplopia or polyopia; may notice iris changes.

Signs Normal or decreased visual acuity, beaten metal appearance of corneal endothelium, corneal edema, increased intraocular pressure, peripheral anterior synechiae, iris changes (see above).

Differential Diagnosis Posterior polymorphous dystrophy, mesodermal dysgenesis syndromes, Fuchs' endothelial dystrophy, iris nevi or melanoma, aniridia, iridodialysis, iridoschisis, trauma.

Evaluation
- Complete ophthalmic history and eye exam with attention to cornea, tonometry, anterior chamber, gonioscopy, iris, lens, and ophthalmoscopy.
- Check visual fields in patients with elevated intraocular pressure or optic nerve cupping to rule out glaucoma.

Management

- Often no treatment necessary.
- May require treatment of increased intraocular pressure (see Primary Open Angle Glaucoma section in Chapter 11).
- May require penetrating keratoplasty or glaucoma surgery.

Prognosis Chronic, progressive process; poor when associated with glaucoma. Essential iris atrophy and iris nevus syndrome may have worse glaucoma than Chandler's syndrome.

Tumors

Cyst

Can be primary (more common; usually peripheral from stroma or iris pigment epithelium) or secondary (usually due to ingrowth of surface epithelium after trauma or surgery); may cause segmental elevation of iris and angle-closure; rarely detaches and becomes free-floating in anterior chamber; may also form at pupillary margin from long-term use of strong miotic medications. Complications include distortion of pupil, occlusion of visual axis, and secondary glaucoma.

Figure 7-36 • Peripheral iris cyst seen as translucent round lesion at the iris periphery.

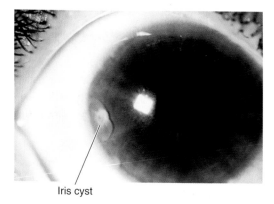

Iris cyst

- May require treatment of increased intraocular pressure (see Primary Open Angle Glaucoma section in Chapter 11).
- Consider surgical excision if vision is affected or secondary glaucoma exists.

Nevus

Single or multiple, flat, pigmented, benign lesions. Pigment spots or freckles occur in 50% of population; rare before 12 years of age. Nevus differentiated from malignant melanoma by size (<3 mm in diameter), thickness (<1 mm thick), and the absence of vascularity, ectropion uveae, secondary cataract, secondary glaucoma, and signs of growth.

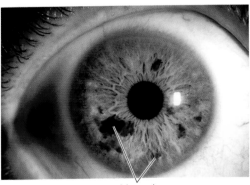

Figure 7-37 • Variably pigmented, small, flat, iris nevi are seen diffusely scattered over the anterior iris surface.

Iris nevi

- Follow with serial anterior segment photographs and clinical examination for any growth that would be suspicious for malignant melanoma.
- Follow for increased intraocular pressure.
- Consider iris fluorescein angiogram to differentiate between nevus and malignant melanoma: nevus has filigree filling pattern that becomes hyperfluorescent early and leaks late or is angiographically silent; malignant melanoma has irregular vessels that fill late.

Nodules

Collections of cells on the iris surface. Several different types:

Brushfield Spots

Ring of small, white-gray, peripheral iris spots associated with Down's syndrome; occurs in 24% of normal individuals (Kunkmann Wolffian bodies).

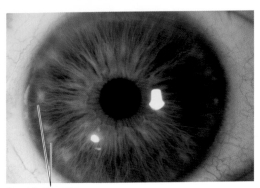

Figure 7-38 • Brushfield spots appear as a ring of peripheral white iris nodules.

Brushfield spots

Lisch Nodules

Bilateral, lightly pigmented, gelatinous, melanocytic hamartomas found in 92% of patients with neurofibromatosis type 1 (NF-1) by age 10; very rare in NF-2; usually involve inferior half of iris; do not involve iris stroma.

Figure 7-39 • Lisch nodules in a patient with neurofibromatosis appear as small, round, lightly colored nodules.

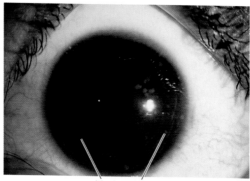

Lisch nodules

Inflammatory Nodules

Composed of monocytes and inflammatory debris; occurs in granulomatous uveitis. Three types:

Berlin Nodules

Nodules in anterior chamber angle.

Busacca Nodules

Nodules on anterior iris surface.

Koeppe Nodules

Nodules at pupillary border.

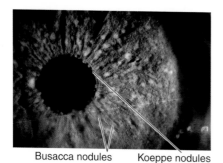

Busacca nodules   Koeppe nodules

Figure 7-40 • Busacca and Koeppe nodules are small, lightly colored collections of inflammatory cells.

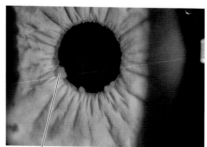

Koeppe nodules

Figure 7-41 • Koeppe nodules at the pupillary border.

Iris Pigment Epithelium Tumors

Very rare tumors of the iris pigment epithelium (adenoma or adenocarcinoma); appear as darkly pigmented, friable nodules.

- Treatment with chemotherapy, radiation, and surgical excision; should be performed by a tumor specialist.

Juvenile Xanthogranuloma

Yellow iris lesions composed of histiocytes; may bleed, causing spontaneous hyphema.

Malignant Melanoma

Dark or amelanotic (pigmentation variable), elevated lesion that usually involves inferior iris and replaces the iris stroma. May be diffuse (associated with heterochromia and secondary glaucoma), tapioca (dark tapioca appearance), ring-shaped, or localized; some have feeder vessels; may involve angle structures; may cause sectoral cataract, hyphema, or secondary glaucoma. 1–3% of all malignant melanomas of the uveal tract involve the iris. Predilection for Caucasians and patients with light irides, rare in African Americans; many patients have history of nevus that undergoes growth. Prognosis good; 4% mortality.

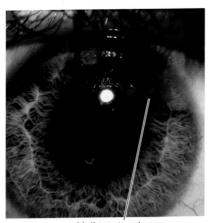

Malignant melanoma

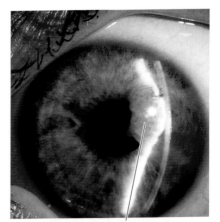

Amelanotic malignant melanoma

Figure 7-42 • Malignant melanoma is seen as a hazy brown confluent patch on this blue iris.

Figure 7-43 • Amelanotic melanoma is visible as a large, pedunculated, vascular mass with obvious elevation as depicted by the bowed appearance of the slit-beam light over the iris surface.

- Consider B-scan ultrasonography or ultrasound biomicroscopy to rule out ciliary body involvement.
- Treatment with chemotherapy, radiation, surgical excision, and enucleation; should be performed by a tumor specialist.

- May require treatment of increased intraocular pressure (see Primary Open Angle Glaucoma section in Chapter 11); glaucoma filtering surgery is not recommended.

Metastatic Tumors

Rare; usually amelanotic, and from primary carcinoma of the breast, lung, or prostate; often found after primary lesion is discovered.

Figure 7-44 • Metastatic carcinoid appearing as an orange-brown peripheral iris lesion.

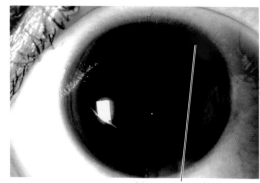

Metastatic carcinoid

- Treatment with chemotherapy, radiation, and surgical excision; should be performed by a tumor specialist.
- May require treatment of increased intraocular pressure (see Primary Open Angle Glaucoma section in Chapter 11); glaucoma filtering surgery is not recommended.

Congenital Anomalies 293
Congenital Cataract 296
Acquired Cataract 300
Posterior Capsular Opacification 306
Aphakia 308
Pseudophakia 309
Exfoliation 310
Pseudoexfoliation Syndrome 311
Pseudoexfoliation Glaucoma 312
Lens-Induced Glaucoma 314
Dislocated Lens 316

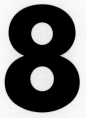

Lens

Congenital Anomalies

Definition Variety of developmental lens abnormalities.

Coloboma

Focal inferior lens flattening due to ciliary body coloboma with absence of zonular support (not a true coloboma); other ocular colobomata (iris) usually exist. Ciliary body tumors may cause a secondary lens "coloboma."

Figure 8-1 • Lens coloboma appears as inferior flattening or truncation of the lens due to lack of zonular attachments when viewed with retroillumination.

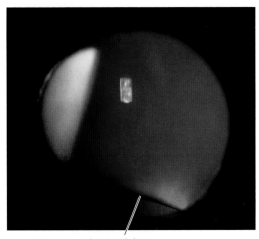

Lens coloboma

Lenticonus

Cone-shaped lens due to bulging from a thin lens capsule; either anteriorly or posteriorly, rarely in both directions.

Anterior

Usually males; bilateral; may be associated with Alport's syndrome (see Congenital Cataract section below).

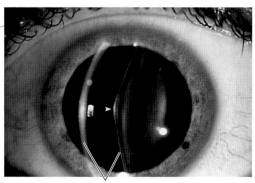

Slit-beam

Figure 8-2 ● Anterior lenticonus in a patient with Alport's syndrome. Note peaked slit-beam as it crosses anterior lens surface (arrowhead).

Posterior

More common; slight female predilection; may have associated cortical lens opacities, may be associated with Lowe's syndrome (see Congenital Cataract section below).

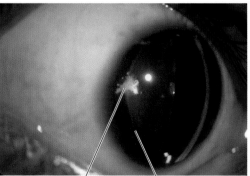

Polar cataract   Posterior lenticonus

Figure 8-3 ● Posterior lenticonus with polar cataract.

Lentiglobus

Globe-shaped lens caused by bulging from thin lens capsule; rare.

Microspherophakia

Small spheric lens; may be an isolated anomaly or part of a syndrome (i.e., dominant spherophakia, Weill-Marchesani syndrome, Lowe's syndrome, Alport's syndrome, Peter's anomaly, rubella).

Mittendorf Dot

A small white spot on the posterior lens capsule that represents a remnant of the posterior tunica vasculosa lentis where the former hyaloid artery attached.

Figure 8-4 • Mittendorf dot demonstrating a small white spot on the posterior lens capsule that represents a remnant of the posterior tunica vasculosa lentis.

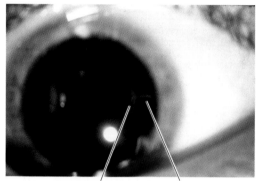

Mittendorf dot   Cloquet's canal

Symptoms Asymptomatic (Mittendorf dot, coloboma); may have decreased vision (lenticonus, lentiglobus, and microspherophakia), diplopia, or symptoms of angle-closure glaucoma (microspherophakia).

Signs Normal or decreased visual acuity; may have amblyopia, strabismus, nystagmus; myopia, and an "oil-droplet" fundus reflex on retroillumination in lenticonus and lentiglobus; may have dislocated lens and increased intraocular pressure in microspherophakia.

Differential Diagnosis See above.

Evaluation

- Complete ophthalmic history and eye exam with attention to cycloplegic refraction, retinoscopy, gonioscopy, lens, and ophthalmoscopy.

Management

- Correct any refractive error.
- Patching or occlusion therapy for amblyopia (see Chapter 12).
- Microspherophakia causing pupillary block is treated with a cycloplegic (scopolamine 0.25% tid or atropine 1% bid); may also require laser iridotomy or lens extraction (see Secondary Angle-Closure Glaucoma section in Chapter 6).

Prognosis Usually good; poorer if amblyopia exists.

Congenital Cataract

Definition Congenital opacity of the crystalline lens usually categorized by location or etiology.

Capsular

Opacity of the lens capsule, usually anteriorly.

Lamellar or Zonular

Central, circumscribed opacity surrounding the nucleus; "sand dollar" appearance.

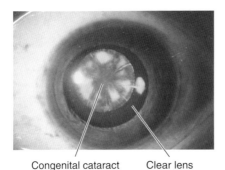

Congenital cataract   Clear lens

Figure 8-5 • Congenital zonular cataract.

Lenticular or Nuclear

Opacity of the lens nucleus.

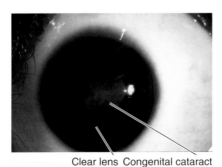

Clear lens Congenital cataract

Figure 8-6 • Congenital nuclear cataract with central white discoid appearance.

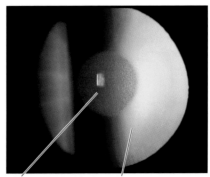

Congenital cataract   Clear lens

Figure 8-7 • Same patient as Figure 8-6 demonstrating congenital nuclear cataract as viewed with retroillumination.

Polar

Central opacity located near the lens capsule, anteriorly or posteriorly.

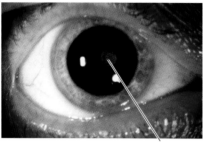

Posterior polar cataract

Figure 8-8 ● Congenital posterior polar cataract.

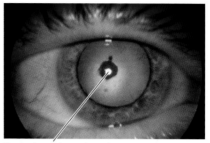

Posterior polar cataract

Figure 8-9 ● Same patient as Figure 8-8 demonstrating congenital polar cataract in retroillumination.

Sutural

Opacity of the Y-shaped sutures in the center of the lens.

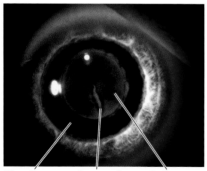

Clear lens   Suture   Congenital cataract

Figure 8-10 ● Congenital cataract with prominent suture lines.

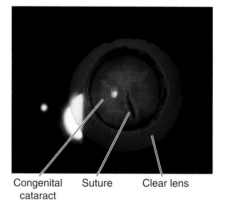

Congenital   Suture   Clear lens
cataract

Figure 8-11 ● Same patient as Figure 8-10 demonstrating congenital sutural cataract in retroillumination.

Etiology

Hereditary or Syndromes

Without chromosomal abnormalities

Autosomal dominant (AD), autosomal recessive (AR), X-linked.

With chromosomal abnormalities

Down's syndrome (snowflake cataracts), Turner's syndrome, and others.

Other syndromes

Craniofacial, central nervous system, skin.

Intrauterine Infections

Congenital rubella syndrome

Cataracts, glaucoma, microcornea, microphthalmos, iris hypoplasia, and retinopathy with characteristic fine, granular, salt-and-pepper appearance (most common finding). Other complications include prematurity, mental retardation, neurosensory deafness, congenital heart disease, growth retardation, hepatosplenomegaly, interstitial pneumonitis, and encephalitis.

Congenital varicella syndrome

Cataracts, chorioretinitis, optic nerve atrophy or hypoplasia, nystagmus, and Horner's syndrome. Systemic findings include hemiparesis, bulbar palsies, dermatomal cicatricial skin lesions, developmental delay, and learning difficulties.

Metabolic

Galactosemia

Bilateral, oil-droplet cataracts from accumulation of galactose metabolites (galactitol) due to hereditary enzymatic deficiency; usually galactose-1-phosphate uridyltransferase, also galactokinase. Associated with mental retardation, hepatosplenomegaly, cirrhosis, malnutrition, and failure to thrive.

Lowe's oculocerebrorenal syndrome (X-linked)

Small discoid lens, posterior lenticonus, and glaucoma. Systemic findings include acidosis, aminoaciduria, renal rickets, hypotonia, mental retardation. Female carriers have posterior, white, punctate cortical opacities and subcapsular, plaquelike opacities.

Alport's syndrome (autosomal dominant)

Basement membrane disease associated with acute hemorrhagic nephropathy, deafness, anterior lenticonus, anterior polar or cortical cataracts, and albipunctatus-like spots in the fundus.

Other metabolic diseases

Hypoglycemia, hypocalcemia (diffuse lamellar punctate opacities), Fabry's disease (spokelike cataracts in 25%), mannosidosis (posterior spokelike opacities).

Ocular Disorders

Persistent hyperplastic primary vitreous, Peter's anomaly, Leber's congenital amaurosis, retinopathy of prematurity, aniridia, posterior lenticonus, tumors.

Other

Birth trauma, idiopathic, and maternal drug ingestion.

Epidemiology Congenital cataracts occur in approximately 1 of 2000 live births. Roughly one-third are isolated, one-third are familial (usually dominant), and one-third are associated with a syndrome; most unilateral cases are not metabolic or genetic.

Symptoms Variable decreased vision; may notice white pupil or eye turn.

Signs Decreased visual acuity, leukocoria, amblyopia; may have strabismus (usually with unilateral cataract), nystagmus (usually does not appear until 2–3 months of age; rarely when cataracts develop after age 6 months), amblyopia; may have other ocular or systemic findings if syndrome exists.

Differential Diagnosis See Leukocoria in Chapter 7.

Evaluation

- Complete ophthalmic history with attention to family history of eye disease, trauma, maternal illnesses and drug ingestion during pregnancy, systemic diseases in the child, and birth problems.
- Complete eye exam with attention to cycloplegic refraction, retinoscopy, tonometry, gonioscopy, lens (size and density of the opacity as viewed with retroillumination), and ophthalmoscopy.
- May require examination under anesthesia.
- Keratometry and biometry when intraocular lens (IOL) implantation is anticipated.
- **Lab tests**: TORCH titers (toxoplasmosis, other infections [syphilis], rubella, cytomegalovirus, and herpes simplex), fasting blood sugar (hypoglycemia), urine reducing substances after milk feeding (galactosemia), calcium (hypocalcemia), and urine amino acids (Lowe's syndrome).
- B-scan ultrasonography if unable to visualize the fundus (can perform through the lids of a crying child).
- Pediatric consultation.

Management

- Dilation (tropicamide 1% [Mydriacyl] with or without phenylephrine 2.5% [Mydfrin] tid) may be used as a temporary measure before surgery to allow light to pass around the cataract; however, surgery should not be delayed.
- If the cataract obscures the visual axis (media opacity >3 mm) or is causing secondary ocular disease (glaucoma or uveitis), cataract extraction should be performed within days to a week after diagnosis in infants because delay may lead to amblyopia; postoperatively, the child requires proper aphakic correction with contact lens or spectacles if bilateral; depending on age and etiology, consider IOL implantation.

Continued

Management—Cont'd

- If the cataract is not causing amblyopia, glaucoma, or uveitis, the child is observed closely for progression.
- Patching or occlusion therapy for amblyopia (see Chapter 12).
- Almost all patients with visually significant, unilateral, congenital cataracts have strabismus and may require muscle surgery after cataract extraction.
- Restrict dietary galactose in galactosemia.

Prognosis Depends on age and duration of visually significant cataract prior to surgery; poor if amblyopia exists.

Acquired Cataract

Definition Lenticular opacity usually categorized by location or etiology.

Cortical Degeneration

Caused by swelling and liquefaction of the cortical fiber cells. Various types:

Spokes and vacuoles

Asymmetrically located, radial, linear opacities and punctate dots.

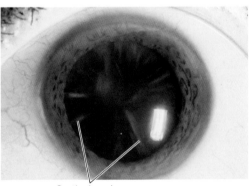

Cortical spokes

Figure 8-12 • Cortical cataract demonstrating white cortical spoking.

Mature cataract

Completely opacified cortex causing the lens to appear white; no red reflex visible from fundus.

Figure 8-13 Mature cataract with white, liquefied cortex.

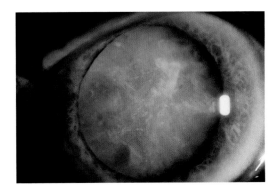

Morgagnian cataract

Mature cataract with dense nucleus displaced inferiorly in completely liquefied, white cortex.

Figure 8-14 Morgagnian cataract demonstrating a dense, brown nucleus sinking inferiorly in a white, liquefied cortex.

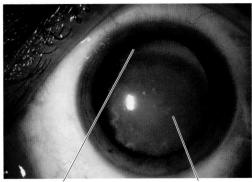

Liquefied cortex   Brunescent nucleus

Hypermature cataract

After morgagnian cataract formation, the lens shrinks, the capsule wrinkles, and calcium deposits can form; proteins may leak into the anterior chamber causing phacolytic glaucoma.

Nuclear Sclerosis

Centrally located lens discoloration/opalescence (yellow-green or brown [brunescent]); caused by deterioration of the central lens fiber cells.

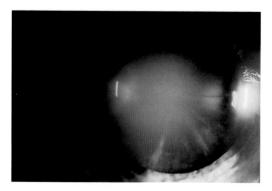

Figure 8-15 Cataract with 2⁺ yellow-green nuclear sclerosis.

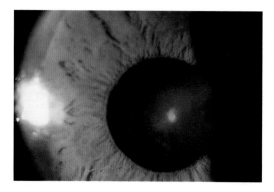

Figure 8-16 Brunescent nuclear sclerotic cataract.

Subcapsular Cataract

Anterior subcapsular

Central fibrous plaque caused by metaplasia of the central zone lens epithelial cells beneath the anterior lens capsule. Medications can cause anterior subcapsular stellate changes; acute angle-closure attacks can cause anterior subcapsular opacities (glaukomflecken) due to lens epithelial necrosis.

Posterior subcapsular

Asymmetric granular opacities with a frosted glass appearance at the posterior surface of the lens; caused by posterior migration of epithelial cells and formation of bladder (Wedl) cells.

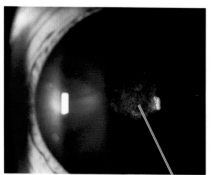

Posterior subcapsular cataract

Figure 8-17 • Posterior subcapsular cataract demonstrating typical white, hazy appearance.

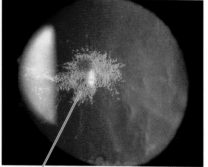

Posterior subcapsular cataract

Figure 8-18 • Posterior subcapsular cataract due to topical steroid use, as viewed with retroillumination.

Etiology

Senile

Most common; due to age-related lens changes (cortical, nuclear, and/or subcapsular).

Systemic Disease

Many different systemic diseases can cause cataracts, including:

Diabetes mellitus

"Sugar" cataracts are cortical or posterior subcapsular opacities that occur earlier in diabetic patients than in age-matched controls, progress rapidly, and are related to poor glucose control more than duration of disease.

Hypocalcemia

Lens opacities are usually small white dots but can aggregate into larger flakes.

Myotonic dystrophy

Central, polychromatic, iridescent, cortical crystals (Christmas tree cataract); may develop a posterior subcapsular cataract later (see Chronic Progressive External Ophthalmoplegia section in Chapter 2).

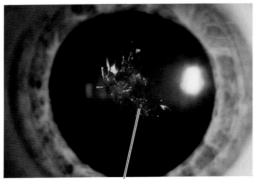

Figure 8-19 • Polychromatic, refractile, cholesterol deposits within the crystalline lens.

"Christmas tree" cholesterol cataract

Wilson's disease

Sunflower cataract due to copper deposition (chalcosis lentis); green-brown surface opacity in the central lens with short stellate processes rather than the full flower petal pattern that occurs in chalcosis (copper foreign body).

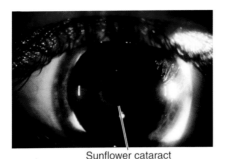

Sunflower cataract

Figure 8-20 • Sunflower cataract in a patient with Wilson's disease.

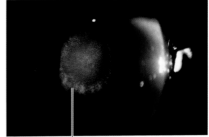

Chalcosis lentis

Figure 8-21 • Sunflower cataract (chalcosis lentis) with green-brown central opacities in the lens (same patient as Figure 5-85 with Kayser-Fleischer ring).

Others

Fabry's disease, atopic dermatitis (anterior subcapsular shieldlike plaque), NF-2 (posterior subcapsular cataracts), and ectodermal dysplasia.

Other Eye Diseases

Uveitis, angle-closure glaucoma (glaukomflecken), retinal detachment, myopia, intraocular tumors, retinitis pigmentosa (posterior subcapsular cataracts), Refsum's disease (posterior subcapsular cataracts), Stickler's syndrome (cortical cataracts), phthisis bulbi.

Toxic

Steroids (posterior subcapsular cataracts), miotic agents, phenothiazines, amiodarone, busulfan; ionizing (X-rays, gamma rays, and neutrons), infrared, ultraviolet, microwave, and shortwave radiation; electricity, and chemicals.

Figure 8-22 Anterior subcapsular star-pattern cataract due to phenothiazine use.

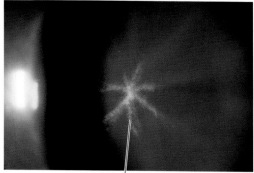

Anterior subcapsular cataract

Trauma

Blunt or penetrating; intraocular foreign bodies (iron, copper); and postoperative (i.e., pars plana vitrectomy, trabeculectomy).

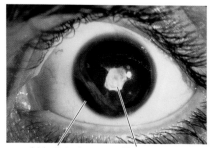

Iridodialysis   Traumatic cataract

Figure 8-23 Dense, white, central cataract due to trauma; also note iridodialysis.

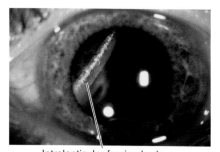

Intralenticular foreign body

Figure 8-24 Intralenticular foreign body.

Epidemiology Senile cataracts represent senescent lens changes related, in part, to ultra-violet B radiation. In the Framingham Eye Study, the prevalence of senile cataracts was 42% in adults 52–64 years old, 73% in 65–74 year olds, and 91% in 75–85 year olds. African American men and women were more likely to have cataracts in every age category. Cataracts are the leading cause of blindness worldwide.

Symptoms Painless, progressive loss of vision, decreased contrast and color sensitivity, glare, starbursts; rarely monocular diplopia.

Signs Decreased visual acuity (distance vision usually affected more than near vision in nuclear sclerosis, and near vision affected more than distance vision in posterior subcapsular), focal or diffuse lens opacification (yellow, green, brown, or white; often best appreciated with retroillumination), induced myopia; intumescent cataracts may cause the iris to bow forward and lead to secondary angle closure (see Chapter 6); hypermature cataracts may leak lens proteins and cause phacolytic glaucoma (see Lens-Induced Glaucoma section).

Differential Diagnosis See above; senile cataract is a diagnosis of exclusion, must rule out secondary causes.

Evaluation
- Complete ophthalmic history with attention to systemic diseases, medications, prior use of steroids, trauma, radiation treatment, other ocular diseases, congenital problems, and functional visual status.
- Complete eye exam with attention to visual acuity, refraction, contrast sensitivity, cornea, gonioscopy, lens, and ophthalmoscopy.
- Consider brightness acuity tester (BAT) and potential acuity meter (PAM) testing (the latter is used to estimate visual potential, especially when posterior segment pathology exists).
- B-scan ultrasonography if unable to visualize the fundus.
- Keratometry and biometry to calculate the IOL implant power before cataract surgery; also consider specular microscopy and pachymetry if cornea guttata or corneal edema exists.

Management

- Cataract extraction and insertion of an IOL is indicated when visual symptoms interfere with daily activities and the patient desires improved visual function, when the cataract causes other ocular diseases (e.g., lens-induced glaucoma, uveitis), or when the cataract prevents examination or treatment of another ocular condition (e.g., diabetic retinopathy, age-related macular degeneration, glaucoma).
- Dilation (tropicamide 1% [Mydriacyl] with or without phenylephrine 2.5% [Mydfrin] tid) may help the patient see around a central opacity in those rare instances when the patient cannot undergo or declines cataract surgery.

Prognosis Very good; success rate for routine cataract surgery is >96%; increased risk of complications for posterior polar and traumatic cataracts, pseudoexfoliation syndrome (see below), ectopia lentis, small pupil, intraoperative floppy iris syndrome (IFIS, caused by alpha-1 adrenergic antagonist drugs [i.e., Flomax]).

Posterior Capsular Opacification (Secondary Cataract)

Definition Clouding of the posterior lens capsule after extracapsular cataract extraction.

Epidemiology After cataract extraction, up to 50% of adult patients may develop posterior capsule opacification; increased incidence in children and patients with uveitis (approaches 100%). IOL material (acrylic) and design (square edge) have reduced the incidence of posterior capsular opacification to less than 10%.

Etiology Epithelial cell proliferation (Elschnig pearls) and fibrosis of the capsule.

Symptoms Asymptomatic or may have decreased vision and glare depending on severity and location with respect to the visual axis.

Signs Posterior capsule opacification; graded on a 1 to 4 scale according to density; may appear as haze, striae, Elschnig pearls, or any combination.

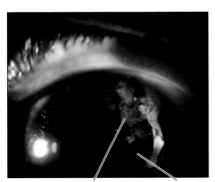

Elschnig pearls   Posterior chamber IOL

Figure 8-25 Secondary cataract composed of Elschnig pearls.

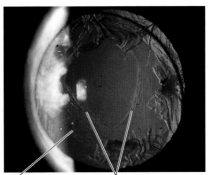

Posterior   Capsular opening
chamber IOL

Figure 8-26 Posterior capsule opening following Nd:YAG laser capsulotomy when viewed with retroillumination. Jagged edges or leaflets of the larger anterior capsulotomy are visible as is the superior edge of the intraocular lens optic from the 12 o'clock to 3 o'clock position.

Evaluation
- Complete ophthalmic history and eye exam with attention to visual acuity, refraction, cornea, tonometry, gonioscopy, IOL position and stability, posterior capsule, and ophthalmoscopy.

Management

- If visually significant, treat with **neodymium:yttrium-aluminum-garnet (Nd:YAG) laser posterior capsulotomy.**

  Procedure parameters: a contact lens is used to stabilize the eye and better focus the beam; the goal is to create a central 3–4 mm opening in the posterior capsule; pupil dilation is usually performed but is not always necessary. Laser energy setting is typically 1–3 mJ and is titrated according to tissue response.

- In young children, a primary posterior capsulotomy and anterior vitrectomy are performed at the time of cataract surgery.

Prognosis Very good; complications of Nd:YAG capsulotomy are rare but include increased intraocular pressure, IOL damage or dislocation, corneal burn, retinal detachment, cystoid macular edema, and hyphema.

Aphakia

Definition Absence of crystalline lens; usually secondary to surgery, rarely traumatic (total dislocation of crystalline lens [Figure 8-37]), or very rarely congenital.

Symptoms Loss of accommodation and decreased uncorrected vision.

Signs Decreased uncorrected visual acuity (usually very high hyperopia), no lens, iridodonesis; may have a visible surgical wound, peripheral iridectomy, vitreous in the anterior chamber, complications from surgery (bullous keratopathy, increased intraocular pressure, iritis, posterior capsule opacification, cystoid macular edema), or evidence of ocular trauma (see appropriate sections).

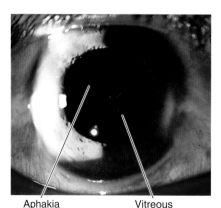

Aphakia   Vitreous

Figure 8-27 • Aphakia demonstrating absence of the crystalline lens. Pigment cells on the anterior vitreous face are visible.

Evaluation

- Complete ophthalmic history with attention to previous ocular surgery or trauma.
- Complete eye exam with attention to refraction, cornea, tonometry, anterior chamber, gonioscopy, iris, lens, and ophthalmoscopy.
- Consider specular microscopy and pachymetry if cornea guttata or corneal edema exists.

Management

- Proper aphakic correction with contact lens; consider aphakic spectacles if bilateral.
- Consider secondary IOL implantation.
- Treat complications if present.

Prognosis Usually good; increased risk of retinal detachment, especially for high myopes and if posterior capsule is not intact.

Pseudophakia

Definition Presence of IOL implant after crystalline lens has been removed; may be inserted primarily or secondarily. There are numerous types of IOLs including: anterior or posterior chamber; rigid or foldable; 1- or 3-piece; loop or plate haptic; round or square edge; polymethylmethacrylate, acrylic, silicone, hydrogel, or collamer; monofocal, multifocal, accommodating, toric, and aspheric.

Symptoms Asymptomatic; may have decreased vision, loss of accommodation, edge glare, monocular diplopia or polyopia, or induced ametropia with decentered or tilted IOL.

Signs IOL implant (may be in anterior chamber, iris plane, capsular bag, or ciliary sulcus with or without suture fixation to iris or sclera); may have a visible surgical wound, peripheral iridectomy, complications from surgery (bullous keratopathy, iris capture, decentered IOL, increased intraocular pressure, iritis, hyphema, opacified posterior capsule, cystoid macular edema).

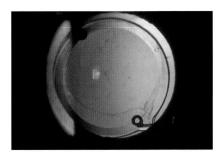

Figure 8-28 • Pseudophakia demonstrating posterior chamber intraocular lens (IOL) well centered in the capsular bag. The anterior capsulorrhexis edge has fibrosed and is visible as a white circle overlying the IOL optic; the edges of the IOL haptics where they insert into the optic are also seen.

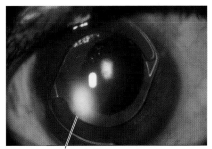

Anterior chamber IOL

Figure 8-29 • Pseudophakia demonstrating anterior chamber intraocular lens in good position above the iris.

Evaluation

• Complete ophthalmic history and eye exam with attention to visual acuity, refraction, cornea, anterior chamber, gonioscopy, iris, IOL position and stability, posterior capsule integrity and clarity, and ophthalmoscopy.

Management

- May require correction of refractive error (usually reading glasses).
- Treat complications if present.

Prognosis Usually good; increased risk of retinal detachment, especially for high myopes and if posterior capsule is not intact.

Exfoliation

Definition True exfoliation is delamination, or schisis, of the anterior lens capsule into sheetlike lamellae.

Etiology Infrared and thermal radiation; also senile form.

Epidemiology Rare; classically occurs in glass blowers.

Symptoms Asymptomatic.

Signs Splitting of anterior lens capsule, appears as scrolls; may have posterior subcapsular cataract.

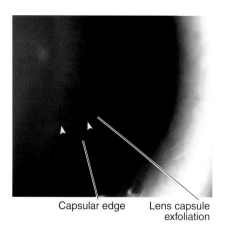

Capsular edge   Lens capsule
exfoliation

Figure 8-30 • True lens exfoliation demonstrating scrolling of split anterior lens capsule (arrowheads).

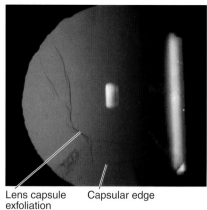

Lens capsule   Capsular edge
exfoliation

Figure 8-31 • Same patient as Figure 8-30, demonstrating appearance of lens capsule exfoliation as viewed with retroillumination.

Differential Diagnosis Pseudoexfoliation syndrome.

Evaluation

- Complete ophthalmic history with attention to infrared and thermal radiation exposure.
- Complete eye exam with attention to lens.

Management

- No treatment recommended.
- Prevention by use of protective goggles.
- May require cataract extraction.

Prognosis Good.

Pseudoexfoliation Syndrome

Definition Pseudoexfoliation is a generalized disorder of elastin formation that results in the abnormal accumulation of small, gray-white fibrillar aggregates (resembling amyloid) on the lens capsule, iris, anterior segment structures, and systemically (may involve the skin, heart, and lungs).

Epidemiology Usually asymmetric, bilateral more often than unilateral. Occurs in all racial groups, common in Scandinavians, South African blacks, Navaho Indians, and Australian aborigines; almost absent in Eskimos. Age-related, rare in individuals under 50 years old, incidence increases after age 60 years (4–6% in patients over 60 years old). Up to 60% develop ocular hypertension or glaucoma (see below); in the United States, 20% have elevated intraocular pressure at initial examination, and 15% develop it within 10 years. Mapped to chromosome 15q24 (LOXL1 gene).

Symptoms Asymptomatic.

Signs Loss of pupillary ruff, iris transillumination defects, pigment deposits on the iris, trabecular meshwork, and anterior to Schwalbe's line (Sampaolesi's line); target pattern of exfoliative material on lens capsule (central disc and peripheral ring with intervening clear area); white exfoliation material is also seen on zonules, anterior hyaloid, iris, and pupillary margin; shallow anterior chamber due to forward displacement of the lens-iris diaphragm; may have phacodonesis, cataract (40%), or signs of glaucoma with increased intraocular pressure, optic nerve cupping, nerve fiber layer defects, and visual field defects.

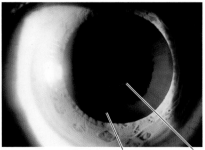

Peripheral ring   Central disc

Figure 8-32 • Exfoliative material on the anterior lens surface in typical pattern of central disc and peripheral ring in a patient with pseudoexfoliation syndrome.

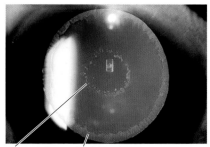

Central disc   Peripheral ring

Figure 8-33 • Central disc and peripheral ring of exfoliative material as seen with retroillumination.

Evaluation

- Complete ophthalmic history and eye exam with attention to tonometry, anterior chamber, gonioscopy, iris, lens, and ophthalmoscopy.
- Check visual fields in patients with elevated intraocular pressure or optic nerve cupping to rule out glaucoma.

Management

- Observe for pseudoexfoliation glaucoma by monitoring intraocular pressure.
- May require treatment of increased intraocular pressure (see Primary Open Angle Glaucoma section in Chapter 11) and pseudoexfoliation glaucoma (see below).

Prognosis Good; poorer if pseudoexfoliation glaucoma develops; increased incidence of complications at cataract surgery due to weak zonules and increased lens mobility.

Pseudoexfoliation Glaucoma

Definition A form of secondary open-angle glaucoma associated with pseudoexfoliation syndrome.

Epidemiology Most common cause of secondary open-angle glaucoma; affects 2% of U.S. population over 50 years old. Up to 60% with pseudoexfoliation syndrome develop ocular hypertension or glaucoma; 50–60% bilateral, often asymmetric; age related (rare in individuals under 50 years old, increases after age 60 years). Mapped to chromosome 15q24 (LOXL1 gene).

Mechanism

(1) Trabecular meshwork (TM) dysfunction due to obstruction by exfoliative material. The exfoliative material may flow into the TM from the anterior chamber, or it may be produced in the TM.

(2) Abnormally weak lamina cribrosa (composed of elastin) that renders the optic nerve more susceptible to elevated IOP.

Symptoms Asymptomatic; may have decreased vision or constricted visual fields in late stages.

Signs Normal or decreased visual acuity, increased intraocular pressure (can be very high and asymmetric); similar ocular signs as in pseudoexfoliation syndrome (see above), optic nerve cupping, nerve fiber layer defects, and visual field defects.

Figure 8-34 Patient with pseudoexfoliation glaucoma demonstrating peripheral ring of exfoliative material on the lens surface with bridging band connecting to the central disc.

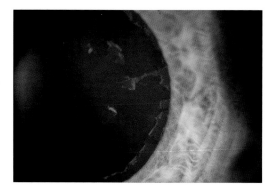

Differential Diagnosis Primary open-angle glaucoma, other forms of secondary open-angle glaucoma.

Evaluation

• Complete ophthalmic history and eye exam with attention to tonometry, anterior chamber, gonioscopy, iris, lens, and ophthalmoscopy.

• Check visual fields.

• Stereo optic nerve photos are useful for comparison at subsequent evaluations.

Management

• Choice and order of topical glaucoma medications depend on many factors, including patient's age, intraocular pressure level and control, and amount and progression of optic nerve cupping and visual field defects. Treatment options are presented in the Primary Open-Angle Glaucoma section (see Chapter 11); more resistant to treatment than primary open-angle glaucoma.

• Laser trabeculoplasty is effective, but action may be short lived.

• May require glaucoma filtering procedure if medical treatment fails.

Prognosis Poorer than primary open-angle glaucoma; increased incidence of angle-closure; lens removal has no effect on progression of disease; increased incidence of complications at cataract surgery due to weak zonules (composed of elastin) and increased lens mobility.

Lens-Induced Glaucoma

Definition Secondary glaucoma due to lens-induced abnormalities.

Etiology/Mechanism

Lens Particle

Retained cortex or nucleus after cataract surgery or penetrating trauma causes inflammatory reaction and obstructs trabecular meshwork; more anterior segment inflammation than phacolytic.

Phacolytic

Lens proteins from hypermature cataract leak through intact capsule and are ingested by macrophages; can occur with intact, dislocated lens; lens proteins and macrophages obstruct trabecular meshwork.

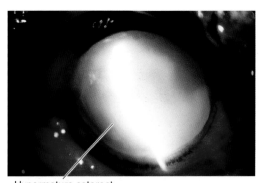

Hypermature cataract

Figure 8-35 • Phacolytic glaucoma demonstrating mature white cataract with anterior chamber inflammation.

Phacomorphic

Enlarged, cataractous lens pushes the iris forward, causing secondary angle-closure (see Chapter 6).

Figure 8-36 • Phacomorphic angle-closure glaucoma due to intumescent cataract pushing the iris forward and thereby obstructing the trabecular meshwork.

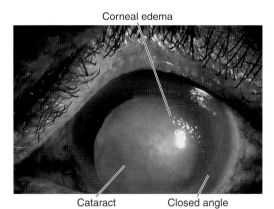

Corneal edema

Cataract   Closed angle

Symptoms Decreased vision, pain, photophobia, red eye; may have halos around lights and other symptoms of angle-closure glaucoma (see Chapter 6); may have constricted visual fields.

Signs Decreased visual acuity, increased intraocular pressure, ciliary injection, anterior chamber cells and flare, peripheral anterior synechiae, cataract or residual lens material, signs of recent surgery or trauma including surgical wounds, sutures, and signs of an open globe (see Chapter 4); may have optic nerve cupping, nerve fiber layer defects, and visual field defects.

Differential Diagnosis See above; other forms of secondary glaucoma, uveitis, endophthalmitis.

Evaluation

- Complete ophthalmic history and eye exam with attention to cornea, tonometry, anterior chamber, gonioscopy, iris, lens, and ophthalmoscopy.
- B-scan ultrasonography if unable to visualize the fundus.
- Check visual fields.

Management

- Topical steroid (prednisolone acetate 1% up to q1h) and cycloplegic (cyclopentolate 1% or scopolamine 0.25% bid to tid).
- Treatment of increased intraocular pressure (see Primary Open-Angle Glaucoma and Angle-Closure Glaucoma sections in Chapters 11 and 6, respectively).
- Definitive treatment consists of surgical lens extraction or removal of retained lens fragments.
- May require glaucoma filtering procedure.

Prognosis Good if definitive treatment is performed early and pressure control is achieved.

Dislocated Lens (Ectopia Lentis)

Definition   Congenital, developmental, or acquired displacement of the crystalline lens; may be incomplete (subluxation) or complete (luxation) dislocation of the lens into the anterior chamber or vitreous.

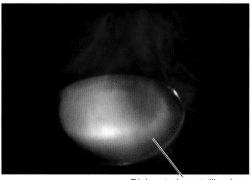

Figure 8-37 ● Dislocated crystalline lens resting on the retina.

Dislocated crystalline lens

Etiology

Ectopia Lentis et Pupillae (Autosomal Recessive)

Associated with oval or slitlike pupils; pupil displacement is in opposite direction of the lens displacement.

Homocystinuria (Autosomal Recessive)

Enzymatic disorder of methionine metabolism with elevated levels of homocystine and methionine; direction of lens displacement is typically down and in; not present at birth; progressive thereafter, with more than 90% having dislocated lenses by the third decade. Patients develop seizures, osteoporosis, mental retardation, and thromboembolism.

Hyperlysinemia

Inability to metabolize lysine; lens subluxation, muscular hypotony, and mental retardation.

Marfan's Syndrome (Autosomal Dominant)

Usually bilateral; occurs in about two-thirds of Marfan's patients due to defective zonules; direction of lens displacement is typically up and out. Other signs include marfanoid habitus with disproportionate growth of extremities, arachnodactyly, joint laxity, pectus deformities, scoliosis, and increasing dilation of the ascending aorta with aortic insufficiency (may cause death). Mapped to chromosome 15q.

Figure 8-38 • Lens subluxed (upward) in a patient with Marfan's syndrome.

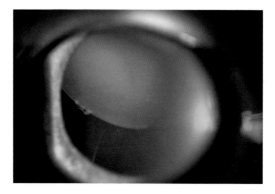

Microspherophakia

Small spheric lens; occurs as an isolated anomaly or as part of a syndrome (i.e., dominant spherophakia, Weill–Marchesani syndrome, Lowe's syndrome, Alpert's syndrome, Peter's anomaly, rubella); direction of lens displacement is often inferiorly or anteriorly.

Simple Ectopia Lentis (Autosomal Dominant)

Often present at birth; lens is small and spheric (microphakic and spherophakic); direction of lens displacement is typically up and out.

Sulfite Oxidase Deficiency (Autosomal Recessive)

Error of sulfur metabolism with ectopia lentis, seizures, and mental retardation.

Other

Aniridia, Ehlers–Danlos syndrome, trauma, syphilis, pseudoexfoliation syndrome, megalocornea.

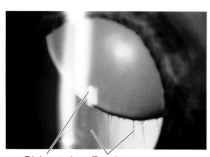

Dislocated   Zonules
crystalline lens

Figure 8-39 • Subluxed lens (up and out) due to trauma. Note broken inferior zonular fibers.

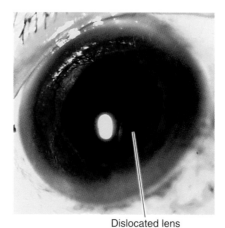

Dislocated lens

Figure 8-40 • Lens subluxed (downward) due to trauma.

Epidemiology Most common cause of lens subluxation or luxation is trauma (up to 50%); associated with cataract and rhegmatogenous retinal detachment. Most frequent cause of heritable lens dislocation is Marfan's syndrome.

Symptoms Asymptomatic; may have decreased vision, diplopia, symptoms of angle-closure glaucoma (see Chapter 6).

Signs Normal or decreased visual acuity, subluxated or luxated lens, phacodonesis, iridodonesis; may have increased intraocular pressure, anterior chamber cells and flare, vitreous in the anterior chamber, iris transillumination defects, angle abnormalities, and other signs of ocular trauma.

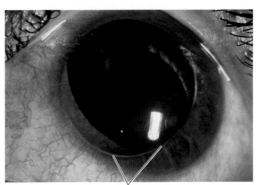

Figure 8-41 Dislocated lens in the anterior chamber. The edge of the clear lens is visible overlying the iris.

Dislocated crystalline lens

Differential Diagnosis See above.

Evaluation

- Complete ophthalmic history and eye exam with attention to visual acuity, refraction, corneal diameter, tonometry, anterior chamber, gonioscopy, iris, and lens.
- Consider B-scan ultrasonography if unable to visualize the fundus.
- **Lab tests**: Venereal Disease Research Laboratory (VDRL) test, fluorescent treponema antibody absorption (FTA-ABS) test, and lumbar puncture if syphilis suspected.
- Medical consultation for systemic diseases.

Management

- Correct any refractive error.
- Consider lens extraction.
- May require treatment of angle-closure glaucoma (see Secondary Angle-Closure Glaucoma section in Chapter 6; miotic agents may exacerbate pupillary block and should be avoided. Microspherophakia causing pupillary block is treated with a cyclo-plegic (scopolamine 0.25% tid or atropine 1% bid); may also require laser iridotomy.
- Treat underlying disorder (e.g., dietary restriction in homocystinuria, IV penicillin for syphilis).

Prognosis Depends on etiology.

Amyloidosis 319
Asteroid Hyalosis 320
Persistent Hyperplastic Primary Vitreous 321
Posterior Vitreous Detachment 323
Synchesis Scintillans 324
Vitreous Hemorrhage 324
Vitritis 326

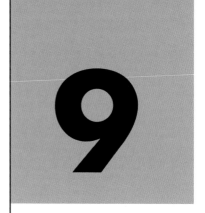

9

Vitreous

Amyloidosis

Definition Group of diseases characterized by abnormal protein production and tissue deposition. Nonfamilial and familial forms; familial amyloidosis (autosomal dominant [AD]) caused by substitution errors in coding of prealbumin. Can be associated with multiple myeloma.

Symptoms Floaters, decreased vision; may have diplopia.

Signs Although any part of the eye can be involved, vitreous involvement is most commonly seen with granular, glass-wool opacities that form in the vitreal cortex, strands attached to the retina, retinal vascular occlusions, cotton wool spots, retinal neovascularization, and

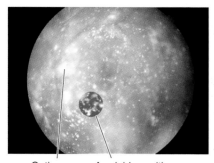

Optic nerve   Amyloid opacities

Figure 9-1 • Amyloidosis demonstrating the characteristic granular, glass-wool opacities in the mid-vitreous cavity that obscures the view of the retina. The optic nerve is barely visible.

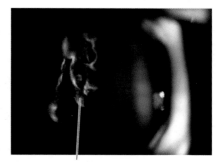

Amyloid opacities in anterior vitreous

Figure 9-2 • Amyloidosis demonstrating the characteristic granular, glass-wool opacities in the anterior vitreous cavity as seen with slit lamp.

compressive optic neuropathy. Other findings include eye lid hemorrhages, ptosis, proptosis, dry eye, corneal deposits, iris stromal infiltrates, and ophthalmoplegia. Systemic findings in nonfamilial forms include polyarthralgias, pulmonary infiltrates, waxy, maculopapular skin lesions, renal failure, postural hypotension, congestive heart failure, and gastrointestinal bleeds. Systemic findings in familial form include autonomic dysfunction, peripheral neuropathies, and cardiomyopathy.

Differential Diagnosis Asteroid hyalosis (see below), vitritis, old vitreous hemorrhage.

Evaluation
- Complete ophthalmic history and eye exam with attention to tonometry, iris, lens, anterior vitreous, Hruby lens, non-contact biomicroscopic or contact lens fundus exam, and ophthalmoscopy.
- **Lab tests:** Complete blood count (CBC), serum protein electrophoresis, liver function tests, chest radiographs, and 12-lead electrocardiogram.
- Diagnosis made on biopsy (dichroism; birefringence with Congo red stain).
- Medical consultation.

Management

- May require systemic treatment.
- No treatment recommended for vitreous involvement unless opacities become so severe that they affect vision, then consider pars plana vitrectomy by a retina specialist; recurs even after vitrectomy.

Prognosis Variable depending on systemic involvement.

Asteroid Hyalosis

Multiple, yellow-white, round, birefringent particles composed of calcium-phosphate soaps attached to the vitreous framework. Common degenerative process in elderly patients over 60 years of age (0.5% of population). Usually asymptomatic, does not cause floaters or interfere with vision, but does affect view of fundus; usually unilateral (75%); associated with diabetes mellitus (30%); good prognosis. Also does not affect FA or OCT so both tests can be used to determine if there are any retinal problems when the asteroid particles impair a direct view of the retina.

Figure 9-3 • Asteroid particles in the anterior vitreous cavity behind the lens. They are best seen using a fine slit-beam at an oblique angle.

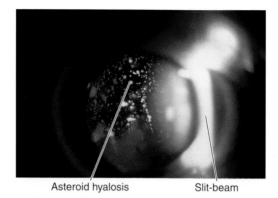

Asteroid hyalosis   Slit-beam

Figure 9-4 • The yellow-white particles of asteroid hyalosis are seen over the optic nerve. The crystals obscure the underlying retina but usually do not affect vision.

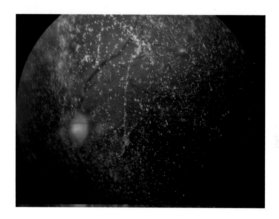

- No treatment usually recommended.

- Consider pars plana vitrectomy if particles become so severe that they affect vision or interfere with the diagnosis or treatment of retinal disorders; should be performed by a retina specialist.

Persistent Hyperplastic Primary Vitreous (Persistent Fetal Vasculature Syndrome)

Definition Sporadic, unilateral (90%), developmental anomaly with abnormal regression of the tunica vasculosa lentis (hyaloid artery) and primary vitreous. Possibly due to abnormality of PAX6 gene.

Symptoms Decreased vision; may have eye turn.

Signs Leukocoria, papillary strands, strabismus, microphthalmos, nystagmus, pink-white retrolenticular/intravitreal membrane often with radiating vessels, "inverted Y" fibrovascular stalk emanating from optic nerve, Mittendorf dot; lens is clear early but becomes cataractous; associated with shallow anterior chamber (AC) (more shallow with age), elongated ciliary processes extending toward membrane, large radial blood vessels that often cover iris; may have angle-closure glaucoma (see Chapter 6), vitreous hemorrhage, or retinal detachment.

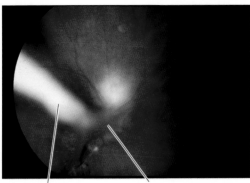

Figure 9-5 • Persistent hyperplastic primary vitreous with fibrovascular stalk emanating from the optic disc.

Fibrovascular stalk   Optic nerve

Differential Diagnosis Leukocoria (see Chapter 7).

Evaluation
- Complete ophthalmic history and eye exam with attention to tonometry, lens, and vitreous; Hruby lens, non-contact biomicroscopic or contact lens fundus exam, and ophthalmoscopy.
- B-scan ultrasonography if unable to visualize the fundus.
- Check orbital computed tomography (CT) scan or magnetic resonance imaging (MRI) for intraocular calcifications.
- Visual evoked potential (VEP) useful to decide whether to operate or not.

Management

- Correct any refractive error.
- Retinal surgery with pars plana vitrectomy, lensectomy, cautery to fibrovascular stalk, and membrane peel advocated early (within first few months of life); lens-sparing surgery considered for patients with clear lenses and eccentric stalks; should be performed by a retina specialist. Contraindications to surgery include severe microphthalmia and clear media with severe retinal dysplasia.
- Nd:YAG laser vitreolysis of traction from optic nerve and peripapillary retina.
- Patching/occlusion therapy for amblyopia (see Chapter 12).

Prognosis Visual outcomes depend on degree of maldevelopment; poor without treatment especially with posterior involvement secondary to glaucoma, recurrent vitreous hemorrhages, and eventually phthisis; earlier treatment improves prognosis.

Posterior Vitreous Detachment

Definition Syneresis (liquefaction) of the vitreous gel that causes dehiscence of the posterior hyaloid from the retina and collapse of the vitreous toward the vitreous base away from the macula and optic disc. Can be localized, partial, or total.

Epidemiology Most commonly caused by aging (53% by 50 years old, 65% by 65 years old); by age 70, majority of the posterior vitreous is liquefied (synchysis senilis); female predilection. Occurs earlier after trauma, vitritis, cataract surgery, neodymium:yttrium-aluminum-garnet (Nd:YAG) laser posterior capsulotomy, and in patients with myopia, diabetes mellitus, hereditary vitreoretinal degenerations, and retinitis pigmentosa.

Symptoms Acute onset of floaters and photopsias, especially with eye movement.

Signs Circular vitreous condensation often over disc (Weiss ring), anterior displacement of the posterior hyaloid, vitreous opacities; may have vitreous pigment cells (tobacco dust), focal intraretinal, preretinal, or vitreous hemorrhage.

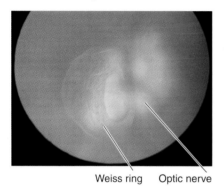

Weiss ring   Optic nerve

Figure 9-6 • Circular Weiss ring seen over the optic nerve in the mid-vitreous cavity.

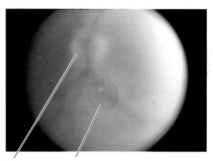

Optic nerve   Weiss ring

Figure 9-7 • Horseshoe-shaped posterior vitreous detachment seen over the optic nerve in the mid-vitreous cavity.

Figure 9-8 • Spectral domain optical coherence tomography of posterior hyaloidal face in a patient with impending PVD.

Detached hyaloid face

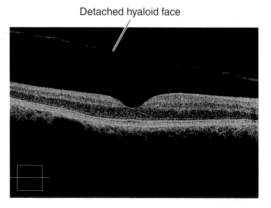

Differential Diagnosis Vitreous hemorrhage (see below), vitritis, fungal cyst.

Evaluation
- Complete ophthalmic history and eye exam with attention to anterior vitreous; Hruby lens, noncontact biomicroscopic or contact lens fundus exam, and ophthalmoscopy with a careful depressed peripheral retinal examination to identify any retinal tears or holes.

Management

- No treatment recommended.
- Instruct patient on retinal detachment warning signs: photopsias, increased floaters, and shadow or shade in peripheral vision/visual field defect; instruct patient to return immediately if RD warning signs occur to rule out retinal tear or detachment.
- Repeat dilated retinal exam 1–3 months after acute posterior vitreous detachment to rule out asymptomatic retinal tear or detachment.
- Treat retinal breaks if present (see Chapter 10).

Prognosis Good; 10–15% risk of retinal break in acute, symptomatic posterior vitreous detachments; 70% risk of retinal break if vitreous hemorrhage is present.

Synchesis Scintillans

Golden brown, refractile cholesterol crystals that are freely mobile within vitreous cavity; associated with liquid vitreous, so the crystals settle inferiorly which is the most dependent area of the vitreous body. Rare, unilateral syndrome that occurs after chronic vitreous hemorrhage, uveitis, or trauma.

Vitreous Hemorrhage

Definition Blood in the vitreous space.

Etiology Retinal break, posterior vitreous detachment, ruptured retinal arterial macroaneurysm, juvenile retinoschisis, familial exudative vitreoretinopathy, Terson's syndrome (blood dissects through the lamina cribrosa into the eye due to subarachnoid hemorrhage and elevated intracranial pressure, often bilateral with severe headache), trauma, retinal angioma, retinopathy of blood disorders, Valsalva retinopathy, and neovascularization from various disorders including diabetic retinopathy, Eales' disease, hypertensive retinopathy, radiation retinopathy, sickle cell retinopathy, and retinopathy of prematurity.

Symptoms Sudden onset of floaters and decreased vision.

Signs Decreased visual acuity, vitreous cells (red blood cells), poor or no view of fundus, poor or absent red reflex; old vitreous hemorrhage appears gray-white.

Figure 9-9 • Vitreous hemorrhage obscures the view of the retina in this diabetic patient. Gravity has layered the blood inferiorly.

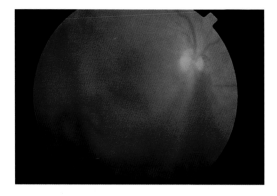

Differential Diagnosis Vitritis, asteroid hyalosis, pigment cells, pars planitis.

Evaluation
- Complete ophthalmic history and eye exam with attention to visual acuity, tonometry, noncontact biomicroscopic or contact lens fundus exam, and careful ophthalmoscopy with a depressed peripheral retinal examination to identify any retinal tears or holes.
- B-scan ultrasonography to rule out retinal tear or detachment if unable to visualize the fundus.

Management

- Conservative treatment and follow for resolution of vitreous hemorrhage, unless associated with a retinal tear or hole which needs to be treated immediately (see Chapter 10).
- Bedrest and elevation of head of bed may settle hemorrhage inferiorly to allow visualization of fundus.
- Avoid aspirin and aspirin-containing products (and other anticoagulants).
- Consider pars plana vitrectomy if there is persistent *idiopathic* vitreous hemorrhage for >6 months, nonclearing diabetic vitreous hemorrhage for >1 month, intractable increased intraocular pressure (ghost cell glaucoma), decreased vision in fellow eye, retinal tear/hole, or retinal detachment; should be performed by a retina specialist.
- Treat underlying medical condition.

Prognosis Usually good.

Vitritis

Inflammation of the vitreous characterized by vitreous white blood cells. Vitritis is a form of uveitis and is associated with anterior uveitis and more commonly intermediate or posterior uveitis; the degree of vitritis is graded on a 1 to 4 scale depending upon how limited the view of the retinal structures is (i.e., 1^+ = few cells with mild obscuration of retina; 2^+ = nerve and vessels visible; 3^+ = only nerve and large vessels visible; 4^+ = nerve and vessels not visible). It is important to distinguish vitritis from other types of cells in the vitreous cavity such as red blood cells (vitreous hemorrhage), pigment cells (retinal tear), and tumor cells (lymphoma, retinoblastoma, choroidal melanoma). The underlying etiology of the inflammation must be determined so that appropriate treatment can be given (see Uveitis sections in Chapters 6 and 10).

Trauma 328
Hemorrhages 331
Cotton-Wool Spot 333
Branch Retinal Artery Occlusion 334
Central Retinal Artery Occlusion 336
Ophthalmic Artery Occlusion 339
Branch Retinal Vein Occlusion 340
Central/Hemiretinal Vein Occlusion 342
Venous Stasis Retinopathy 346
Ocular Ischemic Syndrome 346
Retinopathy of Prematurity 348
Coats' Disease/Leber's Miliary Aneurysms 350
Eales' Disease 352
Idiopathic Juxtafoveal Retinal Telangiectasia 352
Retinopathies Associated with Blood Abnormalities 354
Diabetic Retinopathy 357
Hypertensive Retinopathy 363
Toxemia of Pregnancy 364
Acquired Retinal Arterial Macroaneurysm 365
Radiation Retinopathy 366
Age-Related Macular Degeneration 367
Retinal Angiomatous Proliferation 374
Polypoidal Choroidal Vasculopathy 375
Myopic Degeneration/Pathologic Myopia 377
Angioid Streaks 379
Central Serous Chorioretinopathy 381
Cystoid Macular Edema 383
Macular Hole 385
Epiretinal Membrane/Macular Pucker 388
Myelinated Nerve Fibers 390
Solar/Photic Retinopathy 391
Toxic Maculopathies 392
Lipid Storage Diseases 397
Retinoschisis 400
Retinal Detachment 403
Choroidal Detachment 407
Chorioretinal Folds 408
Chorioretinal Coloboma 409
Proliferative Vitreoretinopathy 410
Intermediate Uveitis/Pars Planitis 411
Neuroretinitis 412
Posterior Uveitis: Infections 414
Posterior Uveitis: White Dot Syndromes 426
Posterior Uveitis: Other Inflammatory Disorders 432
Posterior Uveitis: Evaluation/Management 440
Hereditary Chorioretinal Dystrophies 442
Hereditary Macular Dystrophies 448
Hereditary Vitreoretinal Degenerations 454
Leber's Congenital Amaurosis 458
Retinitis Pigmentosa 459
Albinism 464
Phakomatoses 465
Tumors 468
Paraneoplastic Syndromes 480

10

Retina and Choroid

Trauma

Choroidal Rupture

Tear in choroid, Bruch's membrane, and retinal pigment epithelium (RPE) usually seen after blunt trauma. Acutely, the rupture site may be obscured by hemorrhage; scars form over 3–4 weeks with RPE hyperplasia at the margin of the rupture site. Anterior ruptures are usually parallel to the ora serrata, posterior ruptures are usually crescent-shaped and concentric to the optic nerve. Patient may have decreased vision if commotio retinae or subretinal hemorrhage is present, or if the rupture is located in the macula; increased risk of developing a choroidal neovascular membrane (CNV) during the healing process (months to years after trauma). Good prognosis if the macula is not involved, poor if the fovea is involved.

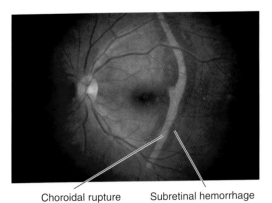

Figure 10-1 • Crescent-shaped, choroidal rupture that is concentric to the optic nerve with surrounding subretinal hemorrhage.

Choroidal rupture   Subretinal hemorrhage

- No treatment recommended, unless CNV occurs.
- Laser photocoagulation of juxtafoveal and extrafoveal CNV; consider photodynamic therapy (PDT) or anti-VEGF agent for subfoveal CNV (experimental).
- Monitor for CNV with Amsler grid.

Commotio Retinae (Berlin's Edema)

Gray-white discoloration of the outer retina due to photoreceptor outer segment disruption following blunt eye trauma; can affect any area of the retina and may be accompanied by hemorrhages or choroidal rupture. Can cause acute decrease in vision if located within the macula that resolves as the retinal discoloration disappears; may cause permanent loss of vision if fovea is damaged, but usually resolves without sequelae. Occasionally, a macular hole can form in the area of commotio with variable prognosis.

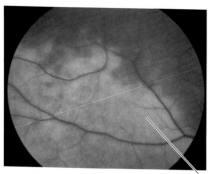

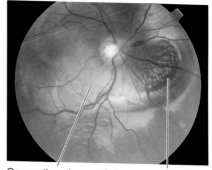

Commotio retinae   Commotio retinae   Subretinal hemorrhage

Figure 10-2 • Gray–white discoloration of the outer retina in a patient with commotio retinae.

Figure 10-3 • Commotio retinae following blunt trauma demonstrating retinal whitening. Note subretinal hemorrhage from underlying choroidal rupture.

- **Fluorescein angiogram:** Early blocked fluorescence in the areas of commotio retinae.
- No treatment recommended.

Purtscher's Retinopathy

Multiple patches of retinal whitening, large cotton-wool spots, and hemorrhages that surround the optic disc following multiple long bone fractures with fat emboli or severe compressive injuries to the chest or head. May have optic disc edema and a relative afferent pupillary defect (RAPD). Usually resolves over weeks to months.

In the absence of trauma, a Purtscher's-like retinopathy may be associated with acute pancreatitis, collagen-vascular disease, leukemia, dermatomyositis, and amniotic fluid embolus.

Figure 10-4 • Multiple patches of retinal whitening, cotton-wool spots, and intraretinal hemorrhages secondary to Purtscher's retinopathy.

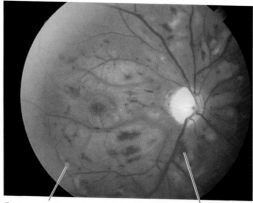

Cotton-wool spot   Subretinal hemorrhage

- **Fluorescein angiogram:** Leakage from retinal vasculature with late venous staining.
- No treatment recommended.

Traumatic Retinal Breaks

Full-thickness tear in the retina, often horseshoe-shaped, that usually occurs along the vitreous base, posterior border of lattice degeneration, or at cystic retinal tufts (areas with strong vitreoretinal adhesions). As most patients are young, the formed vitreous tamponades the tear and prevents a retinal detachment. As the vitreous liquefies over time, the retina can detach.

Giant Retinal Tear

Traumatic retinal break measuring >90° in circumferential extent or >3 clock hours.

Avulsion of Vitreous Base

Separation of vitreous base from ora serrata that is pathognomonic for trauma.

Oral Tear

Tear at the ora serrata due to split of vitreous that has a fish-mouth appearance.

Preoral Tear

Tear at anterior border of vitreous base most often occurs superotemporally.

Retinal Dialysis

Most common form after trauma. Circumferential separation of the retina at the ora serrata, usually in superotemporal (22%) or inferotemporal (31%) quadrant. Risk of retinal detachment increases over time with 10% at initial examination and 80% by 2 years.

Associated with pigmented vitreous cells ("tobacco-dust"), vitreous hemorrhages, operculum (often located over the break), and posterior vitreous detachment. Patients usually report photopsias and floaters that shift with eye movement. Liquefied vitreous can pass through the tear into the subretinal space, causing a retinal detachment even months to years after the tear forms; chronic tears have a ring of pigment around the break.

Horseshoe tear   Retinal vessel   Giant retinal tear

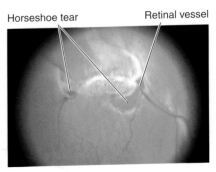
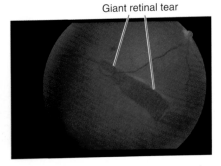

Figure 10-5 • Two horseshoe-shaped retinal tears with a bridging retinal vessel seen across the larger tear.

Figure 10-6 • Very posterior giant retinal tear that extends for more than 3 clock hours

- If symptomatic (photopsias and floaters), treatment with cryopexy along edge of tear (do not treat bare retinal pigment epithelium) or two to three rows of laser photocoagulation demarcation around the tear if no retinal detachment present.

- Retinal surgery required if retinal detachment, retinal dialysis, avulsion of the vitreous base, or giant retinal tear exists; should be performed by a retina specialist.

Chorioretinitis Sclopeteria

Trauma to retina and choroid caused by transmitted shock waves from high-velocity projectile that causes choroidal rupture, retinal hemorrhages, and commotio retinae. Vitreous hemorrhage common. Lesions heal with white fibrous scar and RPE changes. Low risk of retinal detachment in young patients with a formed vitreous.

Figure 10-7 • Chorioretinitis sclopeteria with subretinal hemorrhage and commotio retinae (same patient as Figure 1-6).

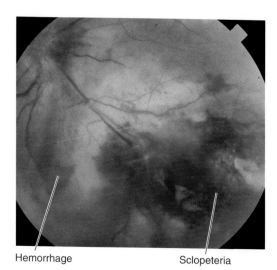

Hemorrhage   Sclopeteria

- No treatment recommended.

Hemorrhages

Preretinal Hemorrhage

Hemorrhage located between the retina and posterior vitreous face (subhyaloid) or under the internal limiting membrane of the retina (sub-ILM). Often amorphous or boat-shaped, with flat upper border and curved lower border, that obscures the underlying retina. Caused by trauma, retinal neovascularization (diabetic retinopathy, radiation retinopathy, breakthrough bleeding from a choroidal neovascular membrane), hypertensive retinopathy, Valsalva retinopathy, posterior vitreous detachment, shaken-baby syndrome, or retinal breaks, and less frequently by vascular occlusion, retinopathy of blood disorders, and leukemia.

Intraretinal Hemorrhage

Bilateral intraretinal hemorrhages are associated with systemic disorders (e.g., diabetes mellitus and hypertension); unilateral intraretinal hemorrhages generally occur in venous occlusive diseases.

Intraretinal hemorrhage: flame and dot/blot

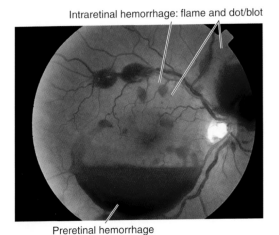

Preretinal hemorrhage

Figure 10-8 • Diabetic retinopathy demonstrating intraretinal and preretinal (boat-shaped configuration due to attached hyaloid containing the blood) hemorrhages.

Subretinal hemorrhage

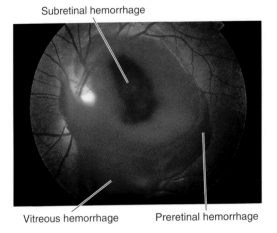

Vitreous hemorrhage   Preretinal hemorrhage

Figure 10-9 • Valsalva retinopathy demonstrating vitreous, preretinal, and subretinal hemorrhages.

Flame-Shaped Hemorrhage

Located in the superficial retina oriented with the nerve fiber layer; feathery borders. Usually occurs in hypertensive retinopathy and vein occlusion; may be peripapillary in glaucoma, especially in normal-tension glaucoma (splinter hemorrhage) and disc edema.

Dot/Blot Hemorrhage

Located in the outer plexiform layer, confined by the anteroposterior orientation of the photoreceptor, bipolar, and Müller's cells; round dots or larger blots. Usually occurs in diabetic retinopathy.

Figure 10-10 • Intraretinal dot and blot hemorrhages in a patient with nonproliferative diabetic retinopathy.

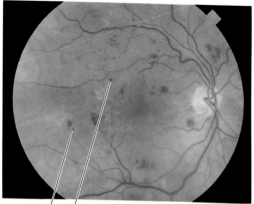

Dot/blot intraretinal hemorrhages

Roth Spot

Hemorrhage with white center that represents an embolus with lymphocytic infiltration. Classically associated with subacute bacterial endocarditis (occurs in 1–5% of such patients); also occurs in leukemia, severe anemia, sickle cell disease, collagen vascular diseases, diabetes mellitus, multiple myeloma, and acquired immunodeficiency syndrome (AIDS) (see Figures 10-40, 10-43).

Subretinal Hemorrhage

Amorphous hemorrhage located under the neurosensory retina or RPE; appears dark and is deep to the retinal vessels. Associated with trauma, subretinal and choroidal neovascular membranes, and macroaneurysms (see Figure 10-70).

All three types of hemorrhages may occur together in several disorders including age-related macular degeneration (AMD), acquired retinal arterial macroaneurysms, Eales' disease, and capillary hemangioma.

Cotton-Wool Spot

Asymptomatic, yellow-white, fluffy lesions in the superficial retina (see Figure 10-4); Nonspecific finding due to multiple etiologies including: retinal ischemia (retinal vascular occlusions, severe anemia, ocular ischemic syndrome), emboli (Purtcher's retinopathy [white blood cell emboli], intravenous drug abuse [talc], cardiac/carotid emboli, deep venous emboli), infections (acquired immunodeficiency syndrome, Rocky Mountain spotted fever, cat scratch fever [*Bartonella henselae*], leptospirosis, onchocerciasis, bacteremia, fungemia), collagen vascular diseases (systemic lupus erythematosus, dermatomyositis, polyarteritis nordosa, scleroderma, giant cell arteritis), drugs (interferon, chemotherapeutic agents), neoplasms (lymphoma, leukemia, metastatic carcinoma, multiple myeloma), retinal traction (epiretinal membrane), trauma (nerve fiber layer laceration, long bone fractures, severe chest compression [white blood cell emboli]), systemic diseases (acute pancreatitis, hypertension, diabetes mellitus, high-altitude retinopathy), and radiation.

• Treat underlying etiology (identified in 95% of cases).

Branch Retinal Artery Occlusion

Definition Disruption of the vascular perfusion in a branch of the central retinal artery (BRAO), leading to focal retinal ischemia.

Etiology Mainly due to embolism from cholesterol (Hollenhorst's plaques), calcifications (heart valves), platelet-fibrin plugs (ulcerated atheromatous plaques due to arteriosclerosis); rarely due to leukoemboli (vasculitis, Purtcher's retinopathy), fat emboli (long bone fractures), amniotic fluid emboli, tumor emboli (atrial myxoma), or septic emboli (heart valve vegetations in bacterial endocarditis or IV drug abuse). The site of the obstruction is usually at the bifurcation of retinal arteries. May result from vasospasm (migraine), compression, or coagulopathies.

Epidemiology Usually occurs in elderly patients (seventh decade); associated with hypertension (67%), carotid occlusive disease (25%), diabetes mellitus (33%), and cardiac valvular disease (25%). CRAO more common (57%) than BRAO (38%) or cilioretinal artery occlusion (5%) (in 32% of eyes, a cilioretinal artery is present).

Symptoms Sudden, unilateral, painless, partial loss of vision, with a visual field defect corresponding to the location of the occlusion. May have history of amaurosis fugax (fleeting episodes of visual loss), prior cerebrovascular accident (CVA), or transient ischemic attacks (TIAs).

Signs Visual field defect with normal or decreased visual acuity; focal, wedge-shaped area of retinal whitening within the distribution of a branch arteriole; 90% involve temporal retinal vessels; emboli (visible in 62% of cases) or Hollenhorst's plaques may be visible at retinal vessel bifurcations. Retinal whitening resolves over several weeks and visual acuity can improve.

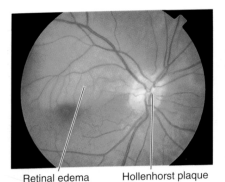

Retinal edema   Hollenhorst plaque

Figure 10-11 • Superior branch artery occlusion with retinal edema extending in a wedge-shaped pattern from the artery occluded by the Hollenhorst plaque.

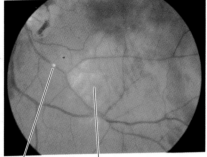

Hollenhorst plaque   Retinal edema

Figure 10-12 • Inferior branch retinal artery occlusion with Hollenhorst plaque and wedge-shaped retinal edema.

Figure 10-13 · Superior branch artery occlusion demonstrating retinal edema.

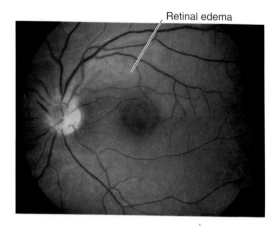

Retinal edema

Figure 10-14 · Fluorescein angiogram of same patient as Figure 10-13 demonstrating no filling of superior retinal vessels and delayed filling of affected veins.

Branch artery occlusion

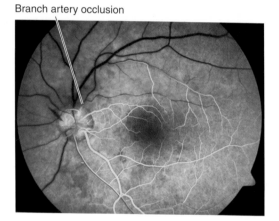

Differential Diagnosis Commotio retinae, branch retinal vein occlusion, CRAO with cilioretinal artery sparing.

Evaluation

- Complete ophthalmic history and eye exam with attention to pupils, non-contact biomicroscopic diopter or contact lens fundus exam, and ophthalmoscopy (retinal vasculature and arteriole bifurcations).

- Check blood pressure.

- **Lab tests:** fasting blood glucose (FBS) and complete blood count (CBC) with differential; consider platelets, prothrombin time/partial thromboplastin time (PT/PTT), protein C, Protein S, antithrombin III, homocysteine, antinuclear antibody (ANA), rheumatoid factor (RF), antiphospholipid antibody, serum protein electrophoresis, hemoglobin electrophoresis, Venereal Disease Research Laboratory (VDRL) test, and fluorescent treponemal antibody absorption (FTA-ABS) test. In patients >50 years old, check erythrocyte sedimentation rate (ESR) to rule out temporal arteritis. If positive, start temporal arteritis treatment immediately (see Chapter 11).

- **Fluorescein angiogram:** Delayed or absent retinal arterial filling in a branch of the central retinal artery; delayed arteriovenous transit time; capillary nonperfusion in wedge-shaped area supplied by the branch artery; staining of occlusion site and vessel wall in late views. When occlusion dissolutes, retinal blood flow is usually restored.
- Consider B-scan ultrasonography or orbital computed tomography (CT) scan to rule out a compressive lesion if the history suggests this etiology.
- Medical consultation for complete cardiovascular evaluation including electrocardiogram, echocardiogram (may require transesophageal echocardiogram to rule out valvular disease), and carotid Doppler studies.

Management

- Same treatment as CRAO (see below) if foveal circulation affected, but this is controversial due to good prognosis and questionable benefit of treatment.

Prognosis Retinal pallor fades and circulation is restored over several weeks. Good if fovea spared; 80% have ≥20/40 vision, but most have some degree of permanent visual field loss. 10% risk in fellow eye.

Central Retinal Artery Occlusion

Definition Disruption of the vascular perfusion in the central retinal artery (CRAO) leading to global retinal ischemia.

Etiology Due to emboli (only visible in 20–40% of cases) or thrombus at the level of the lamina cribosa; other causes include temporal arteritis, leukoemboli in collagen vascular diseases, fat emboli, trauma (through compression, spasm, or direct vessel damage), hypercoagulation disorders, syphilis, sickle cell disease, amniotic fluid emboli, mitral valve prolapse, particles (talc) from IV drug abuse, and compressive lesions; associated with optic disc drusen, papilledema, prepapillary arterial loops, and primary open-angle glaucoma.

Epidemiology Usually occurs in elderly patients; associated with hypertension (67%), carotid occlusive disease (25%), diabetes mellitus (33%), and cardiac valvular disease (25%). CRAO more common (57%) than BRAO (38%) or cilioretinal artery occlusion (5%) (in 32% of eyes, a cilioretinal artery is present). Rarely bilateral.

Symptoms Sudden, unilateral, painless, profound loss of vision; may have history of amaurosis fugax (fleeting episodes of visual loss), prior CVA, or TIAs.

Signs Decreased visual acuity in the count fingers (CF) to light perception (LP) range; RAPD; diffuse retinal whitening and arteriole constriction with segmentation (boxcaring) of blood flow; visible emboli (20–40%) rarely occur in central retinal artery; cherry-red spot in the macula (thin fovea allows visualization of the underlying choroidal circulation). In ciliary retinal artery sparing CRAO (25%), small wedge-shaped area of perfused retina may be present temporal to the optic disc (10% spare the foveola in which case visual acuity improves to 20/50 or better in 80%). *Note*: Ophthalmic artery obstruction usually does not produce a cherry-red spot due to underlying choroidal ischemia.

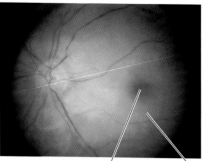

Cherry-red spot   Retinal edema

Figure 10-15 • Central retinal artery occlusion with cherry-red spot in the fovea and surrounding retinal edema.

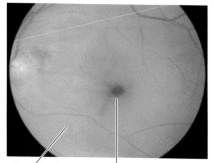

Retinal edema   Cherry-red spot

Figure 10-16 • Central retinal artery occlusion with cherry-red spot.

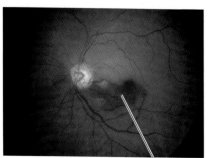

Retinal edema   Patent
                ciliaretinal artery

Figure 10-17 • Cilioretinal artery sparing central retinal artery occlusion with patent ciliaretinal artery allowing perfusion (thus no edema) in a small section of the macula.

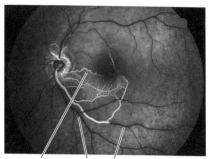

Patent   Absent flow
ciliaretinal artery

Figure 10-18 • Fluorescein angiogram of same patient in Figure 10-17 demonstrating no filling of retinal vessels except in cilioretinal artery and surrounding branches.

Differential Diagnosis Ophthalmic artery occlusion, commotio retinae, cherry-red spot due to inherited metabolic or lysosomal storage diseases, methanol toxicity.

Evaluation

- Complete ophthalmic history and eye exam with attention to pupils, non-contact biomicroscopic or contact lens fundus exam, and ophthalmoscopy (retinal vasculature).
- Check blood pressure.
- **Lab tests:** FBS and CBC with differential; consider platelets, PT/PTT, protein C, protein S, antithrombin III, homocysteine, ANA, RF, antiphospholipid antibody, serum protein electrophoresis, hemoglobin electrophoresis, VDRL, and FTA-ABS. In patients >50 years old, check ESR to rule out arteritic ischemic optic neuropathy.

- **Fluorescein angiogram:** Delayed retinal arterial filling and arteriovenous transit time with normal choroidal filling and perfusion of optic nerve from ciliary branches; prolonged arteriovenous circulation times; extensive capillary nonperfusion.
- **Electrophysiologic testing:** ERG (reduced b wave amplitude, normal a wave).
- Consider B-scan ultrasonography or orbital CT scan to rule out compressive lesion if history suggests compression.
- Medical consultation for complete cardiovascular evaluation including electrocardiogram, echocardiogram (may require transesophageal echocardiogram to rule out valvular disease), and carotid Doppler studies.

Management

OPHTHALMIC EMERGENCY

- Treatment is controversial due to poor prognosis and questionable benefit of treatment. Goal is to move emboli distally to restore proximal retinal blood flow; most maneuvers are aimed at rapid lowering of the intraocular pressure (IOP).
- Treat immediately before starting work-up (if patient presents within 24 hours of visual loss), but best hope is to treat within 90 minutes.
- Digital ocular massage to try and dislodge emboli.
- Systemic acetazolamide (Diamox 500 mg IV or po).
- Topical ocular hypotensive drops: β-blocker (timolol 0.5% 1 gtt q15 min × 2, repeat as necessary).
- **Anterior chamber paracentesis (immediately lowers IOP to 0 mmHg):** This procedure is easily performed at the slit lamp after prepping the eye with topical anesthetic, broad-spectrum antibiotic, and povidone-iodine. A lid speculum is placed, the eye is grasped with forceps at the nasal limbus to prevent movement and provide countertraction, and either a disposable microsurgical knife (15° or MVR blade) or else a 30 gauge 1/2 inch needle on a 1 ml syringe without the plunger, is inserted parallel to the iris through the peripheral cornea at the temporal limbus. If necessary, gentle pressure can be applied to the posterior lip of the paracentesis site so that aqueous can be released in a controlled fashion. Treat with a topical broad-spectrum antibiotic (gatifloxacin [Zymar] or moxifloxacin [Vigamox] qid for 3 days).
- Consider admission to hospital for carbogen treatment (95% oxygen-5% carbon dioxide for 10 minutes q2 h for 24–48 hours) to attempt to increase oxygenation and induce vasodilation.
- Unproven treatments include hyperbaric oxygen, antifibrinolytic drugs, retrobulbar vasodilators, sublingual nitroglycerine, and Nd:YAG laser to dislodge the emboli.
- If arteritic anterior ischemic optic neuropathy (see Chapter 11) suspected: Systemic steroids (methylprednisolone 1 g IV qd in divided doses for 3 days, then prednisone 60–100 mg po qd with a slow taper; decrease by no more than 2.5–5.0 mg/wk).

Prognosis Retinal pallor fades and circulation is restored over several weeks. Poor prognosis; most have persistent severe visual loss with constricted retinal arterioles and optic atrophy. Rubeosis (20%) and disc/retinal neovascularization (2–3%) can rarely occur. Presence of visible embolus associated with increased mortality; most common cause of mortality is myocardial infarction.

Ophthalmic Artery Occlusion

Definition Obstruction at the level of the ophthalmic artery that affects both the retinal and choroidal circulation leading to ischemia more severe than CRAO.

Etiology Usually due to emboli or thrombus, but can be caused by any of the etiologies listed for CRAO.

Epidemiology Usually occurs in elderly patients; associated with hypertension (67%), carotid occlusive disease (25%), diabetes mellitus (33%), and cardiac valvular disease (25%).

Symptoms Sudden, unilateral, painless, profound loss of vision up to the level of light perception or even no light perception.

Signs Marked constriction of the retinal vessels, marked retinal edema often without a cherry red spot (although it may be present); may have RAPD; later, optic atrophy, retinal vascular sclerosis, and diffuse pigmentary changes.

Differential Diagnosis Central retinal artery occlusion, commotio retinae, cherry-red spot due to inherited metabolic or lysosomal storage diseases, methanol toxicity.

Evaluation
- Complete ophthalmic history and eye exam with attention to pupils, non-contact biomicroscopic or contact lens fundus exam, and ophthalmoscopy.
- Check blood pressure.
- **Lab tests:** FBS and CBC with differential; consider platelets, PT/PTT, protein C, protein S, antithrombin III, homocysteine, ANA, RF, antiphospholipid antibody, serum protein electrophoresis, hemoglobin electrophoresis, VDRL, and FTA-ABS. In patients >50 years old, check ESR to rule out arteritic ischemic optic neuropathy.
- **Fluorescein angiogram:** Delayed or absent choroidal *and* retinal vascular filling, extensive capillary nonperfusion.
- **Electrophysiologic testing:** ERG (reduced or absent a and b wave amplitudes).
- Medical consultation for complete cardiovascular evaluation including electrocardiogram, echocardiogram (may require transthoracic echocardiogram to rule out valvular disease), and carotid Doppler studies.

Management

OPHTHALMIC EMERGENCY

• Same treatment as CRAO (see above).

Prognosis Severe visual loss is usually permanent.

Branch Retinal Vein Occlusion

Definition Occlusion of a branch retinal vein (BRVO). Two types:

Non-Ischemic (64%)

<5 disc areas of capillary non-perfusion on fluorescein angiogram.

Ischemic

≥5 disc areas of capillary non-perfusion on fluorescein angiogram.

Etiology Usually caused by a thrombus at arteriovenous crossings where a thickened artery compresses the underlying venous wall; associated with hypertension, coronary artery disease, diabetes mellitus, and peripheral vascular disease; rarely associated with hypercoagulable states (e.g., macroglobulinemia, cryoglobulinemia), hyperviscosity states (polycythemia vera, Waldenström's macroglobulinemia), systemic lupus erythematosus, syphilis, sarcoid, homocystinuria, malignancies (e.g., multiple myeloma, polycythemia vera, leukemia), optic nerve drusen, and external compression. In younger patients, associated with oral contraceptive pills, collagen vascular disease, acquired immunodeficiency syndrome (AIDS), protein S/protein C/antithrombin III deficiency, Factor XII (Hageman factor) deficiency, antiphospholipid antibody syndrome, or activated protein C resistance (factor V Leiden polymerase chain reaction [PCR] assay).

Epidemiology Usually occurs in elderly patients, 60–70 years old; associated with hypertension (50–70%), cardiovascular disease, diabetes mellitus, increased body mass index, and open-angle glaucoma; slight male and hyperopic predilection. Second most common vascular disease after diabetic retinopathy.

Symptoms Sudden, unilateral, painless, visual field loss. Patients may have normal vision, especially when macula is not involved.

Signs Quadrantic visual field defect; dilated, tortuous retinal veins with superficial, retinal hemorrhages, and cotton-wool spots in a wedge-shaped area radiating from an arteriovenous crossing (usually arterial over-crossing where an arteriole and venule share a common vascular sheath). More common superotemporally (60%) than inferotemporally (40%; rare nasally (since usually asymptomatic). The closer the obstruction is to the optic disc, the greater the area of retina involved and more serious the complications. Microaneurysms or macroaneurysms, macular edema (50%), epiretinal membranes (20%), retinal and/or iris/angle neovascularization (very rare), and vitreous hemorrhage may develop; neovascular glaucoma is rare.

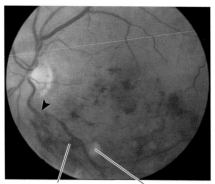

Intraretinal hemorrhage   Cotton-wool spots

Figure 10-19 ● Inferior branch retinal vein occlusion demonstrating wedge-shaped area of intraretinal hemorrhages and cotton wool spots.

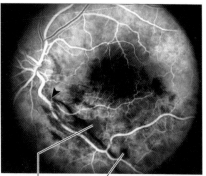

Cotton-wool spots   Intraretinal hemorrhage

Figure 10-20 ● Fluorescein angiogram of same patient as Figure 10-19 demonstrating lack of perfusion in inferior retinal vein with blocking defects from the intraretinal hemorrhages. Site of occlusion is shown with an arrowhead.

Differential Diagnosis Venous stasis retinopathy, ocular ischemic syndrome, hypertensive retinopathy, leukemic retinopathy, retinopathy of anemia, diabetic retinopathy, papilledema, papillophlebitis (in young patients).

Evaluation

- Complete ophthalmic history and eye exam with attention to pupils, tonometry, gonioscopy, non-contact biomicroscopic or contact lens fundus exam, and ophthalmoscopy.
- Check visual fields.
- Check blood pressure.
- **Lab tests:** Fasting blood glucose, glycosylated hemoglobin; consider CBC with differential, platelets, PT/PTT, ANA, RF, angiotensin converting enzyme (ACE), ESR, serum protein electrophoresis, lipid profile, hemoglobin electrophoresis (in African Americans), VDRL, and FTA-ABS depending on clinical situation. In a patient <40 years old and in whom a hypercoagulable state is being considered: check human immunodeficiency virus (HIV) status, functional protein S assay, functional protein C assay, functional antithrombin III assay (type II heparin-binding mutation), antiphospholipid antibody titer, lupus anticoagulant, anticardiolipin antibody titer (IgG and IgM), homocysteine level (if elevated test for folate, B12, and creatinine), Factor XII (Hageman factor) levels, and activated protein C resistance (Factor V Leiden mutation PCR assay); if these tests are normal and clinical suspicion for a hypercoagulable state still exists: add plasminogen antigen assay, heparin cofactor II assay, thrombin time, reptilase time, and fibrinogen functional assay.
- **Fluorescein angiogram:** Delayed retinal venous filling in a branch of the central retinal vein, increased transit time in affected venous distribution, blocked fluorescence in areas of retinal hemorrhages, and capillary nonperfusion (ischemic defined as ≥5 disc areas of capillary nonperfusion) in the area supplied by the involved retinal vein. Retinal edema with cystic changes are not present acutely, but appear later.
- Medical consultation for complete cardiovascular evaluation.

Management

- Quadrantic scatter laser photocoagulation (500 μm spots) when rubeosis (≥2 clock hours of iris or any angle neovascularization), disc/retinal neovascularization, or neovascular glaucoma develops (Branch Vein Occlusion Study-BVOS conclusion); prophylactic laser was not evaluated in BVOS, and is not recommended.
- Macular grid/focal photocoagulation (50–100 μm spots) when macular edema lasts >3 months and vision is <20/40 (BVOS conclusion).
- Experimental options for macular edema include intravitreal 4 mg triamcinolone acetonide [Kenalog], arteriovenous sheathotomy, and intravitreal anti-VEGF agents such as 1.25 mg bevacizumab [Avastin].
- Discontinue oral contraceptives.
- Consider aspirin (80–325 mg po qd).
- Treat underlying medical conditions.

Prognosis

- Good; 50% have ≥20/40 vision unless foveal ischemia or chronic macular edema is present. Risk of another BRVO in same eye is 3% and in fellow eye is 12%.

Central/Hemiretinal Vein Occlusion

Definition Occlusion of the central retinal vein (CRVO). Hemiretinal occlusion (HRVO) occurs when the superior and inferior retinal drainage does not merge into a central retinal vein (20%) and is occluded (more like CRVO than BRVO). Two types:

Non-Ischemic/Perfused (67%)

<10 disc areas of capillary non-perfusion on fluorescein angiogram.

Ischemic/Non-Perfused

=10 disc areas of capillary non-perfusion on fluorescein angiogram.

Etiology Usually caused by a thrombus in the area of the lamina cribosa; associated with hypertension (60%), coronary artery disease, diabetes mellitus, peripheral vascular disease, and primary open-angle glaucoma (40%); rarely associated with hypercoagulable states (e.g., macroglobulinemia, cryoglobulinemia), hyperviscosity states especially in bilateral cases (polycythemia vera, Waldenström's macroglobulinemia), systemic lupus erythematosus, syphilis, sarcoid, homocystinuria, malignancies (e.g., multiple myeloma, polycythemia vera, leukemia), optic nerve drusen, and external compression. In younger patients, associated with oral contraceptive pills, collagen vascular disease, acquired immunodeficiency syndrome (AIDS), protein S/protein C/antithrombin III deficiency, Factor XII (Hageman factor) deficiency, antiphospholipid antibody syndrome, or activated protein C resistance (factor V Leiden polymerase chain reaction [PCR] assay).

Epidemiology Usually occurs in elderly patients (90% are >50 years old); slight male predilection. Ischemic disease is more common in older patients and those with cardiovascular disease. Younger patients can get inflammatory condition termed papillophlebitis or benign retinal vasculitis with benign clinical course.

Symptoms Sudden, unilateral, loss of vision or less frequently history of transient obscuration of vision with complete recovery. Some report pain and present initially with neovascularization of the iris and neovascular glaucoma following a loss of vision 3 months earlier ("90 day glaucoma"). Patients may have normal vision if perfused, especially when the macula is not involved.

Signs Decreased visual acuity ranging from 20/20 to hand motion (HM) with most worse than 20/200 (vision worse in ischemic type; usually >20/200 in non-ischemic); dilated, tortuous retinal veins with superficial, retinal hemorrhages, and cotton-wool spots in all four quadrants extending to periphery; optic disc hyperemia, disc edema, and macular edema common; RAPD (degree of defect correlates with amount of ischemia). Non-ischemic disease rarely produces neovascularization; ischemic disease can produce rubeosis (20% in CRVO, rare in BRVO), disc/retinal neovascularization (border of perfused/nonperfused retina), neovascular glaucoma, and vitreous hemorrhages. Collateral optociliary shunt vessels between retinal and ciliary circulations (50%) occur late. Impending CRVO may have absence of spontaneous venous pulsations (but this can also occur in normal individuals). Transient patchy ischemic retinal whitening may occur early in nonischemic CRVO.

Differential Diagnosis Venous stasis retinopathy, ocular ischemic syndrome, hypertensive retinopathy, leukemic retinopathy, retinopathy of anemia, diabetic retinopathy, radiation retinopathy, and papilledema.

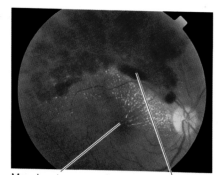

Macular star   Intraretinal hemorrhage

Figure 10-21 • Hemi-retinal vein occlusion with exudates forming partial macular star.

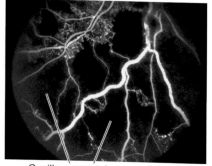

Capillary nonperfusion

Figure 10-22 • Fluorescein angiogram of a patient with a retinal vein occlusion demonstrating peripheral capillary nonperfusion.

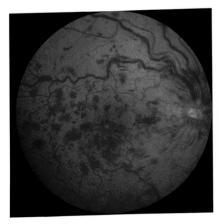

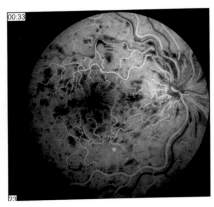

Figure 10-23 • Central retinal vein occlusion demonstrating hemorrhages in all four quadrants.

Figure 10-24 • Fluorescein angiogram demonstrating no filling of the central retinal vein.

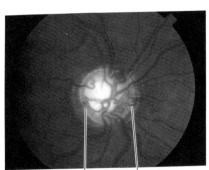

Optociliary shunt vessels

Figure 10-25 • Optociliary shunt vessels in a patient with an old central retinal vein occlusion.

Evaluation

- Complete ophthalmic history and eye exam with attention to visual acuity (worse than 20/400 likely ischemic), pupils (ischemic likely to have RAPD), Golmann visual fields (ischemic cannot see I4e), tonometry, gonioscopy, non-contact biomicroscopic or contact lens fundus exam, and ophthalmoscopy.

- Check blood pressure.

- **Lab tests:** Fasting blood glucose, glycosylated hemoglobin; consider CBC with differential, platelets, PT/PTT, ANA, RF, ACE, ESR, serum protein electrophoresis, lipid profile, hemoglobin electrophoresis (in African American), VDRL, and FTA-ABS depending on clinical situation. In a patient <40 years old and in whom a hypercoagulable state is being considered: check human immunodeficiency virus (HIV) status, functional protein S assay, functional protein C assay, functional antithrombin III assay (type II heparin-binding mutation), antiphospholipid antibody titer, lupus anticoagulant, anticardiolipin antibody titer (IgG and IgM), homocysteine level (if elevated test for folate, B12, and creatinine), Factor XII (Hageman factor) levels, and activated protein C resistance (Factor V Leiden mutation PCR assay); if these tests are normal and clinical suspicion for a hypercoagulable state still exists: add plasminogen antigen assay, heparin cofactor II assay, thrombin time, reptilase time, and fibrinogen functional assay.

- **Fluorescein angiogram:** Delayed retinal venous filling, increased transit time (>20 seconds increases risk of rubeosis), extensive capillary nonperfusion (ischemic defined in CVOS as ≥10 disc areas of capillary nonperfusion), staining of vascular walls, and blocking defects due to retinal hemorrhages. Retinal edema with cystic changes are not present acutely, but appear later.

- **Electrophysiologic testing:** ERG (reduced b wave amplitude [<60% of normal more likely ischemic], reduced b:a wave ratio [<1 associated with increased risk of ischemia and neovascularization], prolonged b wave implicit time).

- Medical consultation for complete cardiovascular evaluation.

Management

- Panretinal laser photocoagulation (PRP) (500 μm spots) when rubeosis (≥2 clock hours of iris or any angle neovascularization), disc/retinal neovascularization, or neovascular glaucoma develops; no benefit to prophylactic PRP (Central Retinal Vein Occlusion Study-CVOS conclusion).

- Focal laser photocoagulation decreases macular edema, but has no effect on visual acuity (CVOS conclusion); trend in CVOS for focal laser to work in younger patients; experimentally, intravitreal 4 mg triamcinolone acetonide [Kenalog] and anti-VEGF agents such as 1.25 mg bevacizumab [Avastin] have been shown to decrease macular edema and transiently improve visual acuity, long-term safety and benefits are not proven.

- Creation of chorioretinal venous anastamosis by intentional rupture of Bruch's membrane with high intensity laser photocoagulation or surgical blade reportedly successful in 1/3 of cases, but still experimental.

- Other experimental surgical options include radial optic neurotomy (RON) and intravenous injection of tissue plasminogen activator (tPA) into the lumen of the central retinal vein.

- Discontinue oral contraceptives and change diuretics to an alternate antihypertensive.

- Consider aspirin (80–325 mg po qd).

- Treat underlying medical condition.

Prognosis Clinical course is variable; evaluate monthly for first 6 months. Nonischemic has better prognosis (10% will completely resolve). Risk of neovascularization depends on amount of ischemia (CVOS conclusion); 16% of nonischemic patients progress to ischemic disease; 60% of ischemic patients develop neovascularization and 33% develop neovascular glaucoma.

Venous Stasis Retinopathy

Milder form of nonischemic central retinal vein occlusion (CRVO) representing patients with better perfusion. Dot/blot/flame hemorrhages, dilated/tortuous vasculature, and microaneurysms occur, usually bilateral; more benign course. Associated with hyperviscosity syndromes including polycythemia vera, multiple myeloma, and Waldenström's macroglobulinemia.

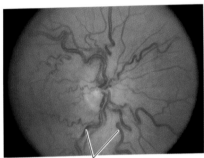 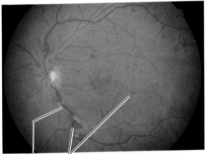

Dilated, tortuous vasculature

Intraretinal hemorrhages
Dilated, tortuous vasculature

Figure 10-26 • Dilated, tortuous, retinal vessels in a patient with hyperviscosity syndrome.

Figure 10-27 • Intraretinal hemorrhages in a patient with venous stasis retinopathy.

Ocular Ischemic Syndrome

Definition Widespread ischemia of both the anterior and posterior segments of the eye due to ipsilateral carotid occlusive disease (less frequently obstruction of the ipsilateral ophthalmic artery), carotid dissection, or arteritis (rare).

Etiology Due to a 90% or greater occlusion of the ipsilateral carotid artery or rarely ophthalmic artery.

Epidemiology Usually occurs in patients aged 50–70 years old (mean = 65 years); 80% unilateral; male predilection (2:1). Associated with atherosclerosis, ischemic heart disease (50%), hypertension (67%), diabetes mellitus (50%), previous stroke (25%), and peripheral arterial disease (20%); rarely due to inflammatory conditions including giant cell arteritis. Blood flow to the eye is relatively unaffected until carotid obstruction exceeds 70%; ocular ischemic syndrome usually does not occur until it reaches 90% (decreasing CRA perfusion by 50%); 50% of patients have complete ipsilateral carotid artery obstruction.

Symptoms Gradual loss of vision (90%) over days to weeks with accompanying dull eye pain/headache (40%) or "ocular angina"; patients may also report amaurosis fugax or a delayed recovery of vision after exposure to bright light due to impaired photoreceptor regeneration.

Signs Gradual or sudden decreased visual acuity ranging from 20/20 to NLP; retinal arterial narrowing and venous dilatation without tortuousity, retinal hemorrhages (80% midperipheral), microaneurysms, macular edema, cotton-wool spots, disc/retinal neovascularization (37%), and spontaneous pulsations of the retinal arteries; anterior segment signs including episcleral injection, corneal edema, anterior chamber cells and flare (keratic precipitates are absent), iris atrophy, chronic conjunctivitis, and rubeosis (66%) are common. Intraocular pressure may be elevated, but may also be normal even with 360° synechia. Light digital pressure on the globe through the eyelid often produces arterial pulsations (does not occur in other disease in differential) and can shut down perfusion of the central retinal artery.

Differential Diagnosis Nonischemic CRVO, venous stasis retinopathy, diabetic retinopathy, hypertensive retinopathy, aortic arch disease, parafoveal telangiectasis, radiation retinopathy, Takayasu's disease.

Evaluation

- Complete ophthalmic history and eye exam with attention to pupils, tonometry, anterior chamber, gonioscopy, non-contact biomicroscopic or contact lens fundus exam, and ophthalmoscopy. Digital pressure on eye causes arterial pulsation.
- Check blood pressure.
- **Fluorescein angiogram:** Delayed arteriovenous transit time (>11 seconds) in 95%; delayed or patchy choroidal filling (>5 seconds) in 60%, arterial vascular staining in 85%.
- **Electrophysiologic testing:** ERG (reduced or absent a wave and b wave amplitudes)
- Medical consultation for complete cardiovascular evaluation including duplex and Doppler scans of carotid arteries (≥90% obstruction of the ipsilateral internal or common carotid arteries).

Management

- Panretinal laser photocoagulation (PRP) (500 μm spots) when anterior or posterior segment neovascularization develops.
- Consider carotid endarterectomy if carotid obstruction exists; more beneficial if performed before rubeosis develops.
- May require treatment of increased intraocular pressure (see Primary Open-Angle Glaucoma section in Chapter 11).
- Glaucoma surgery when anterior chamber angle is closed.

Prognosis Poor prognosis; 5-year mortality rate is 40% mainly due to cardiovascular disease. Sixty percent of patients have count fingers or worse vision at 1 year follow-up; only 25% have better than 20/50 vision. When rubeosis is present, 90% will be count fingers or worse within 1 year. One-third of patients improve vision after carotid endarterectomy, one-third remains unchanged, and one-third worsen despite surgery.

Retinopathy of Prematurity

Definition Abnormal retinal vasculature development in premature infants, especially after supplemental oxygen therapy.

Epidemiology Usually bilateral; associated risk factors include premature birth (<36 weeks' gestation), low birth weight (<750 g: 90% develop ROP and 16% develop threshold disease; 1000–1250 g: 45% develop ROP and 2% develop threshold disease), supplemental oxygen therapy (>50 days), and a complicated hospital course.

Symptoms Asymptomatic; later may have decreased vision.

Signs Shallow anterior chamber, corneal edema, iris atrophy, poor pupillary dilation, posterior synechiae, ectropion uveae, leukocoria, vitreous hemorrhage, retinal detachment, and retrolental fibroplasia; may have strabismus.

International classification of ROP describes the retinal changes in 5 stages:

Stage 1

Thin, circumferential, flat, white, demarcation line develops between posterior vascularized and peripheral avascular retina (beyond line).

Stage 2

Demarcation line becomes elevated and organized into a pink-white ridge, no fibrovascular growth visible.

Stage 3

Extraretinal fibrovascular proliferation from surface of the ridge.

Stage 4

Dragging of vessels, and subtotal traction retinal detachment (4A is macula attached, 4B involves macula).

Stage 5

Total retinal detachment (almost always funnel detachment).

International classification of ROP also describes the extent of retina involved by number of clock hours and location by zone (centered on optic disc, not the fovea because retinal vessels emanate from disc):

Zone 1

Inner zone (posterior pole) corresponding to the area enclosed by a circle around the optic disc with radius equal to twice the distance from the disc to the macula (diameter of 60°).

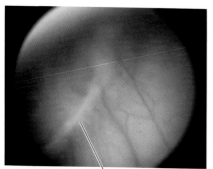

Extraretinal fibrovascular proliferation

Figure 10-28 • Retinopathy of prematurity (ROP) demonstrating extraretinal fibrovascular proliferation along the ridge (Stage 3 ROP).

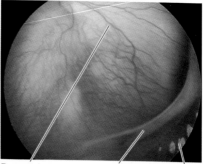

Dragged vessels   Traction RD   Laser spots

Figure 10-29 • Retinopathy of prematurity (ROP) demonstrating dragged vessels, traction retinal detachment, and laser spots anterior to the regressed fibrovascular proliferation (Stage 4a ROP).

Zone 2

The area between Zone 1 and a circle centered on the optic disc and tangent to the nasal ora serrata.

Zone 3

Remaining temporal crescent of retina (last area to become vascularized).

Finally, International classification of ROP defines "Plus" disease:

"Plus" Disease

At least 2 quadrants (usually 6 or more clock hours) of shunted blood causing vascular engorgement in the posterior pole with tortuous arteries, dilated veins, pupillary rigidity due to iris vascular engorgement, and vitreous haze.

Differential Diagnosis Coats' disease, Eales' disease, familial exudative vitreoretinopathy, sickle cell retinopathy, juvenile retinoschisis, persistent hyperplastic primary vitreous, incontinentia pigmenti (Bloch–Sulzberger syndrome), and other causes of leukocoria (see Chapter 7).

Evaluation

- Screen all premature infants at 4–6 weeks chronological age who weighed <1250–1750 g at birth, and larger premature infants on supplemental oxygen for >50 days.
- Complete ophthalmic history with attention to birth history and birth weight.
- Complete eye exam with attention to iris, lens, and ophthalmoscopy (retinal vasculature and retinal periphery with scleral depression).
- Cycloplegic refraction as many develop refractive errors especially myopia.
- Pediatric consultation.

Management

- Treat with ablation of peripheral avascular retina when patient reaches type 1 ROP, defined as: Zone 1, any Stage of ROP with Plus disease; Zone 1, Stage 3 with or without Plus disease; Zone 2, Stage 2 or 3 with Plus disease (Early Treatment of Retinopathy of Prematurity [ETROP] study conclusion).

    Note: this means treating earlier than the older "threshold" definition = Stage 3 Plus disease with at least 5 contiguous or 8 non-contiguous, cumulative clock hours involvement in Zone 1 or 2.

- Indirect argon green or diode laser photocoagulation (500 μm spots) to entire avascular retina in Zone 1 and peripheral Zone 2; laser is at least as effective as cryotherapy (Laser-ROP study conclusion) *or*

- Cryotherapy to entire avascular retina in Zone 2, but not ridge (Cryotherapy for ROP [CRYO-ROP] study conclusion).

- Serial exams with type 2 ROP, defined as Zone 1, Stage 1 or 2 without Plus disease; Zone 2, Stage 3 without Plus disease.

- Tractional retinal detachment or rhegmatogenous retinal detachment (cicatricial ROP, Stages 4–5) require vitreoretinal surgery with pars plana vitrectomy, with/without lensectomy, membrane peel, and possible scleral buckle; should be performed by a retina specialist trained in pediatric retinal disease.

- Follow *very closely* (every 1–2 weeks depending on location and severity of the disease) until extreme periphery is vascularized, then monthly therafter. Beware of "rush" disease defined as Plus disease in Zone 1 or posterior Zone 2. "Rush" disease has a significant risk of rapid progression to Stage 5 within a few days.

- Anti-VEGF agents such as bevacizumab [Avastin] have been used experimentally with positive preliminary results, but safety not proven.

Prognosis Depends on the amount and stage of ROP; 80–90% will spontaneously regress; may develop amblyopia, macular dragging, strabismus; stage 5 disease carries a poor prognosis (functional success in only 3%); may develop high myopia, glaucoma, cataracts, keratoconus, band keratopathy, and retinal detachment.

Coats' Disease/Leber's Miliary Aneurysms

Unilateral (80–95%), idiopathic, progressive, developmental retinal vascular abnormality (telangiectatic and aneurysmal vessels with a predilection for the macula); usually occurs in young males (10:1) <20 years old (two-thirds present before age 10). Retinal microaneurysms, retinal telangiectasia, lipid exudation, "light-bulb" vascular dilatations, capillary nonperfusion and occasionally neovascularization, exudative retinal detachments, and subretinal cholesteol crystals occur primarily in the temporal quadrants, especially on fluorescein angiogram where microaneurysm leakage is common. May present with poor vision, strabismus, or leukocoria. Spectrum of disease from milder form in older patients with equal sex predilection and often bilateral (Leber's miliary aneurysms) to severe form with localized exudative retinal detachments and yellowish subretinal masses, and is included in the differential diagnosis of leukocoria (Coats' disease). Clinical course varies but generally progressive. Rarely associated with systemic disorders including Alport's disease, fascioscapulohumeral dystrophy, muscular dystrophy, tuberous sclerosis, Turner's syndrome, and Senior–Loken syndrome. On histopathologic examination there is loss of vascular endothelium and pericytes with subsequent mural disorganization.

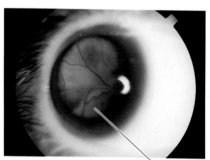

Exudative retinal detachment

Figure 10-30 • Coats' disease demonstrating leukocoria due to exudative retinal detachment.

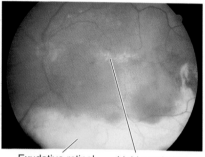

Exudative retinal detachment   Lipid exudation

Figure 10-31 • Coats' disease with massive exudative retinal detachment.

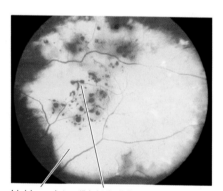

Lipid exudate   "Light-bulb" vascular dilations

Figure 10-32 • Leber's miliary aneurysms demonstrating dilated arterioles with terminal "light-bulbs."

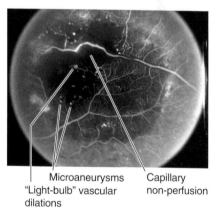

Microaneurysms   Capillary
"Light-bulb" vascular   non-perfusion
dilations

Figure 10-33 • Fluorescein angiogram of same patient as Figure 10-32 demonstrating capillary non-perfusion, microaneurysms, and "light-bulb" vascular dilations.

- **Fluorescein angiogram:** Capillary nonperfusion, microaneurysms, light-bulb vascular dilatations, leakage from telangiectatic vessels, and macular edema.

- Scatter laser photocoagulation to posterior or cryotherapy to anterior areas of abnormal vasculature and areas of nonperfusion when symptomatic. May require multiple treatment sessions. Goal is to ablate areas of vascular leakage and to allow resorption of exudate.

Eales' Disease

Bilateral, idiopathic, peripheral obliterative vasculopathy that occurs in healthy, young adults aged 20–30 years old with male predilection. Patients usually notice floaters and decreased vision and have areas of perivascular sheathing, vitreous cells, peripheral retinal nonperfusion, microaneurysms, intraretinal hemorrhages, white sclerotic ghost vessels, disc/iris/retinal neovascularization, and vitreous hemorrhages. Fibrovascular proliferation may lead to tractional retinal detachments. May have signs of ocular inflammation with keratic precipitates, anterior chamber cells and flare, and cystoid macular edema; variable prognosis. Eales' disease is a diagnosis of exclusion; must rule out other causes of inflammation or neovascularization including BRVO, diabetic retinopathy, sickle cell retinopathy, multiple sclerosis, sarcoidosis, tuberculosis, SLE, and other collagen-vascular diseases.

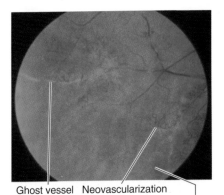

Ghost vessel   Neovascularization
Peripheral non-perfusion

Figure 10-34 • Eales' disease with ghost vessels, peripheral capillary non-perfusion, and neovascularization.

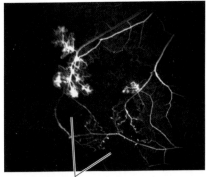

Peripheral non-perfusion

Figure 10-35 • Fluorescein angiogram of patient with Eales' disease demonstrating extensive peripheral nonperfusion and neovascularization.

- **Fluorescein angiogram:** Mid-peripheral retinal nonperfusion with well-demarcated boundary between perfused and nonperfused areas; microaneurysms and neovascularization.
- Scatter laser photocoagulation to nonperfused retina when neovascularization develops. If vitreous hemorrhage obscures view of retina, peripheral cryotherapy can be applied to ablate peripheral avascular retina.
- Consider periocular or systemic steroids for inflammatory component.

Idiopathic Juxtafoveal Retinal Telangiectasia

Group of retinal vascular disorders with abnormal perifoveal capillaries confined to the juxtafoveal region (1–199 μm from center of fovea). Several forms:

Type 1A (Unilateral Congenital Parafoveal Telangiectasia)

Occurs in men in the fourth to fifth decade. Yellow exudate at outer edge of telangiectasis usually temporal to the fovea and 1–2 disc diameters in area; decreased vision ranging from 20/25 to 20/40 from macular edema and exudate. May represent mild presentation of Coats' disease in an adult.

- **Fluorescein angiogram:** Unilateral cluster of telangiectatic vessels with variable leakage; macular edema often with petalloid leakage.

- Consider focal laser photocoagulation to leaking, non-subfoveal vessels.

Type 1B (Unilateral Idiopathic Parafoveal Telangiectasia)

Occurs in middle-aged men. Minimal exudate usually confined to 1 clock hour at the edge of the foveal avascular zone; usually asymptomatic with vision better than 20/25.

Juxtafoveal telangiectasia

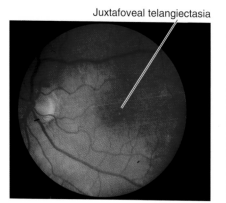

Juxtafoveal telangiectasia

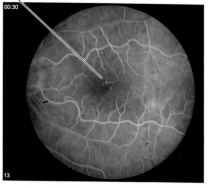

Figure 10-36 ● Juxtafoveal telangiectasia type 1b with mild retinal pigment epithelium changes at edge of fovea.

Figure 10-37 ● Fluorescein angiogram of same patient as Figure 10-36, demonstrating hyperfluorescent leakage from telangiectatic vessels.

- **Fluorescein angiogram:** Unilateral cluster of telangiectatic vessels with variable leakage; macular edema often with petalloid leakage.

- No treatment recommended.

Type 2 (Bilateral Acquired Parafoveal Telangiectasia)

Onset of symptoms in the fifth to sixth decades with equal sex distribution. Symmetric, bilateral, right-angle venules within 1 disc diameter of the central fovea; usually found temporal to the fovea but may surround the fovea; mild blurring of central vision early, slowly progressive loss of central vision over years; blunting or grayish discoloration of the foveal reflex, right-angle retinal venules, and characteristic stellate retinal pigment epithelial hyperplasia/atrophy; leakage from telangiectatic vessels, but no exudates; associated with CNV, hemorrhagic macular detachments, and retinochoroidal anastamosis. May be caused by chronic venous stasis in the macula from unknown reasons.

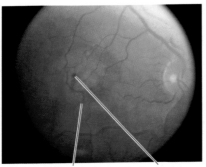

RPE hyperplasia   Intraretinal hemorrhage

Figure 10-38 • Juxtafoveal telangiectasia type 2 with abnormal foveal reflex, intraretinal hemorrhages and retinal pigment epithelium changes.

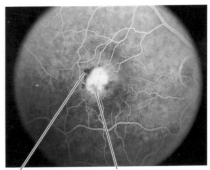

Intraretinal   Vascular leakage
hemorrhage

Figure 10-39 • Fluorescein angiogram of patient shown in Figure 10-38, demonstrating hyperfluorescent leakage from telangiectatic vessels and blockage from the hemorrhages.

- **Fluorescein angiogram:** Bilateral, right-angle venules with variable leakage; macular edema often with petalloid leakage; choroidal neovascularization can develop.
- No treatment recommended unless CNV develops because focal laser photocoagulation to leaking, non-subfoveal vessels does not prevent visual loss.
- Consider focal laser photocoagulation of juxtafoveal and extrafoveal CNV, and photodynamic therapy (PDT) or intravitreal anti-VEGF agents such as 1.25 mg bevacizumab (Avastin) for subfoveal CNV (experimental).

Type 3 (Bilateral Perifoveal Telangiectasis with Capillary Obliteration)

Rare form; occurs in adults in the fifth decade; no sex predilection. Slowly progressive loss of vision due to the marked aneurysmal dilatation and obliteration of the perifoveal telangiectatic capillary network; no leakage from telangiectasis; associated with optic nerve pallor, hyperactive deep tendon reflexes, and other central nervous system symptoms.

- **Fluorescein angiogram:** Aneurysmal dilation of capillary bed with minimal to no leakage; extensive, progressive macular capillary nonperfusion, choroidal neovascularization can develop.
- No treatment recommended unless CNV develops.
- Consider focal laser photocoagulation of juxtafoveal and extrafoveal CNV, and photodynamic therapy (PDT) or intravitreal anti-VEGF agents such as 1.25 mg bevacizumab (Avastin) for subfoveal CNV (experimental).
- Neurology consultation to rule out central nervous system disease.

Retinopathies Associated with Blood Abnormalities

Retinopathy of Anemia

Superficial, flame-shaped, intraretinal hemorrhages, cotton-wool spots, and rarely exudates, retinal edema, and vitreous hemorrhage in patients with anemia (hemoglobin <8 g/100 mL).

Retinopathy is worse when associated with thrombocytopenia. Roth spots are found in pernicious anemia and aplastic anemia.

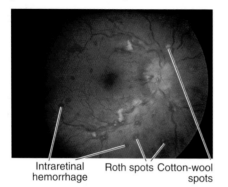

Intraretinal hemorrhage   Roth spots   Cotton-wool spots

Figure 10-40 Retinopathy of anemia demonstrating intraretinal hemorrhages, cotton-wool spots, and Roth spots.

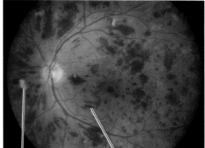

Cotton-wool spots   Flame hemorrhage

Figure 10-41 Retinopathy of anemia demonstrating intraretinal hemorrhages and cotton-wool spots.

- Resolves with treatment of anemia.
- Medical or hematology consultation.

Leukemic Retinopathy

Ocular involvement in leukemia is common (80%). Patients are usually asymptomatic. Characterized by superficial, flame-shaped, intraretinal (24%), preretinal, and vitreous hemorrhages (2%), microaneurysms, Roth spots (11%), cotton-wool spots (16%), dilated/tortuous vessels, perivascular sheathing, and disc edema; rarely direct leukemic infiltrates (3%); direct choroidal involvement appears with choroidal infiltrates, choroidal thickening, and an overlying serous retinal detachment. "Sea fan"-shaped retinal neovascularization can occur late. Retinopathy is due to the associated anemia, thrombocytopenia, and hyperviscosity. Opportunistic infections are also found in patients with leukemia, but are not considered part of leukemic retinopathy.

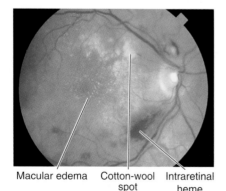

Macular edema   Cotton-wool spot   Intraretinal heme

Figure 10-42 Leukemic retinopathy with macular edema, cotton-wool spots, and intraretinal hemorrhages.

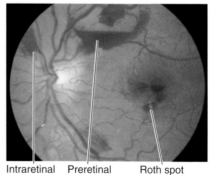

Intraretinal heme   Preretinal heme   Roth spot

Figure 10-43 Leukemic retinopathy with intraretinal and preretinal hemorrhages, cotton-wool spots, and Roth spots.

- **Lab tests:** CBC, platelets, bone marrow biopsy.
- Resolves with treatment of underlying hematologic abnormality.
- Treat direct leukemic infiltrates with systemic chemotherapy to control the underlying problem and/or ocular radiation therapy if systemic therapy fails; should be performed by an experienced tumor specialist.
- Medical or oncology consultation.

Sickle Cell Retinopathy

Nonproliferative and proliferative vascular changes due to the sickling hemoglobinopathies. Results from mutations in hemoglobin (Hb) where the valine is substituted for glutamate at the 6th position in the polypeptide chain (linked to chromosome 11p15) altering Hb conformation and deformability in erythrocytes. This leads to poor flow through capillaries. Proliferative changes (response to retinal ischemia) are more common with Hb SC (most severe) and Hb SThal variants; Hb SS associated with angioid streaks; Hb AS and Hb AC mutations rarely cause ocular manifestations. Patients are usually asymptomatic, but may have decreased vision, visual field loss, floaters, photopsias, scotomas, and dyschromatopsia; more common in people of African and Mediterranean descent. Retinopathy follows an orderly progression:

Stage I

Background (nonproliferative) stage with venous tortuosity, "salmon patch" hemorrhages (pink intraretinal hemorrhages), iridescent spots (schisis cavity with refractile elements), cotton-wool spots, hairpin vascular loops, macular infarction, angioid streaks, black "sunburst" chorioretinal scars, comma-shaped conjunctival and optic nerve head vessels, and peripheral arteriole occlusions.

Stage II

Arteriovenous (AV) anastamosis stage with peripheral "silver-wire" vessels and shunt vessels between arterioles and medium-sized veins at border of perfused and nonperfused retina.

Stage III

Neovascular (proliferative) stage with sea-fan peripheral neovascularization (spontaneously regresses in 60% of cases due to autoinfarction); sea-fans grow along retinal surface in a circumferential pattern and have a predilection for superotemporal quadrant (develops approximately 18 months after formation of AV anastamosis).

Stage IV

Vitreous hemorrhage stage with vitreous traction bands contracting around the sea-fans, causing vitreous hemorrhages (most common in SC variant, 21–23%; SS, 2–3%).

Stage V

Retinal detachment stage with tractional/rhegmatogenous retinal detachments from contraction of the vitreous traction bands.

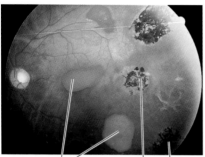

Preretinal hemorrhage   "Sunburst" scars

Figure 10-44 • Nonproliferative sickle cell retinopathy demonstrating preretinal hemorrhage, iridescent spots, and black sunbursts.

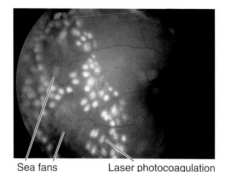

Sea fans   Laser photocoagulation

Figure 10-45 • Proliferative sickle cell retinopathy demonstrating sea-fans following laser treatment.

- **Lab tests:** Sickle cell prep, hemoglobin electrophoresis (hemoglobin C disease and sickle cell trait may have negative sickle cell prep).

- **Fluorescein angiogram:** Capillary nonperfusion near hairpin loops, enlarged foveal avascular zone, peripheral nonperfusion, arteriovenous anastamosis, and sea-fan neovascularization.

- When active peripheral neovascularization develops, scatter laser photocoagulation (500 μm spots) to nonperfused retina.

- If neovascularization persists, then complete panretinal photocoagulation and consider adding direct laser photocoagulation to neovascularization or feeder vessels (increases risk of complications including vitreous hemorrhage).

- The use of triple freeze-thaw cryotherapy for peripheral neovascularization is controversial; should be performed by a retina specialist.

- Retinal surgery for traction retinal detachment and non-clearing, vitreous hemorrhage (>6 months); should be performed by a retina specialist; consider exchange transfusion preoperatively (controversial); avoid scleral buckling to prevent ocular ischemia.

- Medical or hematology consultation.

Diabetic Retinopathy

Definition Retinal vascular complication of diabetes mellitus; classified into nonproliferative diabetic retinopathy (NPDR) and proliferative diabetic retinopathy (PDR).

Epidemiology Leading cause of blindness in US population aged 20–64 years old.

Insulin-Dependent Diabetes (Type I)

Juvenile onset, usually occurs before 30 years of age; most patients are free of retinopathy during first 5 years after diagnosis; 95% of patients with insulin-dependent diabetes mellitus

(IDDM) get DR after 15 years; 72% will develop PDR and 42% will develop CSME; severity worsens with increasing duration of diabetes mellitus.

Non-Insulin-Dependent Diabetes (Type II)

Adult onset, usually diagnosed after 30 years of age; more common form (90%) with optimal control without insulin; DR commonly exists at the time of diagnosis (60%) in non-insulin-dependent diabetes mellitus (NIDDM) with 3% having PDR or CSME at diagnosis of diabetes; 30% will have retinopathy in 5 years and 80% in 15 years. Risk of DR increases with hypertension, chronic hyperglycemia, renal disease, hyperlipidemia, and pregnancy.

Symptoms Asymptomatic, may have decreased or fluctuating vision. Advanced retinopathy can lead to complete blindness.

Signs

Non-Proliferative Diabetic Retinopathy

Grading of NPDR (see Table 10-1) and risk of progression to PDR depends on the amount and location of hard and soft exudates, intraretinal hemorrhages, micro-aneurysms (MA), venous beading and loops, and intraretinal microvascular abnor-malities (IRMA). Cotton-wool spots, dot and blot hemorrhages, posterior subcapsular cataracts, and induced myopia/hyperopia (from lens swelling due to high blood sugar) are common; may have macular edema, which can be clinically significant (CSME). Usually bilateral.

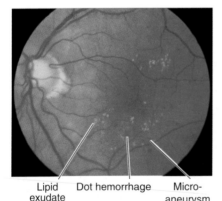

Lipid   Dot hemorrhage   Micro-
exudate   aneurysm

Figure 10-46 • Moderate nonproliferative diabetic retinopathy with intraretinal hemorrhages, microaneurysms, and lipid exudate.

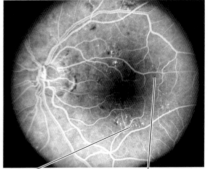

Microaneurysm   Dot hemorrhage

Figure 10-47 • Fluorescein angiogram of same patient as Figure 10-46 demonstrating tiny blocking defects from the intraretinal hemorrhages and spots of hyperfluorescence due to microaneurysms.

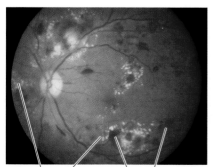

Lipid exudate   Intraretinal hemorrhages

Figure 10-48 • Severe nonproliferative diabetic retinopathy with extensive hemorrhages, microaneurysms, and exudates.

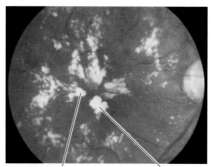

Diffuse macular edema and exudate

Figure 10-49 • Severe nonproliferative diabetic retinopathy with diffuse macular edema and lipid exudate.

Figure 10-50 • Spectral domain optical coherence tomography of diffuse diabetic macular edema with subretinal fluid, intraretinal fluid, and cystoid macular edema.

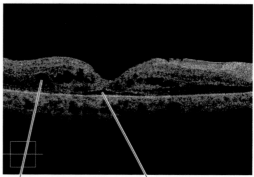

Cystoid macular edema   Subretinal fluid

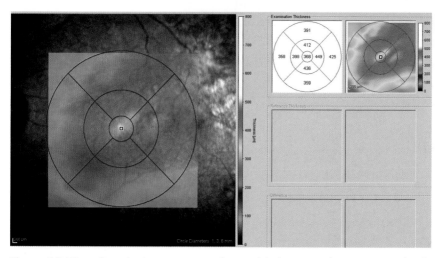

Figure 10-51 • Optical coherence tomography retinal thickness map showing topographically areas of increased retinal thickening in red and white.

Proliferative diabetic retinopathy

Findings of NPDR often present in addition to neovascularization of the disc (NVD) or elsewhere in the retina (NVE), preretinal and vitreous hemorrhages, fibrovascular proliferation on posterior vitreous surface or extending into the vitreous cavity, and tractional retinal detachments; may develop neovascularization of the iris (NVI) and subsequent neovascular glaucoma (NVG). Usually asymmetric, but eventually bilateral.

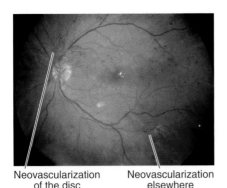

Neovascularization of the disc   Neovascularization elsewhere

Figure 10-52 • Proliferative diabetic retinopathy demonstrating florid neovascularization of the disc and elsewhere.

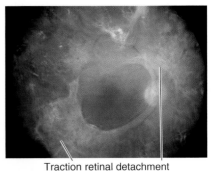

Traction retinal detachment

Figure 10-53 • Proliferative diabetic retinopathy demonstrating neovascularization, fibrosis, and traction retinal detachment.

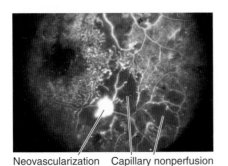

Neovascularization   Capillary nonperfusion

Figure 10-54 • Fluorescein angiogram of patient with proliferative diabetic retinopathy showing extensive capillary nonperfusion, neovascularization elsewhere, and vascular leakage.

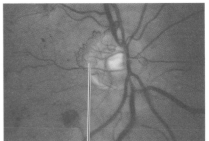

Neovascularization of the disc

Figure 10-55 • Proliferative diabetic retinopathy demonstrating neovascularization of the disc.

Differential Diagnosis Hypertensive retinopathy, CRVO, BRVO, ocular ischemic syndrome, radiation retinopathy, retinopathy associated with blood disorders, Eales' disease, hypertensive retinopathy.

Evaluation

- Complete ophthalmic history and eye exam with attention to tonometry, gonioscopy (NVG), iris (NVI), lens, non-contact biomicroscopic or contact lens fundus exam, and ophthalmoscopy (retinal vascular abnormalities, optic disc [NVD], and mid-periphery [NVE]):

  - IDDM Type I: Examine 5 years after onset of diabetes mellitus, then annually if no retinopathy is detected.

  - NIDDM Type II: Examine at diagnosis of diabetes mellitus, then annually if no retinopathy is detected.

  - During pregnancy: Examine before pregnancy, each trimester, and 3–6 months post partum.

- **Lab tests:** fasting blood glucose, hemoglobin A1C, blood urea nitrogen (BUN), and creatinine.

- B-scan ultrasonography to rule out tractional retinal detachment in eyes when dense vitreous hemorrhage obscures view of fundus.

- **Fluorescein angiogram:** Capillary nonperfusion, microaneurysms, macular edema, and disc/retinal neovascularization.

- **Optical coherence tomography:** Increased retinal thickness, cysts, and subretinal fluid in cases of macular edema; can highlight the presence of posterior hyaloidal traction and traction macular detachment.

- Medical consultation with attention to blood pressure, cardiovascular system, renal status, weight and glycemic control.

Management

- Tight control of blood glucose levels (Diabetes Control and Complications Trial-DCCT conclusion for Type I diabetics and United Kingdom Prospective Diabetes Study-UKPDS conclusion for Type II diabetics).

- Tight blood pressure control (United Kingdom Prospective Diabetes Study-UKPDS conclusion for Type II diabetics).

- Laser photocoagulation using transpupillary delivery and argon green (focal/panretinal photocoagulation) or krypton red laser (panretinal photocoagulation when vitreous hemorrhage or cataract is present), depending on stage of diabetic retinopathy:

- **Clinically significant macular edema (CSME; see Table 10-1):** Macular grid photocoagulation (50–100 μm spots) to areas of diffuse leakage and focal treatment to focal leaks regardless of visual acuity (Early Treatment Diabetic Retinopathy Study-ETDRS conclusion). If foveal avascular zone is enlarged (macular ischemia) on fluorescein angiography then light treatment away from the foveal ischemia can be considered.

- **High-risk (HR) PDR (see Table 10-1):** Scatter panretinal photocoagulation (PRP), 1200–1600 burns, 1 burn width apart (500 μm gray-white spots) in two to three sessions (Diabetic Retinopathy Study-DRS conclusion). Treat inferior/nasal quadrants first to allow further treatment in case of subsequent vitreous hemorrhage during treatment and to avoid worsening macular edema.

Continued

Management—Cont'd

- Additional indications for panretinal photocoagulation: Rubeosis, neovascular glaucoma, widespread retinal ischemia on fluorescein angiogram, NVE alone in Type I IDDM, poor patient compliance, and severe NPDR in a fellow eye or patient with poor outcome in first eye.

- Patients approaching high-risk PDR should have focal treatment to macular edema before panretinal photocoagulation to avoid worsening of macular edema with PRP; if high-risk characteristics exist, do not delay panretinal photocoagulation for focal treatment.

- Pars plana vitrectomy, endolaser, and removal of any fibrovascular complexes in patients with non-clearing vitreous hemorrhage for 6 months or vitreous hemorrhage for >1 month in type 1 IDDM (diabetic retinopathy vitrectomy study-DRVS conclusions); other indications for vitreoretinal surgery include monocular patient with vitreous hemorrhage, bilateral vitreous hemorrhage, diabetic macular edema due to posterior hyaloidal traction, tractional retinal detachment (TRD) with rhegmatogenous component, TRD involving macula, progressive fibrovascular proliferation despite complete PRP, dense premacular hemorrhage or if ocular media are not clear enough for adequate view of fundus to perform PRP; should be performed by a retina specialist.

- Experimental pharmaceutical treatments for refractory, diffuse macular edema include posterior sub-Tenon's injection of 40 mg triamcinolone acetonide, intravitreal 4 mg triamcinolone acetonide, Retisert sustained release (1000 day) implant with fluocinolone acetonide, and intravitreal anti-VEGF injections. The Diabetic Retinopathy Clinical Research network (DRCR.net) reported that laser photocoagulation was superior to intravitreal triamcinolone in patients with CSME.

- Experimental surgical treatment of refractory, diffuse macular edema include pars plana vitrectomy with peeling of posterior hyaloid with/without removal of the internal limiting membrane especially with the presence of a taut, posterior hyaloid exerting traction on the macula.

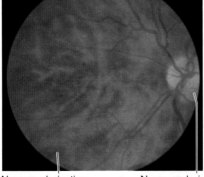

Neovascularization elsewhere   Neovascularization of the disc

Figure 10-56 • Proliferative diabetic retinopathy before laser treatment.

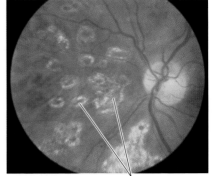

Laser spots

Figure 10-57 • Same patient as Figure 10-56 demonstrating quiescent proliferative diabetic retinopathy following pan-retinal photocoagulation. Note absence of neovascularization.

Prognosis Early treatment allows better control. Good for NPDR without CSME. After adequate treatment, diabetic retinopathy often becomes quiescent for extended periods of time. Focal laser photocoagulation improves vision in 17% of cases (ETDRS conclusion). Complications include cataracts (often posterior subcapsular) and neovascular glaucoma.

Table 10-1 Diabetic Retinopathy Definitions

Clinically Significant Macular Edema (CSME):

Retinal thickening <500 µm from center of fovea *or*
Hard exudates <500 µm from center of fovea with adjacent thickening *or*
Retinal thickening >1 disc size in area < 1 disc diameter from center of fovea

High-Risk (HR) Characteristics of Proliferative Diabetic Retinopathy (PDR)

Neovascularization of the disc (NVD) > standard photo 10A used in DRS (one-quarter to one-third disc area) *or*
Any NVD and vitreous hemorrhage (VH) or preretinal hemorrhage *or*
Neovascularization elsewhere (NVE) > standard photo 7 (one half disc area) and VH or preretinal hemorrhage

Severe Nonproliferative Diabetic Retinopathy (NPDR) 4:2:1 Rule

Diffuse intraretinal hemorrhages and microaneurysms in 4 quadrants *or*
Venous beading in 2 quadrants *or*
Intraretinal microvascular abnormalities (IRMA) in 1 quadrant

---

Hypertensive Retinopathy

Definition Retinal vascular changes secondary to chronic or acutely (malignant) elevated systemic blood pressure.

Epidemiology Hypertension defined as blood pressure >140/90 mmHg; 60 million Americans over 18 years of age have hypertension; more prevalent in African Americans.

Symptoms Asymptomatic; rarely, decreased vision.

Signs Retinal arteriole narrowing/straightening, copper or silver-wire arteriole changes (arteriolosclerosis), arteriovenous crossing changes (nicking), cotton-wool spots, microaneurysms, flame hemorrhages, hard exudates (may be in a circinate or macular star pattern), Elschnig spots (yellow [early] or hyperpigmented [late] patches of retinal pigment epithelium overlying infarcted choriocapillaris lobules), Siegrist streaks (linear hyperpigmented areas over choroidal vessels), arterial macroaneurysms, and disc hyperemia or edema with dilated tortuous vessels (in malignant hypertension).

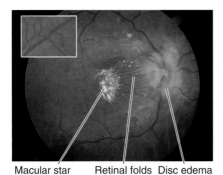

Macular star   Retinal folds Disc edema

Figure 10-58 • Hypertensive retinopathy with disc edema, macular star, and retinal folds in a patient with acute, malignant hypertension. Inset shows arteriovenous nicking.

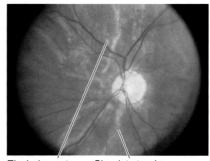

Elschnig spots   Siegrist streaks

Figure 10-59 • Hypertensive retinopathy demonstrating attenuated arterioles, choroidal ischemia, Elschnig spots, and Siegrist streaks.

Differential Diagnosis Diabetic retinopathy, radiation retinopathy, vein occlusion, leukemic retinopathy, retinopathy of anemia, collagen vascular disease, and ocular ischemia syndrome.

Evaluation

- Complete ophthalmic history and eye exam with attention to non-contact biomicroscopic or contact lens fundus exam and ophthalmoscopy (retinal vasculature and arteriovenous crossings).
- Check blood pressure.
- **Fluorescein angiogram:** Retinal arteriole narrowing/straightening, microaneurysms, capillary nonperfusion, and macular edema.
- Medical consultation with attention to cardiovascular and cerebrovascular systems.

Management

- Treat underlying hypertension.

Prognosis Usually good.

Toxemia of Pregnancy

Severe hypertension, proteinuria, edema (pre-eclampsia), and seizures (eclampsia) occur in 2–5% of obstetric patients in the third trimester. Patients have decreased vision, photopsias, and floaters usually just before or after delivery. Signs include focal arteriolar narrowing, cotton-wool spots, retinal hemorrhages, hard exudates, Elschnig spots (RPE changes from choroidal infarction), bullous exudative retinal detachments, neovascularization, and disc edema (all due to hypertensive-related changes).

Figure 10-60 • Toxemia of pregnancy with serous retinal detachment and yellow–white patches.

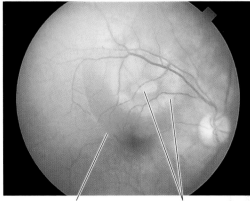

Serous retinal detachment   Exudates

- **Fluorescein angiogram:** Poor choroidal filling, capillary nonperfusion, optic disc leakage, and neovascularization.
- Usually resolves without sequelae after treating hypertension and delivery.
- Emergent obstetrics consultation if presenting to ophthalmologist.

Acquired Retinal Arterial Macroaneurysm

Focal dilatation of retinal artery (>100 μm) often at bifurcation or crossing site; more common in women >60 years old with hypertension (50–70%) or atherosclerosis. Usually asymptomatic, unilateral, and solitary; may cause sudden loss of vision from vitreous hemorrhage; macroaneurysms nasal to the optic disc are less likely to cause symptoms. Subretinal, intraretinal, preretinal, or vitreous hemorrhages (multi-level hemorrhages) from rupture of aneurysm, and surrounding circinate exudates are common. May spontaneously sclerose forming a Z-shaped kink at old aneurysm site.

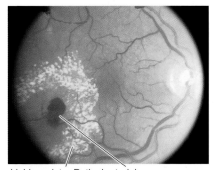

Lipid exudate   Retinal arterial macroaneurysm

Figure 10-61 • Acquired retinal arterial macroaneurysm with circinate exudate.

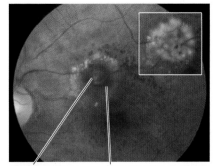

Retinal arterial   Subretinal hemorrhage
macroaneurysm

Figure 10-62 • Acquired retinal arterial macroaneurysm before laser photocoagulation. Inset shows the same lesion after laser treatment.

- **Fluorescein angiogram:** Immediate uniform, focal filling of the macroaneurysm early with late leakage.
- **Indocyanine green angiogram:** Uniform, focal filling of the macroaneurysm; very useful to identify RAM in the presence of intra- and preretinal hemorrhage.
- Most require no treatment, especially in the absence of loss of vision.
- Low-intensity, longer-duration, argon green or yellow laser photocoagulation to microvascular changes around leaking aneurysm if decreased acuity is present (direct treatment controversial because it may cause a vitreous hemorrhage, distal ischemia, or a branch retinal artery occlusion).
- Consider pars plana vitrectomy with surgical evacuation of subretinal hemorrhage (with or without injection of subretinal tissue plasminogen activator) in cases of massive, subfoveal hemorrhage < 10 days old (experimental).
- Medical consultation for hypertension.

Radiation Retinopathy

Definition   Alteration in retinal vascular permeability after receiving local ionizing radiation usually from external beam radiotherapy or plaque brachytherapy.

Etiology   Endothelial cell DNA damage secondary to the radiation leading to progressive cell death and damage to the retinal blood vessels.

Epidemiology   Usually requires >30–35 Gy (3000–3500 rads) total radiation dose; appears 1–2 years after ionizing radiation; diabetics and patients receiving chemotherapy have a lower threshold.

Symptoms   Often asymptomatic until retinopathy involves macula; decreased vision.

Signs   Microaneurysms, telangiectasia, cotton-wool spots, hard exudates, retinal hemorrhages, macular edema, vascular sheathing, disc edema, retinal/disc/iris neovascularization; may have cataract, dry eye disease, lid abnormalities.

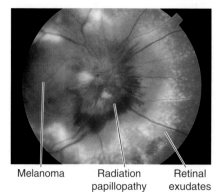

Melanoma   Radiation   Retinal
                papillopathy   exudates

Figure 10-63 • Radiation papillopathy. Note regressed malignant melanoma temporally.

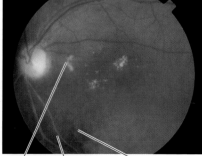

Retinal   Sclerotic   Melanoma
exudates   vessels

Figure 10-64 • Radiation retinopathy with sclerotic vessels overlying regressed malignant melanoma.

Differential Diagnosis Diabetic retinopathy, sickle cell retinopathy, hypertensive retinopathy, retinal vascular occlusion, retinopathy of anemia/thrombocytopenia, and leukemic retinopathy.

Evaluation

- Complete radiation history with attention to radiated field, total dose delivered, and fractionation schedule.
- Complete eye exam with attention to tonometry, gonioscopy, iris, lens, non-contact biomicroscopic or contact lens fundus exam, and ophthalmoscopy.
- **Fluorescein angiogram:** Capillary nonperfusion, macular edema, and neovascularization may be present.

Management

- Treatment based on similar principles used in diabetic retinopathy.
- Focal grid laser photocoagulation (50–100 μm spots) to areas of macular edema.
- Intravitreal 4 mg triamcinolone acetonide [Kenalog] and anti-VEGF agents such as 1.25 mg bevacizumab [Avastin] have been shown to decrease macular edema and transiently improve visual acuity, long-term safety and benefits are not proven.
- Panretinal photocoagulation with 1200–1600 applications (500 μm spots) if neovascular complications develop.

Prognosis Fair; complications include cataract, macular edema/ischemia, optic atrophy, vitreous hemorrhage, and neovascular glaucoma. Two-thirds of patients maintain vision better than 20/200.

Age-Related Macular Degeneration

Definition Progressive degenerative disease of the retinal pigment epithelium, Bruch's membrane, and choriocapillaris. Generally classified into two types: (1) nonexudative or "dry" AMD (85%) and (2) exudative or "wet" AMD characterized by CNV and eventually disciform scarring (15%).

Epidemiology Leading cause of blindness in US population aged >50 years old, as well as the most common cause of blindness in the Western world; 6.4% of patients 65–74 years old and 19.7% of patients >75 years old had signs of AMD in the Framingham Eye Study; more prevalent in Caucasians; slight female predilection. Risk factors include increasing age (>75 years old), positive family history, cigarette smoking, hyperopia, light iris color, hypertension, hypercholesterolemia, female gender, and cardiovascular disease; nutritional factors and light toxicity also play a role in pathogenesis. Associated with variants of genes encoding the alternative complement pathway including complement factor H (CFH) on chromosome 1q31, HTRA1 on chromosome 10q and LOC387715 on chromosome 10q, complement factor B and C2 on chromosome 6p21, and C3. Homozygotes (6×) and heterozygotes (2.5×) for CFH mutations are more likely to develop AMD. Their risk is even greater if they smoke (odds ratio 34 vs. 7.6 in non-smokers), have elevated ESR, and/or have elevated C-reactive protein.

Non-exudative (Dry) Macular Degeneration

Symptoms Initially asymptomatic or may have decreased vision, metamorphopsia early. Advanced atrophic form may have central or pericentral scotoma.

Table 10-2   AREDS Study Definitions

Category 1: Less than 5 small (<63 microns) drusen.

Category 2 (Mild AMD): Multiple small drusen or single or non-extensive intermediate (63–124 microns) drusen; or pigment abnormalities.

Category 3 (Intermediate AMD): Extensive intermediate size drusen or 1 or more large (>125 microns) drusen; or noncentral geographic atrophy.

Category 4 (Advanced AMD): Vision loss (<20/32) due to AMD in 1 eye (either due to central/subfoveal geographic atrophy or exudative macular degeneration).

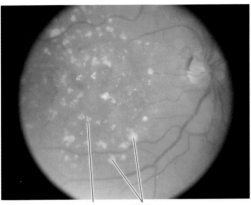

Hard drusen   Soft drusen

Figure 10-65 • Dry, age-related macular degeneration demonstrating drusen and pigmentary changes.

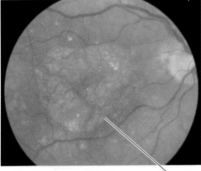

Geographic atrophy

Figure 10-66 • Advanced atrophic, nonexudative, age-related macular degeneration demonstrating subfoveal geographic atrophy.

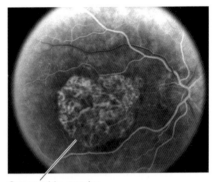

Geographic atrophy

Figure 10-67 • Fluorescein angiogram of same patient as Figure 10-66 demonstrating well-defined window defect corresponding to the area of geographic atrophy.

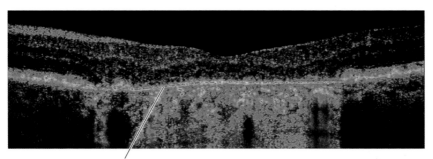

Geographic atrophy

Figure 10-68 • Spectral domain optical coherence tomography of central geographic atrophy. Notice the absence of retinal pigment epithelium in the fovea with increased signal beyond the RPE.

Signs Normal or decreased visual acuity; abnormal Amsler grid (central/paracentral scotomas or metamorphopsia); small, hard drusen, larger, soft drusen, geographic atrophy of the retinal pigment epithelium (RPE), RPE clumping, and blunted foveal reflex.

Differential Diagnosis Dominant drusen, pattern dystrophy, Best's disease, Stargardt's disease, cone dystrophy, and drug toxicity.

Management

- Follow with Amsler grid qd and examine every 6 months; examine sooner if patient experiences a change in vision, metamorphopsia, or change in Amsler grid.
- Supplement with high-dose antioxidants and vitamins (vitamin C, 500 mg; vitamin E, 400 IU; beta carotene, 15 mg; zinc, 80 mg; and copper, 2 mg) for patients with Category 3 (extensive intermediate size drusen, 1 large drusen, noncentral geographic atrophy), or Category 4 (vision loss due to AMD in 1 eye); **Warning**: current smokers should not take beta carotene at such high doses due to increased risk of lung cancer (Age Related Eye Disease Study-AREDS conclusion).
- Consider supplement with lower dose antioxidants (e.g., Centrum Silver, iCaps, Occuvite) for patients with Category 1 (few small drusen), Category 2 (extensive small drusen, few intermediate drusen), and patients with strong family history.
- Supplementation with other vitamins including lutein, bilberry, and Omega-3 fatty acid still unproven but being evaluated in the AREDS2 study.
- Low power, grid, laser photocoagulation to cause resorption of drusen and improve visual acuity (experimental).
- Low vision aids may benefit patients with bilateral central visual loss due to geographic atrophy.

Evaluation
- Complete ophthalmic history and eye exam with attention to Amsler grid and non-contact biomicroscopic or contact lens fundus exam.

- **Fluorescein angiogram:** Window defects from geographic atrophy and punctate hyperfluorescent staining of drusen (no late leakage).

Prognosis   Usually good unless central geographic atrophy or exudative AMD develops. Severe visual loss (defined as loss of >6 lines) occurs in 12% of nonexudative cases; presence of large, soft drusen and focal RPE hyperpigmentation increases risk of developing exudative form (MPS conclusion). Risk of advanced AMD over 5 years varies depending on Category: Category 1 and 2 (1.8%), Category 3 (18%), Category 4 (43%) (AREDS conclusion).

Exudative (Wet) Macular Degeneration

Symptoms   Metamorphopsia, central scotoma, rapid visual loss.

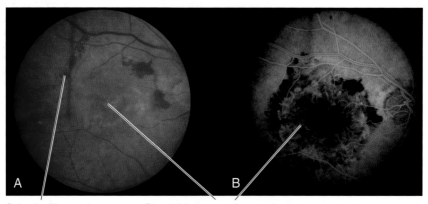

Subretinal hemorrhage   Choroidal neovascular membrane

Figure 10-69 • Exudative age-related macular degeneration with large choroidal neovascular membrane and accompanying subretinal hemorrhage and fibrosis as seen on (A) clinical photo, and (B) flourescein angiogram.

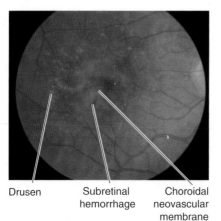

Figure 10-70 • Exudative age-related macular degeneration demonstrating subretinal hemorrhage from choroidal neovascular membrane.

Drusen   Subretinal   Choroidal
               hemorrhage   neovascular
                                membrane

Figure 10-71 • Fluorescein angiogram of same patient as Figure 10-70 demonstrating leakage from the CNV and blocking from the surrounding subretinal blood.

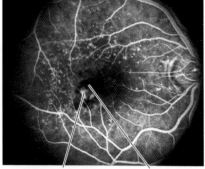

Choroidal neovascular membrane   Hemorrhage

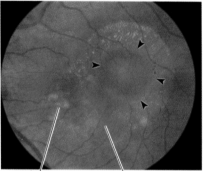

Drusen   Choroidal neovascular membrane

Figure 10-72 • Exudative age-related macular degeneration drusen, pigmentary changes, and an occult choroidal neovascular membrane with associated serous pigment epithelial detachment (arrowheads).

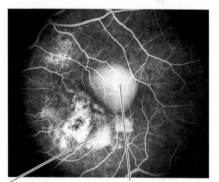

Choroidal neovascular membrane   Serous pigment epithelial detachment

Figure 10-73 • Fluorescein angiogram of same patient as Figure 10-72 demonstrating hyperfluorescent staining of pigmentary changes and drusen, leakage from the CNV and pooling of fluorescein dye within the serous pigment epithelial detachment.

Figure 10-74 • Spectral domain optical coherence tomography of exudative age-related macular degeneration with subretinal pigment epithelium and subretinal fluid from an occult with no classic choroidal neovascular membrane.

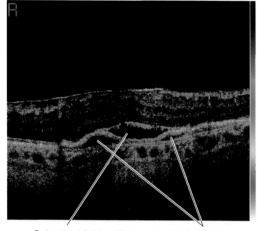

Subretinal fluid   Pigment epithelial detachment

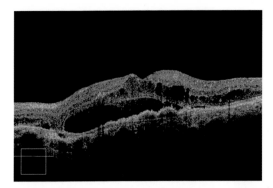

Figure 10-75 • Spectral domain optical coherence tomography of exudative age-related macular degeneration.

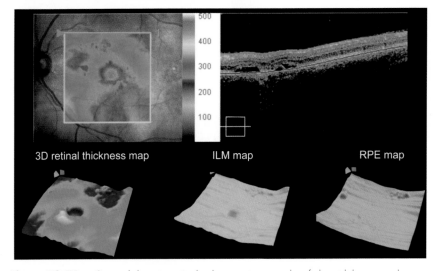

3D retinal thickness map   ILM map   RPE map

Figure 10-76 • Spectral domain optical coherence tomography of choroidal neovascular membrane illustrating advanced segmentation algorithms that shows the increased retinal thickness and elevated retina on the internal limiting membrane (ILM) map.

Signs CNV, lipid exudates, subretinal or intraretinal hemorrhage/fluid, pigment epithelial detachment (PED), and retinal pigment epithelial tears; may have late fibrovascular disciform scars.

Differential Diagnosis Dominant drusen, pattern dystrophy, Best's disease, central serous retinopathy, Stargardt's disease, cone dystrophy, drug toxicity, and choroidal neovascularization from other causes, including presumed ocular histoplasmosis syndrome, angioid streaks, myopic degeneration, traumatic choroidal rupture, retinal dystrophies, inflammatory choroidopathies, and optic nerve drusen.

Evaluation

• Complete ophthalmic history and eye exam with attention to Amsler grid and non-contact biomicroscopic or contact lens fundus exam.

- **Fluorescein angiogram:** Two forms of leakage from CNV: (1) *classic leakage* defined as lacy, network of bright fluorescence during early choroidal filling views that increases in fluorescence throughout the angiogram and leaks beyond its borders in late views; (2) *occult leakage* defined as stippled nonhomogeneous hyperfluorescence at the level of the RPE (best seen on stereoscopic views) that persists through to late views, but the leakage is not as bright as classic lesions (type 1 or fibrovascular PED), or late leakage of undetermined origin (type 2), where the early views show no apparent leakage, but as the angiogram progresses, there is hyperfluorescent stippling at the level of the RPE in late views.

- **Indocyanine green angiogram:** Useful when the CNV is poorly demarcated or obscured by hemorrhage on fluorescein angiogram or if fibrovascular pigment epithelial detachment is present (to identify areas of focal neovascularization or polypoidal choroidal vasculopathy); focal hotspots likely represent retinal angiomatous proliferation (RAP); CNV also appears as plaque of late hyperfluorescence.

- **Optical coherence tomography:** After photodynamic therapy, when the fluorescein angiogram is equivocal between leakage and staining of the CNV or to decide on retreatment with anti-VEGF agents, OCT is useful to delineate the presence and extent of intraretinal and subretinal fluid, as well as the presence of a PED.

Management

- Focal laser photocoagulation with argon green/yellow or krypton red laser and a transpupillary delivery system to form confluent (200–500 µm spots) white burns over the entire CNV depending on size, location, and visual acuity based on the results of the Macular Photocoagulation Study (MPS). *Note*: only patients with a classic, well-defined CNV met eligibility criteria for the MPS study.
  - **Extrafoveal:** Treat entire CNV and 100 µm beyond all boundaries.
  - **Juxtafoveal:** Treat entire CNV and 100 µm beyond on nonfoveal side, and up to CNV border on foveal side. Lesions that are "barely" juxtafoveal or where laser treatment may damage the center of vision should be considered for photodynamic therapy (PDT) or anti-VEGF agents (*Note*: TAP enrollment criteria included subfoveal lesions only, but there was a small subgroup with barely juxtafoveal lesions who responded well to PDT).
  - **Subfoveal:** Although laser photocoagulation was shown to be beneficial, its use in subfoveal lesions has been supplanted by anti-VEGF agents and PDT. Photodynamic therapy with verteporfin (Visudyne) has been shown to prevent visual loss in subfoveal, predominantly classic lesions (>50% of the entire lesion is composed of classic CNV) (Treatment of AMD with Photodynamic Therapy Study-TAP Study conclusion), and in occult lesions with no classic (especially if the lesion is <4 MPS disc areas in size or baseline vision is worse than 20/50) (Verteporfin In Photodynamic therapy Study-VIP Study conclusion). Fluorescein angiograms must be performed within 7 days of PDT treatment to determine lesion size for treatment. PDT retreatment applied as often as every 3 months if fluorescein leakage found from CNV (average 3.4 treatments in year 1, 2.2 in year 2 – TAP conclusion). Patient should avoid direct sunlight or bright indoor light for at least 48 hours after each treatment (drug labeling states 5 days).

Continued

Management—Cont'd

- Anti-VEGF agents (pegaptanib sodium [Macugen], bevacizumab [Avastin], ranibizumab [Lucentis]) have revolutionized management and prognosis of exudative AMD. Among these, Lucentis has been the most effective against all forms of CNV.
- Submacular surgery for removal of CNV or macular translocation have not been promising in regards to vision potential and have largely been abandoned.
- Low vision aids and registration with blind services for patients who are legally blind (<20/200 best corrected visual acuity or <20° visual field in better seeing eye).
- Treatments currently being evaluated in clinical trials include radiation therapy, modulating (feeder) vessel laser photocoagulation, other anti-VEGF agents, and combination therapies.

Prognosis Long term prognosis is not known. CNV may recur or persist after treatment; risk of fellow eye developing CNV is 4–12% annually; 2-year results of Lucentis have shown great promise in stabilizing vision in 90–95% and improving vision in up to 40% of individuals of any CNV type.

Table 10-3   Macular Photocoagulation Study (MPS) Definitions

Extrafoveal: 200–2500 μm from center of foveal avascular zone (FAZ).

Juxtafoveal: 1–199 μm from center of FAZ or choroidal neovascular membrane (CNV) 200–2500 μm from center of FAZ with blood or blocked fluorescence within 1–199 μm of FAZ center.

Subfoveal: Under geometric center of FAZ.

Retinal Angiomatous Proliferation

A CNV in which presumed retinal noevascularization forms a retinal choroidal anastamosis as the retinal vessels grow into the subretinal space. Angiomatous proliferation within the retina is the earliest finding which manifests as focal intraretinal hemorrhages at the site of the neovascularization with an associated pigment epithelial detachment (PED). The lesions are associated with subretinal hemorrhage and exudates. Generally, RAP lesions are more difficult to treat than traditional CNV.

- **Fluorescein angiogram:** To evaluate for polypoidal lesions and differentiate from traditional CNV. RAP lesions appear as focal areas of hyperfluorescence within the pooling of fluorescein dye in the PED. There is often indistinct leakage simulating occult CNV surrounding the RAP lesion.
- **Indocyanine green angiogram:** Ideal for visualizing the focal area of intense hyperfluorescence (hot spot) of a RAP lesion within the hypofluorescent PED. As the RAP lesion anastamoses with the choroidal circulation it may become indistinguishable from an occult CNV.

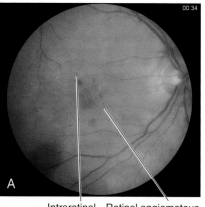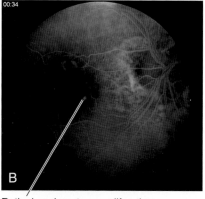

Intraretinal   Retinal angiomatous   Retinal angiomatous proliferation
hemorrhage   proliferation

Figure 10-77 Retinal angiomatous proliferation with intraretinal and subretinal hemorrhage as seen on (A) clinical photo, and (B) fluorescein angiogram demonstrating the focal leakage from the RAP lesion.

Figure 10-78 Spectral domain optical coherence tomography of retinal angiomatous proliferation showing pigment epithelial detachment and cystoid macular edema.

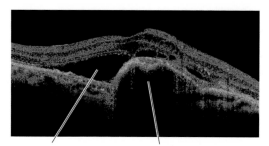

Subretinal fluid   Pigment epithelial detachment

- **Optical coherence tomography:** The PED is present and often the retinal choroidal anastomosis can be visualized on OCT.
- Treat RAP lesions with PDT and anti-VEGF agents such as intravitreal 0.5 mg ranibizumab (Lucentis) or 1.25 mg bevacizumab (Avastin).

Polypoidal Choroidal Vasculopathy

Primary abnormality of the choroidal vasculature characterized by choroidal vessels that end in an aneurysmal bulge. Often unilateral presentation, but bilateral disease consisting of orange-red serosanguineous detachments of the neurosensory retina and RPE with subretinal hemorrhage, retinal pigment epithelial atrophy, and, in late stages, subretinal fibrosis. More common in African Americans and Asians; in Asians, it is more common in males with macular manifestations; in African American patients it is more common in females and peripapillary. Differential diagnosis includes any disease that can produce

CNV and/or exudative maculopathies especially age-related macular degeneration; usually occurs in patients aged 50–65 years old so a CNV diagnosis in these populations should make one consider PCV. Better prognosis and slower course than exudative AMD; may spontaneously regress.

Polypoidal choroidal vasculopathy

Polypoidal choroidal vasculopathy

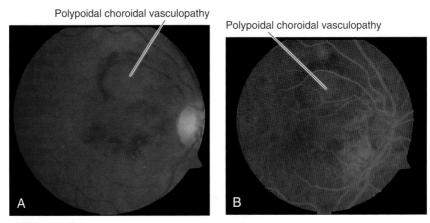

Figure 10-79 • Polypoidal choroidal vasculopathy demonstrating the multiple, orange, serosanguinous pigment epithelial detachments as seen on (A) clinical photo, and (B) fluorescein angiogram.

Polypoidal choroidal vasculopathy

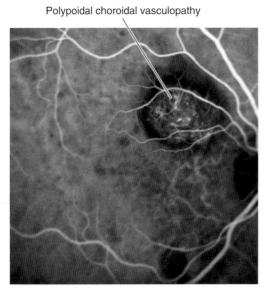

Figure 10-80 • Indocyanine green angiogram of same patient as Figure 10-79 illustrating the polypoidal choroidal lesions.

Figure 10-81 Spectral domain optical coherence tomography of polypoidal choroidal vasculopathy demonstrating the multiple pigment epithelial detachments.

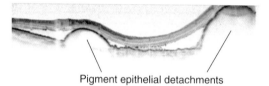

Pigment epithelial detachments

- **Fluorescein angiogram:** To evaluate for polypoidal lesions and differentiate from CNV.
- **Indocyanine green angiogram:** Delineates the polypoidal lesions better than FA. The choroidal vascular abnormalities hyperfluoresce early with a surrounding hypofluorescent area behind the lesions. The polyps are obvious in early frames of the angiogram.
- Observation in cases without foveal hemorrhage or other exudative changes.
- Treat polypoidal lesions with focal laser photocoagulation in juxtafoveal and extrafoveal lesions. PDT and anti-VEGF agents such as intravitreal 0.5 mg ranibizumab (Lucentis) or 1.25 mg bevacizumab (Avastin) have shown benefit in small case series for subfoveal lesions. This is being evaluated in the SUMMIT: MTEVEREST study.

Myopic Degeneration/Pathologic Myopia

Progressive retinal degeneration that occurs in high myopia (≥-6.00 diopters, axial length >26.5 mm) and pathologic myopia (≥-8.00 diopters, axial length >32.5 mm); incidence of 2% in US population. Findings include scleral thinning, posterior staphyloma, lacquer cracks (irregular, yellow streaks), peripapillary, atrophic temporal crescent, tilted optic disc, Fuchs' spots (dark spots due to RPE hyperplasia in macula), "tigroid" fundus due to thinning of RPE allowing visualization of larger choroidal vessels, subretinal hemorrhage (especially near lacquer cracks) and chorioretinal atrophy; increased incidence of posterior vitreous detachment, premature cataract formation, glaucoma, lattice degeneration, giant retinal tears, retinal detachments, macular hole, and CNV. Visual field defects may be present.

Figure 10-82 Myopic degeneration with peripapillary and chorioretinal atrophy.

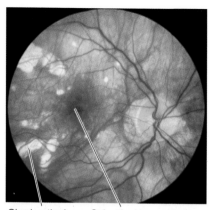

Chorioretinal atrophy   Subretinal hemorrhage

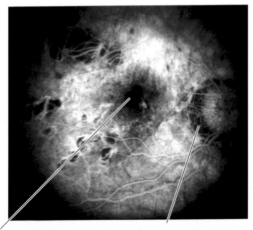

Figure 10-83 ◦ Fluorescein angiogram of same patient as Figure 10-82 demonstrating blocking defect from subretinal hemorrhage and window defects from chorioretinal and peripapillary atrophy.

Subretinal hemorrhage   Peripapillary atrophy

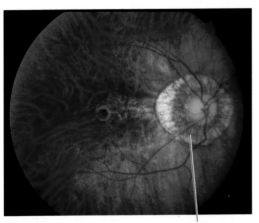

Figure 10-84 ◦ Myopic degeneration with peripapillary atrophy.

Peripapillary atrophy

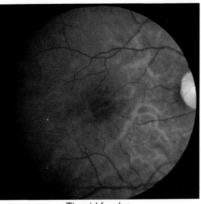

Figure 10-85 ◦ "Tigroid" fundus due to thinning of RPE allowing visualization of larger choroidal vessels.

Tigroid fundus

- **Genetics:** Mapped to chromosome 18p11.31 and 12q21–q23.
- **Fluorescein angiogram:** To evaluate for CNV if suspected clinically. Atrophic areas appear as window defects, lacquer cracks are hyperfluorescent linear areas that stain in late views.
- Correct any refractive error; contact lenses help reduce image minification and prismatic effect of glasses.
- Recommend polycarbonate safety glasses for sports (increased risk of choroidal rupture with minor trauma).
- Follow for signs of complications (CNV, retinal detachment, retinal breaks, macular holes, glaucoma, and cataracts).
- Treat CNV with focal laser photocoagulation per MPS guidelines in extrafoveal lesions (see Age-Related Macular Degeneration section), photodynamic therapy or anti-VEGF agents for juxtafoveal (since laser scar enlargement ["scar creep"] is common in pathologic myopia after laser treatment) and subfoveal lesions (Verteporfin in Photodynamic Therapy Pathologic Myopia Study – VIP-PM conclusion). Bevacizumab (Avastin) and ranibizumab (Lucentis) have shown benefit in case series.
- Treat retinal detachment and macular holes with vitreoretinal surgery performed by a retina specialist.

Angioid Streaks

Definition Full-thickness breaks in calcified, thickened Bruch's membrane with disruption of overlying RPE.

Etiology Idiopathic or associated with systemic diseases (50% of cases) including pseudoxanthoma elasticum (PXE, 60%; redundant skin folds in the neck, gastrointestinal bleeding, hypertension), Paget's disease (8%; extraskeletal calcification, osteoarthritis, deafness, vertigo, increased serum alkaline phosphatase and urine calcium levels), senile elastosis, calcinosis, abetalipoproteinemia, sickle cell disease (5%), thalassemia, hereditary spherocytosis, and Ehlers–Danlos syndrome (blue sclera, hyperextendable joints, elastic skin); also associated with optic disc drusen, acromegaly, lead poisoning, Marfan's syndrome, and retinitis pigmentosa.

Symptoms Usually asymptomatic; may have decreased vision, metamorphopsia if choroidal neovascular membrane develops.

Signs Normal or decreased visual acuity; linear, irregular, deep, dark red-brown streaks radiating from the optic disc in a spoke-like pattern; often have "peau d'orange" retinal pigmentation, peripheral salmon spots, "histo-like" scars, and pigmentation around the streaks; may have subretinal hemorrhage/fluid, retinal pigment epithelial detachments, macular degeneration, and central/paracentral scotomas if CNV develops.

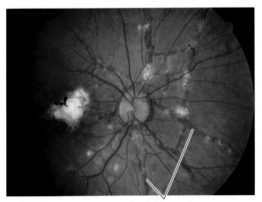

Figure 10-86 • Angioid streaks appear as dark red, branching lines radiating from the optic nerve.

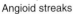

Angioid streaks

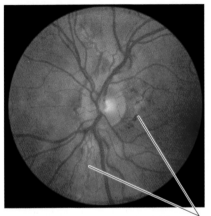

Angioid streaks

Figure 10-87 • Angioid streaks radiating from the optic nerve.

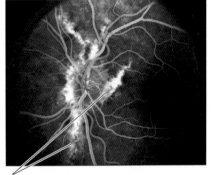

Angioid streaks

Figure 10-88 • Fluorescein angiogram of same patient as shown in Figure 10-87, demonstrating hyperfluorescent window defects corresponding to the angioid streaks.

Differential Diagnosis Age-related macular degeneration, lacquer cracks, myopic degeneration, choroidal rupture, choroidal folds, hypertensive retinopathy (Siegrist streaks), ophthalmic artery occlusion.

Evaluation

- Complete ophthalmic history and eye exam with attention to non-contact biomicroscopic or contact lens fundus exam, and ophthalmoscopy.
- Check Amsler grid to rule out CNV.
- **Lab tests:** sickle cell prep, hemoglobin electrophoresis (sickle cell disease), serum alkaline phosphatase, serum lead levels, urine calcium, stool guaiac, skin biopsy.

- **Fluorescein angiogram:** To evaluate for CNV if suspected clinically. Usually occur along the track of an angioid streak and has granular pattern of hyperfluorescence.
- Medical consultation to rule out systemic diseases including skin biopsy and radiographs.

Management

- Treat CNV with focal photocoagulation similar to MPS guidelines in juxta- and extra-foveal lesions. For subfoveal CNV, PDT and anti-VEGF agents such as intravitreal 0.5 mg ranibizumab (Lucentis) or 1.25 mg bevacizumab (Avastin) have shown benefit.
- Polycarbonate safety glasses because mild blunt trauma can cause hemorrhages or choroidal rupture.
- Treat underlying medical condition.

Prognosis   Good unless CNV develops (high recurrence rates).

Central Serous Chorioretinopathy (Idiopathic Central Serous Choroidopathy

Definition   Idiopathic leakage of fluid from the choroid into the subretinal space (94%), under the RPE (3%), or both (3%) presumably due to RPE or choroidal dysfunction.

Epidemiology   Usually occurs in males (10:1) aged 20–50 years old; in women, tends to occur at a slightly older age. Usually unilateral, but can be bilateral; more common in Caucasians, Hispanics, and Asians; rare in African Americans. Associated with type-A personality, stress, hypochondriasis; also associated with pregnancy, steroid use, hypertension, Cushing's syndrome, systemic lupus erythematosus, and organ transplantation.

Symptoms   Decreased vision, micropsia, metamorphopsia, central scotoma, and mild dyschromatopsia; may be asymptomatic.

Signs   Normal or decreased visual acuity ranging from 20/20 to 20/200 (visual acuity improves with pinhole or plus lenses); induced hyperopia, abnormal Amsler grid (central/paracentral scotomas or metamorphopsia); single or multiple, round or oval-shaped, shallow, serous retinal detachment or pigment epithelial detachment with deep yellow spots at the level of the retinal pigment epithelium; areas of retinal pigment epithelium atrophy may occur at sites of previous episodes. Subretinal fibrin suggests active leakage. Rarely associated with CNV and subretinal fluid.

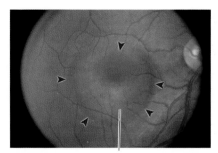

Pigment epithelial detachment

Figure 10-89 • Idiopathic central serous retinopathy with large serous retinal detachment.

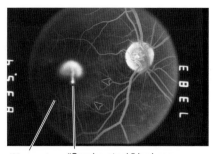

Pigment epithelial detachment   "Smoke-stack" leakage

Figure 10-90 • Fluorescein angiogram of same patient as shown in Figure 10-89, demonstrating classic smoke-stack appearance.

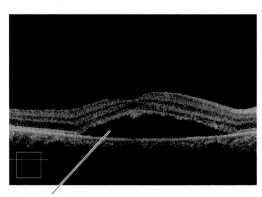

Subretinal fluid

Figure 10-91 • Spectral domain optical coherence tomography of central serous retinopathy. Note the normal foveal depression over the subretinal fluid

Differential Diagnosis Age-related macular degeneration (especially in patients >50 years old), Vogt–Koyanagi–Harada syndrome or other inflammatory choroidal disorders, uveal effusion syndrome, toxemia of pregnancy, optic nerve pit, choroidal tumors, vitelliform macular detachment, pigment epithelial detachment from other causes including CNV.

Evaluation

• Complete ophthalmic history and eye exam with attention to Amsler grid, non-contact biomicroscopic or contact lens fundus examination, and ophthalmoscopy.

• **Fluorescein angiogram:** Focal dot of hyperfluorescence early that leaks in a characteristic smoke-stack pattern (10%) or gradually pools into a pigment epithelial detachment (90%); more than one site may be present simultaneously (30%); often see punctate window defects in other areas in both eyes; recurrent leakage sites are often close to original sites.

- **Indocyanine green angiogram:** Choroidal hyperpermeability.
- **Optical coherence tomography:** Subretinal fluid and often sub-RPE fluid visible. Useful to follow patients for progression/regression.

Management

- No treatment required in most cases; usually resolves spontaneously over 6 weeks.
- Low-intensity direct focal laser photocoagulation or PDT considered for patients who require quicker visual rehabilitation for occupational reasons (monocular, pilots, etc.), poor vision in fellow eye due to central serous retinopathy, no resolution of fluid after several months, recurrent episodes with poor vision, or in severe forms of central serous retinopathy known to have a poor prognosis. Treatment has been shown to reduce duration of symptoms, but not affect final acuity. There have been some reports that photocoagulation reduces the recurrence rate, but others have observed no difference.

Prognosis Good; 94% regain ≥20/30 acuity; 95% of pigment epithelial detachments resolve spontaneously in 3–4 months, acuity improves over 21 months; recurrences common (45%) and usually occur within a year. Recovery of visual acuity is faster following laser treatment but recovery of contrast sensitivity is prolonged and may ultimately be reduced; 5% develop CNV. Prognosis is worse for patients with recurrent disease, multiple areas of detachment, or chronic course.

Cystoid Macular Edema

Definition Accumulation of extracellular fluid in the macular region with characteristic cystoid spaces in the outer plexiform layer.

Etiology Post-surgery (especially in older patients and if the posterior capsule is violated with vitreous loss; CME following cataract surgery is called Irvine–Gass syndrome), post-laser treatment (neodymium:yttrium-aluminum-garnet [Nd:YAG] laser capsulotomy, especially if performed within 3 months of cataract surgery), uveitis, diabetic retinopathy, juxtafoveal/retinal telangiectasia, retinal vein occlusions, retinal vasculitis, epiretinal membrane, hereditary retinal dystrophies (dominant CME, retinitis pigmentosa), medications (epinephrine in aphakic patients, dipivefrin, and prostaglandin analogues), hypertensive retinopathy, AMD, occult rhegmatogenous retinal detachment, intraocular tumors, collagen vascular diseases, hypotony, and chronic inflammation.

Symptoms Decreased or washed-out vision.

Signs Decreased visual acuity, loss of foveal reflex, thickened fovea, foveal folds, intraretinal cystoid spaces, lipid exudates; may have signs of uveitis or surgical complications including open posterior capsule, vitreous to the wound, peaked pupil, or iris incarceration in wound.

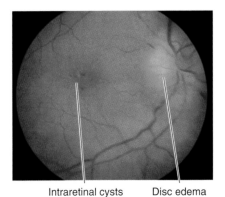

Intraretinal cysts   Disc edema

Figure 10-92 • Cystoid macular edema with decreased foveal reflex, cystic changes in fovea, and intraretinal hemorrhages.

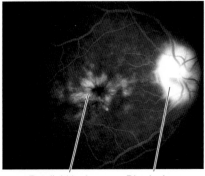

Petalloid leakage   Disc leakage

Figure 10-93 • Fluorescein angiogram of same patient as shown in Figure 10-92 demonstrating characteristic petalloid appearance with optic nerve leakage.

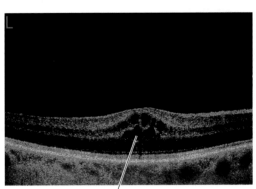

Cystoid macular edema

Figure 10-94 • Spectral domain optical coherence tomography of cystoid macular edema demonstrating intraretinal cystoid spaces and dome-shaped configuration of fovea.

Differential Diagnosis Macular hole (Stage 1), foveal retinoschisis, central serous retinopathy, choroidal neovascular membrane, pseudocystoid macular edema (no leakage on fluorescein angiography).

Evaluation

- Complete ophthalmic history and eye exam with attention to cornea, anterior chamber, iris, lens, non-contact biomicroscopic or contact lens fundus exam, and ophthalmoscopy.

- **Fluorescein angiogram:** Early, perifoveal, punctate hyperfluorescence and characteristic late leakage in a petalloid pattern. *Note*: No leakage occurs in pseudocystoid macular edema from juvenile retinoschisis, nicotinic acid (niacin) maculopathy, Goldmann–Favre disease, and some forms of retinitis pigmentosa.

- **Optical coherence tomography:** Increased retinal thickness with cystoid spaces and loss of normal foveal contour with or without subsensory fluid.

Management

- Treat underlying etiology if possible.
- Discontinue topical epinephrine, dipivefrin, or prostaglandin analogue drops, and nicotinic acid-containing medications. Rarely, diuretics and oral contraceptive pills can cause an atypical CME that resolves on discontinuing medication.
- Topical nonsteroidal anti-inflammatory drugs ([NSAIDs], Voltaren or Acular qid, Nevanac tid, or Xibrom bid) and/or topical steroid (prednisolone acetate 1% qid for 1 month, then taper slowly). One randomized study suggested that combination treatment with NSAID and steroid drops were more effective than either alone.
- Consider posterior sub-Tenon's steroid injection (triamcinolone acetonide 40 mg/mL) in patients who do not respond to topical medications.
- If no response, consider oral NSAIDs (indomethacin 25 mg po tid for 6–8 weeks), oral steroids (prednisone 40–60 mg po qd for 1–2 weeks, then taper slowly), and/or oral acetazolamide (Diamox 250–mg po bid); all are unproven.
- In refractory cases consider intravitreal injection of 4 mg triamcinolone acetonide (experimental).
- If vitreous is present to the wound and vision is <20/80, consider Nd:YAG laser vitreolysis or perform pars plana vitrectomy with peeling of posterior hyaloid (Vitrectomy-Aphakic Cystoid Macular Edema Study conclusion).

Prognosis Usually good; spontaneous resolution in weeks to months (post-surgical); poorer for chronic CME (>6 months), may develop macular hole.

Macular Hole

Definition Retinal hole in the fovea.

Etiology Idiopathic; other risk factors are cystoid macular edema, vitreomacular traction, trauma, post-surgical, myopia, post laser treatment and post-inflammatory.

Epidemiology Senile (idiopathic) macular holes (83%) usually occur in women (3:1) aged 60–80 years old; traumatic holes rare (5%); 25–30% bilateral.

Symptoms Decreased vision, metamorphopsia, and less commonly central scotoma.

Signs Decreased visual acuity ranging from 20/40 in Stage 1 to 20/100 to HM in Stage 3/4; retinal detachments rare except in high myopes. Fundus findings can be classified into 4 stages:

Stage 1

Premacular hole (impending hole) with foveal detachment, absent foveal reflex, macular cyst (1A = yellow spot, 100–200 µm in diameter, 1B = yellow ring, 200–300 µm in diameter).

Stage 2

Early, small, full-thickness hole either centrally within the ring or eccentrically at the ring's margin.

Stage 3

Full-thickness hole (≥400 µm) with yellow deposits at level of retinal pigment epithelium (Klein's tags), operculum, cuff of subretinal fluid, cystoid macular edema, and positive Watzke–Allen sign (subjective interruption of slit beam on biomicroscopy).

Stage 4

Stage 3 and posterior vitreous detachment (PVD).

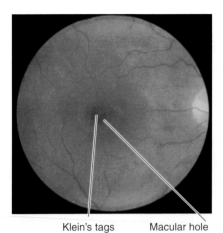

Klein's tags   Macular hole

Figure 10-95 • Macular hole with multiple yellow spots (Klein's tags) at the base of the hole.

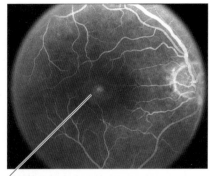

Macular hole

Figure 10-96 • Fluorescein angiogram of same patient in Figure 10-95 demonstrating early hyperfluorescence of the hole that does not leak in late views.

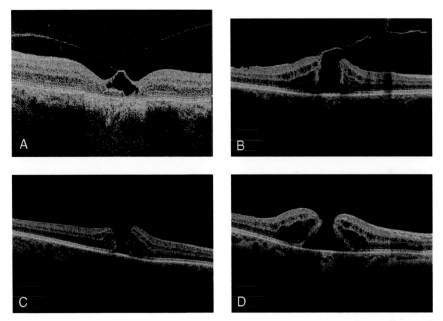

Figure 10-97 • Optical coherence tomography demonstrating cross sectional image of all stages (1–4 [A–D, respectively]) of macular hole formation and the full-thickness retinal defect characteristic of stage 3 and 4 holes.

Differential Diagnosis Epiretinal membrane with pseudo-hole, solar retinopathy, central serous retinopathy, AMD, vitreomacular traction syndrome, cystoid macular edema, solitary druse, lamellar hole.

Evaluation

- Complete ophthalmic history and eye exam with attention to visual acuity, Amsler grid, Watzke–Allen test, non-contact biomicroscopic or contact lens fundus exam, and ophthalmoscopy.

- **Optical coherence tomography:** Full-thickness defect in retina with or without traction on edges of hole; can differentiate lamellar holes and cysts from true macular holes; useful for staging holes and for surgical planning.

- **Fluorescein angiogram:** Hyperfluorescent window defect in the central fovea.

Management

- No treatment recommended for Stage 1 holes because spontaneous hole closure can occur, but 50% progress necessitating surgery.

- Pars plana vitrectomy, membrane peel, gas fluid exchange, and gas injection with 7–14 days prone positioning for Stage 2–4 holes of recent onset (<1 year) and reduced visual acuity in the range of 20/40 to 20/400; should be performed by a retina specialist.

Prognosis Good for recent onset holes; surgery has successful anatomic results in 60–95% depending on duration, of which 73% have improved acuity; preoperative visual acuity is inversely correlated with the absolute amount of visual improvement; poor for holes >1 year's duration.

Epiretinal Membrane/Macular Pucker

Definition Cellular proliferation along the internal limiting membrane and retinal surface. Contraction of this membrane causes the retinal surface to become wrinkled (pucker/cellophane maculopathy).

Etiology Risk factors include prior retinal surgery, intraocular inflammation, retinal vascular occlusion, sickle retinopathy, vitreous hemorrhage, trauma, macular holes, intraocular tumors such as angiomas and hamartomas, telangiectasis, retinal arterial macroaneurysms, retinitis pigmentosa, laser photocoagulation, PVD, retinal break, and cryotherapy; often idiopathic.

Epidemiology Incidence increases with increasing age; occurs in 2% of population >50 years old and in 20% >75 years old; 20–30% bilateral, although often asymmetric. Slight female predilection (3:2); diabetes has been found to be associated with idiophathic ERMs.

Symptoms Asymptomatic with normal or near-normal vision; mild distortion or blurred vision; less commonly, macropsia, central photopsia, or monocular diplopia if macular pucker exists.

Signs Normal or decreased visual acuity; abnormal Amsler grid; thin, translucent membrane appears as mild sheen (cellophane) along macula; may have dragged or tortuous vessels, retinal striae, pseudo-holes, foveal ectopia, and cystoid macular edema. Occasionally multiple punctate hemorrhages occur in the inner retina.

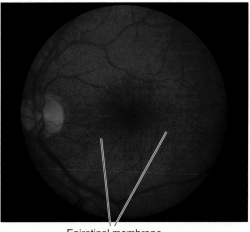

Epiretinal membrane

Figure 10-98 • Cellophane epiretinal membrane with retinal striae.

Figure 10-99 • Epiretinal membrane with dragged vessels.

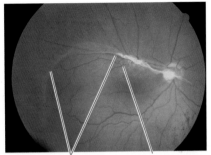

Epiretinal membrane   Dragged vessels

Figure 10-100 • Spectral domain optical coherence tomography of epiretinal membrane with increased retinal thickening.

Epiretinal membrane

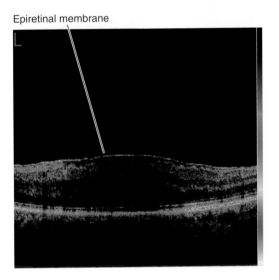

Figure 10-101 • Spectral domain optical coherence tomography of pseudohole due to an epiretinal membrane. Since the defect is not full thickness, this is not a macular hole.

Pseudohole   Epiretinal membrane

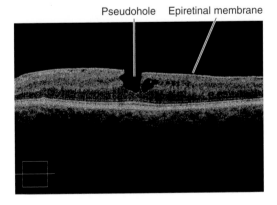

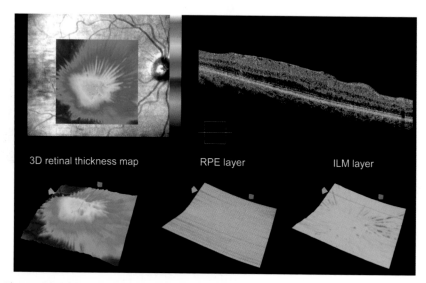

3D retinal thickness map   RPE layer   ILM layer

Figure 10-102 • Spectral domain optical coherence tomography of epiretinal membrane illustrating advanced segmentation algorithms that shows the increased retinal thickness and surface wrinkling on the ILM (internal limiting membrane) map.

Differential Diagnosis Traction retinal detachment from diabetic retinopathy, sickle cell retinopathy, or radiation retinopathy; choroidal folds.

Evaluation

- Complete ophthalmic history and eye exam with attention to non-contact biomicroscopic or contact lens fundus exam, and ophthalmoscopy.
- Consider optical coherence tomography to evaluate retinal thickening and traction.

Management

- Treatment rarely required unless visual changes become problematic.
- Pars plana vitrectomy and membrane peel in patients with reduced acuity (e.g., <20/50) or intractable symptoms; should be performed by a retina specialist.

Prognosis Good; 75% of patients have improvement in symptoms and acuity after surgery.

Myelinated Nerve Fibers

Abnormal myelination of ganglion cell axons anterior to the lamina cribosa; appears as yellow-white patches with feathery borders in the superficial retina (nerve fiber layer). Typically unilateral (80%) and occurs adjacent to the optic nerve, but can be located anywhere in the posterior pole. Obscures underlying retinal vasculature and can be confused with cotton-wool spots, astrocytic hamartomas, commotio retinae, or rarely retinal artery occlusion if extensive. Patients are usually asymptomatic, but scotomas corresponding to the areas of myelination can be demonstrated on visual fields; slight male predilection.

Figure 10-103 • Myelinated nerve fibers demonstrating fluffy white appearance extending from optic nerve and partially obscuring disc margins and retinal vessels.

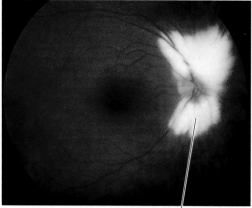

Myelinated nerve fibers

- No treatment required.
- Consider visual fields.

Solar/Photic Retinopathy

Bilateral decreased vision ranging from 20/40 to 20/100, metamorphopsia, photophobia, dyschromatopsia, after-images, scotomas, headaches, and orbital pain 1–4 hours after unprotected, long-term sun gazing. Retinal damage ranges from no changes to a yellow spot with surrounding pigmentary changes in the foveolar region in the early stages. Late changes include lamellar holes or depressions in the fovea. Vision can improve over 3–6 months, with residual scotomas and metamorphopsia. Similar problems may occur from unprotected viewing of lasers, welding arcs, and extended exposure to operating microscope lights (unilateral).

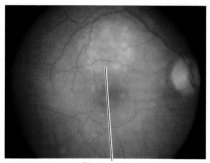

Phototoxicity

Figure 10-104 • Photic retinopathy demonstrating retinal edema secondary to operating-room microscope over-exposure.

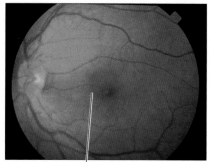

Solar retinopathy

Figure 10-105 • Solar retinopathy. Note pigmentary changes in the macula.

- No effective treatment.

Toxic (Drug) Maculopathies

Aminoglycosides (Gentamicin/Tobramicin/Amikacin)

Aminoglycosides may be toxic when delivered into the eye by any technique including sub-conjunctival injection without apparent scleral perforation, diffusion through cataract wound from subconjunctival injection, or when used with a collagen corneal shield. Gentamicin (Garamycin) demonstrates more toxicity than amikacin (Amikin) or tobramycin (Nebcin). Toxicity, due to occlusion of the retinal capillaries by granulocytes, has occurred at doses as low as 0.1 mg of gentamicin or 0.2 mg of amikacin. Leads to acute, severe, permanent visual loss. Retinal toxic reaction with marked retinal whitening (especially in macula), arteriolar attenuation, venous beading, and widespread retinal hemorrhages; optic atrophy and pigmentary changes occur later. Poor visual prognosis.

- **Fluorescein angiogram:** Sharp zones of capillary nonperfusion corresponding to the areas of ischemic retina.
- No effective treatment.

Canthaxanthine (Orobronze)

The carotenoid pigment canthaxanthine is prescribed for photosensitivity disorders and vitiligo. Toxicity produces characteristic refractile yellow spots in a wreath-like pattern around the fovea (gold-dust retinopathy). Usually asymptomatic or causes mild metamorphopsia and decreased vision while this oral tanning agent is being taken. Occurs with cumulative doses >35 g.

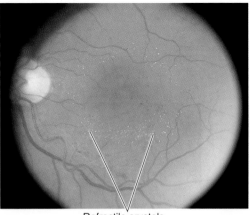

Figure 10-106 • Crystalline maculopathy due to canthaxanthine.

Refractile crystals

- Check visual fields (central 10°).
- Decrease or discontinue the medication if toxicity develops.

Chloroquine (Aralen)/Hydroxychloroquine (Plaquenil)

Quinolines were first used as an antimalarial agent in World War II and now are used to treat rheumatologic disorders such as systemic lupus erythematosis, rheumatoid arthritis, and for short-term pulse treatment for graft versus host disease, as well as amoebiasis. Toxicity produces central/paracentral scotomas, blurry vision, nyctalopia, photopsias, dyschromatopsia, photophobia, and, in late stages, constriction of visual fields, loss of color vision, decreased vision, and absolute scotomas. Early retinal changes include loss of foveal reflex and abnormal macular pigmentation (reversible); "bull's eye" maculopathy (not reversible), peripheral bone spicules, vasculature attenuation, and disc pallor appear later; late stages can appear similar to end-stage retinitis pigmentosa. May also develop eyelash whitening and whorl-like subepithelial corneal deposits (cornea verticillata, vortex keratopathy). Doses >3.5 mg/kg/day or 300 g total (chloroquine), and >6.5 mg/kg/day (<400 mg/day appears safe) or 700 g total (hydroxychloroquine) may produce the maculopathy; total daily dose seems more critical than total accumulative dose; in patients with renal insufficiency, lower doses are required. Quinolines are stored to a greater degree in lean body tissues than in fat; dosages based on actual, rather than ideal, body weight will lead to overdoses in obese patients; often progresses after medications are discontinued because the drug concentrates in the eye. Hydroxychloroquine appears safer since it does not readily cross the blood–retinal barrier (toxicity rarely occurs with use <7 years).

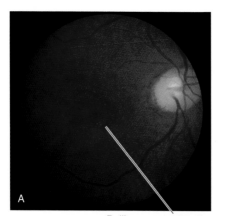
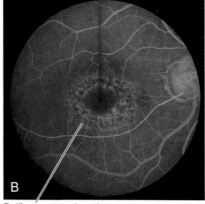

Bull's eye maculopathy   Bull's eye maculopathy

Figure 10-107 • Bull's eye maculopathy due to Plaquenil toxicity as seem on (A) clinical photo, and (B) fluorescein angiogram demonstrating same pattern with a circular window defect.

Figure 10-108 • Optical coherence tomography of same patient as Figure 10-107 demonstarting thinning of the retina in the area of the bull's eye.

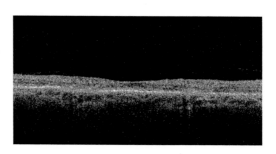

- Differential diagnosis of "bull's eye" maculopathy includes cone dystrophy, AMD, Stargardt's disease/fundus flavimaculatus, Spielmeyer–Vogt disease, albinism, fenestrated sheen macular dystrophy, central areolar choroidal dystrophy, benign concentric annular macular dystrophy, clofazimine toxicity, fucosidosis.

- Check visual acuity, red Amsler grid and visual fields (central 10° with red test object) at baseline and every 6 months (chloroquine) or 12 months (hydroxychloroquine) while patient is taking medications; color fundus photographs (especially if abnormalities seen) and color vision (preferably including the blue-yellow axis) are optionally checked; patients with drug use >5 years with high fat level body habitus, renal or liver disease, and age >60 years old especially if frail or extremely thin are at higher risk of developing toxicity and should be checked more frequently.

- Low-risk patients (defined as nonobese individuals under age 60 years old, using less than 3 mg/kg/day of chloroquine or 6.5 mg/kg/day of hydroxychloroquine for fewer than 5 years, and without concomitant renal, hepatic, or retinal disease) require no additional screening evaluations.

- **Fluorescein angiogram:** Hypofluorescence with ring of hyperfluorescence corresponding to the bull's eye lesion, often visible before fundus lesion.

- **Electrophysiologic testing:** Electrooculogram (EOG) (normal early, reduced [<1.6] light-peak/dark-trough [Arden] ratio later).

- Decrease or discontinue the medication if toxicity develops.

Chlorpromazine (Thorazine)

Patients have pigment deposition in eyelids, cornea, lens, and retina with toxic doses >1200–1400 mg/day for at least 1 year.

- Decrease or discontinue the medication if toxicity develops.

Deferoxamine (Desferal)

Chelator of iron and aluminum that is prescribed for patients undergoing multiple blood transfusions. Toxicity causes decreased vision, nyctalopia, and visual field loss. The most common initial finding is a subtle gray macular discoloration, although a bull's eye lesion may develop; a generalized pigmentary disturbance develops over weeks, which may persist despite drug discontinuation. Toxicity may occur after a single dose.

- Decrease or discontinue the medication if toxicity develops.

Interferon-alpha

Interferon-alpha antiviral agents used to treat hepatitis cause vascular occlusion due to presumed immune-complex deposition. Toxicity causes cotton-wool spots, intraretinal hemorrhages, cystoid macular edema, capillary nonperfusion, and rarely vascular occlusion.

- Decrease or discontinue the medication if toxicity develops.

Methoxyflurane (Penthrane)

This inhaled anesthetic that is rarely used today may cause irreversible renal failure, partly through calcium oxalate crystalline deposition and retinal toxicity with yellow-white crystalline deposits in the posterior pole and along the arterioles. Methoxyflurane is metabolized to oxalate which binds calcium to form insoluble calcium oxalate salts that are permanent.

- No effective treatment.

Figure 10-109 Methoxyflurane toxicity demonstrating crystalline deposits along the retinal arterioles.

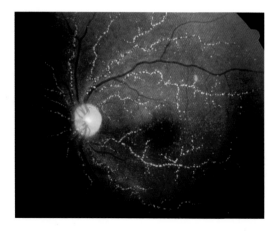

Niacin

Used to treat hypercholesterolemia. May produce decreased vision and metamorphopsia due to pseudocystoid macular edema (nicotinic acid maculopathy) caused by intracellular edema of Müller's cells.

- **Fluorescein angiogram:** Early, perifoveal, punctate hyperfluorescence as in CME but no leakage.
- **Optical coherence tomography:** Cystoid spaces.
- Decrease or discontinue the medication if toxicity develops.

Quinine (Quinamm)

A quinolin, used to treat benign muscle cramps, which acutely causes retinal edema with venous engorgement and a cherry red spot, progressing to RPE mottling, retinal vascular attenuation and optic atrophy; although the end stage resembles a vascular occlusion, the toxic effects appear to concentrate within the neurosensory retina. Toxicity causes generalized neurologic symptoms and blurred vision, visual field loss, photophobia; acute overdose (single dose >4 g) may cause permanent blindness.

- No effective treatment.

Figure 10-110 Bull's eye maculopathy due to quinine toxicity.

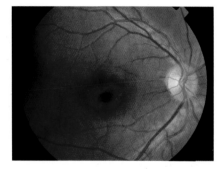

Sildenafil (Viagra)

This selective phosphodiesterase 5 (PDE-5) inhibitor commonly prescribed for erectile dysfunction, demonstrates cross-activity with the PDE-6 receptors in the photoreceptor layer. Produces reversible changes in color perception including a blue or blue-green tint or central haze of vision (may be pink or yellow); changes in light perception including darker colors appearing darker, increased perception of brightness, and flashing lights within 15–30 minutes of ingesting drug that peaks within 1–2 hours; may also have photophobia and conjunctival hyperemia; resolves within 1 hour at doses <50 mg, 2 hours with 100 mg, and 4–6 hours for 200 mg. The drug modifies the transduction cascade in photoreceptors (blocks PDE-5 10× more than PDE-6 leading to interference in cGMP); occurs in 3% of patients taking a dose of 25–50 mg; 11% of patients taking 100 mg dose, and in 40–50% taking >100 mg; incidence the same for all ages. No permanent visual effects have been reported; long-term effects not known. Use with extreme caution in patients with retinitis pigmentosa and congenital stationary night blindness. There have been some reports of ischemic optic neuropathy, although no true association or causal relationship has been determined.

- **Electrophysiologic testing:** Electroretinogram (ERG) mildly reduced photopic and scotopic b-wave amplitudes and less than 10% decrease in photopic a and b-wave implicit times during acute episode, reverts back to normal over time, no permanent effects seen.
- Decrease or discontinue the medication if toxicity develops.
- No effective treatment of ischemic optic neuropathy.

Tadalafil (Cialis)/Vardenafil (Levitra)

Similar to sildenafil, there have been some reports of ischemic optic neuropathy, although no true association or causal relationship has been determined. The FDA has advised patients to discontinue the use of these medications if they experience sudden or decreased vision loss in one or both eyes.

- No effective treatment of ischemic optic neuropathy.

Talc

Magnesium silicate (talc) has no medicinal value, but serves as a vehicle for several oral medications, including methylphenidate (Ritalin) and methadone. Refractive yellow deposits near or in arterioles occurs in IV drug abusers; similar findings occur in IV drug abusers injecting suspensions of crushed methylphenidate (Ritalin) tablets. Talc particles smaller than an erythrocyte will clear the pulmonary capillary network and enter the arterial system. Repeated intravenous injection appears to induce shunt formation, allowing larger particles access to the ophthalmic artery.

- No effective treatment.

Tamoxifen (Nolvadex)

Used to treat metastatic breast adenocarcinoma. Produces refractile yellow-white crystals scattered throughout the posterior pole in a donut-shaped pattern, mild cystoid macular edema, and retinal pigmentary changes later; may develop whorl-like, white, subepithelial corneal deposits. Usually asymptomatic, but may cause mild decreases in vision and dyschromatopsia. Occurs with doses >30 mg/day, at the initial higher dosage levels crystals often occur, but can resolve with lowering dose.

- **Fluorescein angiogram:** Characteristic petalloid leakage from CME.
- **Optical coherence tomography:** Cystoid spaces from CME.
- Decrease or discontinue the medication if toxicity develops.

Thioridazine (Mellaril)

Phenothiazine, introduced in 1952 for the treatment of psychoses, may produce nyctalopia, decreased vision, ring/paracentral scotomas, and brown discoloration of vision. Pigment granularity/clumping in the midperiphery appears first (reversible), then progresses and coalesces into large areas of pigmentation (salt and pepper pigment retinopathy) or chorioretinal atrophy with short-term, high-dose use. A variant, termed nummular retinopathy, with chorioretinal atrophy posterior to the equator occurs with chronic use. Late stages can appear similar to end-stage retinitis pigmentosa or tapetoretinal degeneration with arteriolar attenuation, optic atrophy, and widespread pigmentary disturbances. Doses >800 mg/day (300 mg recommended) can produce retinopathy; total daily dose seems more critical than total accumulative dose; may progress after medication is withdrawn because the drug is stored in the eye.

Figure 10-111 • Diffuse pigmentary retinopathy in end-stage thioridazine toxicity

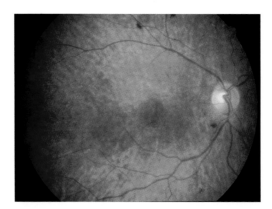

- Check vision, color vision and visual fields every 6 months while on medication.
- **Electrophysiologic testing:** Electroretinogram (ERG) (normal early; reduced amplitude and abnormal dark adaptation later).
- **Fluorescein angiogram:** Salt and pepper pattern of hypofluorescent spots and hyperfluorescent window defects; nummular pattern produces large areas of RPE loss.
- Decrease or discontinue the medication if toxicity develops.

Lipid Storage Diseases

Sphingolipid storage diseases cause accumulation of ceramide in liposomes, especially in retinal ganglion cells, giving a characteristic cherry-red spot in the macula.

Farber's Disease (Glycolipid) (Autosomal Recessive)

Mild cherry-red spot, failure to thrive, subcutaneous nodules, hoarse cry, progressive arthropathy, and early mortality by 6–18 years of age.

Mucolipidosis (Mucopolysaccharidoses) (Autosomal Recessive)

Cherry-red spot, nystagmus, myoclonus, corneal clouding, optic atrophy, cataracts, Hurler-like facies, hepatosplenomegaly, and failure to thrive.

Niemann–Pick Disease (Ceramide Phosphatidyl Choline) (Autosomal Recessive)

Prominent cherry-red spot, corneal stromal opacities, splenomegaly, bone marrow foam cells, and hyperlipidemia.

Sandhoff's Disease (Gangliosidosis Type II) (Autosomal Recessive)

Prominent cherry-red spot and optic atrophy with associated lipid-storage problems in the kidney, liver, pancreas, and other gastrointestinal organs.

Tay–Sachs Disease (Gangliosidosis Type I) (Autosomal Recessive)

Prominent cherry-red spot, blindness, deafness, convulsions; mainly occurs in Ashkenazic Jewish children.

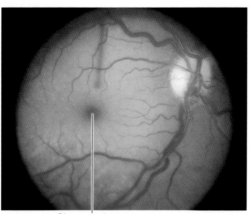

Figure 10-112 • Cherry-red spot in an infant with Tay–Sachs disease.

Cherry-red spot

Peripheral Retinal Degenerations

Lattice Degeneration

Occurs in 7–10% of general population; more common in myopes; 33–50% bilateral. Oval, circumferential area of retinal thinning and overlying vitreous liquefaction found anterior to the equator; appears as criss-crossing, white lines (sclerotic vessels) with variable overlying retinal pigmentation that clusters in the inferior and superior peripheral retina. Atrophic holes (25%) common; retinal tears can occur with posterior vitreous separation pulling on the atrophic, thinned retina; increased risk of retinal detachment.

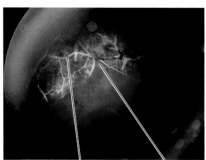

Sclerotic vessels   Lattice degeneration

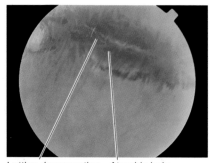

Lattice degeneration   Atrophic hole

Figure 10-113 Lattice degeneration demonstrating retinal pigment epithelium changes and characteristic linear branching pattern.

Figure 10-114 Atrophic retinal hole within an area of lattice degeneration.

- Asymptomatic lattice degeneration and atrophic holes do not require treatment; consider prophylactic treatment in patients with high myopia, aphakia, history of retinal detachment in the fellow eye, or strong family history of retinal detachment. Prophylactic treatment before cataract extraction or LASIK is controversial.

- Symptomatic lesions (photopsias/floaters) should receive prophylactic treatment with either cryopexy or two to three rows of laser photocoagulation around lattice degeneration and holes.

Pavingstone (Cobblestone) Degeneration

Occurs in 22–27% of general population; 33% bilateral. Appears as round, discrete, yellow–white spots 1/2 to 2 disc diameters in size with darkly pigmented borders found anterior to the equator adjacent to ora; correspond to areas of thinned outer retina with loss of choriocapillaris and retinal pigment epithelium; usually found inferiorly; normal vitreous over lesions. May protect against retinal detachment due to adherence of thinned retina and choroid. Increased incidence with age and myopia.

Figure 10-115 Yellow–white, pavingstone lesions with pigmented borders characteristic of peripheral cobblestone degeneration.

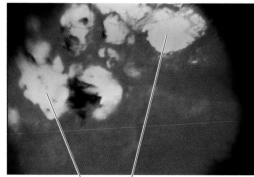

Cobblestone degeneration

- No treatment recommended.

Peripheral Cystoid Degeneration

Clusters of tiny intraretinal cysts (Blessig-Iwanoff cysts) in the outer plexiform layer just posterior to ora serrata. The bubble-like cysts can coalesce and progress to typical degenerative retinoschisis; no increased risk of retinal detachment.

- No treatment recommended.

Snail Track Degeneration

Chains of fine, white dots that occur circumferentially in the peripheral retina; associated with myopia. Atrophic holes may develop in the areas of degeneration increasing the risk of retinal detachment.

- Asymptomatic snail track degeneration, atrophic holes, and tears do not require treatment; consider prophylactic treatment in patients with high myopia, aphakia, history of retinal detachment in the fellow eye, or strong family history of retinal detachment. Prophylactic treatment before cataract extraction is controversial.
- Symptomatic lesions (photopsias/floaters) should receive prophylactic treatment with either cryopexy or two to three rows of laser photocoagulation around tears or holes.

Retinoschisis

Definition Splitting of the retina. Two types:

Acquired

Senile, degenerative process with splitting between the inner nuclear and outer plexiform layers.

Juvenile

Congenital process with splitting of the nerve fiber layer.

Epidemiology

Acquired

More common; occurs in 4–7% of general population especially in patients >40 years old; 50–75% bilateral often symmetric; also associated with hyperopia.

Juvenile (X-Linked Recessive)

Onset in first decade; may be present at birth. Mapped to XLRS1/Retinoschisin gene on chromosome Xp22 that codes proteins necessary for cell–cell adhesion; rarely autosomal; 98% bilateral.

Acquired

Usually asymptomatic and nonprogressive, may have visual field defect with sharp borders.

Juvenile

Decreased vision (often due to vitreous hemorrhage), or may be asymptomatic.

Acquired

Bilateral, smooth, convex, elevated schisis cavity usually in inferotemporal quadrant (70%); height of elevation constant even with change in head position; white dots (Gunn's dots), "snowflakes" or "frosting" and sheathed retinal vessels (sclerotic in periphery) occur in the elevated inner retinal layer; outer layer breaks are common, large, well-delineated, have rolled margins and appear pock-marked on scleral depression; inner layer breaks, vitreous hemorrhage, and rhegmatogenous retinal detachments are rare; intact outer retinal layer whitens with scleral depression; cystoid degeneration at the ora serrata; absolute scotoma.

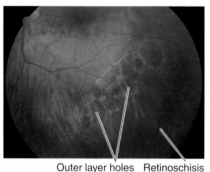

Outer layer holes   Retinoschisis

Figure 10-116 • Acquired retinoschisis with outer layer breaks.

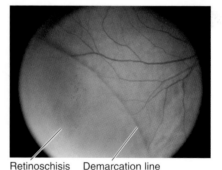

Retinoschisis   Demarcation line

Figure 10-117 • Acquired retinoschisis with evident demarcation line at edge of elevated schisis cavity.

Juvenile

Slowly progressive decreased visual acuity ranging from 20/25 to 20/80; nystagmus and strabismus often occur; foveal schisis with fine, radiating folds from fovea (occur in 100% of cases), spoke-like foveal cysts, pigment mottling, and microcystic foveal elevation (looks like cystoid macular edema but does not stain on fluorescein angiogram) common; may have vitreous hemorrhage, vitreous veils, retinal vessels bridging inner and outer layers; peripheral retinoschisis (50%) with peripheral pigmentation and loss of retinal vessels, especially in inferotemporal quadrant, often found.

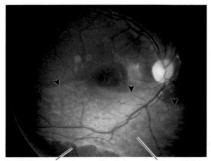

Bridging vessel   Peripheral retinoschisis

Figure 10-118 • Juvenile retinoschisis with foveal and peripheral schisis. Note bridging retinal vessel.

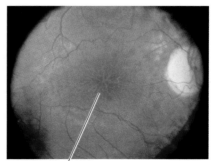

Foveal retinoschisis

Figure 10-119 • Foveal retinoschisis with fine, radiating folds and spoke-like cysts in a patient with juvenile retinoschisis.

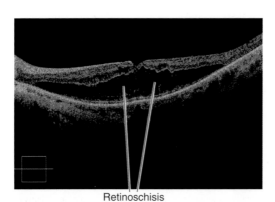

Retinoschisis

Figure 10-120 • Spectral domain optical coherence tomography of foveal retinoschisis.

Differential Diagnosis Retinal detachment, Goldmann–Favre disease, hereditary macular disease. Differentiating features from retinal detachment include no underlying RPE degeneration, blanching of RPE with laser treatment (no blanching with RD), no tobacco dust, and absolute scotoma (relative scotoma with RD).

Evaluation

- Complete ophthalmic history and eye exam with attention to color vision, non-contact biomicroscopic or contact lens fundus exam, ophthalmoscopy, and depressed peripheral retinal exam.

- **Color vision:** Initial tritan defect followed by deutan-tritan defect (less severe than for cone-rod dystrophy).

- **Electrophysiologic testing (in juvenile cases):** Electroretinogram (ERG) (select decrease in b-wave amplitude, normal a-wave; Schubert–Bornsheim tracing or electronegative ERG), electrooculogram (EOG) (normal in mild cases to subnormal in advanced cases), and dark adaptation (normal to subnormal).

- **Visual fields:** Absolute scotomas corresponding to areas of schisis.

- **Fluorescein angiogram:** Macular cysts in foveal schisis do not leak fluorescein.
- **Optical coherence tomography:** Macular cysts occur in foveal schisis; can also differentiate retinoschisis from retinal detachment.

Management

- No treatment recommended; follow closely if breaks are identified.
- Children with juvenile retinoschisis should be counseled to avoid physical activity since even minor trauma can lead to vitreous hemorrhage and/or retinal detachment.
- If symptomatic rhegmatogenous retinal detachment occurs, may require retinal surgery to repair; should be performed by a retina specialist.
- If vitreous hemorrhage occurs, treat conservatively (occlusive patching in child); rarely, pars plana vitrectomy required.

Prognosis Good; usually stationary for years.

Retinal Detachment

Separation of the neurosensory retina from the retinal pigment epithelium. Three types:

Rhegmatogenous Retinal Detachment

Definition From Greek rhegma = rent; retinal detachment due to full-thickness retinal break (tear/hole/dialysis) that allows vitreous fluid access to subretinal space.

Etiology Lattice degeneration (30%), posterior vitreous detachment (especially with vitreous hemorrhage), myopia, trauma (5–10%), and previous ocular surgery (especially with vitreous loss) increased risk of rhegmatogenous retinal detachments; retinal dialysis and giant retinal tears (>3 clock hours in extent) more common after trauma.

Symptoms Acute onset of photopsias, floaters ("shade" or "cob-webs"), shadow or curtain across visual field, decreased vision; may be asymptomatic.

Signs Undulating, mobile, convex retina with corrugated folds; clear subretinal fluid that does not shift with body position; retinal break usually seen; may have "tobacco-dust" (Shafer's sign: pigment cells in the vitreous), vitreous hemorrhage, or operculum; usually lower intraocular pressure in the affected eye and may have RAPD; chronic rhegmatogenous retinal detachments (RRD) may have pigmented demarcation lines, intraretinal cysts, fixed folds, or subretinal precipitates. Configuration of detachment helps localize retinal break:

(1) **Superotemporal/nasal detachment:** break within 1–1.5 clock hours of highest border.
(2) **Superior detachment that straddles 12 o'clock:** break between 11 and 1 o'clock.
(3) **Inferior detachment with one higher side:** break within 1–1.5 clock hours of highest border.
(4) **Inferior detachment equally high on either side:** break between 5 and 7 o'clock.

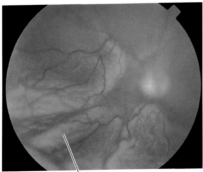

Rhegmatogenous retinal detachment

Figure 10-121 • Rhegmatogenous retinal detachment demonstrating corrugated folds.

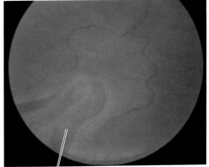

Horseshoe retinal tear

Figure 10-122 • Same patient as Figure 10-121 demonstrating peripheral horseshoe tear that caused the rhegmatogenous retinal detachment.

Differential Diagnosis Retinoschisis, choroidal detachment.

Evaluation

- Complete ophthalmic history and eye exam with attention to visual acuity, pupils, ophthalmoscopy, and depressed peripheral retinal exam to identify any retinal breaks.
- **B-scan ultrasonography:** If unable to visualize the fundus; smooth, convex, freely mobile retina appears as highly reflective echo in the vitreous cavity that is attached at the optic nerve head and ora serrata; retinal tears can be visualized in the periphery.

Management

- **Asymptomatic, not threatening macula:** Very rarely can be followed closely by a retina specialist; however, most should be treated (see below).
- **Symptomatic:** Pneumatic retinopexy or retinal surgery with scleral buckle/cryotherapy, with or without pars plana vitrectomy, drainage of subretinal fluid, endolaser, and/or other surgical maneuvers. Macular threatening ("Mac on") rhegmatogenous retinal detachment is treated emergently (within 24 hours); if macula is already detached ("Mac off"), treat urgently (within 48 to 96 hours).

Prognosis Variable (depends on underlying etiology); 5–10% of rhegmatogenous retinal detachment repairs develop proliferative vitreoretinopathy (PVR).

Serous (Exudative) Retinal Detachment

Definition Nonrhegmatogenous retinal detachment (not secondary to a retinal break) due to subretinal transudation of fluid from tumor, inflammatory process, vascular lesions, or degenerative lesions.

Etiology Vogt–Koyanagi–Harada syndrome, Harada's disease, idiopathic uveal effusion syndrome, choroidal tumors, central serous retinopathy, posterior scleritis, hypertensive retinopathy, Coats' disease, optic nerve pit, retinal coloboma, and toxemia of pregnancy.

Symptoms Usually asymptomatic until serous retinal detachment involves macula; may have acute onset of photopsias, floaters ("shade" or "cob-webs"), shadow across visual field, or decreased vision.

Signs Smooth, serous elevation of retina; subretinal fluid shifts with changing head position; there is no retinal break by definition; mild RAPD may be observed.

Figure 10-123 Exudative retinal detachment secondary to malignant melanoma.

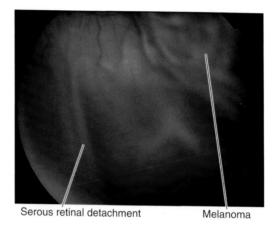

Serous retinal detachment　　　　Melanoma

Differential Diagnosis Retinoschisis, choroidal detachment, rhegmatogenous retinal detachment

Evaluation
- Complete ophthalmic history and eye exam with attention to visual acuity, pupils, ophthalmoscopy, and depressed peripheral retinal exam to identify any retinal breaks.
- **B-scan ultrasonography:** If unable to visualize the fundus, smooth, convex, freely mobile echos that shifts with changing head position; retina appears as highly reflective echo in the vitreous cavity that is attached at the optic nerve head and ora serrata.

Management

- Treat underlying condition; rarely requires surgical intervention.

Prognosis Variable (depends on underlying etiology).

Traction Retinal Detachment

Definition Nonrhegmatogenous retinal detachment (not secondary to a retinal break) due to fibrovascular or fibrotic proliferation and subsequent contraction pulling retina up.

Etiology Diabetic retinopathy, sickle cell retinopathy, retinopathy of prematurity, proliferative vitreoretinopathy, toxocariasis, and familial exudative vitreoretinopathy.

Symptoms May be asymptomatic if traction retinal detachment does not involve macula; acute onset of photopsias, floaters ("shade" or "cob-webs"), shadow across visual field, or decreased vision.

Signs Smooth, concave, usually localized, does not extend to the ora serrata; usually with fibrovascular proliferation; may have pseudo-holes or true holes in a combined traction–rhegmatogenous detachment that progresses more rapidly than traction retinal detachment (TRD) alone; if a retinal tear develops detachment may become convex.

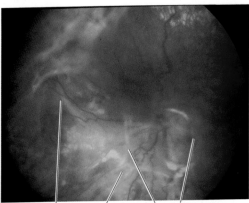

Figure 10-124 • Traction retinal detachment due to proliferative vitreoretinopathy following penetrating ocular trauma.

Retinal detachment   Preretinal traction

Differential Diagnosis Retinoschisis, choroidal detachment, rhegmatogenous retinal detachment.

Evaluation

- Complete ophthalmic history and eye exam with attention to visual acuity, pupils, ophthalmoscopy, and depressed peripheral retinal exam to identify any retinal breaks.
- **B-scan ultrasonography**: If unable to visualize the fundus; usually has tented appearance with vitreous adhesions; retina appears as highly reflective echo in the vitreous cavity that is attached at the optic nerve head and ora serrata.

Management

- Observation unless traction retinal detachment threatens the macula or becomes a combined traction-rhegmatogenous retinal detachment.
- Vitreoretinal surgery to release the vitreoretinal traction depending on clinical situation should be performed by a retina specialist.

Prognosis Variable (depends on underlying etiology).

Choroidal Detachment

Smooth, bullous, orange–brown elevation of retina and choroid; usually extends 360° around the periphery in a lobular configuration, the ora serrata is visible without scleral depression. Two forms:

Choroidal Effusion

Often asymptomatic with decreased intraocular pressure, may have shallow anterior chamber. Associated with acute ocular hypotony, post-surgical (excessive filtration through filtering bleb, wound leak, cyclodialysis cleft, post-scleral buckling surgery), posterior scleritis, Vogt–Koyanagi–Harada syndrome, trauma (open globe), intraocular tumors, or uveal effusion syndrome.

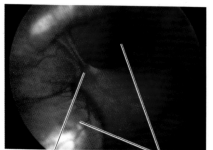
Optic nerve   Choroidal detachment

Figure 10-125 • Choroidal detachment demonstrating smooth elevations of eye wall.

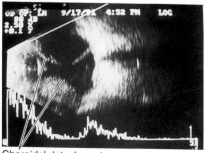
Choroidal detachment

Figure 10-126 • B-scan ultrasound demonstrating choroidal detachment.

Choroidal Hemorrhage

Causes pain (often severe), decreased vision, red eye, intraocular inflammation, and increased intraocular pressure. Classically occurs acutely during anterior segment surgery, but may be delayed up to 1–7 days after surgery or trauma especially in patients with hypertension or taking anticoagulants.

- **B-scan ultrasonography:** Smooth, convex, elevated membrane limited in the equatorial region by the vortex veins and anteriorly by the scleral spur; appears thicker and less mobile than retina.

- Treat intraoperative choroidal hemorrhage with immediate closure of surgical wound and if massive hemorrhage, perform sclerotomies to allow drainage of blood, to close surgical wound; total intraoperative drainage is usually not possible.

- Topical cycloplegic (atropine 1% bid) and steroid (prednisolone acetate 1% qid).

- May require treatment of increased intraocular pressure (see Primary Open-Angle Glaucoma section in Chapter 11).

- Consider surgical drainage when appositional or "kissing" (temporal and nasal choroid touch), severe intraocular pressure elevation despite maximal medical treatment, or corneal decompensation; visual results in appositional choroidal hemorrhage are very poor.

- Treat underlying condition.

Chorioretinal Folds

Definition   Folds of the choroid and retina.

Etiology   Compression of the sclera produces a series of folds in the inner choroid, Bruch's membrane, RPE, and retina. This may be idiopathic or occur secondarily due to tumors (choroidal, orbital), hypotony, inflammation (posterior scleritis, idiopathic orbital inflammation, thyroid-related ophthalmopathy, and autoimmune disorders), choroidal neovascular membranes, papilledema, and extraocular hardware (scleral buckle, radiotherapy plaque, orbital implants for fractures).

Symptoms   Asymptomatic or may have metamorphopsia or decreased vision if folds involve fovea.

Signs   Normal or decreased visual acuity; may have true or induced hyperopia and abnormal Amsler grid (metamorphopsia); chorioretinal folds appear as curvilinear, parallel, or circular oriented alternating light and dark bands, usually in the posterior pole or temporal fundus; the crest of the fold is pale and broad, while the trough between the folds is darker and narrower; idiopathic folds are usually bilateral and symmetric; while unilateral folds are more common with tumors and external lesions. May have signs of the underlying etiology (i.e. scleral injection, wound leak, proptosis, choroidal lesion, optic disc swelling).

Differential Diagnosis   Retinal folds, which are usually due to epiretinal membranes (thinner, subtler, irregular folds that do not appear on fluorescein angiography), optic disc swelling (Paton's lines), rhegmatogenous or traction retinal detachments, ROP, toxocariasis, and congenital.

Evaluation
- Complete ophthalmic history and eye exam with attention to refraction (hyperopia), non-contact biomicroscopic or contact lens fundus examination, and ophthalmoscopy.
- **Fluorescein angiogram:** Characteristic alternating bands of hyper- and hypofluorescence that correspond to the peaks (where the RPE is stretched) and troughs (where the RPE is compressed) of the folds, respectively.
- **Optical coherence tomography:** Scans perpendicular to the direction of the folds show the hollows and bulges of the folds.
- Consider lab tests (CBC, RF, ANA, C-ANCA) for suspected autoimmune disease.
- Consider B-scan ultrasonography for posterior scleritis and to rule out a tumor.
- Consider orbital CT scan for suspected retrobulbar mass, idiopathic orbital inflammation, and thyroid-related ophthalmopathy.
- May require medical consultation depending on the etiology.

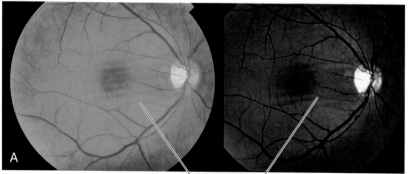

Chorioretinal folds

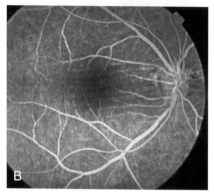

Figure 10-127 • Idiopathic chorioretinal folds radiating from optic disc on (A) color photo and red free image. Fluorescein angiogram (B) shows characteristic hyper- and hypofluorescent lines.

Management

- Treat underlying etiology.

Prognosis Depends on underlying etiology.

Chorioretinal Coloboma

Defect in retina, retinal pigment epithelium, and choroid due to incomplete closure of the embryonic fissure; usually located inferonasally. Variable size, may involve macula; appears as yellow–white lesion with pigmented margins. Associated with other ocular colobomata; increased risk of retinal detachment and CNV at margin of coloboma.

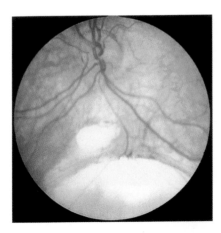

Figure 10-128   Inferior chorioretinal coloboma.

Proliferative Vitreoretinopathy

Fibrotic membranes composed of retinal pigment epithelial, glial, and inflammatory cells that form after retinal detachment or retinal surgery (8–10%); the membranes contract and pull on the retinal surface (6–8 weeks after surgery); may be preretinal or subretinal; primary cause of redetachment after successful retinal detachment surgery. Risk factors include previous retinal surgery, vitreous hemorrhage, choroidal detachment, giant retinal tears, multiple retinal breaks, penetrating trauma, excessive cryotherapy, and failure to reattach the retina at primary surgery. Final anatomic reattachment rate is 72–96%, variable visual prognosis (14–37% achieve > 20/100 vision).

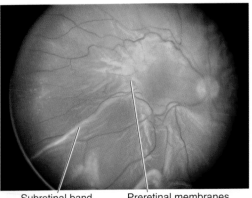

Figure 10-129   Retinal detachment with proliferative vitreoretinopathy demonstrating retinal folds and dragged vessels.

Subretinal band   Preretinal membranes

- Retinal surgery to remove preretinal and subretinal fibrotic membranes and reattach retina using silicone oil or intraocular C3F8 gas injection (The Silicone Oil Study conclusions); occasionally requires retinectomy to reattach retina; should be performed by a retina specialist.

Intermediate Uveitis/Pars Planitis

Definition Intermediate uveitis is an inflammation primarily limited to the vitreous cavity that usually involves the pars plana and ciliary body of unknown etiology. Pars planitis is a form of intermediate uveitis, classically with vitritis, pars plana exudate, and peripheral retinal vasculitis of unknown etiology.

Epidemiology Occurs in children and young adults; average age 23–28 years old; 75–90% bilateral; associated with multiple sclerosis (up to 15%) and sarcoidosis. No sexual predilection; rare in African Americans and Asians. Represents roughly 5–8% of all uveitis cases with an incidence between 2 and 5:100,000.

Symptoms Decreased vision, floaters; no red eye, pain, or photophobia.

Signs Decreased visual acuity, fibrovascular exudates especially along the inferior pars plana ("snow-banking"), extensive vitreous cells (100% of cases), vitreous cellular aggregates ("snowballs") inferiorly, minimal anterior chamber cells and flare, posterior vitreous detachment, peripheral vasculitis, and cystoid macular edema (85% of cases); may develop neovascularization and vitreous hemorrhage in the pars plana exudate.

Figure 10-130 • Pars planitis demonstrating snowballs in the vitreous cavity.

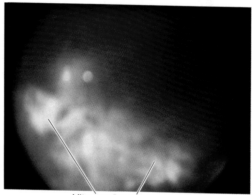

Vitreous "snowballs"

Differential Diagnosis Sarcoidosis, multiple sclerosis, Lyme disease, Behçet's disease, masquerade syndromes (especially lymphoma), syphilis, tuberculosis, cat-scratch disease, leptospirosis, Whipple's disease, HTLV-1 associated uveitis, posterior uveitis, amyloidosis, familial exudative vitreoretinopathy, Irvine-Gass syndrome (cystoid macular edema after cataract extraction), toxocariasis, toxoplasmosis, Candidiasis, fungal endophthalmitis, Eales' disease, VKH, and retinoblastoma.

Evaluation

- Complete ophthalmic history and eye exam with attention to anterior chamber, anterior vitreous, non-contact biomicroscopic or contact lens fundus exam, and ophthalmoscopy (cystoid macular edema and retinal periphery).

- **Fluorescein angiogram:** Petalloid leakage from cystoid macular edema occurs in late views.
- **Lab tests:** are used to rule out other causes from differentital diagnosis although HLA-DR2 sometimes associated. ACE, chest radiographs, and serum lysozyme (sarcoidosis), CBC (masquerade syndromes), VDRL, FTA-ABS, Lyme titers, toxocariasis and toxoplasmosis IgG and IgM serology (infection).
- CT-scan of the chest to rule out mediastinal lymphadenopathy.
- Consider brain MRI or lumbar puncture to rule out multiple sclerosis if high level of suspicion.

Management

- Posterior sub-Tenon's steroid injection (triamcinolone acetonide 40 mg/mL) when vision is affected by cystoid macular edema or severe inflammation.
- Oral steroids (prednisone 1 mg/kg po qd pulse with rapid taper to 10–15 mg/day) if unable to tolerate injections or in severe bilateral cases; check PPD and controls, blood glucose, and chest radiographs before starting systemic steroids.
- Add H2-blocker (ranitidine [Zantac] 150 mg po bid) when administering systemic steroids.
- Consider topical steroid (prednisolone acetate 1% q2–6 h) and cycloplegic (scopolamine 0.25% bid to qid) if severe inflammation or macular edema exists (minimal effect).
- Consider intravitreal steroid injection or implant in severe cases.
- Cryotherapy to the peripheral retina reserved for neovascularization. Pars plana vitrectomy is controversial to treat difficult cases.
- Consider immunosuppressive agents (Cyclosporine [Neoral], Azathioprine, Methotrexate, Cytoxan) for recalcitrant cases (see Posterior Uveitis management section).

Prognosis Fifty-one percent of patients will achieve 20/30 vision; 10–20% may have self-limited disease; 40–60% will have a smoldering, chronic course with episodic exacerbations and remissions. Macular edema generally determines visual outcome. Zero tolerance to inflammation and aggressive treatment of active inflammation is a key factor in determining a good outcome.

Neuroretinitis (Leber's Idiopathic Stellate Neuroretinitis)

Definition Optic disc edema and macular star formation with no other systemic abnormalities.

Etiology Due to pleomorphic Gram-negative bacillus *Bartonella henselae* (formerly known as *Rochalimaea*); associated with cat-scratch disease.

Symptoms Mild, unilateral decreased vision, rarely pain with eye movement; may have viral prodrome (52%) with fever, malaise, lymphadenopathy, upper respiratory, gastrointestinal, or urinary tract infection.

Signs Decreased visual acuity, visual field defects (cecocentral/central scotomas), RAPD, optic disc edema with macular star, peripapillary exudative retinal detachment, vitreous cells, rare anterior chamber cells and flare, yellow–white lesions at level of retinal pigment epithelium.

Figure 10-131 • Leber's idiopathic stellate neuroretinitis demonstrating optic disc edema and partial macular star.

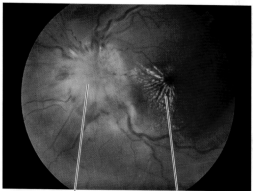

Disc edema   Macular star

Differential Diagnosis Hypertensive retinopathy, diabetic retinopathy, anterior ischemic optic neuropathy (AION), retinal vein occlusion, syphilis, diffuse unilateral subacute neuroretinitis (DUSN), acute macular neuroretinopathy, viral retinitis, sarcoidosis, toxocariasis, toxoplasmosis, tuberculosis, papilledema.

Evaluation

- Complete ophthalmic history and eye exam with attention to pupils, non-contact biomicroscopic and contact lens fundus exam, and ophthalmoscopy.
- **Lab tests:** VDRL, FTA-ABS, PPD and controls, indirect fluorescent antibody test for *Bartonella henselae* (*Rochalimaea*).
- Check blood pressure.
- **Fluorescein angiogram:** Leakage from optic disc capillaries, no perifoveal leakage.

Management

- No treatment necessary.
- Use of systemic antibiotics (doxycycline, tetracycline, ciprofloxacin, trimethoprim [Bactrim]) and steroids are controversial.

Prognosis Good; 67% regain ≥20/20 vision, and 97% >20/40 vision; usually spontaneous recovery; disc edema resolves over 8–12 weeks, macular star over 6–12 months; optic atrophy may develop.

Posterior Uveitis: Infections

Acute Retinal Necrosis

Fulminant retinitis/vitritis due to the herpes zoster virus (HZV), herpes simplex virus (HSV), or, rarely, cytomegalovirus (CMV). Occurs in healthy, as well as immunocompromised, patients; slight male predilection (2:1 over females). Patients have pain, decreased vision, and floaters after a recent herpes simplex or zoster infection. Starts with small, well-demarcated, areas of retinal necrosis outside the vascular arcades that spread rapidly and circumferentially into large, confluent areas of white, retinal necrosis with retinal vascular occlusions and small satellite lesions; 36% bilateral (BARN); associated with granulomatous anterior uveitis and retinal vasculitis. In the cicatricial phase (1–3 months later), retinal detachments (50–75%) with multiple holes and giant tears are common; poor visual prognosis (only 30% achieve >20/200 vision).

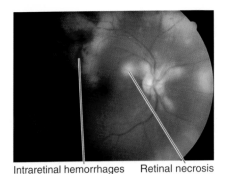

Intraretinal hemorrhages   Retinal necrosis

Figure 10-132 • Acute retinal necrosis demonstrating hemorrhage and yellow–white patches of necrosis.

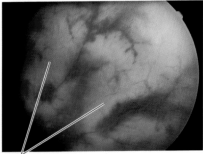

Retinal necrosis

Figure 10-133 • Same patient as Figure 10-132, 2 days later demonstrating rapid progression with confluence of lesions.

- **Lab tests:** HZV and HSV (type 1 and 2) immunoglobulin G and M titers or PCR.
- Systemic antiviral (acyclovir 5–10 mg/kg IV in three divided doses qd until resolution of the retinitis then acyclovir [Zovirax] 800 mg po 5×/day or famciclovir [Famvir] 500 mg po or valacyclovir [Valtrex] 1 g po tid for 1–2 months); follow blood urea nitrogen (BUN) and creatinine levels for nephrotoxicity.
- 24 hours after acyclovir started, oral steroids (prednisone 60–100 mg po qd for 1–2 months with slow taper); check PPD and controls, blood glucose, and chest radiographs before starting systemic steroids.
- Add H2-blocker (ranitidine [Zantac] 150 mg po bid) when administering systemic steroids.

- Topical steroid (prednisolone acetate 1% q2–6 h) and cycloplegic (homatropine 5% bid) in the presence of active inflammation.

- If treatment fails, fulminant course, or patient is HIV-positive, then consider IV ganciclovir and/or foscarnet, as well as intravitreal ganciclovir injections (see doses in Cytomegalovirus section).

- Role of anticoagulation is controversial.

- Consider three to four rows of laser photocoagulation to demarcate active areas of retinitis and necrosis to prevent retinal breaks and retinal detachments (controversial).

- Laser demarcation or retinal surgery for retinal detachments; usually requires use of silicon oil.

- Medical consultation.

Candidiasis

Endogenous endophthalmitis caused by fungal Candida species (*C. albicans* or *C. tropicalis*) with white, fluffy, chorioretinal infiltrates and overlying vitreous haze; vitreous "puff-balls," anterior chamber cells and flare, hypopyon, Roth spots, and hemorrhages occur less often. Occurs in IV drug abusers, debilitated patients especially on hyperalimentation, and immunocompromised patients.

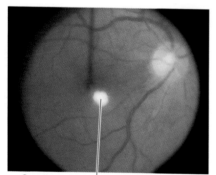
Candida albicans chorioretinal infiltrate

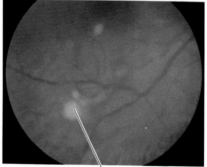
Candida albicans vitreous "puff-ball"

Figure 10-134 ○ Candidiasis demonstrating white fluffy, chorioretinal infiltrate.

Figure 10-135 ○ Vitreous "puff-ball" due to *Candida albicans* endogenous endophthalmitis.

- **Lab tests:** Sputum, urine, blood, and stool cultures for fungi.

- Systemic antifungal (fluconazole 100 mg po bid or amphotericin B 0.25–1.0 mg/kg IV over 6 h) if disseminated disease is present.

- If moderate-to-severe inflammation, pars plana vitrectomy and intraocular injection of antifungal (amphotericin B 0.005 mg/0.1 mL) and steroid (dexamethasone 0.4 mg/0.1 mL).

- Topical steroid (prednisolone acetate 1% qid) and cycloplegic (scopolamine 0.25% bid to qid).

- Medical consultation to treat systemic source of infection.

Cysticercosis

Subretinal or intravitreal, round, mobile, translucent, yellow–white cyst due to *Cysticercus cellulosae*, the larval form of the tapeworm *Taenia solium*. Asymptomatic until the parasite grows and causes painless, progressive, decreased vision and visual field defects; produces cystic subretinal or intravitreal lesions (cysticercus); worm death may incite an inflammatory response. May also have central nervous system (CNS) involvement with seizures, hydrocephalus, and headaches.

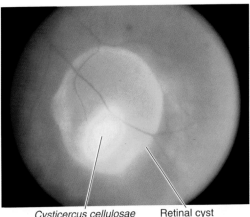

Figure 10-136 • Cysticercosis with cyst surrounding the tapeworm.

Cysticercus cellulosae   Retinal cyst

- **Lab tests:** Enzyme-linked immunosorbent assay (ELISA) for anticysticercus immunoglobulin G.
- **B-scan ultrasonography:** Highly reflective echoes from the cyst walls and often the worm within the cystic space.
- No antihelminthic medication is effective for intraocular infection.
- Consider direct laser photocoagulation of worm.
- Pars plana vitrectomy for removal of intravitreal cysticercus.
- Neurology consultation to rule out CNS involvement.

Cytomegalovirus

Hemorrhagic retinitis with thick, yellow–white retinal necrosis, vascular sheathing (severe sheathing with frosted-branch appearance may occur outside the area of retinitis), mild anterior chamber cells and flare, vitreous cells, and retinal hemorrhages. Brush-fire appearance with indolent, granular, yellow advancing border and peripheral, atrophic region is also common. Less, commonly, cytomegalovirus (CMV) retinitis may present with a clinical picture of frosted branch angiitits. Retinal detachments (15–50%) with multiple, small, peripheral breaks commonly occur in atrophic areas. Usually asymptomatic, but may have floaters, paracentral scotomas, metamorphopsia, and decreased acuity; bilateral on presentation in 40%; 15–20% become bilateral after treatment. Most common retinal infection in AIDS (15–46%) especially when CD4 <50 cells/mm^3.

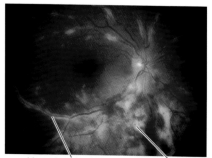

Vascular sheathing   Retinal necrosis

Figure 10-137 • Cytomegalovirus
retinitis demonstrating patchy necrotic lesions,
hemorrhage, and vascular sheathing.

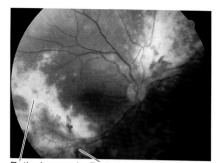

Retinal necrosis Retinal hemorrhage

Figure 10-138 • Cytomegalovirus retinitis
with larger areas of necrosis and hemorrhage.

- **Lab tests:** HIV antibody test, CD4 count, HIV viral load, urine for CMV; consider CMV PCR assay.
- If first episode, induction therapy with either:
  - Ganciclovir (Cytovene 5–7.5 mg/kg IV bid for 2–4 weeks then maintenance with 5–10 mg/kg IV qd); follow CBC for neutropenia (worsened by zidovudine [formerly AZT]) and thrombocytopenia; if bone marrow suppression is severe, add recombinant granulocyte colony stimulating factor (G-CSF) (filgrastim [Neupogen]) or recombinant granulocyte-macrophage colony stimulating factor (GM-CSF) (sargramostim [Leukine]).
  - Foscarnet (Foscavir, 90 mg/kg IV bid or 60 mg/kg IV tid for 2 weeks, then maintenance with 90–120 mg/kg IV qd); infuse slowly with 500–1000 mL normal saline or 5% dextrose; push liquids to avoid dehydration; follow electrolytes (potassium, phosphorus, calcium, and magnesium), BUN, and creatinine for nephrotoxicity; avoid other nephrotoxic medications.
  - *Note*: Foscarnet–Ganciclovir CMV Retinitis Trial showed equal efficacy between foscarnet and ganciclovir; possible survival advantage with IV foscarnet.
  - Cidofovir (Vistide, 3–5 mg/kg IV every week for 2 weeks, then maintenance with 3–5 mg/kg IV q2 wk) and probenecid (1 g po before infusion, 2 mg po after infusion); does not work in patients with ganciclovir resistance; follow BUN and creatinine for nephrotoxicity.
- Alternatively, combination of intravitreal surgical implantation of a ganciclovir implant (Vitrasert: 1 µg per hour, lasts ~6–8 months) and oral ganciclovir (1000–2000 mg po tid) for systemic CMV prophylaxis; good choice in new onset, unilateral cases; do not use in recurrent cases; should be performed by a retina specialist.
- Recurrence/progression can be re-induced with same regimen or new drug regimen (mean time to relapse ~60 days in Foscarnet–Ganciclovir CMV Retinitis Trial). In the era of highly active antiretroviral therapy (HAART), there is a much longer period of remission prior to reactivation.
- Treatment failures should be induced with new drug or a combination of drugs (use lower dosages due to the higher risk of toxic side effects); combination treatment is effective against disease progression (Cytomegalovirus Retreatment Trial conclusion).

- Intravitreal injections can be used if there is an intolerance to antiviral therapy or progressive retinitis despite systemic treatment (should be performed by a retina specialist):
  - Ganciclovir (Cytovene, 200–2000 µg/0.1 mL 2 to 3 times a week for 2–3 weeks then maintenance with 200–2000 µg/0.1 mL once a week).
  - Foscarnet (Foscavir, 2.4 mg/0.1 mL or 1.2 mg/0.05 mL 2 to 3 times a week for 2–3 weeks, then maintenance with 2.4 mg/0.1 mL 1 to 2 times a week).
  - Vitravene (165–330 µg a week for 3 weeks, then every 2 weeks for maintenance).
- Follow monthly with serial photography (60°, nine peripheral fields) to document inactivity/progression.
- Retinal detachments that threaten the macula with no macular retinitis may be treated with pars plana vitrectomy, endolaser, and gas or silicon oil tamponade; peripheral shallow detachments may be followed closely (especially inferiorly) or demarcated with two to three rows of laser photocoagulation; should be performed by a retina specialist.
- Medical consultation.

Diffuse Unilateral Subacute Neuroretinitis

Unilateral, indolent, multifocal, diffuse pigmentary changes with gray–yellow outer retinal lesions that reflect the movement of a subretinal nematode: *Ancylostoma caninum* (dog hook-worm, 400–1000 µm, endemic in southeastern United States, South America, and the Caribbean) or *Baylisascaris procyonis* (raccoon intestinal worm, 400–2000 µm, endemic in northern and mid-western United States). Movement of the worm is believed to cause destruction of photorecepter outer segments. Occurs in healthy patients with decreased vision (often out of proportion to retinal findings); usually minimal intraocular inflammation; may have RAPD. Chronic infection causes irreversible poor vision (20/200 or worse), visual field defects, optic nerve pallor, chorioretinal atrophy, and narrowed retinal vessels in a retinitis pigmentosa-like pattern. Poor prognosis without treatment; variable prognosis with treatment if worm can be killed.

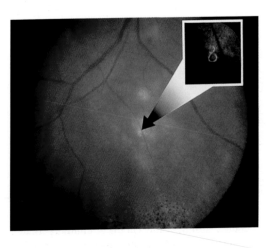

Figure 10-139 • Diffuse unilateral subacute neuroretinitis demonstrating subretinal nematode (inset).

- Complete history with attention to travel and animal exposure.
- **Fluorescein angiogram:** Lesions hypofluorescent early and stain late, perivascular leakage, and disc staining; more advanced disease shows widespread window defects.

- **Lab tests:** Stool for ova and parasites, CBC with differential (eosinophilia sometimes present), LDH and SGOT sometimes elevated.
- **Electrophysiologic testing:** ERG (subnormal, loss of b-wave) helps differentiate from optic nerve abnormalities.
- Most effective treatment is direct laser photocoagulation of the worm. Surgical subretinal removal of the worm is controversial and very difficult.
- Systemic antihelminthic medications (thiabendazole, diethylcarbamazine, pyrantel pamoate) are controversial and often not effective; steroids usually added since worm death may increase inflammation.

Human Immunodeficiency Virus

Asymptomatic, nonprogressive, microangiopathy characterized by multiple cotton-wool spots (50–70%), Roth spots (40%), retinal hemorrhages, and microaneurysms in the posterior pole that resolves without treatment within 1–2 months. Occurs in up to 50% of patients with HIV infection.

Figure 10-140 Human immunodeficiency virus retinopathy demonstrating cotton-wool spots and one intraretinal hemorrhage.

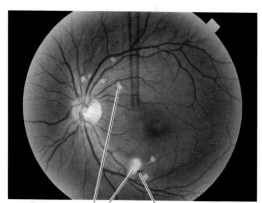

Cotton-wool spots   Intraretinal hemorrhage

- **Lab tests:** HIV antibody test, CD4 count, HIV viral load.
- No treatment necessary.
- Medical consultation.

Pneumocystis carinii Choroidopathy

Asymptomatic, unifocal or multifocal, round, creamy, yellow choroidal infiltrates located in the posterior pole caused by disseminated infection from the opportunistic organism *Pneumocystis carinii*. Infiltrates enlarge slowly with minimal vitreous inflammation; may be bilateral; resolution takes weeks to months after therapy is initiated. Has become very rare with the elimination of aerosolized pentamidine prophylaxis in AIDS patients.

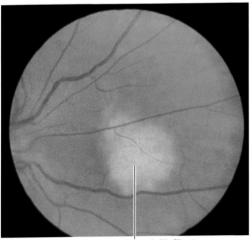

Figure 10-141 • Round, creamy, yellow choroidal infiltrate from *Pneumocystis carinii* choroidopathy.

Pneumocystis carinii infiltrate

- **Lab tests:** Induced sputum or bronchoalveolar lavage (BAL) for histopathologic staining.
- **Fluorescein angiogram:** Early hypofluorescence with late staining of lesions.
- Systemic antibiotics (trimethoprim 20 mg/kg and sulfamethoxazole 100 mg/kg divided equally IV qid) or pentamidine isothionate (slow infusion 4 mg/kg IV qd) for 14–21 days.
- Medical consultation.

Presumed Ocular Histoplasmosis Syndrome

Small, round, yellow–brown, punched-out chorioretinal lesions ("histo spots") in midperiphery and posterior pole, and juxtapapillary atrophic changes caused by the dimorphic fungus, *Histoplasma capsulatum*. Endemic in the Ohio and Mississippi river valleys. Histo spots occur in 2–3% of the population in endemic areas; rare in African Americans. Usually asymptomatic; no vitritis; macular disciform lesions can occur due to CNV. Better visual prognosis than CNV due to age-related macular degeneration, 30% recurrence rate; associated with HLA-B7.

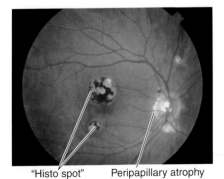

"Histo spot"   Peripapillary atrophy

Figure 10-142 • Presumed ocular histoplasmosis syndrome demonstrating macular and peripapillary lesions.

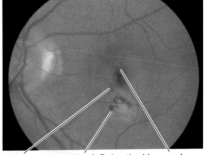

CNV   "Histo spot" Subretinal hemorrhage

Figure 10-143 • Presumed ocular histoplasmosis syndrome demonstrating CNV and a "histo" spot.

- Check Amsler grid.
- **Lab tests:** Histoplasmin antigen skin testing (not necessary).
- **Fluorescein angiogram:** Early hypofluorescence and late staining of histo spots, also identifies CNV if present.
- Extra and juxtafoveal CNV (see Table 10-3) can be treated with focal laser photocoagulation (MPS-OHS conclusion). Subfoveal CNV should not be treated with laser (14% regress spontaneously).
- Consider combination treatment with PDT (Visudyne in Ocular Histoplasmosis [VOH] Study conclusion) and intravitreal 4 mg triamcinolone acetonide or anti-VEGF agents (experimental) for subfoveal CNV.
- Removal of CNV with subretinal surgery was evaluated in the Subretinal Surgery Trials (Group H); however, up to 50% recur within 1 year (experimental).
- Oral steroids (prednisone 60–100 mg po qd with slow taper) and/or intravitreal steroid injection (4 mg triamcinolone acetonide) are controversial.

Progressive Outer Retinal Necrosis Syndrome

Multifocal, patchy, retinal opacification that starts in the posterior pole and spreads rapidly to involve the entire retina due to the herpes zoster virus (HZV); minimal anterior chamber cells and flare, vitreous cells, or retinal vasculitis (differentiates from acute retinal necrosis). Occurs in severely immunocompromised patients; poor response to therapy; may develop retinal detachments.

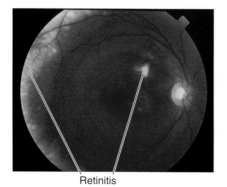

Retinitis

Figure 10-144 • Progressive outer retinal necrosis with multifocal retinal opacification.

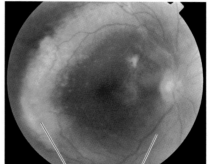

Progressive outer retinal necrosis

Figure 10-145 • Same patient as Figure 10-144, 7 days later with a massive increase in retinal necrosis. The posterior pole lesion has become atrophic.

- **Lab tests:** HZV immunoglobulin G and M titers.
- Systemic antiviral (acyclovir 5–10 mg/kg IV in divided doses tid until resolution of retinitis then acyclovir [Zovirax] 800 mg po 5×/day or famciclovir [Famvir] 500 mg po or valacyclovir [Valtrex] 1 g po tid for 1–2 months); follow BUN and creatinine for nephrotoxicity.

- 24 hours after acyclovir started, oral steroids (prednisone 60–100 mg po qd for 1–2 months with slow taper); check PPD and controls, blood glucose, and chest radiographs before starting systemic steroids.
- Add H2-blocker (ranitidine [Zantac] 150 mg po bid) when administering systemic steroids.
- Topical steroid (prednisolone acetate 1% q2–6 h) and cycloplegic (scopolamine 0.25% bid to qid) in the presence of active inflammation.
- If treatment fails or fulminant course, consider IV ganciclovir and/or foscarnet, as well as intravitreal ganciclovir injections (see CMV section for doses).
- Laser demarcation or retinal surgery for retinal detachments; usually requires use of silicon oil.
- Medical consultation.

Rubella

Congenital syndrome classically characterized by congenital cataracts, glaucoma, and rubella retinopathy with salt-and-pepper pigmentary changes; also associated with microphthalmia, iris transillumination defects, bilateral deafness, congenital heart disease, growth retardation, and bone and dental abnormalities. Eighty percent bilateral; vision is generally good (20/25); may rarely develop choroidal neovascular membrane (CNV).

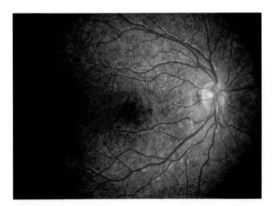

Figure 10-146 Rubella retinopathy demonstrating salt-and-pepper fundus appearance.

- **Fluorescein angiogram:** Mottled hyperfluorescence.
- Electrophysiologic testing: ERG and EOG are normal.

Syphilis (Luetic Chorioretinitis)

Extensive iritis/retinitis/vitritis (panuveitis) occurs in secondary syphilis (6 weeks to 6 months after primary infection) due to the spirochete *Treponema pallidum*. Signs include anterior chamber cells and flare, keratic precipitates, vitritis, multifocal, yellow-white chorioretinal infiltrates, salt-and-pepper pigmentary changes, flame-shaped retinal hemorrhages, and vascular sheathing; called "great mimic," since it can resemble many other retinal diseases; associated with sectoral interstitial keratitis, papillitis, and rarely CNV. Variant called acute syphilitic posterior placoid chorioretinitis (ASPPC) with large, placoid, yellow lesions with faded centers. Mucocutaneous manifestations of secondary syphilis are often evident.

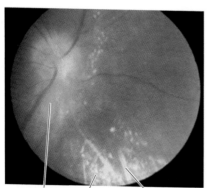

Chorioretinal infiltrates   Vascular sheathing

Figure 10-147 • Multifocal, yellow–white chorioretinal infiltrates and vascular sheathing patient with luetic chorioretinitis

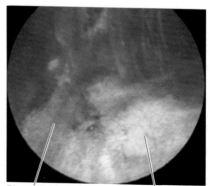

Pigmentary changes   Chorioretinal infiltrate

Figure 10-148 • Late luetic chorioretinitis with pigmentary changes and resolving chorioretinal infiltrate.

- **Lab tests:** Rapid Plasma Reagin (RPR, reflects current activity) or Venereal Disease Research Laboratory (VDRL, reflects current activity) and fluorescent treponemal antibody absorption (FTA-ABS) or microhemagglutination for *Treponema pallidum* (MHA-TP) tests.
- Lumbar puncture for VDRL, FTA-ABS, total protein, and cell counts to rule out neurosyphilis.
- Penicillin G (2.4 million U IV q4h for 10–14 days then 2.4 million U IM every week for 3 weeks); tetracycline if patient is allergic to penicillin.
- Long-term tetracycline (250–500 mg po qd) or doxycycline (100 mg po qd) in HIV-positive or immunocompromised patients.
- Follow serum RPR or VDRL to monitor treatment efficacy.
- Medical consultation.

Toxocariasis

Unilateral, multifocal, subretinal, yellow-white granulomas caused by the second-stage larval form of the roundworm *Toxocara canis*. Associated with papillitis, serous/traction retinal detachments, dragged macula and retinal vessels, vitritis, dense vitreous infiltrates, and chronic endophthalmitis; gray–white chorioretinal scars remain after active infection. Usually occurs in children (included in differential diagnosis of leukocoria) and young adults; associated with pica (eating dirt) and close contact with puppies; children with visceral larva migrans do not develop ocular involvement.

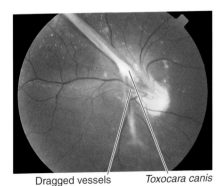

Dragged vessels   *Toxocara canis*
                          granuloma

Figure 10-149 • Toxocariasis
demonstrating fibrous attachment of peripheral
granuloma to optic nerve with dragged retina
and vessels.

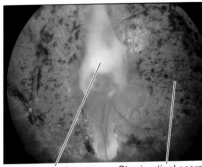

Toxocara canis   Chorioretinal scars
granuloma

Figure 10-150 • End stage infection
with *Toxocara canis* demonstrating diffuse
chorioretinal scarring, dragged vessels, and
granuloma.

- **Lab tests:** ELISA for Toxocara antibody titers.
- Topical steroid (prednisolone acetate 1% q2–6 h) and cycloplegic (scopolamine 0.25% bid to qid) for active anterior segment inflammation.
- Posterior sub-Tenon's steroid injection (triamcinolone acetonide 40 mg/mL) and oral steroids (prednisone 60–100 mg po qd) for severe inflammation; check PPD and controls, blood glucose, and chest radiographs before starting systemic steroids.
- Add H2-blocker (ranitidine [Zantac] 150 mg po bid) when administering systemic steroids.
- Systemic antihelminthic medications (thiabendazole, diethylcarbamazine, pyrantel pamoate) controversial, since worm death may increase inflammation.
- Retinal surgery for retinal detachment (successful in 70–80%).

Toxoplasmosis

Acquired (eating poorly cooked meat) or congenital (transplacental transmission; accounts for 90% of ocular disease) necrotizing retinitis caused by the parasite *Toxoplasma gondii*. Congenital toxoplasmosis appears as an atrophic, chorioretinal scar (often located in the macula) with gray–white punctate peripheral lesions; associated with microphthalmia, nystagmus, strabismus, intracranial calcifications, convulsions, microcephaly, and hydrocephalus. Acquired toxoplasmosis (especially in immunocompromised patients) and re-activated congenital lesions present with decreased vision, photophobia, floaters, vascular sheathing, full-thickness retinal necrosis, fluffy yellow–white retinal lesion (solitary in acquired and adjacent to old scars in congenital), overlying vitreous reaction, and anterior chamber cells and flare. May have peripapillary form with disc edema and no chorioretinal lesions (simulating optic neuritis). Treatment is usually reserved for vision-threatening lesions. Frequently reactivates (up to 50% by 3 years); poorer prognosis with larger lesions, recurrence, longer duration, and proximity to fovea and nerve.

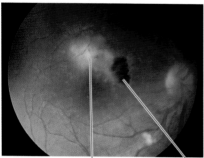

Toxoplasma gondii retinitis   Chorioretinal scar

Figure 10-151 • Toxoplasmosis demonstrating active, fluffy white lesion adjacent to old, darkly pigmented scar.

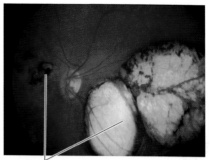

Chorioretinal scar

Figure 10-152 • Congenital toxoplasmosis demonstrating inactive chorioretinal macular and peripapillary scars.

- **Lab tests:** ELISA or indirect immunofluorescence assay (IFA) for *Toxoplasma* immunoglobulin G or M (definitive test) except in immunocompromised patients; elevated IgM indicates acquired active disease, elevated IgG is common in population (>4× elevation may indicate active disease).

- **Posterior pole lesions (involving macula and optic nerve) or sight-threatening lesions:** Pyrimethamine (Daraprim, 75–200 mg po loading dose then 25–50 mg po qd for maintenance up to 4–6 weeks), folinic acid (leucovorin 5 mg po qd), and one of the following: sulfadiazine (2 g po loading dose, then 0.5–1 g po qid for maintenance), clindamycin (300 mg po qid), clarithromycin (0.5 g po bid), Azithromycin (250 mg po qd), or atovaquone (750 mg po tid); give plenty of fluids to prevent sulfadiazine renal crystals.

- **Peripheral lesions:** clindamycin (300 mg po qid) and trimethoprim-sulfamethoxazole (Bactrim, 1 double-strength tablet po bid). *Note*: Immunocompetent patients may not require treatment.

- Treat with antibiotic combinations for 4–6 weeks; immunocompromised patients may require indefinite treatment and should be treated regardless of location of lesion with either trimethoprim-sulfamethoxazole (Bactrim, 1 double-strength tablet po bid) or doxycycline (100 mg po qid); may also consider prophylactic treatment in patients with frequent recurrences.

- If lesion is near the optic disc, in posterior pole, or if there is intense vitritis, may add oral steroids (prednisone 20–80 mg po qd for 1 week, then taper) 24 hours after starting antimicrobial therapy (never start steroids alone); check PPD and controls, blood glucose, and chest radiographs before starting systemic steroids.

- Add H2-blocker (ranitidine [Zantac] 150 mg po bid) when administering systemic steroids.

- No subconjunctival or sub-Tenon's steroid should be given secondary to risk of acute retinal necrosis.

Tuberculosis

Multifocal (may be focal), light-colored choroidal granulomas caused by the bacilli *Mycobacterium tuberculosis*. May present as endophthalmitis; usually associated with constitutional symptoms including malaise, night sweats, and pulmonary symptoms.

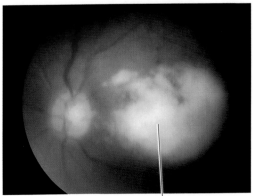

Figure 10-153 • Tuberculosis with choroidal tubercle appearing as a large white subretinal mass.

Choroidal granuloma

- **Lab tests:** Positive PPD skin test and chest radiographs.
- Isoniazid (INH, 300 mg po qd) and rifampin (600 mg po qd) for 6–9 months; follow liver function tests for toxicity.
- Consider adding pyrazinamide (25–35 mg/kg po qd) for first 2 months.
- Medical consultation for systemic evaluation.

Posterior Uveitis: White Dot Syndromes

Group of inflammatory disorders that produce discrete yellow–white retinal lesions mainly in young adults; differentiated by history, appearance, laterality, and fluorescein angiogram findings.

Acute Macular Neuroretinopathy

Acute onset of paracentral scotomas usually in 20–30-year-old females (89%) following a viral prodrome (68%). Vision is often normal but may be decreased; usually presents with bilateral (68%) cloverleaf or wedge-shaped, brown–red lesions in the posterior pole with no vitreous cells. Recovery of the visual field defect is rare.

- Check Amsler grid.
- **Fluorescein angiogram:** Minimal hypofluorescence of the lesions.
- No effective treatment.

Acute Posterior Multifocal Placoid Pigment Epitheliopathy

Rapid loss of central or paracentral vision in 20–30-year-old (mean 29 years), healthy adults after a flu-like, viral prodrome; no sex predilection. Usually bilateral, but asymmetric;

Table 10-4 White Dot Syndromes

	APMPPE	MEWDS	Serpiginous	Birdshot	Multifocal Choroiditis with Panuveitis	PIC
Age (years)	20–40	20–30	30–50	40–60	30–40	20–30
Sex	F = M	F > M	F = M	F > M	F > M	Female
Laterality	Bilateral	Unilateral	Bilateral	Bilateral	Bilateral	Bilateral
HLA	B7, DR2	None	B7	A29	None	None
Vitritis	Mild	Mild	Mild	Chronic, moderate	Chronic, moderate	None
Lesions	Large, geographic, gray-white, shallow pigmented scars within 1–2 weeks	Small, soft, gray-white dots; no scarring	Active, geographic, gray-white patches; deep scars with fibrosis	Deep, creamy spots; indistinct margins; yellow scars without pigmentation	100–200 μm white-yellow spots; mixture of old scars and new spots	100–200 μm yellow spots; punched-out scars
Macula	Rare CNV	Granularity	Subretinal scars 25% CNV	CME rare CNV rare	CME 35% CNV rare	Atrophic scars 40% CNV
Prognosis	Good	Good	Poor	Fair	Fair	Good
Treatment	None	None	Steroids Laser CNV	Steroids? Cyclosporine	Steroids? Laser CNV	Steroids? Laser CNV

multiple, round, discrete, large, flat gray–yellow, placoid lesions scattered throughout the posterior pole at the level of retinal pigment epithelium that later develop into well-demarcated retinal pigment epithelium scars; minimal vitreous cell; may have associated disc edema, cerebral vasculitis, headache, dysacousia, and tinnitus. Spontaneous resolution with late visual recovery within 1–6 months (80% regain ≥ 20/40 vision); recurrences rare.

APMPPE lesions

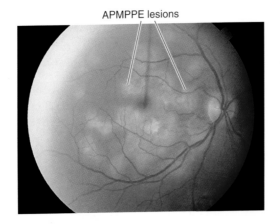

Figure 10-154 ● Acute posterior multifocal placoid pigment epitheliopathy demonstrating multiple posterior pole lesions.

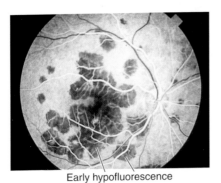

Early hypofluorescence

Figure 10-155 ● Fluorescein angiogram of same patient as Figure 10-154 demonstrating early hypofluorescence of the lesions.

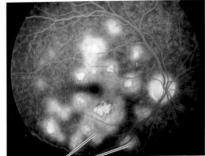

Late staining

Figure 10-156 ● Fluorescein angiogram of same patient as Figure 10-154 demonstrating late staining of the lesions.

- **Fluorescein angiogram:** Early hypofluorescence and late staining of the placoid lesions.
- **Indocyanine green angiogram:** Early and late hypofluorescence.
- No treatment necessary, but if macular (sight-threatening) lesions occur, steroids may be helpful.

Acute Retinal Pigment Epitheliitis (Krill's Disease)

Rare cause of acute, moderate, visual loss in young adults; no sex predilection; no viral prodrome. Discrete clusters of hyperpigmented spots (300–400 μm) with hypopigmented halos at the level of the retinal pigment epithelium in the perifoveal region; usually unilateral with no vitritis. Spontaneous resolution with recovery of visual acuity within 7–10 weeks; recurrences possible.

- **Fluorescein angiogram:** Blockage from the central spot and hyperfluorescence corresponding to the halo.
- No effective treatment.

Birdshot Choroidopathy (Vitiliginous Chorioretinitis)

Multiple, small, discrete, ovoid, creamy yellow–white spots scattered like a birdshot blast from a shotgun in the midperiphery (spares macula); often in a vascular distribution; associated with mild vitritis, mild anterior chamber cells and flare (in 25% of cases), cystoid macular edema, and disc edema. Usually bilateral, occurs in 50–60-year-old females (70%), and almost exclusively in Caucasians; associated with HLA-A29 (90–98%). Patients have mild blurring of vision and floaters. Chronic, slowly progressive, recurring disease with variable visual prognosis; choroidal neovascular membranes, epiretinal membranes, and macular cysts/holes are late complications.

Figure 10-157 ● Birdshot choroidopathy/vitiliginous chorioretinitis demonstrating scattered fundus lesions.

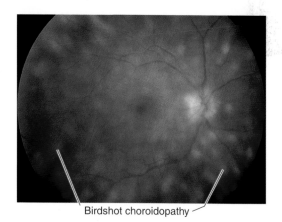

Birdshot choroidopathy

- **Fluorescein angiogram:** Mild hyperfluorescence, early and late staining of lesions; active lesions may hypofluoresce early. Late views show profuse vascular incompetence with leakage and secondary retinal staining.
- **Electrophysiologic testing:** ERG (subnormal) and EOG (subnormal); can monitor course of disease with serial ERG and can be used to monitor systemic immunomodulatory therapy.
- Treatment is reserved for patients with decreased visual acuity, significant inflammation, or complications including cystoid macular edema.
- Despite historically poor responses to steroids, initial improvement can occur with oral steroids (prednisone 60–100 mg po qd); check PPD and controls, blood glucose, and chest radiographs before starting systemic steroids.
- Add H2-blocker (ranitidine [Zantac] 150 mg po bid) when administering systemic steroids.

- Consider sub-Tenon's steroid injection (triamcinolone acetonide 40 mg/mL) in patients with severe inflammation or cystoid macular edema.
- Cyclosporine (2–5 mg/kg/d) can dramatically improve vitritis and cystoid macular edema; should only be administered by a specialist trained in inflammatory diseases.

Multifocal Choroiditis and Panuveitis/Subretinal Fibrosis and Uveitis Syndrome

Spectrum of disorders causing blurred vision, metamorphopsia, paracentral scotomas, and photopsias. Mainly occurs in 30–40-year-old (mean 36 years), healthy, Caucasian (86%), females (3:1 over males); etiology unknown. Usually unilateral symptoms with bilateral (80%) fundus findings including small (100–200 μm), round, discrete, yellow–white spots and minimal signs of intraocular inflammation; lesions develop into atrophic scars or subretinal fibrosis; choroidal neovascular membranes and macular edema are late complications. Recurrences common; poor visual prognosis.

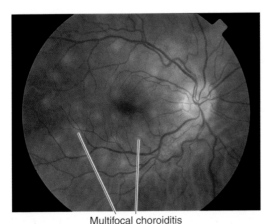

Figure 10-158 • Multifocal choroiditis demonstrating small deep spots in the macula.

Multifocal choroiditis

- **Fluorescein angiogram:** Early hyperfluorescence and late staining of the lesions.
- Treatment with steroids is controversial.

Punctate Inner Choroidopathy

Acute onset of blurred vision, metamorphopsia, paracentral scotomas, and photopsias. Mainly occurs in 20–30-year-old (mean 27 years), healthy, myopic (mean –6 diopters) females (>90%); unknown etiology. Usually unilateral symptoms with bilateral fundus findings including small (100–200 μm), round, discrete, yellow–white spots and minimal to no signs of intraocular inflammation; lesions develop into atrophic scars over 1 month; scars progressively pigment and enlarge; choroidal neovascular membranes and macular edema are common, late complications. Recurrences common; good visual prognosis unless CNV or macular edema occur.

- **Fluorescein angiogram:** Early hyperfluorescence and late staining of the lesions.
- Treatment with steroids is controversial.

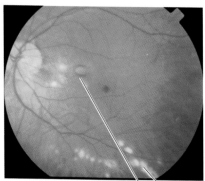

Punctate inner choroidopathy

Figure 10-159 • Punctate inner choroidopathy with small, round, yellow spots in the macula and punched out, atrophic scars along the inferior arcade.

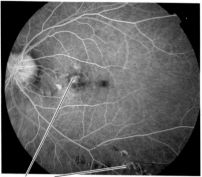

Punctate inner choroidopathy

Figure 10-160 • Fluorescein angiogram of same patient as Figure 10-159 demonstrating hyperfluorescence of the active lesions and window defects of the atrophic scars.

- Consider focal laser photocoagulation of juxtafoveal and extrafoveal CNV, and photodynamic therapy (PDT) or anti-VEGF agents such as 1.25 mg bevacizumab (Avastin) for subfoveal CNV (experimental).

Multiple Evanescent White Dot Syndrome

Sudden, unilateral, acute visual loss with paracentral/central scotomas and photopsias. Mainly occurs in 20–30-year-old (mean 28 years), healthy females (4:1 over males) after a viral prodrome (occurs in 50% of cases); cause unknown. Multiple, small (100–200 μm), discrete, gray–white spots at the level of the retinal pigment epithelium in the posterior pole sparing the fovea (spots appear and disappear quickly); may have RAPD, foveal granularity, mild vitritis, mild anterior chamber cells and flare, optic disc edema, and an enlarged blind spot. Spontaneous resolution with recovery of vision in 3–10 weeks; white dots disappear first followed by improvement in vision; recurrences rare (10%).

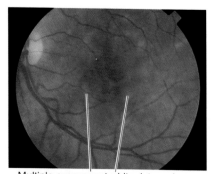

Multiple evanescent white dot syndrome

Figure 10-161 • Multiple evanescent white dot syndrome demonstrating faint white spots.

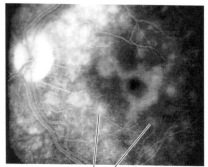

Early hyperfluorescence

Figure 10-162 • Same patient as Figure 10-161 demonstrating late fluorescein angiogram appearance.

- Check Amsler grid or visual fields (central 10°).
- **Fluorescein angiogram:** Early, punctate hyperfluorescence in a wreath-like pattern and late staining of the lesions and optic nerve.
- **Indocyanine green angiogram:** Early and late hypofluorescence.
- **Visual fields:** Paracentral/central scotomas.
- **Electrophysiologic testing:** ERG (reduced a wave).
- No treatment recommended.

Acute Idiopathic Blind Spot Enlargement Syndrome

Subset of MEWDS (see above) that occurs in young females with enlargement of the blind spot and no optic disc edema and no visible fundus lesions; usually no RAPD exists. May represent MEWDS after lesions have faded.

- Check Amsler grid or visual fields (central 10°).
- **Visual fields:** Enlarged blind spot.
- No treatment recommended.

Posterior Uveitis: Other Inflammatory Disorders

Behçet's Disease

Triad of aphthous oral ulcers, genital ulcers, and bilateral nongranulomatous uveitis; also associated with erythema nodosum, arthritis, vascular lesions, HLA-B5 (subtypes Bw51 and B52) and HLA-B12. The uveitis (see Chapter 6) is severe and recurring, causing hypopyon, iris atrophy, posterior synechiae, optic disc edema, attenuation of arterioles, severe vitritis, cystoid macular edema, and an occlusive retinal vasculitis with retinal hemorrhages and edema. Patients have photophobia, pain, red eye, and decreased vision. Lab tests are positive for antinuclear antibody (ANA), elevated erythrocyte sedimentation rate (ESR)/C-reactive protein/acute phase reactants/serum proteins, but are not diagnostic. Poor visual prognosis; frequent relapses are common; ischemic optic neuropathy is a late complication.

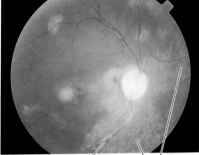

Vasculitis   Chorioretinal atrophy

Figure 10-163 • Behçet's disease demonstrating old vasculitis with sclerosed vessels and chorioretinal atrophy.

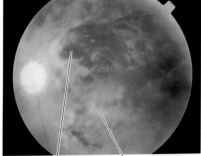

Retinal hemorrhages   Retinal edema

Figure 10-164 • Behçet's disease demonstrating acute vasculitis with hemorrhage.

Figure 10-165 • Behçet's disease demonstrating aphthous oral ulcers on tongue.

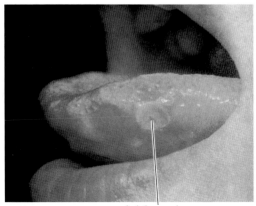

Aphthous ulcer

- **Lab tests:** Behçetine skin test (prick skin with sterile needle, the formation of a pustule within a few minutes is a positive result), ESR, ANA, C-reactive protein, serum haplotyping.
- **Fluorescein angiogram:** Extensive vascular leakage early with late staining of vessel walls.
- Topical steroid (prednisolone acetate 1% q2–6 h).
- Colchicine (600 mg po bid) is controversial.
- **Mild:** oral steroids (prednisone 60–100 mg po qd); check PPD and controls, blood glucose, and chest radiographs before starting systemic steroids.
- Add H2-blocker (ranitidine [Zantac] 150 mg po bid) when administering systemic steroids.
- **Severe:** sub-Tenon's steroid injection (triamcinolone acetonide 40 mg/mL), oral steroid (prednisone 60–100 mg po qd), and either chlorambucil (0.1 mg/kg/d) cyclophosphamide (1–2 mg/kg/d IV) or cyclosporine (2–7 mg/kg/d); should be administered by a specialist trained in inflammatory diseases (see Management section).
- Medical consultation.

Idiopathic Uveal Effusion Syndrome

Bullous serous retinal detachment (with shifting fluid), serous choroidal and ciliary body detachments, mild vitritis, leopard spot retinal pigment epithelium pigmentation, and dilated conjunctival vessels. Occurs in healthy, middle-aged males; patients have decreased vision, metamorphopsia, and scotomas. Chronic, recurrent course.

- **B-scan ultrasonography:** Thickening of the sclera.
- **Fluorescein angiogram:** No discrete leak under serous retinal detachment.
- Steroids and antimetabolites are not effective.
- Consider decompression of vortex veins and scleral resection in nanophthalmic eyes.
- Surgery to create partial-thickness scleral windows is controversial.

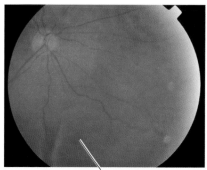

Serous retinal detachment

Figure 10-166 Bullous serous retinal detachment in a patient with idiopathic uveal effusion syndrome that shifts with changes in head position.

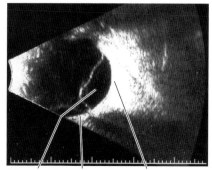

Serous retinal   Choroidal   Scleral thickening
detachment   detachment

Figure 10-167 B-scan ultrasound of same patient as Figure 10-166 demonstrating serous retinal detachment with shifting fluid, shallow peripheral choroidal detachment, and diffuse scleral thickening.

Masquerade Syndromes

Systemic and ophthalmologic diseases can mimic uveitis. These should always be considered in the differential diagnosis of uveitis, because they can be life-threatening. The masquerade syndromes can be divided by etiology: malignancies, endophthalmitis and noninfectious/nonmalignant.

Malignancies

Intraocular Lymphoma

This rare and lethal malignancy is commonly a non-Hodgkin's large B cell lymphoma of the eye and the CNS; occurs in later adulthood (median age of 50 to 60 years old); sex distribution is not clear. The most common symptoms are blurred vision and floaters associated with vitritis. The vitreous has large clumps of cells and the fundus examination is significant for multifocal, large, yellow, sub-retinal and sub-RPE infiltrative lesions.

- A high level of suspicion is essential in order to make the diagnosis of this condition.

- Complete neurological evaluation should be performed in search of CNS involvement including magnetic resonance imaging (MRI) and CNS cytology.

- Diagnostic pars plana vitrectomy in cases where diagnosis is in doubt. An undilute vitreous biopsy (approximately 1 cc) should be performed in the eye with vitritis and sent for cytology, flow-cytometry analysis for B and T cell markers and kappa/lambda light chains. Other ancillary tests include the measurement of IL-6 and IL-10 (high IL10 and high ratio of IL10 to IL6 are suggestive of intraocular lymphoma).

- The treatment of primary intraocular lymphoma is controversial and includes intravitreal methotrexate (400 µg in 0.1 ml twice weekly for 1 month, then weekly for 1 month, then monthly for a year) and orbital radiation in cases without CNS involvement. However, most patients develop CNS involvement, which is usually treated with chemotherapy with blood–brain barrier disruption or high dose systemic methotrexate.

- Medical and oncology consultation.

Other Malignancies

Other malignancies that can present as a masquerade uveitis include: leukemias, malignant melanoma, retinoblastoma, and metastatic tumors.

Endophthalmitis

Chronic postoperative endophthalmitis and endogenous endophthalmitis can present as a masquerade syndrome (see Chapter 6).

Non-Malignant/Non-Infectious

These forms of masquerade syndromes are a group of disorders characterized by the presence of intraocular cells secondary to non-inflammatory conditions. Although rare, the following disorders should be considered: rhegmatogenous retinal detachment, retinitis pigmentosa, intraocular foreign body, ocular ischemic syndrome, and juvenile xanthogranuloma.

Posterior Scleritis

Inflammation of the sclera posteriorly. Produces orange–red elevation of the choroid and retinal pigment epithelium by the thickened choroid with overlying serous retinal detachments, choroidal folds, vitritis, and optic disc edema; scleral thickening can cause induced hyperopia, proptosis, limitation of ocular motility, and angle-closure glaucoma (anterior rotation of ciliary body with forward displacement of the lens-iris diaphragm). Usually occurs in 20–30-year-old females; 20–30% bilateral. Patients have pain, photophobia, and decreased vision. Associated with collagen vascular diseases, rheumatoid arthritis, relapsing polychondritis, inflammatory bowel disease, Wegener's granulomatosis, and syphilis.

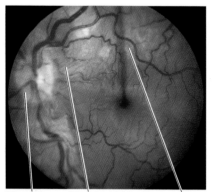

Disc edema   Choroidal folds   Serous retinal detachment

Figure 10-168 • Posterior scleritis with orange-red choroidal elevation superiorly, serous retinal detachments, vitritis, and mild optic disc edema.

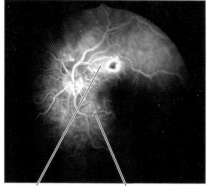

Serous retinal detachment   Punctate hyperfluorescence

Figure 10-169 • Fluorescein angiogram of same patient as Figure 10-168 demonstrating punctate hyperfluorescence and early pooling into the serous retinal detachments.

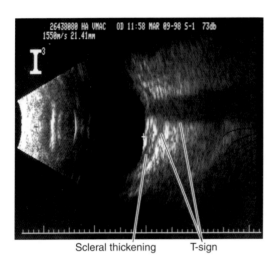

Scleral thickening   T-sign

Figure 10-170 • B-scan ultrasound of same patient as Figure 10-168 demonstrating scleral thickening and the characteristic peripapillary T-sign.

- **B-scan ultrasonography:** Diffuse scleral thickening (echolucent space between choroid and Tenon's capsule), and edema with medium reflectivity in Tenon's space, T-sign in the peripapillary region from scleral thickening around echolucent optic nerve.

- **Fluorescein angiogram:** Punctate hyperfluorescence early with pooling late within serous retinal detachments.

- Oral steroids (prednisone 60–100 mg po qd); if severe, consider high-dose IV steroids; check PPD and controls, blood glucose, and chest radiographs before starting systemic steroids.

- Oral nonsteroidal anti-inflammatory drugs (NSAIDs; indomethacin 25–50 mg po tid)

- Add H2-blocker (ranitidine [Zantac] 150 mg po bid) when administering systemic steroids or NSAIDs.

- Sub-Tenon's steroid injection (triamcinolone acetonide 40 mg/mL) sometimes required.

- Consider immunosuppressive therapy (azathioprine, cyclosporine) in refractory cases; should be administered by a specialist trained in inflammatory diseases.

- Medical consultation.

Sarcoidosis

Granulomatous panuveitis with retinal vasculitis, vascular sheathing, periphlebitis (candle wax drippings), vitreous snowballs or string of pearls, yellow–white retinal/choroidal granulomas, anterior chamber cells and flare, mutton fat keratic precipitates, Koeppe/Busacca iris nodules, and macular edema. Disc/retinal neovascularization (often in sea-fan configuration) and epiretinal membranes are late complications. The disease is more severe in young African Americans (incidence 82:100,000), but can occur in elderly, Caucasian women; bimodal age distribution with peaks at 20–30 years old and 50–60 years old; chronic, relapsing course (72%). Ocular findings occur in 25–75% of patients with sarcoidosis while 94% have lung findings; patients present first with ocular complaints in only 2–3% of cases, 15–40% present with respiratory complaints; African Americans more likely to develop ocular complications. Systemic findings include hilar adenopathy, pulmonary parenchymal involvement, pulmonary fibrosis, erythema nodosum, subcutaneous nodules, lupus pernio (purple lupus), lymphadenopathy; may also have CNS, bone, connective tissue, cardiac, renal, and sinus involvement. Pathologic hallmark is non-caseating granulomas. Most patients are asymptomatic; can have chronic, potentially fatal course.

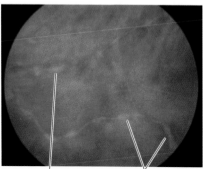

Vascular sheathing   "Candle-wax drippings"

Figure 10-171 • Sarcoidosis with periphlebitis and vascular sheathing.

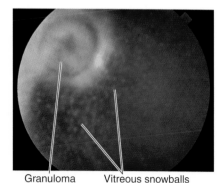

Granuloma   Vitreous snowballs

Figure 10-172 • Sarcoidosis demonstrating peripheral granuloma with overlying vitritis and vitreous snowballs.

- **Lab tests:** ACE, chest radiographs, serum lysozyme, sickle cell prep/hemoglobin electrophoresis (to rule-out sickle cell anemia); consider CT-scan of the chest to rule out mediastinal lymphadenopathy; consider Gallium scan, Kneim–Silzbach skin test/reaction.
- **Fluorescein angiogram:** Early hyperfluorescence and late leakage from vascular permeability and macular edema.
- Oral steroids (prednisone 60–100 mg po qd); check PPD and controls, blood glucose, and chest radiographs before starting systemic steroids.
- Add H2-blocker (ranitidine [Zantac] 150 mg po bid) when administering systemic steroids.
- Sub-Tenon's steroid injection (triamcinolone acetonide 40 mg/mL) when macular edema is severe; topical steroids reserved for only anterior disease.
- Laser photocoagulation to areas of capillary nonperfusion when neovascularization persists or progresses after steroid treatment.
- Consider immunosuppressive therapy (hydroxychloroquine; methotrexate; chlorambucil; azathioprine) in refractory cases; should only be administered by a specialist trained in inflammatory diseases.
- Medical consultation.

Serpiginous Choroidopathy (Geographic Helicoid Peripapillary Choroidopathy)

Bilateral, asymmetric uveitis with peripapillary, well-circumscribed, gray–white active lesions, which extend centrifugally from the disc in a pseudopodal, serpiginous pattern leaving chorioretinal scars in areas of previous involvement; skip lesions common; mild vitritis. Patients have paracentral scotomas and decreased vision. Usually bilateral, slight male predilection, and occurs in the fifth to seventh decades; etiology unknown; associated with HLA-B7. Chronic, recurrent disease with fair visual prognosis (severe visual loss rare); CNV develops in 25%.

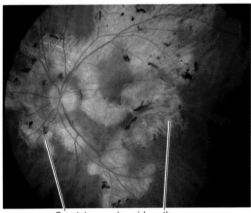

Figure 10-173 Serpiginous choroidopathy demonstrating typical pattern of atrophic scarring extending from the optic nerve.

Serpiginous choroidopathy

- **Fluorescein angiogram:** Hypofluorescence early and late staining beginning at the borders of the lesion and spreading centrally.
- **Indocyanine green angiogram:** Early and late hypofluorescence.
- Oral steroids (prednisone 1 mg/kg/day po) and sub-Tenon's steroid injection (triamcinolone acetonide 40 mg/mL) are controversial (consider when macula threatened).
- Consider immunosuppressive therapy (azathioprine 5 mg/kg/day, cyclosporine 1.5 mg/kg/day) in refractory cases; should only be administered by a specialist trained in inflammatory diseases.
- Laser photocoagulation, photodynamic therapy, or anti-VEGF agents for CNV depending on location in relation to the fovea.

Sympathetic Ophthalmia

Rare, bilateral, immune-mediated, mild-to-severe granulomatous uveitis that occurs typically 2 weeks to 3 months (80%) after penetrating trauma or surgery, although there are reported cases even decades later. Scattered, multifocal, yellow-white subretinal infiltrates (Dalen–Fuchs nodules, 50%) with overlying serous retinal detachments, vitritis, and papillitis. Associated with inflammation in sympathizing (fellow) eye and worsened inflammation in exciting (injured) eye (keratic precipitates are an ominous sign); may have meningeal signs, poliosis, and alopecia (as in Vogt–Koyanagi–Harada syndrome). Patients have transient visual obscurations, photophobia, pain, and blurred vision. Male predilection (probably reflects increased incidence of trauma in this group); associated with HLA-A11. Chronic, recurring course; good prognosis (65% achieve >20/60 vision after treatment); spares choriocapillaris unlike VKH.

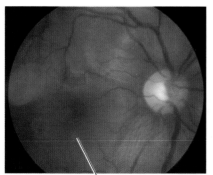

Serous retinal detachment

Figure 10-174 • Early sympathetic ophthalmia demonstrating serous retinal detachment.

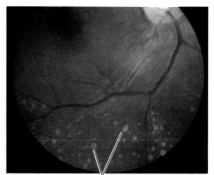

Dalen-Fuchs nodules

Figure 10-175 • Dalen–Fuchs nodules in a patient with sympathetic ophthalmia.

- Check for previous history of penetrating surgery or trauma.

- **Fluorescein angiogram:** Pinpoint areas of hyperfluorescence with central hypofluorescence and patchy areas of choriocapillaris hypoperfusion leakage late from optic nerve.

- Moderate-to-high-dose oral steroids (prednisone 60–200 mg po qd); check PPD and controls, blood glucose, and chest radiographs before starting systemic steroids.

- Add H2-blocker (ranitidine [Zantac] 150 mg po bid) when administering systemic steroids.

- Sub-Tenon's steroid injection (triamcinolone acetonide 40 mg/mL).

- Topical steroid (prednisolone acetate 1% q2–6 h) and cycloplegic (scopolamine 0.25% bid to qid).

- Consider immunosuppressive therapy (azathioprine, methotrexate, chlorambucil); should be administered by a specialist trained in inflammatory diseases.

- No proven benefit from enucleating exciting eye, but this option should be considered in eyes with no light perception (NLP) vision, since removal of the eye within 2 weeks of injury may prevent sympathetic ophthalmia.

Vogt–Koyanagi–Harada Syndrome/Harada's Disease

Bilateral inflammatory disorder with yellow–white exudates at the level of the retinal pigment epithelium, bullous serous retinal detachments (75%, shifting fluid often present) and focal retinal pigment epithelial detachments; associated with anterior chamber cells and flare, mutton fat keratic precipitates, posterior synechiae, vitritis, choroidal folds, choroidal thickening, Dalen–Fuchs-like nodules, and optic disc hyperemia (Harada's disease); may have systemic manifestations including meningeal signs (headache, nausea, stiff neck, deafness, tinnitus), poliosis, alopecia, dysacousis, and vitiligo (Vogt–Koyanagi–Harada [VKH] syndrome); late retinal pigment epithelial changes result in yellow–orange ("sunset glow") fundus. Patients have decreased vision and photophobia. Occurs in pigmented individuals (Native Americans, African Americans, Asians, and Hispanics) 20–40 years old; slight female predilection (60%); associated with HLA-DR4, HLA-DRw53, HLA-DQw7, HLA-DQw3, and HLA-Bw54. Recurrences common; good visual prognosis.

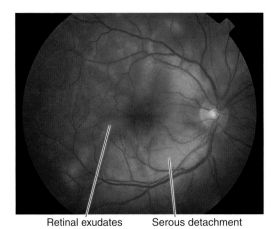

Figure 10-176 ● Vogt–Koyanagi–Harada syndrome with multiple serous retinal detachments.

Retinal exudates   Serous detachment

- **B-scan ultrasonography:** Low reflectivity and choroidal thickening with overlying serous retinal detachment.
- **Fluorescein angiogram:** Pinpoint areas of hyperfluorescence and delayed choroidal fluorescence.
- Moderate-to-high-dose oral steroids (prednisone 60–200 mg po qd, then taper slowly); check PPD and controls, blood glucose, and chest radiographs before starting systemic steroids.
- Add H2-blocker (ranitidine [Zantac] 150 mg po bid) when administering systemic steroids.
- Topical steroid (prednisolone acetate 1% q2–6 h) and cycloplegic (scopolamine 0.25% bid to qid) in the presence of active anterior segment inflammation.
- Sub-Tenon's steroid injection (triamcinolone acetonide 40 mg/mL) sometimes required.
- Cyclosporine (2–7 mg/kg/d) or immunosuppressive agents for refractory cases; should be administered by a specialist trained in inflammatory diseases.

Posterior Uveitis: Evaluation/Management

Evaluation

- Complete ophthalmic history and eye exam with attention to visual acuity, pupils, tonometry, anterior chamber, vitreous cells, non-contact biomicroscopic or contact lens fundus exam, and ophthalmoscopy.
- Consider work-up as clinical examination and history dictate (see below).
- **Lab tests:** Basic testing recommended for intermediate and posterior uveitis with a negative history, review of systems and medical examination: CBC, ESR, Rapid Plasma Reagin (RPR; syphilis) or VDRL (syphilis), microhemagglutination for treponema pallidum (MHA-TP; syphilis) or FTA-ABS (syphilis), Lyme titer, PPD (tuberculosis) and controls, serum lysozyme, ACE (sarcoidosis).

- **Other labs tests that should be ordered according to history and/or evidence of granulomatous inflammation:** ANA, RF (juvenile rheumatoid arthritis), ELISA for Lyme immunoglobulin M (IgM) and immunoglobulin G (IgG), HIV antibody test, chest radiographs (sarcoidosis, tuberculosis), sacroiliac radiographs (ankylosing spondylitis), gallium scan (sarcoidosis), urinalysis.
- **Special diagnostic lab tests:** HLA typing (HLA-A29: Birdshot Choroidopathy), in the presence of vasculitis: ANCA (Wegener's granulomatosis, polyarteritis nodosa), Raji cell and C1q binding assays for circulating immune complexes (SLE, systemic vasculitides), complement proteins: C3, C4, total complement (SLE, cryoglobulinemia, glomerulonephritis), soluble IL-2 receptor.
- Medical consultation.

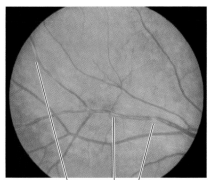

Retinal vasculitis

Figure 10-177 ● Retinal vasculitis with sheathing of retinal vessels.

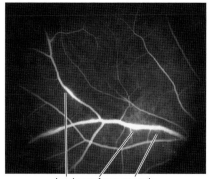

Leakage from vessels

Figure 10-178 ● Fluorescein angiogram of same patient as Figure 10-177 showing retinal vascular leakage.

Management

- Consider oral steroids (prednisone 60–100 mg po qd); check PPD and controls, blood glucose, and chest radiographs before starting systemic steroids.
- Add H2-blocker (ranitidine [Zantac] 150 mg po bid) when administering systemic steroids.
- Consider posterior sub-Tenon steroid injection (triamcinolone acetonide 40 mg/mL) or intravitreal steroid injection (triamcinolone acetonide 4 mg/ 0.1 mL).
- If the uveitis becomes steroid dependent then consider a step-ladder approach to treat with steroid-sparing agents that would eventually allow the tapering or minimal use of topical and systemic corticosteroids:

Management—Cont'd

Nonsteroidal anti-inflammatory drugs: diclofenac (Voltaren) 75 mg po bid or diflusinal (Dolobid) 250 mg po bid. Other nonselective NSAIDs that can be used as a second line of therapy include indomethacin (Indocin SR) 75 mg po bid or naproxen (Naprosyn) 250 mg po bid. In patients with a known history of gastritis or peptic ulceration, the use of COX-2 selective inhibitor should be considered (celecoxib (Celebrex) 100 mg po bid).

Immunosuppressive chemotherapy: should be managed by a uveitis specialist or in coordination with a medical specialist familiar with these agents; indications include Behçet's disease, sympathetic ophthalmia, VKH, serpiginous choroidopathy, rheumatoid necrotizing scleritis and/or PUK, Wegener's granulomatosis, polyarteritis nodosa, relapsing polychondritis, JRA, or sarcoidosis unresponsive to conventional therapy. Methotrexate is most commonly used first.

    Antimetabolites: azathioprine 1–3 mg/kg/day, methotrexate 0.15 mg/kg/day, mycophenolate mofetil (CellCept) 1–2 g po qd ("off-label" use for autoimmune ocular inflammatory diseases).

    Inhibitors of leukocyte signaling: cyclosporine 2.5–5.0 mg/kg/day, tacrolimus (Prograf) 0.1–0.15 mg/kg/day.

    Alkylating agents: cyclophosphamide 1–3 mg/kg/day, chlorambucil 0.1 mg/kg/day.

    Biologic agents: TNF-alpha inhibitors (infliximab [Remicade], etanercept [Enbrel], adalimumab [Humira]).

    Other agents: dapsone 25–50 mg bid or tid, colchicine 0.6 mg po bid for Behçet's disease is controversial.

Hereditary Chorioretinal Dystrophies

Central Areolar Choroidal Dystrophy (Autosomal Dominant)

Starts as mild, non-specific retinal pigment epithelial granularity and mottling in the fovea; progresses to a round, well-defined area of geographic atrophy with loss of the choriocapillaris; the area of atrophy slowly enlarges with large choroidal vessels visible underneath; usually bilateral and symmetric. Symptoms appear in third to fifth decades with decreased vision (20/25–20/200).

- **Genetics:** Linked to RDS/peripherin gene on chromosome 6p and CACD gene on chromosome 17p13.
- **Color vision:** Moderate protan-deutan defect.
- **Electrophysiologic testing:** ERG (photopic: normal to slightly subnormal; scotopic: normal), EOG (normal to slightly subnormal), and dark adaptation (normal).
- **Fluorescein angiogram:** Early lesions may show faint RPE transmission defects within the fovea; later well-circumscribed hyperfluorescent window defects that correspond to the areas of atrophy.
- **Visual fields:** Large central scotoma in late stages.
- No effective treatment.

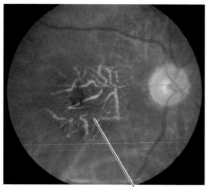

Central areolar choroidal dystrophy

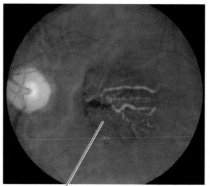

Central areolar choroidal dystrophy

Figure 10-179 • Central geographic atrophy in a patient with central areolar choroidal dystrophy.

Figure 10-180 • Left eye of same patient as Figure 10-179 demonstrating similar central geographic atrophy.

Choroideremia (X-linked recessive)

Progressive, bilateral, diffuse atrophy of the choriocapillaris and overlying retinal pigment epithelium with scalloped edges and large choroidal vessels visible underneath; spares macula until late. Affected males have nyctalopia, photophobia, and constricted visual fields in late childhood; female carriers have normal vision, visual fields, color vision, and ERG, but may show pigmentary retinal changes. Poor prognosis with legal blindness by 50–60 years of age.

- **Genetics:** Mapped to chromosome Xq21 (encodes for a component of rab geranyl-geranyl transferase, an enzyme involved in membrane metabolism).
- Check color vision.

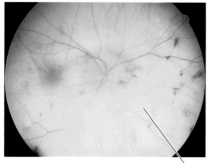

Choroideremia

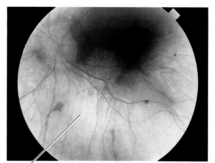

Choroideremia

Figure 10-181 • Choroideremia demonstrating late stage with complete atrophy of the RPE and visible choroidal vessels.

Figure 10-182 • Choroideremia demonstrating scalloped border of atrophic changes near macula. Radial choroidal vessels are easily seen inferiorly.

- **Electrophysiologic testing:** ERG (markedly reduced).
- **Fluorescein angiogram:** Absent choroidal flush with large choroidal vessels visible underneath with scalloped borders.
- **Visual fields:** Constricted.
- No effective treatment.

Congenital Stationary Night Blindness

Group of bilateral, nonprogressive disorders with reduced night vision (rods) and normal day vision (cones). Patients have normal acuity, color vision, and full visual fields, but have reduced acuity with low light levels (nyctalopia), paradoxical pupillary response, absent Purkinje shift, and reduced rod ERG by first decade. Two categories:

Without Fundus Changes

Nougaret's Disease (Autosomal Dominant)

Night blindness but no reduction in central vision; onset at birth. Retina totally normal ophthalmoscopically.

- **Genetics:** Associated with GNAT1 gene on chromosome 3p21.
- **Electrophysiologic testing:** Photopic ERG (normal), scotopic ERG (subnormal, no rod a-wave), EOG (normal).

Riggs Type (Autosomal Recessive)

Rare; some residual rod function, no myopia. Retina totally normal ophthalmoscopically.

- **Electrophysiologic testing:** Photopic ERG (normal), scotopic ERG (subnormal, some rod a-detectable), EOG (normal).

Schubert-Bornschein type (X-linked recessive)

May have some residual rod function (type 2, incomplete form) or no rod function (type 1, complete form); non-progressive. May have nystagmus; distinguished from dominant Nougaret type by presence of myopia and by mode of inheritance; carriers are asymptomatic. Retina usually normal, but may show myopic changes, some pigment washout and some fine pigmentary changes in the periphery.

- **Genetics:** Type 1 (complete) linked to NYX gene on chromosome Xp11.4; Type 2 (incomplete) linked to CACNA1F gene on chromosome Xp11.23.
- **Electrophysiologic testing:** Photopic ERG (normal), scotopic ERG (minimal to no rod function depending on type), and dark adaptation (may be abnormal).
- **Fluorescein angiogram:** Usually normal but may show minor window transmission defects.

With Fundus Changes

Fundus Albipunctatus (Autosomal Recessive)

Distinctive, discreet, yellow–white (50 μm) deep dots located in the midperipheral retina, sparing the macula. Not all lesions fluoresce on fluorescein angiogram (unlike drusen); stationary unlike retinitis punctata albescens.

Figure 10-183 ● Fundus albipunctatus demonstrating small white spots in the posterior pole sparing the central macula.

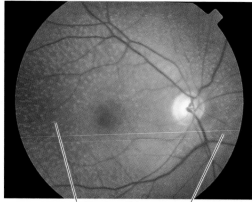

Fundus albipunctatus

- **Genetics:** Associated with RDH5 gene on chromosome 12q13-q14; gene encodes 11-*cis* retinol dehydrogenase 5, an RPE microsomal enzyme involved in photoreceptor transduction.
- **Electrophysiologic testing:** Delayed cone and rod adaptation; a and b wave amplitudes increase slowly with dark adaptation and reach normal levels after about 3 hours.

Kandori's Flecked Retina Syndrome (Autosomal Recessive)

Irregularly shaped, deep yellow spots usually found in the equatorial region. Fewer and larger spots than fundus albipunctatus (may be variant).

Oguchi's Disease (Autosomal Recessive)

Diffuse golden–brown/yellow or gray retinal discoloration in light that returns to normal retinal color (orange–red) with prolonged (2–12 hours) dark adaptation (Mizuo phenomenon); onset at birth.

Figure 10-184 ● Oguchi's disease demonstrating characteristic golden retinal sheen.

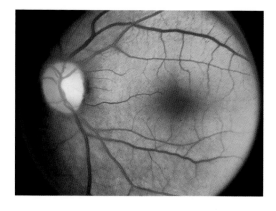

- **Genetics:** Mapped to Oguchi1/Arrestin/SAG gene on chromosome 2q37.1 and Oguchi2 gene on chromosome 13q34 encoding rhodopsin kinase (RHOK).
- **Electrophysiologic testing:** Photopic ERG (normal), scotopic ERG (reduced, no b wave, a wave increases with dark adaptation time), and dark adaptation (no rod phase).
- **Fluorescein angiogram:** Normal.
- No effective treatment.

Crystalline Retinopathy of Bietti (Autosomal Recessive)

Glittering, yellow–white, refractile spots scattered throughout fundus (located in inner and outer layers of retina) with multiple areas of geographic atrophy. Associated with crystals in the perilimbal anterior corneal stroma. Patients have slowly progressive decreased vision beginning in fifth decade.

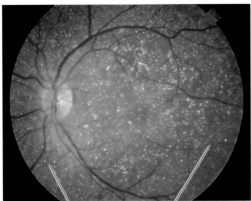

Figure 10-185 Crystalline retinopathy of Bietti demonstrating refractile fundus lesions.

Bietti's crystalline retinopathy

- **Electrophysiologic testing:** ERG (reduced).
- **Fluorescein angiogram:** Patchy areas of blocked fluorescence and window defects corresponding to the areas of atrophy; crystals hyperfluorescence early.
- No effective treatment.

Gyrate Atrophy (Autosomal Recessive)

Progressive, bilateral retinal degeneration with well-circumscribed, scalloped areas of chorioretinal atrophy that enlarge and coalesce starting anteriorly and spreading posteriorly. Patients develop nyctalopia, constricted visual fields, and decreased vision by the second decade. Abnormal laboratory studies including hypolysinemia, hyperornithinuria, and increased plasma ornithine levels (10–20 times normal) due to deficiency of the mitochondrial matrix enzyme, ornithine aminotransferase. Associated with posterior subcapsular cataracts and high myopia.

- **Genetics:** Associated with numerous mutations in OAT gene on chromosome 10q26 that encodes ornithine aminotransferase.
- **Lab tests:** Plasma ornithine levels, also consider urine ornithine levels and plasma lysine levels.

Figure 10-186 • Gyrate atrophy demonstrating coalescence of well-circumscribed atrophic patches.

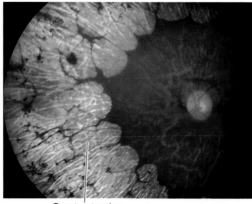

Gyrate atrophy

- **Electrophysiologic testing:** ERG (reduced) and dark adaptation (prolonged).
- **Fluorescein angiogram:** Window defects corresponding to the areas of atrophy.
- Restrict dietary arginine and protein; vitamin B6 (pyridoxine 300–500 mg po QD) therapy may be helpful.

Progressive Cone Dystrophy (AD>AR>X-linked)

Profound cone dysfunction with normal rod function. Often develop "bull's eye" macular pigment changes, patchy atrophy in the posterior pole, vascular attenuation, and temporal pallor or optic atrophy. Patients have slowly progressive loss of central vision (worse during day), dyschromatopsia, and photophobia that develops in the first to third decades. Called cone degeneration when not inherited. Poor prognosis with vision deteriorating to the 20/200 level by fourth decade.

- **Genetics:** Cone dystrophy mapped to several loci including: COD1/RPGR gene on chromosome Xp21.1 encoding retinitis pigmentosa GTPase regulator; COD2 gene linked to chromosome Xq27; COD3/GUCA1A/GCAP1 gene on chromosome 6p21.1 encoding guanylate cyclase activating protein.
- **Color vision:** Severe deutan-tritan defect out of proportion to visual acuity; no color perception.

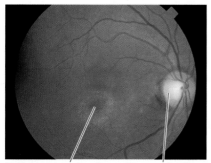

Bull's eye maculopathy   Temporal pallor

Figure 10-187 • Progressive cone dystrophy with bull's eye appearance and temporal optic atrophy.

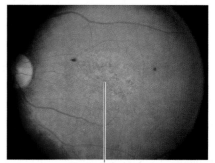

Central atrophy

Figure 10-188 • Progressive cone dystrophy with patchy atrophy in the posterior pole.

- **Electrophysiologic testing:** Photopic ERG (markedly reduced to non-recordable), scotopic ERG (can be normal, often subnormal), and EOG (normal to subnormal), dark adaptation (cone segment: abnormal; rod segment: normal [may be subnormal to abnormal later in disease]).
- **Fluorescein angiogram:** Hypofluorescence with ring of hyperfluorescence corresponding to the "bull's eye" lesion; diffuse, irregular window defects throughout posterior pole and often midperiphery.
- **Visual fields:** Central scotomas, peripheral fields usually intact; may get midperipheral relative scotomas late.
- No effective treatment; dark glasses may help photophobia.

Rod Monochromatism (Achromatopsia) (Autosomal Recessive)

Total absence of cone function with normal rod function. Patients have poor central vision (<20/200), achromatopsia (no color perception), congenital nystagmus, and photophobia from birth. May have normal macula, but often develop similar pigmentary changes as progressive cone dystrophy with granular changes and "bull's eye" maculopathy. Nonprogressive; poor prognosis with vision deteriorating to the 20/200 level by fourth decade.

- **Genetics:** Linked to ACHM1 gene on chromosome 14; ACHM2/CNGA3 gene encoding a cone photoreceptor cGMP-gated cation channel alpha subunit; ACHM3/CNGB3 gene encoding cone cGMP-gated cation channel beta 3 subunit.
- **Color vision:** No color perception; all colors appear as shades of gray.
- **Electrophysiologic testing:** Photopic ERG (absent, non-recordable), scotopic ERG (usually normal, may be subnormal), flicker fusion frequency (generally below 20 Hz), EOG (normal), dark adaptation (cone segment: abnormal and may be absent; rod segment: normal).
- **Fluorescein angiogram:** Normal, or may show window defects in areas of pigmentary changes.
- **Visual fields:** Central scotomas, peripheral fields intact.
- No effective treatment; dark glasses may help photophobia.

Hereditary Macular Dystrophies

Adult Foveomacular Vitelliform Dystrophy (Autosomal Dominant)

Bilateral, symmetric, round, slightly elevated, yellow–orange lesions with surrounding darker border and pigment clumping. Onset between 30 and 50 years of age with minimally affected vision and metamorphopsia (often unilateral symptoms, but bilateral disease). Smaller lesions than Best's disease, no disruption or layering of the yellow pigment, and occurs in older patients; good prognosis.

Best's Disease (Autosomal Dominant)

Uncommon hereditary macular dystrophy due to abnormality of the RPE with high phenotypic variability first described by Franz Best in 1905. Usually starts asymptomatically (75% better than 20/40) with yellow, round, subretinal vitelliform macular lesion ("egg-yolk" lesion) in early childhood (5–10 years), but age of onset is variable. Various stages:

Figure 10-189 • Adult foveomacular vitelliform dystrophy demonstrating central round yellow lesion.

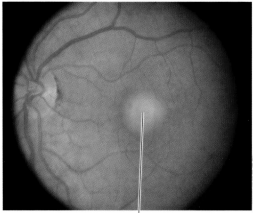

Adult foveomacular vitelliform lesion

Stage 0 (Previtelliform)

Average age at onset is 6 years old, normal macula, abnormal EOG, normal vision.

Stage 1 (Previtelliform)

Normal clinically, normal vision, fluorescein angiogram shows RPE window defects.

Stage 2 (Vitelliform)

Age 3–15 years old, classic "egg yolk" appearance clinically, mild visual loss, fluorescein angiogram shows blocking defects.

Stage 2a (Vitelliruptive)

"Scrambled-egg" stage as the cysts break apart with irregular subretinal spots, mild visual loss, fluorescein angiogram shows nonhomogenous blocking and hyperfluorescence.

Stage 3 (Pseudohypopyon)

Age 8–38 years old, fluid level with yellow vitelline material as the subretinal material layers, mild visual loss, fluorescein angiogram blocks in area of pseudohypopyon, hyperfluorescent above it.

Stage 4a (Atrophic)

Age >40 years old, greater visual loss (>20/100), atrophy of RPE.

Stage 4b (Cicatricial)

Macular scarring.

Stage 4c (Neovascular)

CNV develops.

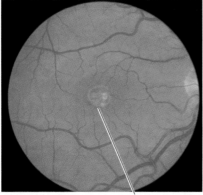

"Sunny-side up" egg-yolk lesion

Figure 10-190 • Small egg-yolk lesion in a 7-year-old boy with Best's disease

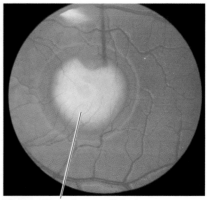

"Sunny-side up" egg-yolk lesion

Figure 10-191 • Left eye of same patient as Figure 10-190 demonstrating characteristic "sunny side up" egg-yolk lesion.

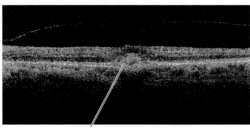

Foveal vitelliform lesion

Figure 10-192 • Spectral domain optical coherence tomography of vitelliform lesion.

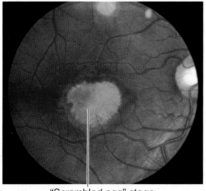

"Scrambled egg" stage

Figure 10-193 • Best's disease demonstrating "scrambled egg" lesion in the macula.

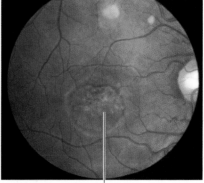

Atrophic scar

Figure 10-194 • Same patient as Figure 10-193, 5 years later demonstrating atrophic lesion in central macula.

Usually bilateral, slowly progressive, and occurs in Caucasians who are slightly hyperopic. Variable vision loss, deteriorates slowly and may be stable for years (75–88% have >20/40 vision in one eye up to age 50 years old); cannot predict visual function from fundus appearance; tritan color deficiency; incidental trauma can lead to visual loss. Good prognosis with vision ranging from 20/30 to 20/100 unless CNV develops.

- **Genetics:** Mapped to VMD2 gene on chromosome 11q12-q13.1; Bestrophin protein function still unknown.
- **Color vision:** Color defects proportional to degree of visual loss.
- **Electrophysiologic testing:** ERG (normal, but foveal or multifocal ERG may have reduced amplitudes), EOG (markedly abnormal in all stages even in otherwise normal appearing carriers, Arden (light-peak/dark-trough ratio <1.5), and dark adaptation (normal).
- **Fluorescein angiogram:** Blockage by vitelliform lesion; transmission when cyst ruptures; irregular RPE transmission and staining depending on presence of pigmentary disturbance, choroidal neovascularization and scarring.
- **Visual fields:** Relative central scotoma early; more dense scotomas may be noted following degeneration and organization of lesion.
- No effective treatment unless CNV forms.

Butterfly Pattern Dystrophy (Autosomal Dominant)

Bilateral, subtle RPE mottling in younger patients; symmetric, gray–yellow, butterfly-shaped lesions in central macula with surrounding halo of depigmentation in older patients; may develop choroidal neovascular membrane. Onset between 20 and 50 years of age with mild decrease in vision (20/25 to 20/40) and slow progression. Relatively good prognosis unless CNV develops.

- **Genetics:** Linked to RDS/peripherin gene on chromosome 6p21.1-cen encoding peripherin.
- **Color vision:** Normal.
- **Electrophysiologic testing:** ERG (photopic: normal to subnormal; scotopic: normal to subnormal), EOG (usually normal, but can be markedly subnormal), and dark adaptation (normal).
- **Fluorescein angiogram:** Hypofluorescent blocking defects by pigment and lipofuscin, window defects corresponding to the areas of the atrophy; hyperfluorescent leakage from CNV if present.
- **Visual fields:** Relative central scotoma; normal peripheral fields.
- No effective treatment.

Dominant Drusen (Doyne's Honeycomb Dystrophy, Malattia Leventinese) (Autosomal Dominant)

Asymptomatic, unless degenerative changes occur in the macula. Bilateral, symmetric, round, yellow–white deposits (nodular thickening of the retinal pigment epithelium basement membrane) scattered throughout the posterior pole and nasal to the optic disc. Occurs by age 20–30 years old. The lesions coalesce (forming a honeycomb appearance), enlarge, or disappear. May be associated with pigment clumping, RPE pigmentary disturbance, RPE detachment, chorioretinal atrophy, and choroidal neovascular membrane.

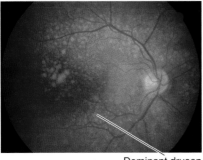

Dominant drusen

Dominant drusen

Figure 10-195 • Dominant drusen demonstrating abundant yellow lesions in the posterior pole.

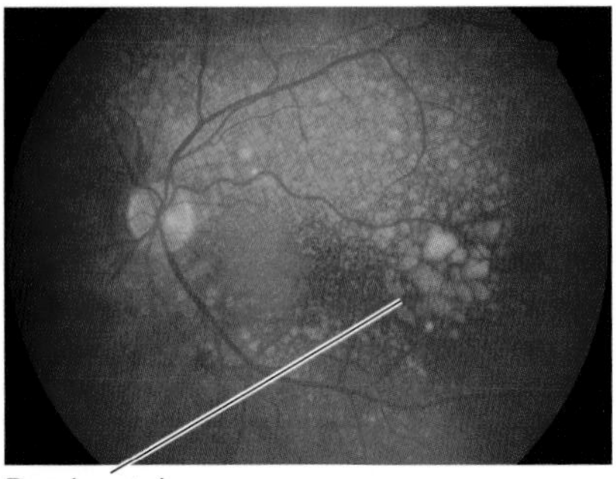

Figure 10-196 • Left eye of same patient as Figure 10-195.

- **Genetics:** Mapped to EFEMP1 gene on chromosome 2p16–p21; produces an extracellular matrix protein.
- **Color vision:** Normal.
- **Electrophysiologic testing:** ERG (normal), EOG (subnormal in late stages), and dark adaptation (normal).
- **Fluorescein angiogram:** Early blockage and late hyperfluorescent staining of drusen; irregular dye transmission, leakage and pooling within macula depending on degree of associated degenerative change; hyperfluorescent leakage from CNV if present.
- **Visual fields:** Normal; central scotoma if macular degeneration present.
- No effective treatment.

North Carolina Macular Dystrophy (Lefler-Wadsworth-Sidbury Dystrophy) (Autosomal Dominant)

Yellow spots (drusen) appear in early childhood (first decade) and progress to chorioretinal atrophy, macular staphyloma or "colobomas," and peripheral drusen. Normal central vision early unless atrophic macular "coloboma" forms; possible progression to 20/200 or worse vision late in patients who develop choroidal neovascular membranes; typically nonprogressive. Three grades:

Grade I

Drusen-like lesions and pigment dispersion in fovea.

Grade II

Confluent drusen-like lesions in fovea.

Grade III

Atrophy of RPE and choriocapillaris within central macula.

- **Genetics:** Linked to MCDR1 gene on chromosome 6q14–q16.2 at same location as clinically distinct dominant progressive bifocal chorioretinal atrophy.
- **Color vision:** Normal.
- **Electrophysiologic testing:** ERG (normal), EOG (normal), dark adaptation (normal).

- **Fluorescein angiogram:** Grades I and II: RPE transmission defects and late staining of drusen-like lesions; Grade III: nonperfusion of choriocapillaris.
- **Visual fields:** Central scotoma; normal peripheral fields.
- No effective treatment.

Pseudoinflammatory Macular Dystrophy (Sorsby's Dystrophy) (Autosomal Dominant)

Bilateral, symmetric, choroidal atrophy with decreased vision, nyctalopia, and tritone dyschromatopsia; occurs in 40–50-year-old patients. Three early patterns seen: disciform maculopathy with drusenoid deposits, disciform maculopathy without deposits, and chorioretinal atrophy. All patterns lead to end-stage pattern of progressively enlarging chorioretinal atrophy from the macula outward. May develop choroidal neovascular membrane. Poor prognosis with final vision in hand motion range.

- **Genetics:** Linked to SFD/TIMP-3 gene cloned on chromosome 22q12.1-q13.2 encoding tissue inhibitor of metalloproteinase-3 (TIMP-3).
- Check color vision.
- **Electrophysiologic testing:** ERG (subnormal in advanced stages), EOG (subnormal in advanced stages), and dark adaptation (delayed).
- **Fluorescein angiogram:** Hyperfluorescent window defects in areas of atrophy and hyperfluorescent leakage from CNV if present.
- No effective treatment.

Sjögren Reticular Pigment Dystrophy (Autosomal Recessive)

Hyperpigmented fishnet/reticular pattern at the level of the retinal pigment epithelium that starts centrally and spreads peripherally. Usually asymptomatic with good vision.

- **Electrophysiologic testing:** ERG (normal), EOG (lower limit of normal), and dark adaptation (normal).
- **Fluorescein angiogram:** Hypofluorescence of the fishnet-reticulum over normal background fluorescence in early views.
- No effective treatment.

Stargardt's Disease/Fundus Flavimaculatus (Autosomal Recessive>Autosomal Dominant)

Most common hereditary macular dystrophy. Onset in first to second decade. Bilateral, deep, symmetric, yellow pisciform (fish-tail shaped) flecks (yellow flecks are groups of enlarged RPE cells packed with a granular substance with ultrastructural, autofluorescent and histochemical properties consistent with lipofuscin) at the level of the retinal pigment epithelium and scattered throughout the posterior pole. Spectrum of disease: fundus flavimaculatus (no macular dystrophy; occurs in adults) to Stargardt's disease ("bull's eye" atrophic maculopathy with "beaten bronze" appearance, patchy areas of atrophy; occurs in late childhood/adolescence). "Salt and pepper" pigmentary changes in periphery may develop late; no sex predilection; patients have bilateral decreased vision even before fundus changes appear. Poor prognosis with vision deteriorating to the 20/200 level by third decade and stable or continued slowly progressive loss of vision therafter. Autosomal dominant form has more benign course with milder color and night vision changes, no photophobia, later onset, and generally less severe clinical course.

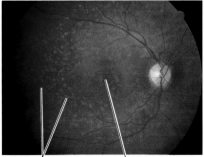

Pisciform flecks   "Bull's eye" maculopathy

Figure 10-197 • Stargardt's disease demonstrating pisciform flecks along the vascular arcades and pigmentary changes in the fovea.

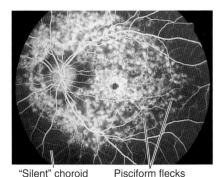

"Silent" choroid   Pisciform flecks

Figure 10-198 • Fluorescein angiogram of same patient as Figure 10-197 demonstrating hyperfluorescence of the lesions and the characteristic "silent" choroid.

- **Genetics:** Mapped to STGD1/ABCA4 gene on chromosome 1p21-p22 associated with autosomal recessive Stargardt's disease; autosomal dominant Stargardt's disease linked to STGD4 gene on chromosome 4p and to STGD3/ELOVL4 gene on chromosome 6q14 encoding a photoreceptor-specific component of a polyunsaturated fatty acid elongation system; fundus flavimaculatus mapped to ABCA4 gene on chromosome 1p21-p13.

- **Color vision:** May be abnormal with mild to moderate deutan-tritan defects as disease progresses.

- **Electrophysiologic testing:** ERG (usually normal, but 1/3 may have photopic abnormalities), EOG (normal to subnormal), and dark adaptation (usually normal, mildly elevated in late stages).

- **Fluorescein angiogram:** Generalized decreased choroidal fluorescence (dark or "silent" choroid sign), hyperfluorescent spots that do not correspond to the flecks seen clinically, flecks demonstrate early blockage and late hyperfluorescent staining, and window defects corresponding to the areas of the macular atrophy.

- **Optical coherence tomography:** Loss of photoreceptor layers corresponding to macular atrophic areas.

- **Visual fields:** May be normal, or develop central scotoma late.

- No effective treatment. Targeting the vitamin A cycle may potentially lower lipofuscin levels and A2E accumulation.

Hereditary Vitreoretinal Degenerations

Familial Exudative Vitreoretinopathy (Autosomal Dominant>Autosomal Recessive)

Rare, slowly progressive, bilateral, peripheral vascular developmental disorder; similar in appearance to retinopathy of prematurity, but without premature birth, low birth weight, and supplemental oxygen; asymmetric with no associated systemic diseases. Premature arrest of retinal angiogenesis or retinal vascular differentiation with incomplete peripheral retinal vasculature.

Stage 1

Starts with peripheral avascularity, white with/without pressure, vitreous bands, peripheral cystoid degeneration, microaneurysms, telangiectasia, straightened vessels, and vascular engorgement especially in the temporal periphery. Asymptomatic in 73% of cases, but may have strabismus and nystagmus. Progression to stage 2 may or may not occur.

Stage 2

Dilated, tortuous peripheral vessels, neovascularization, fibrovascular proliferation, subretinal/intraretinal exudation, dragging of disc and macula, falciform retinal folds, and localized retinal detachments. Get "dragged disc" and ectopic macula. Visual loss after second to third decade is rare unless degeneration progresses to stage 3.

Stage 3

Cicatrization causes traction (rare) and/or rhegmatogenous retinal detachments (10–20%); retinal folds, fibrotic scaffolding and massive subretinal exudates; secondary findings include vitreous hemorrhage, band keratopathy, posterior synechia, iris atrophy, secondary cataract, and neovascular glaucoma; retinal detachments common in third to fourth decade; retinal detachments difficult to repair (recurrent retinal detachments and proliferative vitreoretinopathy).

Figure 10-199 Familial exudative vitreoretinopathy demonstrating fibrovascular proliferation, exudates, and cicatrization.

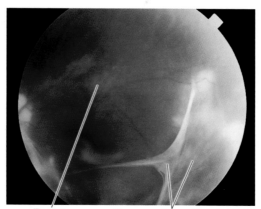

Exudate   Fibrovascular proliferation

- **Genetics:** Phenotypes linked to chromosome 11q13-q23 (EVR1 gene locus; FZD4 gene; AD), chromosome 11q13-q14 (EVR1 gene locus; LRP5 gene; AR), chromosome 11p13-p12 (EVR3 gene; AD); chromosome 11q (EVR4 gene locus; AD); 100% penetrance with variable expressivity; sporadic cases have been described.

- **Fluorescein angiogram:** Peripheral nonperfusion past vascularized retina; at border area, arteriovenous anastamoses form and leak fluorescein.

- Prophylactic laser treatment of the avascular retina is controversial; most retina specialists laser treat avascular retinal periphery when extraretinal vascularization occurs.

- Retinal surgery for retinal detachments; should be performed by a retina specialist.

Enhanced S-cone Syndrome/Goldmann–Favre Syndrome (Autosomal Recessive)

Extremely rare, bilateral vitreotapetoretinal degeneration with foveal and peripheral retinoschisis (similar to juvenile retinoschisis), "optically empty" vitreous cavity, condensed vitreous veils, attenuation of retinal vessels, peripheral pigmentary (bone spicules) changes, subretinal dot-like flecks in peripheral retina, lattice degeneration, progressive cataracts, and waxy optic disc pallor. No sex predilection (unlike juvenile retinoschisis). Patients have nyctalopia and constricted visual fields from early childhood. Reduced vision becomes evident with age. Goldmann–Favre refers to the severe end of the disease spectrum.

- **Genetics:** Phenotypes linked to NR2E3 or PNR gene on chromosome 15q23.
- **Electrophysiologic testing:** ERG (scotopic does not reveal any rod-driven responses; large, slow waveforms are detected in response to bright flashes; photopic is more sensitive to blue than to red or white stimuli) and EOG (abnormal, reduced light peak; *Note*: helps differentiate from juvenile retinoschisis).
- **Fluorescein angiogram:** No leakage from foveal schisis.
- Consider prophylactic treatment of any retinal breaks/tears.
- Retinal surgery for retinal detachments; should be performed by a retina specialist.

Marshall Syndrome

Rare degeneration with pronounced facial dysmorphism; less frequent risk of retinal detachments.

Snowflake Degeneration (Autosomal Dominant)

Rare degeneration with yellow–white deposits in peripheral retina associated with white without pressure, sheathing of retinal vessels, vitreous degeneration, and cataracts; increased risk of retinal detachments.

- No treatment recommended.
- Retinal surgery for retinal detachments; should be performed by a retina specialist.

Wagner/Jansen/Stickler Vitreoretinal Dystrophies (Autosomal Dominant)

All have "optically empty" vitreous cavity with thick, transvitreal and preretinal membranes/strands, retinal perivascular pigmentary changes (60%), and lattice-like degeneration; associated with myopia, glaucoma, and posterior subcapsular cataracts. Occurs in 1:10,000 cases.

Wagner Disease

No systemic associations and no increased risk of retinal detachments.

- **Genetics:** Linked to WGN1 gene on chromosome 5q13-q14; additional phenotype linked to mutation in exon 2 of COL2A1 gene on chromosome 12q13.11-q13.2, the candidate gene for Stickler syndrome. This exon is present in vitreous collagen mRNAs, but absent in cartilage mRNAs, thus accounting for the lack of systemic manifestations associated with Stickler's.

Jansen Disease

No systemic associations, but patients do have an increased risk of retinal detachments; often bilateral retinal detachments.

Stickler Syndrome

Also known as hereditary progressive arthro-ophthalmopathy; associated with systemic abnormalities and connective tissue disorders including Marfanoid habitus, facial hypoplasia, flat nasal bridge, anteverted nares, Pierre Robin sequence, cleft palate, neurosensory hearing loss, skeletal abnormalities (90%) including hyperextensible joints, degenerative joint disease in third or fourth decade, and spondyloepiphyseal dysplasia of vertebrae, hip, and shoulder. Ocular abnormalities include congenital progressive high myopia (75–90%) in first decade, cataract (30–80%) often with wedge or fleck-shaped cortical opacities, angle abnormalities including prominent iris processes, hypoplastic iris root, and open angle glaucoma; and increased risk of retinal breaks (75%) and retinal detachments often bilateral (42–50%). Three types:

Type 1

Most common (75% of patients); membranous vitreous.

Type 2

Severe hearing loss; beaded vitreous.

Type 3

Least common.

Figure 10-200 • Stickler vitreoretinal dystrophy with pigmented demarcation lines from a chronic retinal detachment.

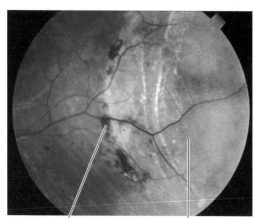

Demarcation line   Chronic retinal detachment

• **Genetics:** Linked to genes encoding collagen type II and XI precursors; type 1 linked to COL2A1 gene on chromosome 12q13.11-q13.2 for collagen type II alpha1 chain; type 2 linked to COL11A1 gene on chromosome 1p21 for collagen type XI alpha1; type 3 linked to COL11A2 gene on chromosome 6p21.3 for collagen type XI alpha2 chain.

- **Electrophysiologic testing:** ERG (reduced) and EOG (normal).
- Genetic counseling.
- ENT or orthopedic evaluation (cleft palate repair, hearing aids, joint replacement).
- Retinal surgery for retinal detachments (increased risk of PVR from abnormal adherence between vitreous and retina); prophylactic laser photocoagulation controversial; should be performed by a retina specialist.

Leber's Congenital Amaurosis (Autosomal Recessive)

Group of hereditary disorders with onset at birth or early childhood of severe visual impairment, sluggish pupils, nyctalopia, light sensitivity (50%), and nystagmus. May have range of fundus abnormalities from no fundus changes (most common especially early in life) to progressive retinal pigment epithelial granularity, vascular attenuation, tapetal sheen, yellow flecks, "salt-and-pepper" fundus, macular "colobomas," chorioretinal atrophy, or a retinitis pigmentosa appearance. Associated with high hyperopia, oculodigital sign, mental retardation (37%), deafness, seizures, skeletal abnormalities, posterior subcapsular cataracts, keratoconus, and renal/muscular abnormalities.

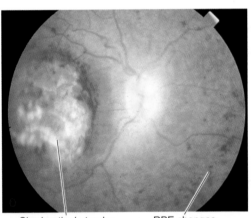

Figure 10-201 Leber's congenital amaurosis demonstrating granular and RP-like pigmentary changes, attenuated vessels, and a macular scar.

Chorioretinal atrophy   RPE changes

- **Genetics:** RPE65/LCA2 gene on chromosome 1p31 accounts for up to 16% of Leber's congenital amaurosis (LCA), encoding protein essential in vitamin A metabolism; RPGRIP1 gene on chromosome 14q11 encodes RPGR-interacting protein 1 and accounts for 6% of LCA; LCA1 and LCA4 genes on chromosome 17p13.1 encode arylhydrocarbon-interacting receptor protein-like 1 and account for approximately 15% of LCA; CRX gene on chromosome 19q13.3 encodes cone-rod otx-like photoreceptor homeobox transcription factor and accounts for 3% of LCA.
- **Color vision:** Abnormal.
- **Electrophysiologic testing:** ERG (markedly reduced, absent) EOG (abnormal).
- **Visual fields:** Constricted.
- No effective treatment.

Retinitis Pigmentosa

Definition Group of hereditary, progressive retinal degenerations (rod-cone dystrophies) that result from abnormal production of photoreceptor proteins. There are more than 29 loci associated with various phenotypes of RP with more being discovered daily.

Atypical forms

Retinitis Pigmentosa Inversus

Macula and posterior pole are affected differentially; confused with hereditary macular disorders. Central and color vision are reduced earlier than normal, and pericentral ring/central scotomas occur.

Retinitis Pigmentosa Sine Pigmento

Descriptive term to describe patients with symptoms of retinitis pigmentosa, but who fail to show pigmentary fundus changes. Occurs in up to 20% of cases; associated with more pronounced cone dysfunction.

Retinitis Punctata Albescens (Autosomal Recessive)

Multiple, punctate white (50–100 µm) spots at the level of the retinal pigment epithelium scattered in the midperiphery with attenuated vessels and bone spicules. Slowly progressive (differentiates from fundus albipunctatus).

Sector Retinitis Pigmentosa

Subtype with pigmentary changes limited to one retinal area that generally does not enlarge; usually infero-nasal quadrants. Relatively good ERG responses.

Forms Associated with Systemic Abnormalities

Abetalipoproteinemia (Bassen-Kornzweig Syndrome) (Autosomal Recessive)

Associated with ataxia, steatorrhea, erythrocyte acanthocytosis, growth retardation, neuropathy, and lack of serum beta-lipoprotein causing intestinal malabsorption of fat-soluble vitamins (A, D, E, K), triglycerides, and cholesterol; minimal pigmentary changes early.

- **Genetics:** MTP gene cloned on chromosome 4q24 produces microsomal triglyceride transfer protein.
- Treat with vitamin A (15,000 IU po QD), vitamin E (100 IU/kg po QD), vitamin K (0.15 mg/kg po QD), omega-3 fatty acids (0.10 gm/kg po QD), and dietary fat restriction.

Alstrom's Disease (Autosomal Recessive)

Associated with cataracts, deafness, obesity, renal failure, acanthosis nigricans, baldness, and hypogenitalism; early and profound visual loss.

- **Genetics:** ALMS1 gene cloned on chromosome 2p13.

Cockayne's Syndrome

Associated with band keratopathy, cataracts, dwarfism, deafness, intracranial calcifications, and psychosis.

Kearns–Sayre Syndrome (Autosomal Recessive)

Associated with chronic, progressive external ophthalmoplegia, ptosis, cardiac conduction defects (arrhythmias, heart block, cardiomyopathy), and other abnormalities (see Chapter 2). "Ragged red" fibers found histologically on muscle biopsy.

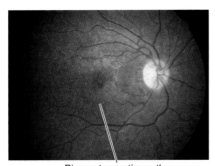

Pigmentary retinopathy

Figure 10-202 • Kearns–Sayre syndrome with pigmentary retinopathy

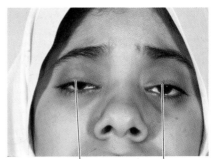

Ptosis due to CPEO

Figure 10-203 • Same patient as Figure 10-202 demonstrating chronic progressive external ophthalmoplegia with ptosis. This patient also could not move her eyes.

Laurence–Moon/Bardet–Biedl Syndromes (Autosomal Recessive)

Characterized by pigmentary retinopathy with early macular involvement (often bull's eye); salt-and-pepper appearance to frank bone spicules. Two syndromes: Bardet–Biedl (polydactyly in 75% and syndactyly in 14%) and Laurence–Moon (spastic paraplegia, no polydactyly/syndactyly). Both include short stature, congenital obesity (above 95th

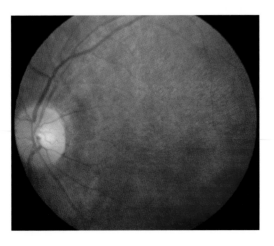

Figure 10-204 • Diffuse pigmentary changes in a patient with Laurence–Moon syndrome.

percentile), hypogenitalism (74–96%; sterility in males), partial deafness (5%), renal abnormalities (46–95%), and mental retardation (41–85%); minimal pigmentary changes early; severe vision loss in almost all patients by age 30 years old. Very common in the Middle East especially among Bedouins (1:13,500); normal (1:100,000).

- **Genetics:** Heterogeneous with 11 genes; linked to BBS1 gene on chromosome 11q13 (TRIM32 an E3 ubiquitin ligase); BBS2 gene on chromosome 16q21; BBS3 gene on chromosome 3p13-p12; BBS4 gene on chromosome 15q22.3-q23; BBS5 gene on chromosome 2q31; and BBS6 gene on chromosome 20p12. BBS proteins assist microtubule-related transport and cellular organization processes.

Neuronal Ceroid Lipofuscinosis (Batten Disease) (Autosomal Recessive)

Associated with seizures, dementia, ataxia, and mental retardation; infantile (Hagberg–Santavuori syndrome), juvenile, or adult onset. Conjunctival biopsy shows granular inclusions with autofluorescent lipopigments that also accumulate in neurons causing the retinal and CNS degeneration.

Refsum's Disease (Autosomal Recessive)

Associated with ichthyosis, EKG abnormalities, anosmia, deafness, progressive peripheral neuropathy, cerebellar ataxia, hypotonia, hepatomegaly, mental retardation, and elevated CSF protein; minimal pigmentary changes early. Defect in fatty acid metabolism due to phytanic acid oxidase deficiency; causes elevated plasma phytanic acid, pipecolic acid, and very long-chain fatty acid levels.

- **Genetics:** Associated with PNYH gene cloned on chromosome 10p15.3-p12.2 that encodes phytanoyl-CoA hydroxylase; infantile Refsum's associated with PEX1 gene on chromosome 7q21-q22 encoding peroxisome biogenesis factor 1.
- Treat by restricting dietary phytanic acid (animal fats and milk products) and phytol (leafy green vegetables); follow serum phytanic acid levels.

Usher's Syndrome (Autosomal Recessive)

Associated with congenital, neurosensory hearing loss. Most common syndrome associated with retinitis pigmentosa (5%). Four types:

Type I

Total deafness with no vestibular function.

Type II

Partial deafness with normal vestibular function, most common type (67%), better vision.

Type III *(Hallgren's syndrome)*

Deafness, vestibular ataxia, psychosis.

Type IV

Deafness and mental retardation.

Note: controversial if Types III and IV are forms of Usher's syndrome or separate genetic entities.

- **Genetics:** USH2A gene on chromosome 1q41 associated with autosomal recessive Usher's syndrome; produces usherin, a basement membrane protein in the retina and inner ear; numerous additional loci including 10q21-22; 11p15.1; 11q13.5; 14q32; 17q34-q35; 21q21.
- Protect ears against loud noises; avoid ototoxic medications, such as aminoglycosides.

Epidemiology Most common hereditary degeneration (1:5000); can have any inheritance pattern: AR (25%), AD (20%, usually with variable penatrance, later onset, milder course), X-linked (9%, more severe, carriers also affected), isolated (38%), and undetermined (8%).

Symptoms Nyctalopia, dark adaptation problems, photophobia, progressive constriction of visual fields ("tunnel vision"), dyschromatopsia, photopsias, and slowly, progressive, decreased central vision starting at approximately age 20 years old.

Signs Decreased visual acuity, constricted visual fields, decreased color vision (tritanopic); classic fundus appearance with dark pigmentary clumps in the midperiphery and perivenous areas (bone spicules), attenuated retinal vessels, cystoid macular edema, fine pigmented vitreous cells, and waxy optic disc pallor; associated with posterior subcapsular cataracts (39–72%), high myopia, astigmatism, keratoconus, and mild hearing loss (30%, excluding Usher's patients). Fifty percent of female carriers with X-linked form have golden reflex in posterior pole.

Differential Diagnosis Congenital rubella syndrome, syphilis, thioridazine/chloroquine drug toxicity, carcinoma-associated retinopathy, congenital stationary night blindness, vitamin A deficiency, atypical cytomegalovirus or herpes virus chorioretinitis, trauma, diffuse unilateral subacute neuroretinitis, gyrate atrophy, bear tracks, congenital hypertrophy of the retinal pigment epithelium (CHRPE).

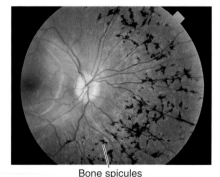

Bone spicules

Figure 10-205 • Retinitis pigmentosa demonstrating characteristic bone-spicule pigmentary changes.

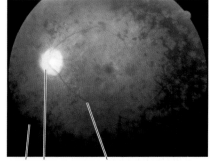

Bone   Waxy pallor   Attenuated vessels
spicules

Figure 10-206 • Retinitis pigmentosa demonstrating dense retinal pigment epithelium changes, optic disc pallor, and attenuated retinal vessels.

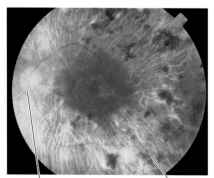

Waxy pallor   Chorioretinal atrophy

Figure 10-207 • Retinitis pigmentosa with diffuse chorioretinal atrophy and early optic disc pallor.

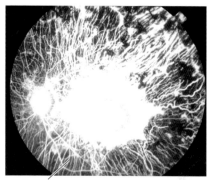

Chorioretinal atrophy

Figure 10-208 • Fluorescein angiogram of same patient as Figure 10-207 demonstrating the diffuse chorioretinal atrophy.

Evaluation

- Complete ophthalmic history with attention to consanguinity, family history, and hearing.
- Complete eye exam with attention to refraction, pupils, cornea, lens, vitreous cells, and ophthalmoscopy.
- **Lab tests:** Plasma ornithine levels, fat-soluble vitamin levels (especially vitamin A), serum lipoprotein electrophoresis (Bassen–Kornzweig syndrome), serum cholesterol/triglycerides, VDRL, FTA-ABS, peripheral blood smears (acanthocytosis), serum phytanic acid levels (Refsum's disease).
- **Color vision (Farnsworth panel D15):** Normal except very late in the disease.
- **Electrophysiologic testing:** ERG (markedly reduced/absent; decreases 10% per year, abnormal in 90% of female carriers in X-linked, subnormal scotopic amplitudes precede reduction of photopic amplitudes), EOG (abnormal), dark adaptation (elevated rod and cone thresholds).
- **Visual fields:** Mid-peripheral ring scotoma; progresses to total loss except for central islands that disappear at the very end of the disease process.

Management

- No effective treatment except in forms with treatable systemic diseases (abetalipoproteinemia, Refsum's disease).
- Correct any refractive error; prescribe dark glasses.
- Low vision consultation for visual aids.
- For common forms of retinitis pigmentosa (age >18 years old): vitamin A (15,000 IU po qd of palmitate form) slows reduction of ERG amplitudes and avoid vitamin E; follow liver function tests and serum retinol levels annually. *Note:* controversial and not tested in atypical forms of RP. The use of vitamin A in younger patients is even more controversial: age 6–10 years old, vitamin A (5,000 IU po qd of palmitate form), 10–15 years, vitamin A (10,000 IU po qd of palmitate form); check with pediatrician before starting high dose vitamin A therapy.

Continued

Management—Cont'd

- Systemic acetazolamide (Diamox 500 mg IV or po) for cystoid macular edema is controversial.
- Cataract surgery may be indicated depending on retinal function; check potential acuity meter (PAM) when considering cataract extraction.

Prognosis Poor, usually legally blind by fourth decade.

Albinism

Ocular Albinism (X-linked/Autosomal Recessive)

Congenital disorder of melanogenesis limited to the eye; decreased number of melanosomes (although each melanosome is fully pigmented). Patients have decreased vision and photophobia; signs include nystagmus, strabismus, high myopia, diffuse iris transillumination, foveal hypoplasia, and fundus hypopigmentation.

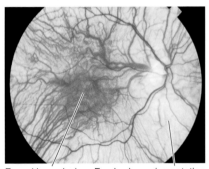

Foveal hypoplasia   Fundus hypopigmentation

Figure 10-209 • Fundus hypopigmentation in a patient with albinism. The deep choroidal vasculature is clearly visible.

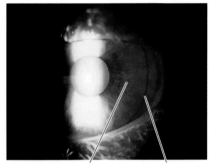

Transillumination defects   Lens equator

Figure 10-210 • Albinism demonstrating diffuse iris transillumination. Note that the equator of the crystalline lens is visible as a dark line near the peripheral iris.

Oculocutaneous Albinism (Autosomal Recessive>Autosomal Dominant)

Systemic problem with decreased melanin in all melanosomes. Two forms: tyrosinase positive (some pigmentation) and tyrosinase negative (no pigmentation). These patients lack pigmentation of the hair, skin, and eyes. Potentially lethal variants of oculocutaneous albinism include Chédiak–Higashi (AR; reticuloendothelial incompetence with neutropenia, anemia, thrombocytopenia, recurrent infections, leukemia, and lymphoma) and Hermansky–Pudlak (AR; clotting disorders and bleeding tendencies secondary to platelet abnormalities).

- No effective treatment.
- Medical and hematology consultation to rule out potentially lethal variants.

Phakomatoses

Group of congenital, mainly heritable, syndromes with multiple tumorous growths both ocular and systemic; commonly have incomplete penetrance and variable expressivity. Phako = "motherspot" (birthmark).

Angiomatosis Retinae (von Hippel-Lindau Disease) (Autosomal Dominant)

Retinal capillary hemangioblastomas (45–60%), cystic cerebellar hemangioblastoma (60%, most common cause of death), renal cell carcinoma, pheochromocytoma, liver, pancreas, and epididymis cysts (if only retinal findings = von Hippel disease). Earliest manifestations are retinal (95% by age 10 years old); bilateral in 50%.

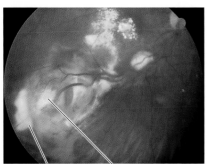

Exudate   Retinal angioma

Figure 10-211 Angiomatosis retinae (von Hippel–Lindau disease) demonstrating retinal capillary hemangioma with feeder and draining vessels, and surrounding exudates.

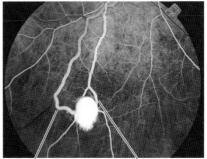

Draining vessel   Feeder vessel

Figure 10-212 Fluorescein angiogram of a patient with retinal angioma demonstrating fluorescein filling from feeder vessel and drainage via drainage vessel.

- **Genetics:** Linked to chromosome 3p25-p26; mutation in the VHL tumor suppressor gene that regulates cell growth and controls VEGF expression.
- Head, upper cervical spinal cord, and abdominal CT scan or MRI.
- Medical consultation.

Ataxia Telangiectasia (Louis-Bar Syndrome) (Autosomal Recessive)

Progressive cerebellar ataxia (first symptom), telangiectasia of the skin (especially around face, ears, and neck) and bulbar conjunctiva, ocular motility abnormalities; also associated with seborrheic dermatitis, mental retardation, thymus gland hypoplasia with reduced T-cell immunity. High incidence of malignancies (33%) including lymphoma and leukemia, and humoral/cellular immunodeficiency with increased risk of infections especially chronic respiratory infections. Poor prognosis with death by adolescence.

- **Genetics:** Linked to ATM gene on chromosome 11q22-q23; thought to encode protein vital to DNA repair.
- Medical consultation.

Encephalotrigeminal Angiomatosis (Sturge–Weber Syndrome)

Diffuse, flat, dark red, "tomato catsup" choroidal hemangioma (40–50%), congenital facial angioma (nevus flammeus or "port wine stain" = essential for diagnosis), ipsilateral intracranial hemangioma, nevus flammeus involving the eyelid (suspect glaucoma if upper eyelid involved), large anomalous blood vessels in the conjunctiva and episclera, and congenital, ipsilateral glaucoma (30%). May have mental retardation, convulsions, and cerebral calcifications. Sporadic, no hereditary pattern; no associated malignancies. Variable prognosis depending on CNS involvement.

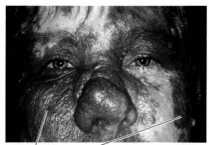

Nevus flammeus

Figure 10-213 • Encephalotrigeminal angiomatosis (Sturge–Weber syndrome) demonstrating nevus flammeus.

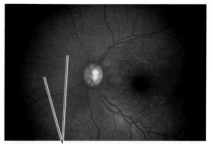

Diffuse choroidal hemangioma

Figure 10-214 • Encephalotrigeminal angiomatosis demonstrating tomato-catsup fundus appearance of a diffuse choroidal hemangioma.

- Head and orbital CT scan.
- May require treatment of increased intraocular pressure (see Primary Open-Angle Glaucoma section in Chapter 11).
- Neurology consultation if intracranial lesions exist.

Neurofibromatosis (von Recklinghausen's Disease) (Autosomal Dominant)

Disorder of the neuroectodermal system. Two forms (see Chapter 3).

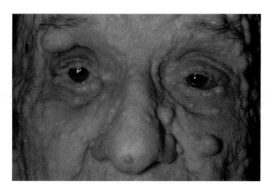

Figure 10-215 • Neurofibromatosis (von Recklinghausen's disease) demonstrating facial neurofibromas.

Anomalous anastamosis between the arterial and venous systems of the retina, brain (20–30% have intracranial arteriovenous malformations causing mental status changes or hemiparesis; 30% cause visual fields defects including homonymous hemianopia), orbit, and facial bones (pterygoid fossa, mandible, and maxilla). Usually unilateral (96%) racemose angiomas that appear as intertwined tangles of dilated vessels; may cause visual loss due to retinal or vitreous hemorrhage. Sporadic, no hereditary pattern. Early mortality due to intracranial arteriovenous malformations.

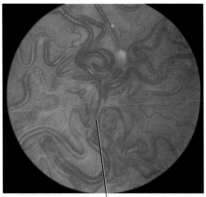

Retinal vascular arteriovenous malformation

Figure 10-216 Racemose hemangiomatosis (Wyburn–Mason syndrome) demonstrating retinal vascular arteriovenous malformation (AVM) with dilated, tortuous vessels.

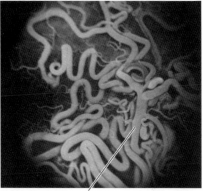

Retinal vascular arteriovenous malformation

Figure 10-217 Fluorescein angiogram of same patient as Figure 10-216 demonstrating the retinal vascular arteriovenous malformation filled with fluorescein dye. Note: line points at same vessel in both pictures.

- Head and orbital CT scan.
- Neurology consultation if intracranial lesions exist.
- Asymptomatic retinal lesions do not require treatment.
- Consider laser photocoagulation around lesions (direct treatment dangerous) if symptomatic.

Triad of seizures (infantile spasms, 80–93%), mental retardation (50–60%), and adenoma sebaceum (85%, a misnomer for angiofibromas, a red–brown papular malar rash). Primary criteria include: facial angiofibromas (adenoma sebaceum), subungal angiofibromas, cortical tuber, subependymal hamartomas and multiple retinal hamartomas. Secondary criteria include: infantile spasms (25%), cutaneous shagreen patch (fibromatous skin infiltration especially on lower back and forehead; 25%), ash-leaf spots (hypopigmented skin macules seen best with ultraviolet "Wood's" lamp; 80%), skin tags (molluscum fibrosum pendulum), bilateral renal angiomyolipomata or cysts (80%), cystic lung disease, cardiac rhabdomyoma, calcified CNS astrocytic hamartomas ("brain stones" in cerebellum, basal ganglia, and posterior fossa), or a first-degree relative with tuberous sclerosis. Poor prognosis with 75% mortality prior to age 20 years old.

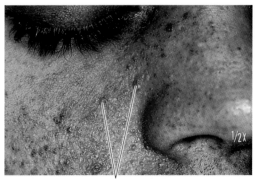

Figure 10-218 • Tuberous sclerosis (Bourneville's disease) demonstrating adenoma sebaceum.

Adenoma sebaceum

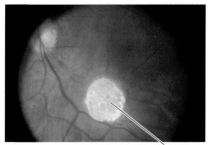

Astrocytic hamartoma

Figure 10-219 • Tuberous sclerosis demonstrating astrocytic hamartoma with mulberry appearance.

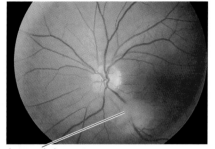

Astrocytic hamartoma

Figure 10-220 • Tuberous sclerosis demonstrating astrocytic hamartoma with smooth appearance.

- **Genetics:** Linked to TSC1 gene on chromosome 9q34 encoding hamartin and TSC2 gene on chromosome 16p13.3 encoding tuberin, a GTP-ase activating protein.
- Medical and neurology consultation.

Tumors

Benign Choroidal Tumors

Choroidal Hemangioma

Vascular tumor. Two forms:

(1) Usually unilateral, well-circumscribed, solitary; round, slightly elevated (<3 mm), orange–red lesion located in the posterior pole often with an overlying serous retinal detachment. Occurs in fourth decade. No extraocular associations.

(2) Diffuse, reddish, choroidal thickening described as "tomato-catsup" fundus (reddish thickening overlying dark fundus). Occurs in children with Sturge–Weber syndrome (see Fig. 10-214).

Usually asymptomatic, but both types can cause exudative retinal detachments (50%). Reduced vision, metamorphopsia, micropsia from foveal distortion due to underlying tumor or accumulation of subretinal fluid.

Figure 10-221 • Choroidal hemangioma (discrete type) appearing as an elevated orange lesion in the macula.

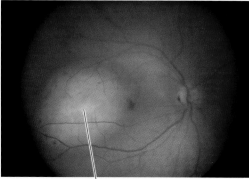

Choroidal hemangioma

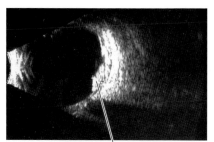

Choroidal hemangioma

Figure 10-222 • B-scan ultrasound of same patient as Figure 10-221 demonstrating elevated mass with underlying thickened choroid.

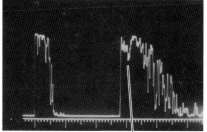

High internal reflectivity

Figure 10-223 • A-scan ultrasound of same patient as Figure 10-221 with high internal reflectivity.

- **B-scan ultrasonography:** Mass with moderate elevation, thickened choroid, and high internal reflectivity, often with overlying serous retinal detachment.

- **Fluorescein angiogram:** Early filling of intrinsic tumor vessels or feeder vessels, progressive hyperfluorescence during the transit views, and late leakage (multiloculated pattern); circumscribed lesions have defined vascular pattern.

- **Indocyanine green angiogram:** Circumscribed hemangiomas: early hyperfluorescence with relative late hypofluorescence, or "washout" phenomenon. Diffuse hemangioma: early hyperfluorescence with late hypofluorescence of the lesion and persistent hot spots of hyperfluorescence along the vascular channels.

- Observe if asymptomatic especially if extrafoveal without subretinal fluid; long-standing subfoveal lesions with poor chance of recovery of vision are also observed.

- Decision to treat is individualized based on extent of symptoms, loss of vision, and potential for visual recovery; aim of treatment is to induce tumor atrophy with resolution of subretinal fluid and tumor-induced foveal distortion without destroying function of overlying retina; goal is not to obliterate tumor.

- Treatment of circumscribed hemangiomas includes laser photocoagulation (moderately intense, white reaction on the tumor surface to eliminate serous exudation), photodynamic therapy with verteporfin using standard treatment parameters, transpupillary thermotherapy, or I-125 plaque brachytherapy.

- Visual loss can be progressive and irreversible; poor visual acuity results may be expected despite resolution of fluid exudates from chronic macular edema and photoreceptor loss.

Choroidal Nevus

Dark gray–brown pigmented, flat or slightly elevated lesion (<2 mm); often with overlying drusen and a hypopigmented ring around the base. Usually nonprogressive, but can grow during puberty; growth in an adult should be watched carefully. Multiple nevi may occur in patients with neurofibromatosis. Characteristics of suspicious nevi include growth, tumor thickness (>2 mm), presence of visual symptoms, overlying orange pigment, subsensory fluid, and proximity to the optic nerve head. Ten percent of suspicious nevi progress to malignant melanoma.

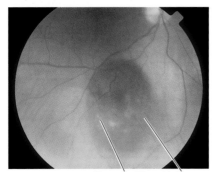

Drusen Choroidal nevus

Figure 10-224 • Large choroidal nevus (nevoma) with overlying drusen.

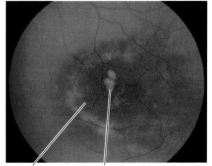

Choroidal nevus   Drusen

Figure 10-225 • Flat choroidal nevus with overlying drusen indicating chronicity.

- **B-scan ultrasonography:** Flat to slightly elevated lesion, choroidal discontinuity, and medium to high internal reflectivity.
- Follow with serial photographs, ultrasonography, and clinical examination for any growth that would be suspicious for malignant melanoma at 1, 3, 6, 9, and 12 months, and then on an annual or semi-annual basis if there is no growth.

Choroidal Osteoma

Slightly elevated, well-circumscribed, peripapillary, orange–red (early) to cream-colored (late) benign tumor with small vascular networks on the surface. Eighty to ninety percent unilateral; typically occurs in younger patients who may be asymptomatic or have decreased vision, paracentral scotomas, and metamorphopsia, although well documented in older patients; slight female predilection. Consists of mature cancellous bone; growth may occur over years, and may spontaneously resolve. Choroidal neovascular membrane common at tumor margins; variable prognosis.

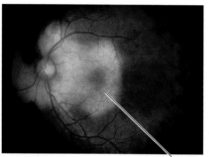

Choroidal osteoma

Figure 10-226 • Choroidal osteoma with orange, placoid appearance.

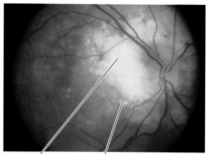

Choroidal osteoma   Calcification

Figure 10-227 • Choroidal osteoma with calcification.

- **B-scan ultrasonography:** Calcification, orbital shadowing, and a high reflective spike from the tumor surface.

- **Fluorescein angiogram:** Irregular hyperfluorescence and late staining of the tumor; the vascular networks may appear hypofluorescent against the hyperfluorescent tumor.

- Orbital radiographs and CT scan show the calcifications within the tumor.

- Treat CNV with laser photocoagulation for juxta- and extrafoveal lesions, often requires multiple sessions; for subfoveal CNV consider anti-VEGF agents and/or photodynamic therapy.

Benign Retinal Tumors

Astrocytic Hamartoma

Yellow–white, well-circumscribed, elevated lesion that may contain nodular areas of calcification and/or clear cystic spaces; classically has mulberry appearance but may have softer, smooth appearance (see Figs 10-219 and 10-220). Multiple lesions common in tuberous sclerosis. Usually do not grow. Rare cases of exudative retinal detachment have been reported.

- **Fluorescein angiogram:** Variable vascularization within tumor that leaks in late views.

- No treatment necessary.

Capillary Hemangioma

Benign vascular tumor arising from the inner retina and extending toward the retinal surface. Two forms:

(1) Sporadic, nonhereditary, and unilateral; no systemic associations; usually no feeder vessels.

(2) Hereditary, bilateral (50%), multifocal, and associated with multiple systemic abnormalities (von Hippel-Lindau syndrome); classically has dilated feeder and draining vessels.

Both forms initially appear as a red, pink, or gray lesion that later grows as proliferation of capillary channels within the tumor progresses. These new capillaries leak fluid, leading to exudates and serous retinal detachments. Associated with preretinal membranes.

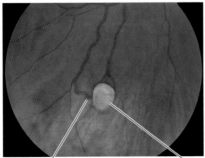

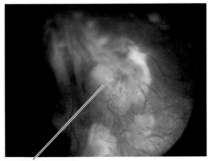

Draining vessel   Retinal angioma   Retinal angioma

Figure 10-228 • Retinal angioma with feeder and draining vessels in patient with von Hippel–Lindau syndrome (see Figure 10-212 for fluorescein angiogram).

Figure 10-229 • Capillary hemangioma in a patient with von Hippel disease demonstrating the characteristic pink lesion with a dilated, tortuous, feeder vessel; there is also some surrounding exudate.

- **Fluorescein angiogram:** Early filling of tumor in arterial phase with late leakage.
- No treatment recommended for sporadic tumor unless vision is affected.
- Consider cryotherapy, photocoagulation, and plaque brachytherapy for hereditary tumors; should be performed by an ophthalmic oncologist.
- Medical consultation for hereditary form for evaluation of systemic capillary hemangiomas.

Cavernous Hemangioma

Rare, vascular tumor composed of clumps of saccular, intraretinal aneurysms filled with dark venous blood ("cluster-of-grapes" appearance). Fine, gray epiretinal membranes may cover the tumor. Typically unilateral; occurs in second to third decade, slight female predilection (60%). Usually no exudation occurs, retinal/vitreous hemorrhages rare; commonly asymptomatic and nonprogressive.

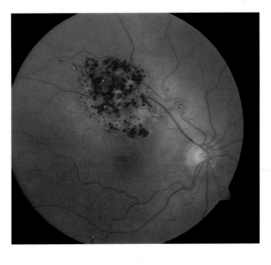

Figure 10-230 • Cavernous hemangioma with "cluster-of-grapes" appearance.

Figure 10-231 • Flourescein angiogram of same patient as Figure 10-230 showing fluorescein fluid levels within the aneurysms.

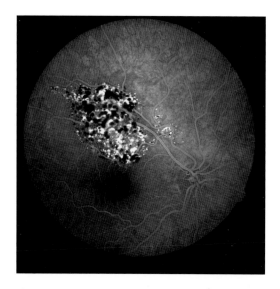

Figure 10-232 • Optical coherence tomography of same patient as Figure 10-230 showing irregular retinal surface from the saccular aneurysms that shadow beyond.

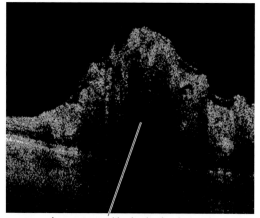

Aneurysms with shadowing beyond

- **Fluorescein angiogram:** Hyperfluorescent saccules with fluid levels; "layering" effect.
- No treatment necessary.

Congenital Hypertrophy of the Retinal Pigment Epithelium

Flat or slightly elevated, round, solitary, dark brown-to-black pigmented lesion with sharp borders, scalloped edges, and central hypopigmented lacunae. Vast majority are stationary, although enlargement has been documented. Bilateral, multifocal CHRPE lesions (>4 lesions) occur in familial adenomatous polyposis (Gardner's syndrome [AD]: triad of multiple intestinal polyps, skeletal hamartomas, and soft tissue tumors).

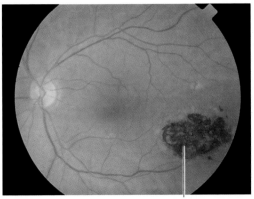

Figure 10-233 Congenital hypertrophy of the retinal pigment epithelium with hypopigmented lacunae.

CHRPE

- No treatment necessary if no growth.
- Several reported cases of nodular growth within an area of the CHRPE lesion associated with retinal exudates and cystoid macular edema. Consider plaque brachytherapy in these cases (experimental).

Bear Tracks

Multifocal variant of CHRPE clustered in one quadrant with appearance of animal tracks. Polar bear tracks are another variant in which the lesions are hypopigmented. Familial cases have been reported.

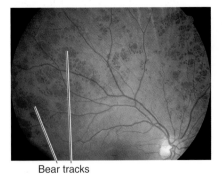

Bear tracks

Figure 10-234 Bear tracks demonstrating multifocal congenital hypertrophy of the retinal pigment epithelium clusters.

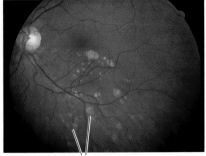

Polar bear tracks

Figure 10-235 Polar bear tracks demonstrating hypopigmented lesions.

- No treatment necessary.

Combined Hamartoma of Retinal Pigment Epithelium and Retina

Slightly elevated, dark gray (variable pigmentation) lesion with poorly defined, feathery borders often associated with a fine glial membrane on the surface of the tumor; dilated, tortuous retinal vessels common. Can occur in a peripapillary location (46%) or in the posterior pole; causes decreased vision, metamorphopsia, and strabismus in children and young adults. Choroidal neovascular membrane and subretinal exudation are late complications. Bilateral cases associated with neurofibromatosis type 2 (NF-2). Variable prognosis.

Figure 10-236 ◦ Combined hamartoma of retinal pigment epithelium (RPE) and retina demonstrating gray appearance with feathery borders.

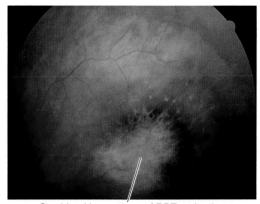

Combined hamartoma of RPE and retina

- **Fluorescein angiogram:** Early filling of the dilated, tortuous retinal vessels with late leakage.
- Consider pars plana vitrectomy with membrane peel if epiretinal membrane results in significant visual distortion; should be performed by a retina specialist.
- Laser photocoagulation if CNV develops.

Malignant Tumors

Note: Treatment and work-up for tumors of the retina and choroid should be performed by a multidisciplinary team composed of an internist, an oncologist, and an ophthalmic oncology specialist. Therefore, in-depth discussions of management for these tumors are beyond the scope of this book, and treatment is best relegated to the physicians caring for the patient.

Choroidal Malignant Melanoma

Most common primary intraocular malignancy in adults. Focal, darkly pigmented or amelanotic, dome- or collar-button-shaped (break through Bruch's membrane) tumor usually associated with overlying serous retinal detachment and lipofuscin (orange spots); commonly have episcleral sentinel vessels. Collaborative Ocular Melanoma Study (COMS) classified lesions by size: small, medium, and large (see below). Most common sites of metastasis: liver, lung, bone, skin, and central nervous system. Factors predictive of metastasis: presence of epithelioid cells (Callender classification), high number of mitoses, extrascleral extension, increased tumor thickness, ciliary body involvement, tumor growth, and proximity to optic disk.

Collaborative Ocular Melanoma Study (COMS) results:

- **Small lesions (1–2.5 mm apical height, 5–16 mm basal diameter):** 204 patients with tumors not large enough to be randomized were followed in the COMS trial; 6% all-cause mortality at 5 years, 14.9% all cause mortality at 8 years; 1% melanoma mortality at 5 years, 3.8% at 8 years.

- **Medium lesions (2.5–10 mm apical height and ≤16 mm longest basal diameter):** 1317 patients with medium tumors were randomized to enucleation versus Iodine-125 brachytherapy; 34% all-cause mortality for enucleation and 34% all cause mortality for Iodine-125 brachytherapy at 10 years; metastatic mortality in 17% after enucleation and 17% after Iodine-125 brachytherapy at 10 years.

- **Large lesions (apical height ≤2 mm and >16 mm longest basal diameter *or* >10 mm apical height, regardless of basal diameter *or* >8 mm apical height if <2 mm from the optic disk):** 1003 patients with large tumors all received enucleation and were randomized to pre-enucleation external beam radiation (PERT) or not; 61% all-cause mortality for enucleation, 61% all-cause mortality for PERT/enucleation at 10 years; metastasis in 62% histologically confirmed at time of death; additional 21% suspected based on imaging and ancillary testing. Metastatic mortality in 39% after enucleation and 42% after PERT/enucleation at 10 years.

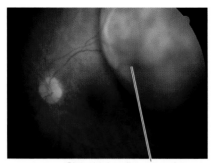

Choroidal malignant melanoma

Figure 10-237 • Choroidal malignant melanoma demonstrating elevated dome-shaped tumor.

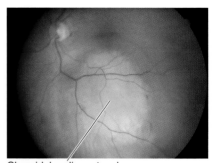

Choroidal malignant melanoma

Figure 10-238 • Choroidal amelanotic melanoma demonstrating hypopigmented subretinal mass.

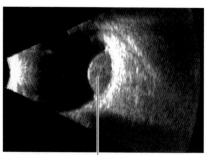

Choroidal malignant melanoma

Figure 10-239 • B-scan ultrasound of same patient as Figure 10-238 demonstrating dome-shaped choroidal mass.

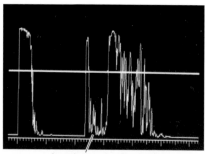

Low internal reflectivity

Figure 10-240 • A-scan ultrasound of same patient as Figure 10-238 demonstrating low internal reflectivity.

- **B-scan ultrasonography:** Collar-button-shaped (27% in COMS) or dome-shaped (60% in COMS) mass >2.5 mm (95%), low to medium (5–60% spike height) internal reflectivity (84% in COMS), regular internal structure, solid consistency, echo attenuation, acoustic hollowness within the tumor, choroidal excavation, and orbital shadowing.

- **Fluorescein angiogram:** May demonstrate double circulation due to intrinsic tumor circulation in large tumors, late staining of lesion with multiple pinpoint hyperfluorescent hot spots; not useful unless the intrinsic circulation is documented.

- Medical and oncology consultation for systemic work-up.

Choroidal Metastasis

Most common intraocular malignancy in adults; creamy yellow–white lesions with mottled pigment clumping (leopard spots); low to medium elevation; often with overlying serous retinal detachment; predilection for posterior pole; may be multifocal and bilateral (20%). Two-thirds of metastatic lesions come from a known primary; primary not detected in 17%. Most common primary tumors for females are breast (metastasis late), lung, GI and pancreas, skin melanoma, and other rare sources; for males are lung (metastasis early), unknown primary, GI and pancreas, prostate, renal cell, and skin melanoma. Ocular involvement is by hematogenous spread; rapid growth; very poor prognosis (median survival is 8.5 months from the time of diagnosis).

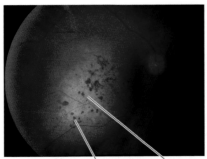

"Leopard spots" Choroidal metastasis

Figure 10-241 • Choroidal metastasis with leopard-spot appearance (lung carcinoma).

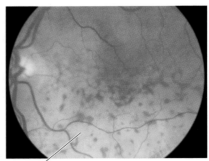

Choroidal metastasis

Figure 10-242 • Metastatic breast carcinoma with yellow, creamy posterior pole lesion.

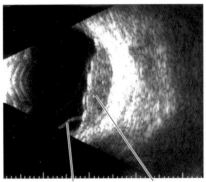

Serous retinal   Choroidal metastasis
detachment

Figure 10-243 • B-scan ultrasound of a patient with choroidal metastasis demonstrating elevated choroidal mass with irregular surface and overlying serous retinal detachment.

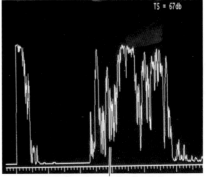

Medium internal reflectivity

Figure 10-244 • A-scan ultrasound of same patient as Figure 10-243 demonstrating medium internal reflectivity.

- **Lab tests:** Liver function tests, serum chemistry analysis, isotope bone scan, and chest radiographs.
- **B-scan ultrasonography:** Flat or mildly elevated mass with irregular surface, medium to high internal reflectivity, serous retinal detachment usually visible, no orbital shadowing or acoustically silent zone.
- **Fluorescein angiogram:** Early hypofluorescence with pinpoint hyperfluorescence in the venous phase that increases in later views.
- Enucleation, laser photocoagulation, radiation therapy, brachytherapy, and chemotherapy are all used; should be performed by an experienced tumor specialist.
- Oncology consultation for metastatic work-up if no known primary site.

Primary Intraocular Lymphoma (Reticulum Cell Sarcoma)

Bilateral (80%) anterior uveitis, vitritis, retinal vasculitis, cystoid macular edema, creamy yellow pigment epithelial detachments, hypopigmented retinal pigment epithelial lesions with overlying serous retinal detachments, and disc edema. Occurs in sixth to seventh decades; mimics uveitis (masquerade syndrome [see p. 434]). Patients have decreased vision and floaters; associated with central nervous system involvement and dementia. Poor prognosis, with death within 2 years of diagnosis.

- **Fluorescein angiogram:** Early staining of pigment epithelial detachments with late pooling; window defects occur in areas of atrophy.
- Consider diagnostic pars plana vitrectomy to obtain vitreous biopsy for histopathologic and cytologic analysis; should be performed by a retina specialist.
- Lumbar puncture for cytology.
- Head MRI.
- Treatment with chemotherapy and radiation should be performed by an oncologist.
- Medical and oncology consultation.

Retinoblastoma

Globular, white–yellow, elevated mass or masses with calcifications that may grow toward the vitreous (endophytic) causing vitreous seeding, or toward the choroid (exophytic) causing retinal detachment, or diffusely infiltrating within the retina. Most common primary intraocular malignancy in children (1 in 15–20,000 live births or approximately 300 cases/year in the US). Ninety percent diagnosed by 5 years of age. 70% are unilateral, 40% heritable, 95% sporadic (25% germinal, 75% somatic), and 5% familial (AD). Mapped to chromosome 13q14. Children present with leukocoria (50%), strabismus (18%), intraocular inflammation, and decreased vision. Risk factors for poor prognosis include optic nerve invasion, extraocular extension, and delay in diagnosis. Prognosis is usually good, with long-term survival approaching 85–90%; 25–30% of children with heritable retinoblastoma may develop a secondary malignancy.

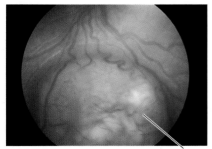

Retinoblastoma

Figure 10-245 • Retinoblastoma demonstrating discrete round tumor.

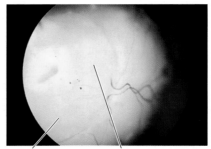

Retinoblastoma   Serous retinal detachment

Figure 10-246 • Retinoblastoma demonstrating exophytic growth with a serous retinal detachment.

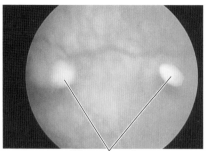

Vitreous seeding

Figure 10-247 • Retinoblastoma demonstrating endophytic growth with vitreous seeding.

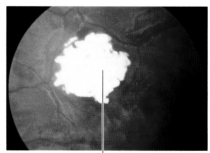

Retinoblastoma

Figure 10-248 • Retinoblastoma demonstrating discrete round tumor.

- Examination under anesthesia required for ophthalmoscopy and treatment.
- B-scan ultrasonography and CT scan to detect calcifications (80%).
- Head and orbital MRI to evaluate for extraocular extension and trilateral retinoblastoma (bilateral with pinealblastoma or parasellar mass).
- Enucleation, cryotherapy, laser photocoagulation, external beam radiation therapy, brachytherapy, and chemotherapy are all used to treat retinoblastoma; should be performed by an experienced ophthalmic oncologist.
- Oncology consultation.

Paraneoplastic Syndromes

Bilateral Diffuse Uveal Melanocytic Proliferation Syndrome

Rare paraneoplastic disorder consisting of diffuse uveal thickening with multiple, faint, yellow–orange spots or slightly elevated, pigmented lesions scattered throughout the fundus ("giraffe-skin" fundus). Occurs in elderly patients with a systemic malignancy who have progressive decreased vision; bilateral, shallow serous retinal detachments may occur late. Poor prognosis, with death within 2 years of diagnosis.

- **B-scan ultrasonography:** Diffuse uveal thickening.
- **Fluorescein angiogram:** Orange spots appear hyperfluorescent.
- **Electrophysiologic testing:** ERG (markedly reduced).
- No effective ocular treatment; treat underlying malignancy.
- Oncology consultation.

Carcinoma-Associated Retinopathy

Sudden onset of nyctalopia, decreased vision (can progress to no light perception [NLP] over months to years), dyschromatopsia, and visual field changes in patients >50 years old who have a systemic malignancy (notably small-cell lung carcinoma). Patients develop a retinal pigment degeneration with narrowed retinal vessels and vitreous cells. Poor prognosis.

- **Electrophysiologic testing:** ERG (markedly reduced).
- **Lab tests:** Antibody against recoverin.
- No effective treatment.
- Oncology consultation.

Cutaneous Melanoma-Associated Retinopathy

Subset of carcinoma-associated retinopathy (CAR) with similar symptoms and fundus findings; paraneoplastic syndrome associated with cutaneous melanoma. Antibodies to bipolar cells cause a selective loss of b-wave on ERG.

- **Electrophysiologic testing:** ERG (markedly reduced with selective loss of b-wave).
- **Lab tests:** Antibody against bipolar cell.
- No effective treatment.
- Oncology consultation.

Papilledema 483
Idiopathic Intracranial Hypertension 485
Optic Neuritis 486
Anterior Ischemic Optic Neuropathy 488
Traumatic Optic Neuropathy 491
Other Optic Neuropathies 493
Congenital Anomalies 496
Tumors 501
Chiasmal Syndromes 505
Congenital Glaucoma 508
Primary Open-Angle Glaucoma 509
Secondary Open-Angle Glaucoma 517
Normal (Low) Tension Glaucoma 520

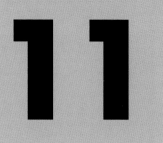

11

Optic Nerve and Glaucoma

Papilledema

Definition Optic disc swelling caused by elevated intracranial pressure (ICP).

Etiology Elevated ICP occurs in a variety of settings including: congenitally; with intracranial neoplasm or other mass; infection (meningitis, encephalitis); or subdural or subarachnoid hemorrhage. Often no cause is identified (idiopathic intracranial hypertension or pseudotumor cerebri; see below).

Symptoms Initially asymptomatic, visual loss and dyschromatopsia occur with chronic papilledema; may have headache, nausea, emesis, transient visual obscurations (lasting seconds), diplopia, altered mental status, or other neurologic deficits.

Signs Normal or decreased visual acuity and color vision, red desaturation, enlarged blind spot proportional to degree of edema, bilateral (rarely unilateral) optic disc edema with blurred disc margins, disc hyperemia, reduced physiologic cup, thickened nerve fiber layer obscuring retinal vessels, peripapillary nerve fiber layer hemorrhages, cotton-wool spots, exudates, retinal folds (Paton's lines), and absent venous pulsations (absent in 20% of normal individuals); may have cranial nerve VI palsy, vascular attenuation, visual field defects, decreased visual acuity and optic atrophy (occurs late with axonal loss). Foster–Kennedy syndrome refers to the finding of unilateral papilledema with contralateral optic atrophy and anosmia, due to an olfactory groove meningioma resulting in compression on one side (atrophy) and elevated ICP causing edema of the other disc.

Papilledema   Retinal hemorrhages

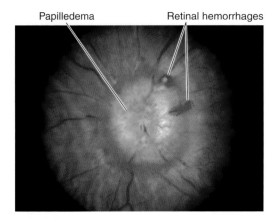

Figure 11-1 • Papilledema due to an intracranial tumor. There is marked edema of the nerve head with blurring of the disc margins 360° and two flame-shaped hemorrhages.

Differential Diagnosis Optic disc edema without elevated ICP is due to malignant hypertension, diabetic papillitis, anemia, central retinal vein occlusion, neuroretinitis, uveitis, optic neuritis, anterior ischemic optic neuropathy, Leber's optic neuropathy, hypotony, infiltration (lymphoma, leukemia), optic nerve mass, pseudopapilledema (e.g., optic nerve drusen).

Evaluation

- Complete ophthalmic history, neurologic exam, and eye exam with attention to visual acuity, color vision, pupils, and ophthalmoscopy.
- Check visual fields.
- Emergent neuroimaging: magnetic resonance imaging (MRI) to rule out intracranial processes; consider angiography (MRA/CTA) if MRI is normal.
- Lumbar puncture (after MRI) to check opening pressure and composition of cerebrospinal fluid.
- **Lab tests:** to identify etiology of disc edema if ICP is not elevated on LP: fasting blood sugar, complete blood count (CBC), erythrocyte sedimentation rate (ESR), C reactive protein (CRP), antinuclear antibody (ANA), antineutrophil cytoplasmic antibodies (ANCA), angiotensin converting enzyme (ACE).
- Check blood pressure.
- Neurology consultation.

Management

- Treat underlying etiology.

Prognosis Depends on etiology.

Idiopathic Intracranial Hypertension (Pseudotumor Cerebri)

Definition Disorder of unknown etiology that meets the following criteria: 1) signs and symptoms of increased intracranial pressure, 2) high cerebrospinal fluid pressure (>200 mmH$_2$O in nonobese and >250 mmH$_2$O in obese patient) with normal composition, 3) normal neuroimaging studies, 4) normal neurologic examination findings (except papilledema or cranial nerve VI palsy), and 5) no identifiable cause, such as an inciting medication (modified Dandy criteria).

Etiology Idiopathic; may be associated with vitamin A, tetracycline, oral contraceptive pills (due to hypercoaguability and dural sinus thrombosis), nalidixic acid, lithium, or steroid use or withdrawal; also associated with dural sinus thrombosis, radical neck surgery, middle ear disease (which may cause dural sinus thrombosis), recent weight gain, chronic obstructive pulmonary disease, and pregnancy. Idiopathic intracranial hypertension is a diagnosis of exclusion.

Epidemiology Usually occurs in obese 20–45-year-old females (2:1).

Symptoms Asymptomatic; may have headache, transient visual obscurations (lasting seconds), intracranial noises (whooshing), diplopia, pulsatile tinnitus, dizziness, nausea, and emesis.

Signs Normal or decreased visual acuity, color vision, and contrast sensitivity; bilateral optic disc edema; may have cranial nerve VI palsy (30%) or visual field defect.

Figure 11-2 • Idiopathic intracranial hypertension demonstrating papilledema.

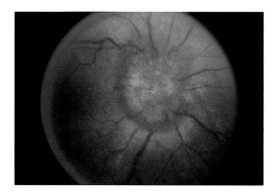

Differential Diagnosis Rule out other causes of papilledema and optic disc edema (see Papilledema section).

Evaluation
- Complete ophthalmic history, neurologic exam, and eye exam with attention to visual acuity, color vision, pupils, motility, and ophthalmoscopy.
- Check visual fields (enlarged blind spot, generalized constriction).
- Emergent head and orbital CT scan or MRI to rule out intracranial processes.
- Lumbar puncture to check opening pressure and composition of cerebrospinal fluid.
- Check blood pressure.
- Neurology consultation.

Management

- If the patient is obese, initiate a weight-loss program.
- Discontinue vitamin A, tetracycline, oral contraceptive pills, nalidixic acid, lithium, or steroid use.
- No further treatment recommended unless patient exhibits progressive visual loss, visual field defects, or intractable headaches.
- Systemic acetazolamide (Diamox) 500–2000 mg po qd.
- Consider systemic diuretics (furosemide [Lasix] 60–120 mg po divided q6h), follow visual field, visual acuity, and color vision.
- Oral steroids (prednisone 60–100 mg po qd) are controversial; check purified protein derivative (PPD) and controls, blood glucose, and chest radiographs before starting systemic steroids.
- Add H_2-blocker (ranitidine [Zantac] 150 mg po bid) or proton pump inhibitor when administering systemic steroids.
- Consider surgery for progressive visual loss despite maximal medical therapy (optic-nerve sheath fenestration, lumboperitoneal shunt).

Prognosis Usually self-limited over 6–12 months; variable if visual loss has occurred.

Optic Neuritis

Definition The term optic neuritis refers to inflammation of the optic nerve.

Papillitis

Inflammation is anterior, optic disc swelling present.

Retrobulbar

Inflammation is behind the globe, no optic disc swelling; more common.

Devic's Syndrome

Bilateral optic neuritis with transverse myelitis.

Etiology Demyelination is most common cause, others include vasculitic, infectious, and autoimmune.

Epidemiology Demyelinative optic neuritis usually occurs in 15–45-year-old females. The majority of patients with multiple sclerosis (MS) have evidence of optic neuritis; this approaches 100% in postmortem pathologic studies; optic neuritis is the initial diagnosis in 20% of MS cases; conversely, roughly 50–60% of patients with isolated optic neuritis will eventually develop MS. *Note:* optic neuritis in children is usually bilateral, postviral (i.e., mumps, measles), and less likely to be associated with MS.

Symptoms Subacute visual loss (usually progresses for 1–2 weeks followed by recovery over the following 3 months), pain on eye movement, dyschromatopsia, diminished sense of brightness; may have previous viral syndrome, or phosphenes (light flashes) on eye movement or with loud noises.

Signs Decreased visual acuity ranging from 20/20 to no light perception, visual field defect (most often central or paracentral scotoma, but any pattern of field loss can occur), decreased color vision and contrast sensitivity, relative afferent pupillary defect (RAPD); may have optic disc swelling (35%), mild vitritis, altered depth perception (Pulfrich's phenomenon), and increased latency and decreased amplitude of visual evoked response.

Differential Diagnosis Intraocular inflammation, malignant hypertension, diabetes mellitus, cat-scratch disease, optic perineuritis, sarcoidosis, syphilis, tuberculosis, collagen vascular disease, Leber's optic neuropathy, optic nerve glioma, orbital tumor, anterior ischemic optic neuropathy, central serous retinopathy, multiple evanescent white dot syndrome, acute idiopathic blind spot enlargement syndrome.

Evaluation
- Complete ophthalmic history, neurologic exam, and eye exam with attention to visual acuity, color vision, Amsler grid, contrast sensitivity, pupils, motility, and ophthalmoscopy.
- Check visual fields.
- If patient does not carry the diagnosis of MS, then obtain an MRI of the head and orbits to evaluate periventricular white matter for demyelinating lesions or plaques (best predictor of future development of MS).
- **Lab tests:** unnecessary for typical case of optic neuritis. When atypical features exist: ANA, ACE, Venereal Disease Research Laboratory (VDRL) test, fluorescent treponemal antibody absorption (FTA-ABS) test, ESR; consider *Bartonella henselae* if optic nerve swollen and exposure to kittens.
- Check blood pressure.
- Consider lumbar puncture to rule out intracranial processes.
- Neuro-ophthalmology consultation.

Management

- If MRI is positive, consider systemic steroids (methylprednisolone 250 mg IV q6h for 3 days, followed by prednisone 1 mg/kg/day for 11 days and rapid taper 20 mg/day on day 12 and 10 mg/day on days 13–15). The Optic Neuritis Treatment Trial (ONTT) showed that this regimen led to visual recovery 2 weeks faster than other treatments; however, no difference in final visual acuity, and a decreased incidence of MS over the ensuing 2 years but no difference after 3 years. *Note:* do not use oral steroids alone, because this led to an increased risk of recurrent optic neuritis (ONTT conclusion).
- Check PPD and controls, blood glucose, and chest radiographs before starting systemic steroids.
- Add H_2-blocker (ranitidine [Zantac] 150 mg po bid) or proton pump inhibitor when administering systemic steroids.
- The CHAMPS study group showed that patients receiving weekly intramuscular interferon β-1a (Avonex) following steroid therapy for a first episode of optic neuritis associated with at least two lesions on MRI greater than 3 mm had a reduction in onset of clinical MS over 3 years and improvement or less worsening of MRI lesions.

Prognosis Good in cases of demyelination; visual acuity improves over months; final acuity depends on severity of initial visual loss; 70% of patients will recover 20/20 vision; permanent subtle color vision and contrast sensitivity deficits are common; even after recovery, patient may have blurred vision with increased body temperature or exercise (Uhthoff's symptom). Approximately 30% will have another attack in either eye, and 30–50% of patients with isolated optic neuritis will develop MS over 5–10 years.

Anterior Ischemic Optic Neuropathy

Definition Ischemic infarction of anterior optic nerve due to occlusion of the posterior ciliary circulation just behind the lamina cribrosa.

Etiology Optic nerve infarction is encountered in different settings, but is often divided into two categories:

Arteritic

Occurs in the setting of giant cell arteritis ([GCA] temporal arteritis).

Nonarteritic

Occurs in several settings but is most often "spontaneous" without an identifying precipitating factor.

Epidemiology

Arteritic

Usually occurs in patients >55 years old (mostly over 70), the fellow eye is involved in 75% of cases within 2 weeks without treatment; associated with polymyalgia rheumatica.

Nonarteritic

Usually occurs in middle-aged patients; fellow eye involved in up to 40% of cases; associated with hypertension (40%), diabetes mellitus (30%), ischemic heart disease (20%), hypercholesterolemia (70%), and smoking (50%); arteriosclerotic changes are found in optic disc vessels.

Symptoms Acute, unilateral, painless visual loss (arteritic > nonarteritic) and dyschromatopsia.

Arteritic

May also have headache, fever, malaise, weight loss, scalp tenderness, jaw claudication, amaurosis fugax, diplopia, polymyalgia rheumatica symptoms (joint pain), and eye pain.

Signs Normal or decreased visual acuity, decreased color vision, RAPD, central or altitudinal visual field defect (usually inferior and large), swollen optic disc (pallor or atrophy after 6–8 weeks), fellow nerve often crowded with a small or absent cup, fellow nerve may be pale from prior episode (pseudo Foster–Kennedy syndrome; more common than true Foster–Kennedy [see above]).

Arteritic

May also have swollen, tender, temporal artery, cotton-wool spots, branch or central retinal artery occlusion, ophthalmic artery occlusion, anterior segment ischemia, cranial nerve palsy (especially cranial nerve VI); optic disc cupping occurs late; choroidal infarcts can be seen on fluorescein angiogram.

Figure 11-3 • Anterior ischemic optic neuropathy with disc edema and flame hemorrhages.

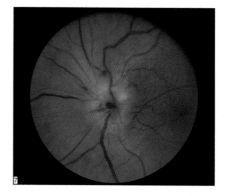

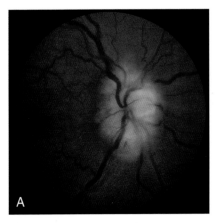 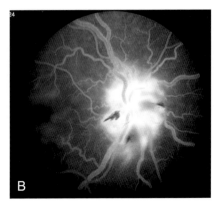

Figure 11-4 • Anterior ischemic optic neuropathy with (A) disc edema and (B) late leakage on fluorescein angiogram.

Differential Diagnosis Malignant hypertension, diabetes mellitus, retinal vascular occlusion, compressive lesion, collagen vascular disease, syphilis, herpes zoster; also migraine, postoperative, massive blood loss, normal (low) tension glaucoma.

Evaluation
- Complete ophthalmic history with attention to erectile dysfunction drugs, amiodarone, and obstructive sleep apnea.
- Complete eye exam with attention to visual acuity, color vision, Amsler grid, pupils, and ophthalmoscopy.
- Check visual fields.
- **Lab tests:** STAT ESR (to rule out arteritic form; ESR > [age/2] in men and > [(age + 10)/2] in women is abnormal), CBC (low hematocrit, high platelets), fasting blood glucose, C reactive protein (CRP), VDRL, FTA-ABS, ANA.
- Check blood pressure.
- **Arteritic:** consider temporal artery biopsy (beware; can get false-negative results from skip lesions); will remain positive up to 2 weeks after starting corticosteroids.
- Consider fluorescein angiogram: choroidal nonperfusion in arteritic form.
- Medical consultation.

Management

ARTERITIC
- Systemic steroids (methylprednisolone 1 g IV qd in divided doses for 3 days, then prednisone 60–100 mg po qd with a slow taper; decrease by no more than 2.5–5.0 mg/wk) started before results of biopsy known to prevent ischemic optic neuropathy in fellow eye; follow ESR, CRP, and symptoms carefully.

Management—Cont'd

- Check PPD and controls, blood glucose, and chest radiographs before starting systemic steroids.
- Add H_2-blocker (ranitidine [Zantac] 150 mg po bid) or proton pump inhibitor when administering systemic steroids.

NONARTERITIC
- Consider daily aspirin.

Prognosis Worse for the arteritic form associated with GCA in which visual recovery is rare. Roughly 10% with NAION will progress and slightly greater than 42% will improve (≥3 Snellen lines, but some of this perceived improvement may represent learning to scan with the remaining visual field as opposed to true axonal recovery).

Traumatic Optic Neuropathy

Definition Damage to the optic nerve (intraocular, intraorbital, or intracranial) from direct or indirect trauma.

Etiology

Direct Injuries

Orbital or cerebral trauma that transgresses normal tissue planes to disrupt the anatomic integrity of the optic nerve (e.g., penetrating injury or bone fragment).

Indirect Injuries

Forces transmitted at a distance from the optic nerve; the mechanism of injury may involve transmission of energy through the cranium, resulting in elastic deformation of the sphenoid bone, and thus a direct transfer of force to the canalicular portion of the nerve.

Optic Nerve Avulsion

Dislocation of the nerve at its point of attachment with the globe. Usually occurs with deceleration injuries causing anterior displacement of the globe.

Epidemiology Occurs in 3% of patients with severe head trauma and 2.5% of patients with midface fractures.

Symptoms Acute visual loss, dyschromatopsia, pain from associated injuries.

Signs Decreased visual acuity ranging from 20/20 to no light perception, RAPD, decreased color vision, visual field defect, optic nerve usually appears normal acutely with optic atrophy developing later; may have other signs of ocular trauma. Hemorrhage at the location of the optic disc occurs with optic nerve avulsion.

Optic nerve avulsion

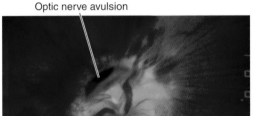

Figure 11-5 • Traumatic optic nerve avulsion.

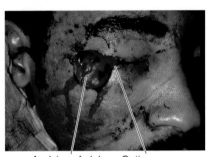

Figure 11-6 • Traumatic avulsion of the globe. The entire globe is extruded from the orbit but still attached to the optic nerve.

Avulsion of globe   Optic nerve

Differential Diagnosis Commotio, open globe, retinal detachment, Terson's syndrome, Purtscher's retinopathy, macular hole, vitreous hemorrhage.

Evaluation
- Check for associated life-threatening injuries.
- Complete ophthalmic history, neurologic exam, and eye exam with attention to mechanism of injury, visual acuity, color vision, pupils, motility, tonometry, anterior segment, and ophthalmoscopy.
- Orbital CT scan with thin coronal images through the canal to assess location and extent of damage, mechanism of injury, and associated trauma.
- Check visual fields.
- Medical or neurology consultation may be required for associated injuries.

Management

- Consider megadose systemic steroids (methylprednisolone 30 mg/kg IV initial dose, then starting 2 hours later 15 mg/kg every 6 hours for 1–3 days); controversial because dosage, length of treatment, and efficacy are unproved.
- Consider surgical decompression if there is no improvement or there is radiographic evidence of optic canal fracture.

Prognosis Usually poor, depends on degree of optic nerve damage; 20–35% improve spontaneously.

Other Optic Neuropathies

Definition Variety of processes that cause unilateral or bilateral optic nerve damage and subsequent optic atrophy. Atrophy of axons with resultant disc pallor occurs 6–8 weeks after injury anterior to the lateral geniculate nucleus.

Figure 11-7 • Optic atrophy demonstrating pale nerve. The optic nerve pallor is most striking in the inferotemporal region of the disc (arrowhead).

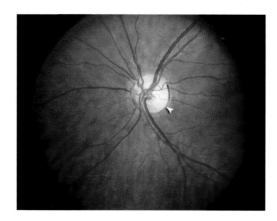

Etiology

Compressive

Neoplasm (orbit, suprasellar), thyroid-related ophthalmopathy, hematoma.

Hereditary

Isolated

Leber's Hereditary Optic Neuropathy Typically occurs in 10- to 30-year-old males (9:1). Rapid, severe visual loss that starts unilaterally, but sequentially involves fellow eye usually within 1 year but can be within days to weeks. Optic nerve hyperemia and swollen nerve fiber layer with small, peripapillary, telangiectatic blood vessels that do not leak on fluorescein angiography (optic nerve also does not stain). Mitochondrial DNA mutation – mothers transmit defect to all sons (50% affected) and all daughters are carriers (10% affected). Three common mutations in the mitochondrial genome at nucleotide positions 3460, 11778, and 14484 have been identified.

Dominant Optic Atrophy (Kjer or Juvenile Optic Atrophy) Most common hereditary optic neuropathy, prevalence of 1:12,000 to 1:50,000; highly variable age of onset (mean around 4 to 6 years of age). Mild, insidious loss of vision (ranging from 20/20 to 20/800), tritanopic dyschromatopsia; slight progression; nystagmus rare; a wedge of pallor is seen on the temporal aspect of the disc (temporal excavation). Mapped to chromosome 3q28-q29 (OPA1 gene, 18q12.2-q12.3 (OPA4 gene), and 22q12-q13 (OPA5 gene).

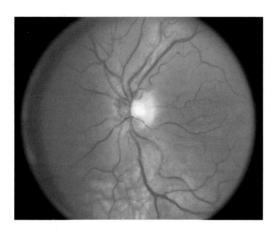

Figure 11-8 • Leber's hereditary optic neuropathy with optic nerve pallor.

Other

- **Recessive optic atrophy (Costeff syndrome):** mapped to OPA6 gene on chromosome 8q21-q22.
- **X-linked optic atrophy:** mapped to OPA2 gene on chromosome Xp11.4-p11.2.

With syndrome

DIDMOAD (Wolfram's Syndrome) Diabetes insipidus, diabetes mellitus, optic atrophy, and deafness. Early onset, rapid progression. Mitochondrial DNA inheritance. Mapped to chromosome 4p16.1 (WFS1 gene) and 4q22-q24 (WFS2 gene).

Complicated hereditary infantile optic atrophy (Behr's syndrome) Occurs between 1 and 8 years of age; male predilection. Moderate visual loss; no progression; associated with nystagmus in 50%, increased deep tendon reflexes, spasticity, hypotonia, ataxia, urinary incontinence, pes cavus, and mental retardation. Mapped to chromosome 19q13 (OPA3 gene).

Other Various syndromic hereditary optic neuropathies often with deafness and other systemic findings.

Infectious

Toxoplasmosis, toxocariasis, cytomegalovirus, tuberculosis.

Infiltrative

Sarcoidosis, malignancy (lymphoma, leukemia, carcinoma, plasmacytoma, metastasis).

Ischemic

Radiation.

Nutritional

Various vitamin deficiencies including B_1 (thiamine), B_2 (riboflavin), B_6 (pyridoxine), B_{12} (cobalamin), and folic acid.

Toxic

Most commonly due to ethambutol; rarer causes include isoniazid, chloramphenicol, streptomycin, arsenic, lead, methanol, digitalis, chloroquine, quinine, and tobacco-related or alcohol-related amblyopia.

There are anecdotal reports of an ischemic-like optic neuropathy occurring with the use of erectile dysfunction drugs (i.e., sildenafil, vardenafil, tadalafil) and amiodarone. Whether a true causative relationship exists remains to be determined; however, patients with ischemic optic neuropathy should probably be instructed to avoid such medications if possible. Additionally, rare reports of optic neuropathy following LASIK and epi-LASIK have been described possibly related to increased intraocular pressure from the suction ring.

Symptoms Decreased vision, dyschromatopsia, visual field loss.

Signs Unilateral or bilateral decreased visual acuity ranging from 20/20 to 20/400, decreased color vision, and decreased contrast sensitivity; RAPD if optic nerve damage is asymmetric (if symmetric damage, RAPD may be absent); optic disc pallor, retinal nerve fiber layer defects, visual field defects (central or cecocentral scotomas); abnormal visual evoked response; retrobulbar mass lesions may cause proptosis and motility deficits.

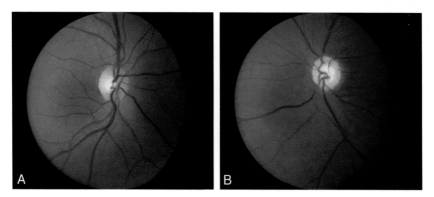

Figure 11-9 • Patient with optic atrophy OS demonstrating (A) normal optic nerve OD and (B) pallor of the nerve head OS.

Differential Diagnosis As above; normal tension glaucoma.

Evaluation
- Complete ophthalmic history, neurologic exam, and eye exam with attention to visual acuity, color vision, pupils, motility, exophthalmometry, and ophthalmoscopy.
- Check visual fields.
- Head and orbital CT scan or MRI to rule out intracranial processes or mass lesion.

- Consider lab tests: CBC; vitamin B_1, B_2, B_6, B_{12}, and folate levels; toxin screen; ELISA for *Toxoplasma* and *Toxocara* antibody titers, HIV antibody test, CD4 count, HIV viral load, urine CMV, purified protein derivative (PPD) and controls.
- Consider medical or oncology consultation.

Management

- Treatment depends on etiology.

COMPRESSIVE

- Oral steroids (prednisone 60–200 mg po qd) and surgical decompression for thyroid-related ophthalmopathy.
- Consider surgical resection for some tumors.

HEREDITARY

- No effective treatment.
- Genetic counseling.
- Molecular screening may add prognostic value.

INFECTIOUS

- May require systemic antiinfectives.

INFILTRATIVE

- Leukemic optic nerve infiltration occurs in children and is an ophthalmic emergency that requires radiation therapy to salvage vision. Do not initiate steroids prior to oncology evaluation with bone marrow biopsy if leukemia is possible.

NUTRITIONAL

- Consider vitamin B_1 (thiamine 100 mg po bid), vitamin B_{12} (1 mg IM q month), folate (0.1 mg po qd), or multivitamin (qd) supplementation.

TOXIC

- Discontinue offending toxic agent.

Prognosis Depends on etiology; poor once optic atrophy has occurred.

Congenital Anomalies

Definition Variety of developmental optic nerve abnormalities.

Figure 11-10 • Anomalous optic nerve. Note the atypical configuration of the vessels (arrowhead) as they emerge from the nerve head.

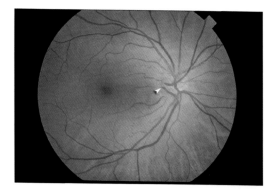

Aplasia

Very rare, no optic nerve or retinal vessels present.

Dysplasias

Coloboma

Spectrum of large, abnormal-appearing optic discs due to incomplete closure of the embryonic fissure; usually located inferonasally; associated with other ocular colobomata. May be associated with systemic defects including congenital heart defects, double aortic arch, transposition of the great vessels, coarctation of the aorta, and intracranial carotid anomalies.

Figure 11-11 • Optic nerve coloboma demonstrating large abnormal disc that appears elongated inferiorly with irregular pattern of vessels.

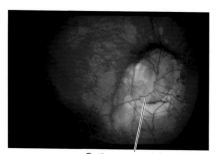

Optic nerve coloboma

Hypoplasia

Small discs, "double ring" sign (peripapillary ring of pigmentary changes). Unilateral cases usually idiopathic; bilateral cases associated with midline abnormalities, endocrine dysfunction, and maternal history of diabetes mellitus or drug use (dilantin, quinine, alcohol, LSD) during pregnancy.

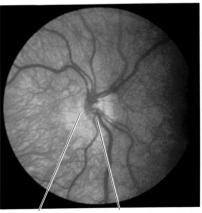

Figure 11-12 • Optic nerve hypoplasia demonstrating "double ring" sign or peripapillary ring of pigmentary changes.

"Double ring" sign   Optic nerve hypoplasia

Morning Glory Syndrome

Large, unilateral, excavated disc with central, white, glial tissue surrounded by elevated pigment ring; may represent a form of optic nerve coloboma. Female predilection (2:1); usually severe visual loss; may develop a localized serous retinal detachment; associated with midline facial defects and forebrain anomalies. May be associated with the papillorenal syndrome, a PAX2 gene mutation.

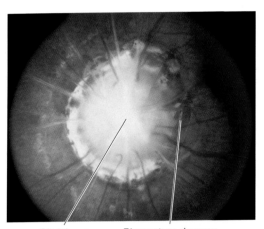

Figure 11-13 • Morning glory syndrome demonstrating characteristic appearance with central white glial tissue, surrounding pigmentary changes, and straightened spokelike vessels radiating from disc.

Glial tissue   Pigmentary changes

Optic Nerve Drusen

Superficial or buried hyaline-like material in the substance of the nerve anterior to the lamina cribrosa; may calcify. 75% bilateral; may be hereditary (AD); associated with retinitis pigmentosa; may develop visual field defects usually inferonasal or arcuate scotomas.

Figure 11-14 • Optic nerve drusen (arrowheads). Multiple drusen are evident as elevated, chunky, refractile nodules.

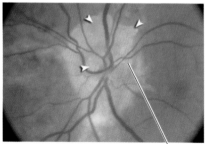

Optic nerve drusen

Figure 11-15 • Optic nerve drusen demonstrating autofluorescence when fluorescein filters are in place through a fundus camera. The multiple drusen are quite evident as small, round bumps. This view is obtained without injecting any fluorescein dye.

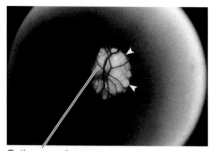

Optic nerve drusen

Figure 11-16 • Orbital CT of optic nerve drusen demonstrating calcification

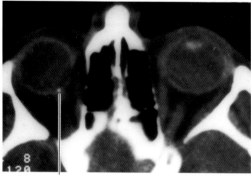

Optic nerve drusen

Pit

Depression in optic disc, 0.1–0.7 disc diameter, usually located temporally; appears gray–white; 85% unilateral. Peripapillary retinal pigment epithelium changes in 95%; 40% develop localized serous retinal detachment in teardrop configuration extending from the pit into papillomacular retina; source of subretinal fluid (cerebrospinal fluid vs. liquefied vitreous) is controversial; retinal detachments often resolve spontaneously.

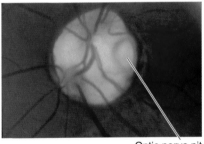

Optic nerve pit

Figure 11-17 • Optic nerve pit demonstrating round depression in neural rim at typical temporal location.

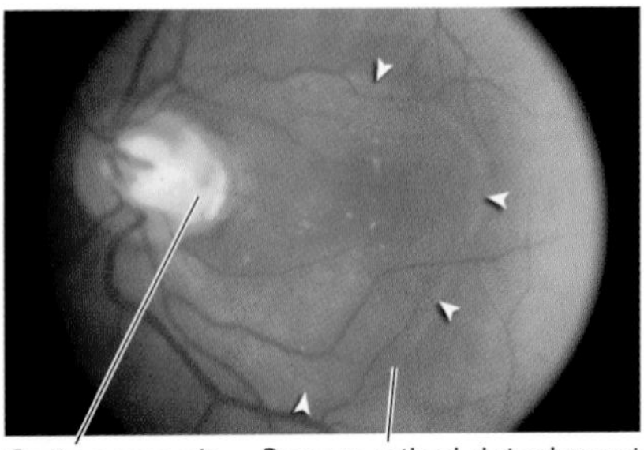

Optic nerve pit   Serous retinal detachment

Figure 11-18 • Optic nerve pit with serous retinal detachment (arrowheads).

Optic pit   Macular schisis

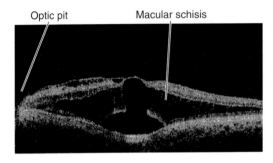

Figure 11-19 • Spectral domain optical coherence tomography of optic nerve pit with serous macular detachment.

Septo-Optic Dysplasia (De Morsier Syndrome)

Syndrome of optic disc hypoplasia, absence of septum pellucidum, agenesis of corpus callosum, and endocrine problems; may have see-saw nystagmus. Associated with mutations in the HESX-1 gene.

Tilted Optic Disc

Displacement of one side of optic disc peripherally with oblique insertion of retinal vessels. Associated with high myopia (may have visual field defect that is usually felt to be refractive in nature with a staphyloma adjacent to the optic disc); can cause bitemporal visual field defects that do not respect the vertical midline.

Symptoms Asymptomatic; may have decreased vision, metamorphopsia, or visual field loss.

Signs Normal or decreased visual acuity, abnormal appearing optic disc, variety of visual field defects; may have RAPD. Drusen can be visualized on B-scan ultrasonogram, CT scan, and MRI, and autofluorescence occurs on fluorescein angiogram.

Differential Diagnosis See above; optic disc drusen may give appearance of papilledema (pseudopapilledema).

Evaluation

- Complete ophthalmic history and eye exam with attention to visual acuity, color vision, pupils, and ophthalmoscopy.
- Check visual fields.
- **Fluorescein angiogram:** serous retinal detachment with early punctate fluorescence and late filling may be seen with optic pits; optic nerve drusen autofluoresce with only filter in place before any fluorescein administration.
- Consider B-scan ultrasonography to identify buried drusen.
- Head and orbital CT scan for dysplasias.
- Endocrine consultation for hypoplasia.

Management

- No treatment usually required.
- May require polycarbonate protective lenses if amblyopia or decreased visual acuity present.
- Laser photocoagulation to demarcate serous retinal detachments associated with optic pits (controversial); may also consider pars plana vitrectomy, peeling of posterior hyaloid, air-fluid exchange, and long-acting gas tamponade if laser fails (controversial).
- Treat any underlying endocrine abnormalities.

Prognosis Most congenitally anomalous discs are not associated with progressive visual loss. Decreased vision from compression, choroidal neovascularization, or central retinal artery or vein occlusion can occur rarely with optic nerve drusen; basal encephalocele can occur in any of the dysplasias.

Tumors

Definition Variety of intrinsic neoplasms (benign and malignant) that may affect the optic nerve anywhere along its course.

Angioma (von Hippel Lesion)

Retinal capillary hemangioma (see Chapter 10); benign lesion that may involve the optic nerve. May be associated with intracranial (especially cerebellar) hemangiomas (von Hippel-Lindau syndrome) (see Figs 10-211, 10-228, and 10-229).

Astrocytic Hamartoma

Benign, yellow–white lesion that occurs in tuberous sclerosis and neurofibromatosis (see Chapter 10); may be smooth or have nodular, glistening, "mulberry-like" appearance; may be isolated, multiple, unilateral, or bilateral (see Figs 10-219 and 10-220).

Combined Hamartoma of Retina and Retinal Pigment Epithelium

Rare, peripapillary tumor composed of retinal, retinal pigment epithelial, vascular, and glial tissue. May cause epiretinal membranes with macular traction or edema (see Chapter 10; Fig. 10-236).

Glioma

Two types:

Glioblastoma multiforme

Rare, malignant tumor found in adults who develop rapid, occasionally painful visual loss, with chiasmal extension the fellow eye may be involved. Aggressive tumor with blindness in months and death within 6–9 months if not completely excised; may have central retinal artery or central retinal vein occlusion as tumor compromises blood supply. Enlargement of optic canal present on CT scan; endocrine or neurologic deficits may appear if tumor invades other structures.

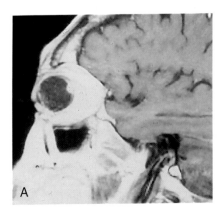 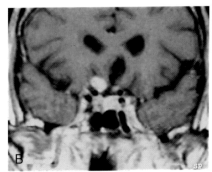

Figure 11-20 • MRI (T1) of optic nerve glioma (glioblastoma multiforme) demonstrating involvement of the right optic nerve which appears as a hyperintense enlargement (A) intraocularly at the nerve head, and (B) intracranially along the course of the nerve.

Juvenile pilocytic astrocytoma

Most common intrinsic neoplasm of the optic nerve accounting for 65% of such tumors; benign. Two distinct growth patterns: *intraneural glial proliferation* (most common, growth occurs within individual fascicles) and *perineural arachnoidal gliomatosis* (PAG; characterized by florid invasion of the leptomeninges with relative sparing of the nerve itself). 90% occur in the first and second decades with peak between 2 and 6 years of age. Causes gradual, unilateral, progressive, painless proptosis, decreased vision, RAPD, and optic disc edema; optic atrophy or strabismus may develop later; chiasmal involvement in 50% of cases. Orbital CT scan shows fusiform enlargement of the optic nerve; histologically characterized by Rosenthal fibers, pilocytic astrocytes, and myxomatous differentiation. Associated with neurofibromatosis type 1 in 25–50% of cases.

Melanocytoma

Benign, darkly pigmented tumor located over or adjacent to the optic disc, usually jet black with fuzzy borders; rarely increases in size. More common in African Americans. Malignant transformation is exceedingly rare.

Figure 11-21 • Melanocytoma. This darkly pigmented tumor is obscuring most of the optic nerve head inferiorly.

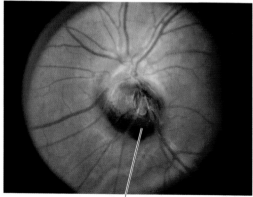

Melanocytoma

Meningioma

Rare, histologically benign tumor arising from optic nerve sheath arachnoid tissue or from adjacent meninges. Usually occurs in middle-aged females (3:1) in the third to fifth decades. Signs include unilateral proptosis, painless decreased visual acuity and color vision, RAPD, opticociliary shunt vessels, and optic nerve edema or atrophy; may grow rapidly during pregnancy and involute after delivery; optic nerve pallor and opticociliary shunt vessels occur later. Orbital CT scan demonstrates tubular enlargement of the optic nerve, hyperostosis, and calcification resulting in the "train-track" sign seen on axial views and "double ring" appearance seen on coronal views. Histologic features include whorl pattern and psammoma bodies (meningocytes that form whorls around hyalinized calcium salts).

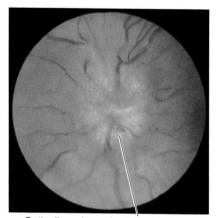

Optic disc edema due to meningioma

Figure 11-22 • Meningioma producing optic disc edema.

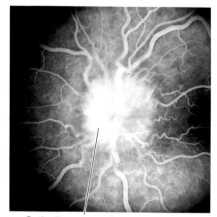

Optic disc edema due to meningioma

Figure 11-23 • Fluorescein angiogram of same patient as Figure 11-22 demonstrating leakage of fluorescein from the optic disc.

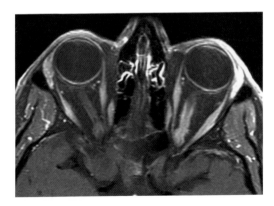

Figure 11-24 • MRI (T1) of optic nerve sheath meningioma demonstrating tubular enlargement of the left optic nerve with "train track" sign.

Symptoms Asymptomatic; may have decreased vision, dyschromatopsia, metamorphopsia with distortion of the posterior globe.

Signs Normal or decreased visual acuity and color vision, RAPD, proptosis, motility disturbances, increased intraocular pressure, optic nerve or peripapillary lesion, optic disc swelling or pallor, visual field defect; opticociliary shunt vessels in meningioma; angiomas may rarely cause vitreous or retinal hemorrhage.

Differential Diagnosis See above.

Evaluation
- Complete ophthalmic history, neurologic exam, and eye exam with attention to visual acuity, color vision, pupils, exophthalmometry, tonometry, and ophthalmoscopy.
- Check visual fields.
- B-scan ultrasonography to evaluate course of optic nerve.
- Fluorescein angiogram to rule out retinal angiomas.
- Head and orbital CT scan or MRI (also to rule out intracranial lesions): optic nerve enlargement, train track sign (ringlike calcification of outer nerve), or bony erosion of optic canal.

Management

- Treatment depends on etiology and is controversial; younger patients with meningiomas or gliomas are treated more aggressively.
- May require treatment of increased intraocular pressure (see Primary Open-Angle Glaucoma section).
- Consider laser photocoagulation of angiomas (see Chapter 10).
- Treatment of malignant tumors with chemotherapy, radiation, or surgery should be performed by a tumor specialist.

Prognosis Good for benign lesions, variable for meningiomas, and poor for malignant lesions.

Chiasmal Syndromes

Definition Variety of optic chiasm disorders that cause visual field defects.

Epidemiology Mass lesions in 95% of cases, usually pituitary tumor. Most lesions are large, because chiasm is 10 mm above the sella turcica (microadenomas do not cause field defects); may occur acutely with pituitary apoplexy secondary to hemorrhage or necrosis.

Symptoms Asymptomatic; may have headache, decreased vision, dyschromatopsia, visual field loss, diplopia, or vague visual complaints; systemically decreased libido, malaise, galactorrhea or inability to conceive may be present.

Signs Normal or decreased visual acuity and color vision; may have RAPD, optic atrophy, visual field defect (junctional scotoma, bitemporal hemianopia, incongruous homonymous hemianopia), or signs of pituitary apoplexy (severe headache, ophthalmoplegia, and decreased visual acuity).

Figure 11-25 • Optic atrophy demonstrating "bow-tie" appearance of pallor in the horizontal meridian (arrowheads).

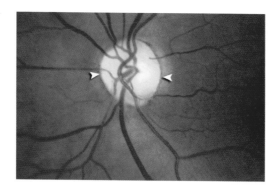

Differential Diagnosis Pituitary tumor, pituitary apoplexy, meningioma, aneurysm, trauma, sarcoidosis, craniopharyngioma, chiasmal neuritis, glioma, ethambutol.

Evaluation
- Complete ophthalmic history, endocrine history, and eye exam with attention to visual acuity, color vision, pupils, and ophthalmoscopy.
- Check visual fields with attention to vertical midline.
- Head and orbital CT scan or MRI (emergenDt if pituitary apoplexy suspected).
- **Lab tests:** consider checking hormone levels.

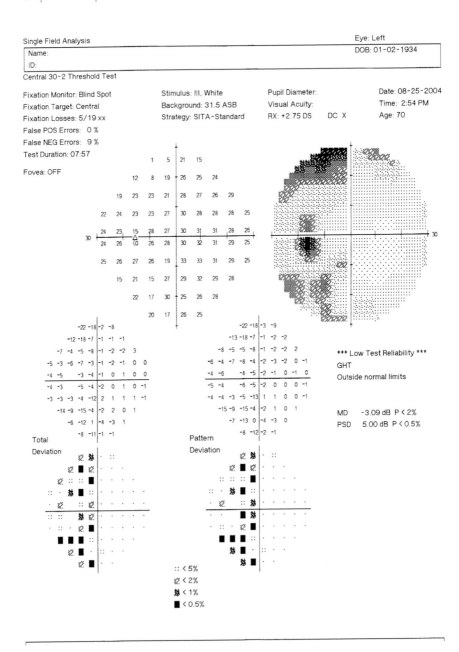

A

Figure 11-26 • A and B Humphrey visual fields of a patient with a pituitary tumor demonstrating bitemporal hemianopic field defects.

Continued

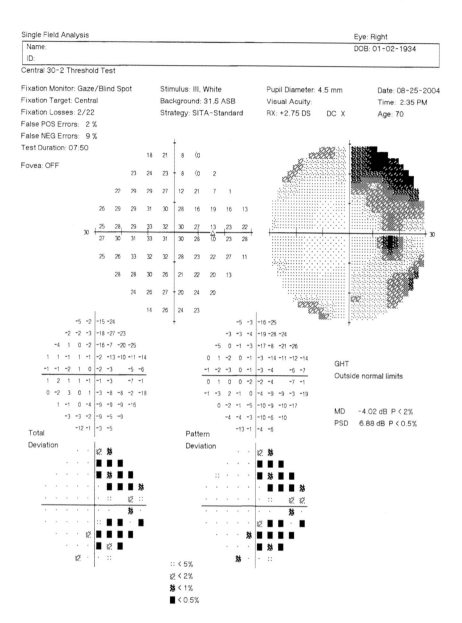

Single Field Analysis

Eye: Right

Name:
ID:

DOB: 01-02-1934

Central 30-2 Threshold Test

Fixation Monitor: Gaze/Blind Spot
Fixation Target: Central
Fixation Losses: 2/22
False POS Errors: 2 %
False NEG Errors: 9 %
Test Duration: 07:50

Fovea: OFF

Stimulus: III, White
Background: 31.5 ASB
Strategy: SITA-Standard

Pupil Diameter: 4.5 mm
Visual Acuity:
RX: +2.75 DS   DC X

Date: 08-25-2004
Time: 2:35 PM
Age: 70

GHT
Outside normal limits

MD   -4.02 dB P < 2%
PSD   6.88 dB P < 0.5%

Total Deviation

Pattern Deviation

:: < 5%
✗ < 2%
❋ < 1%
■ < 0.5%

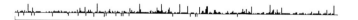

B

© 2005 Carl Zeiss Meditec
HFA II 750-1895-12.5/14.0

Figure 11-26—Cont'd

Management

- Treatment depends on etiology.
- Pituitary lesions that require surgery, radiation therapy, bromocriptine, hormone replacement should be managed by a neurosurgeon or internist or both.
- Systemic steroids and surgical decompression for pituitary apoplexy.

Prognosis Depends on etiology; pituitary tumors have a fairly good prognosis.

Congenital Glaucoma

Definition Congenital: onset of glaucoma from birth to 3 months of age (infantile, 3 months to 3 years; juvenile, 3 to 35 years).

Epidemiology Incidence of 1 in 10,000 births. Three forms: approximately one-third primary, one-third secondary, one-third associated with systemic syndromes or anomalies.

Primary

Seventy percent bilateral, 65% male, multifactorial inheritance, 40% at birth, 85% by 1 year of age. Mapped to chromosome 1p36 (GLC3B gene) and 2p22-p21 (GLC3A gene, CYP1B1 gene). A mutation in the CYP1B1 gene accounts for ~ 85% of congenital glaucoma.

Secondary

Inflammation, steroid induced, lens induced, trauma, tumors.

Associated syndromes

Mesodermal dysgenesis syndromes, aniridia, persistent hyperplastic primary vitreous, nanophthalmos, rubella, nevus of Ota, Sturge–Weber syndrome, neurofibromatosis, Marfan's syndrome, Weill–Marchesani syndrome, Lowe's syndrome, mucopolysaccharidoses.

Mechanism

Primary

Developmental abnormality of the angle (goniodysgenesis) with faulty cleavage and abnormal insertion of ciliary muscle. Associated with mutations in CYP1B1 gene, a member of the cytochrome p450 gene family.

Symptoms Epiphora, photophobia, blepharospasm.

Signs Decreased visual acuity, myopia (primary or secondary to pressure induced change), amblyopia, increased intraocular pressure, corneal diameter >12 mm by 1 year of age, corneal edema, Haab's striae (breaks in Descemet's membrane horizontal or concentric to limbus; see Figure 5-66), optic nerve cupping (may reverse with treatment), buphthalmos (enlarged eye).

Differential Diagnosis Nasolacrimal duct obstruction, megalocornea, high myopia, proptosis, birth trauma, congenital hereditary endothelial dystrophy of the cornea, sclerocornea, metabolic diseases.

Evaluation

- Complete ophthalmic history and eye exam with attention to retinoscopy, tonometry, corneal diameter, gonioscopy, and ophthalmoscopy.
- May require examination under anesthesia. *Note:* intraocular pressure affected by anesthetic agents (transiently increased by ketamine; decreased by inhalants).
- Check visual fields in older children.

Management

- Treatment is primarily surgical but depends on the type of glaucoma, intraocular pressure level and control, and amount and progression of optic nerve cupping and visual field defects (older children); should be performed by a glaucoma specialist; treatment options include:
  - **Medical (temporize before surgery):** topical β-blocker (timolol maleate [Timoptic] or betaxolol [Betoptic S] bid) or carbonic anhydrase inhibitor (dorzolamide [Trusopt] tid, brinzolamide [Azopt] tid, or acetazolamide [Diamox] 15 mg/kg/d po), or both. Miotic agents may be associated with a paradoxical increase in intraocular pressure; brimonidine [Alphagan] may be associated with infant death.
  - **Surgical:** goniotomy, trabeculotomy; also trabeculectomy, glaucoma drainage implant, cycloablation.
- Correct any refractive error (myopia).
- Patching or occlusion therapy for amblyopia (see Chapter 12).

Prognosis Usually poor; best for primary congenital form and onset between 1 and 24 months of age.

▎Primary Open-Angle Glaucoma

Definition Progressive, bilateral, optic neuropathy with open angles, typical pattern of nerve fiber bundle visual field loss, and increased intraocular pressure (IOP >21 mmHg) not caused by another systemic or local disease (see Secondary Open-Angle Glaucoma section).

Epidemiology Occurs in 2–5% of population >40 years old; risk increases with age; most common form of glaucoma (60–70%); no sex predilection. Risk factors are increased intraocular pressure, increased cup:disc ratio, thinner central corneal thickness (less than ~550 μm by ultrasound or ~520 μm by optical pachymetry), race (African Americans are 3–6 times more likely to develop primary open-angle glaucoma [POAG] than Caucasians; POAG also occurs earlier, is six times more likely to cause blindness, and is the leading cause of blindness in African Americans), increased age, and positive family history in first-degree relatives (parents, siblings). Inconsistently associated factors include myopia, diabetes mellitus, hypertension, and cardiovascular disease. Mapped to chromosome 2qcen-q13 (GLC1B gene), 2p15-p16 (GLC1H gene), 3q21-q24 (GLC1C gene),

5q22 (GLC1G gene), 7q35-q36 (GLC1F gene), 8q23 (GLC1D gene), 10p14 (GLC1E gene, OPTN gene). A mutation in the OPTN gene accounts for ~ 17% of POAG.

Mechanism

Elevated Intraocular Pressure

Mechanical resistance to outflow (at juxtacanalicular meshwork), disturbance of trabecular meshwork collagen, trabecular meshwork endothelial cell dysfunction, basement membrane thickening, glycosaminoglycan deposition, narrowed intertrabecular spaces, collapse of Schlemm's canal. A subgroup of patients has been identified with mutations of the myocilin glycoprotein. This protein is also mutated in patients with autosomal dominant juvenile open-angle glaucoma (GLC1A, MYOC/TIGR gene), which has been mapped to chromosome 1q23-q25.

Optic Nerve Damage

Various theories:

Mechanical

Compression of optic nerve fibers against lamina cribrosa with interruption of axoplasmic flow.

Vascular

Poor optic nerve perfusion or disturbed blood flow autoregulation.

Other pathways leading to ganglion cell necrosis or apoptosis

Excitotoxicity (glutamate), neurotrophin starvation, autoimmunity, abnormal glial-neuronal interactions (TNF), defects in endogenous protective mechanisms (heat shock proteins).

Symptoms Asymptomatic; may have decreased vision or constricted visual fields in late stages.

Signs Normal or decreased visual acuity, increased intraocular pressure, optic nerve cupping, splinter hemorrhages at optic disc, retinal nerve fiber layer defects, visual field defects.

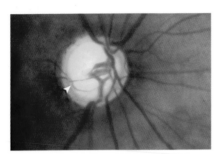

Figure 11-27 • Optic nerve cupping due to primary open-angle glaucoma. Note the extreme degree of disc excavation and course of the vessels at the poles and temporally as they travel up and over the rim giving a "bean pot" configuration (arrowhead).

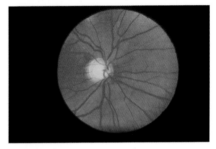

Figure 11-28 • Physiologic cupping. Although the cup is large, there is a healthy rim of neural tissue 360°.

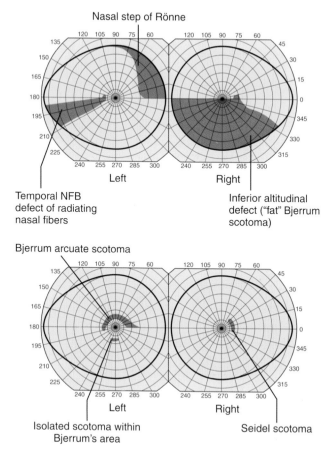

Figure 11-29 • Composite diagram depicting different types of field defects. NFB, nerve fiber bundle.

Differential Diagnosis Secondary open-angle glaucoma, normal tension glaucoma, ocular hypertension, optic neuropathy, physiologic cupping.

Evaluation

- Complete ophthalmic history and eye exam with attention to cornea, tonometry, anterior chamber, gonioscopy, iris, lens, and ophthalmoscopy.

- Check corneal pachymetry (IOP measurement by applanation tonometry may be artifactually high or low for thicker or thinner than average corneas, respectively).

- Check visual fields: visual field defects characteristic of glaucoma include paracentral scotomas (within central 10° of fixation), arcuate (Bjerrum) scotomas (isolated, nasal step of Ronne, or Seidel [connected to blind spot]), and temporal wedge.

- Stereo optic nerve photos are useful for comparison at subsequent evaluations.

- Optic nerve head analysis: various methods including confocal scanning laser ophthalmoscopy (HRT, TopSS), optical coherence tomography (OCT), scanning laser polarimetry (Nerve Fiber Analyzer, GDx), and optic nerve blood flow measurement (color Doppler imaging and laser Doppler flowmetry).

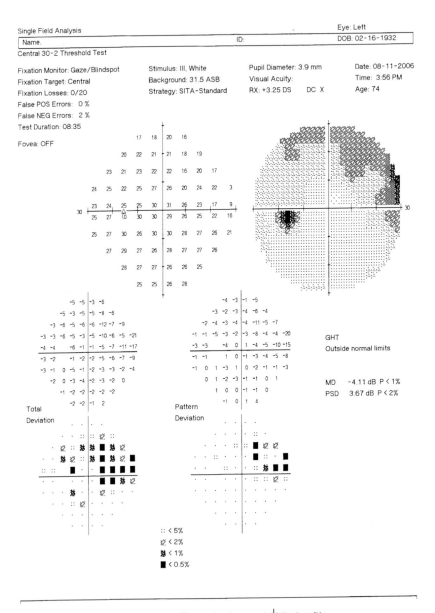

© 1994-2000 Humphrey Systems
HFA II 750-1895-12.5/12.5

Figure 11-30 • Humphrey visual field of the left eye demonstrating superior nasal step defect.

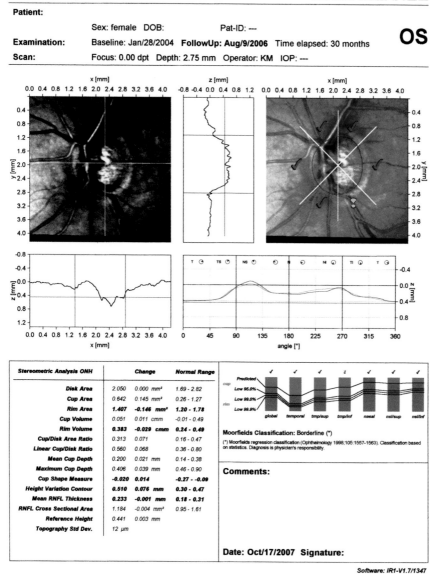

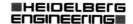

Figure 11-31 • Heidelberg Retinal Tomograph (HRT) of same patient as Figure 11-30 demonstrating inferotemporal nerve fiber layer thinning (yellow exclamation point).

STRATUS OCT
RNFL Thickness Average Analysis Report - 4.0.7 (0132)

ZEISS

	Scan Type: Fast RNFL Thickness (3.4)
	Scan Date: 10/17/2007
DOB: NA, Female	Scan Length: 10.87 mm

OD

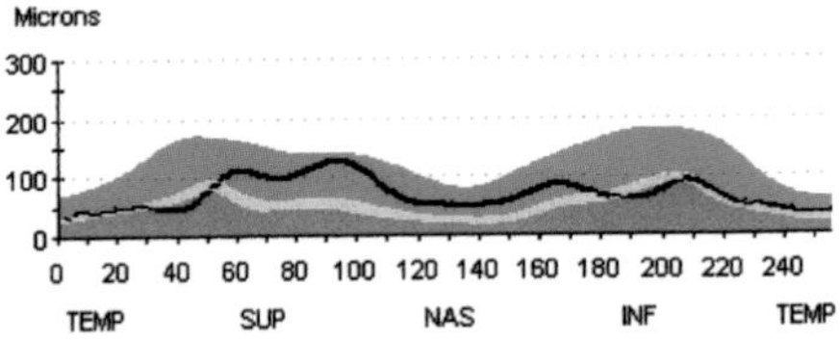

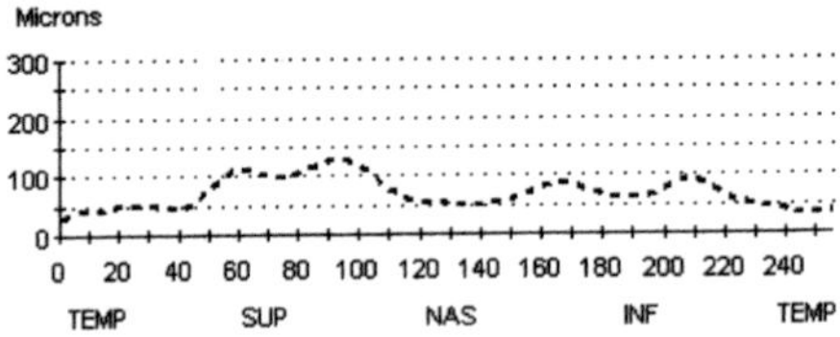

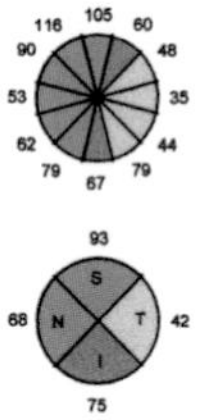

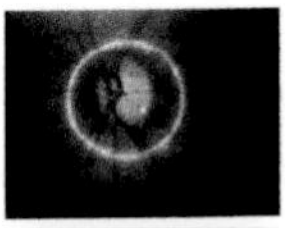

OS

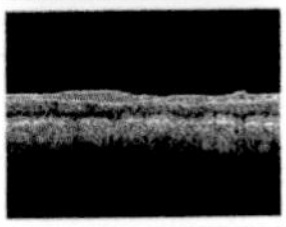

Signal Strength (Max 10)	10

	OD (N=0)	OS (N=3)	OD-OS
Imax/Smax	0.00	0.74	-0.74
Smax/Imax	0.00	1.35	-1.35
Smax/Tavg	0.00	2.98	-2.98
Imax/Tavg	0.00	2.20	-2.20
Smax/Navg	0.00	1.85	-1.85
Max-Min	0.00	95.00	-95.00
Smax	0.00	126.00	-126.00
Imax	0.00	94.00	-94.00
Savg	0.00	93.00	-93.00
Iavg	0.00	75.00	-75.00
Avg.Thick	0.00	69.74	-69.74

----- **OS**

OS	Scans used	1, 2, 3

Normal distribution Percentiles	100%
	95%
	5%
	1%
	0%

Signature:

Physician:

Figure 11-32 • Stratus optical coherence tomography evaluation of same patient as Figure 11-30 demonstrating inferotemporal nerve fiber layer thinning (red and yellow quadrants).

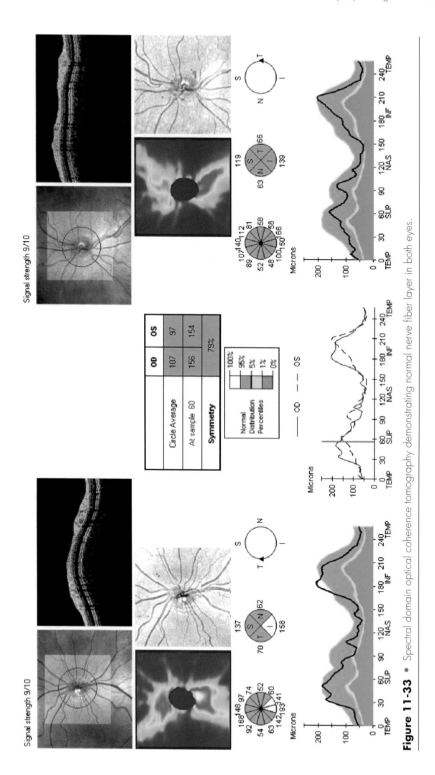

Figure 11-33 • Spectral domain optical coherence tomography demonstrating normal nerve fiber layer in both eyes.

Management

- Choice and order of treatment modality depend on many factors, including patient's age, intraocular pressure level and control, and amount and progression of optic nerve cupping and visual field defects. Treatment options include:
  - **Observation:** intraocular pressure checks every 3–6 months, visual field examination every 6–12 months, gonioscopy and optic nerve evaluation yearly.
  - **Medical:** topical β-blockers traditionally have been the first line of treatment; however, the topical prostaglandin analogues have become first-line drugs and have a better safety profile. If intraocular pressure is not controlled, additional medications can be added. Follow-up (after intraocular pressure stabilization) at 3–4 weeks after changing treatment to evaluate efficacy. Treatment options include single agent or combination therapy with the following medications:
    - Topical prostaglandin analogue (latanoprost [Xalatan], travopost [Travatan], or bimatoprost [Lumigan] qd); increases uveoscleral outflow.
    - Topical β-blocker (timolol maleate [Timoptic], betaxolol hydrochloride [Betoptic S] selective β_1-blocker, levobunolol hydrochloride [Betagan], metipranolol [OptiPranolol], carteolol hydrochloride [Ocupress] bid, or timolol gel [Timoptic XE] qd); decreases aqueous production; check for history of cardiac and pulmonary disease before prescribing.
    - Topical α-adrenergic agonist (brimonidine tartrate [Alphagan-P] tid, apraclonidine hydrochloride [Iopidine] tid, or dipivefrin hydrochloride [Propine] bid); decreases aqueous production.
    - Topical carbonic anhydrase inhibitor (dorzolamide hydrochloride [Trusopt], or brinzolamide [Azopt] tid); decreases aqueous production.
    - Topical cholinergic medication (pilocarpine qid, carbachol tid, or phospholine iodide bid); increases outflow through trabecular meshwork.
    - Systemic carbonic anhydrase inhibitor (acetazolamide [Diamox] or methazolamide [Neptazane] qd to qid); decreases aqueous production; rarely used due to systemic side effects.
  - **Laser:** trabeculoplasty, sclerostomy, cyclophotocoagulation:
    - *Argon laser trabeculoplasty procedure parameters:* 0.1 sec duration, 50 μ spot size, 600–1200 mW power, approximately 50 spot applications per 180°, a contact lens is used to stabilize the eye and better focus the beam, spots are placed on the pigmented trabecular meshwork, and the power setting is adjusted until a slight blanching of tissue is observed.
    - *Selective laser trabeculoplasty procedure parameters:* 0.7–0.9 mJ power, time and spot size (400 μm) are fixed, approximately 50 confluent spot applications per 180°, spots are placed to straddle the trabecular meshwork, and the power setting is adjusted until a small bubble is produced.
  - **Surgical:** trabeculectomy, glaucoma drainage implant, cycloablation.

Figure 11-34 • Conjunctival filtering bleb following glaucoma surgery (trabeculectomy), demonstrating typical appearance of a well-functioning, thin, cystic, avascular bleb. Note the curve of the slit-beam at the inferior portion of the elevated bleb (arrowhead).

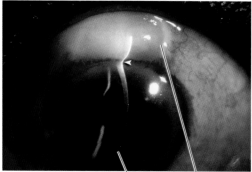

Slit-beam   Filtering bleb

Prognosis Variable; depends on extent of optic nerve damage since visual loss is permanent. Usually good if detected early and intraocular pressure is controlled adequately; worse in African Americans.

Secondary Open-Angle Glaucoma

Definition Open-angle glaucoma caused by a variety of local or systemic disorders.

Etiology Pseudoexfoliation syndrome (see Chapter 8), pigment dispersion syndrome (see Chapter 7), uveitis, lens induced (see Chapter 8), intraocular tumors, trauma, and drugs; also elevated episcleral venous pressure (orbital mass, thyroid-related ophthalmopathy, arteriovenous fistulas, orbital varices, superior vena cava syndrome, Sturge–Weber syndrome, idiopathic), retinal disease (retinal detachment, retinitis pigmentosa, Stickler's syndrome), systemic disease (pituitary tumors, Cushing's syndrome, thyroid disease, renal disease), postoperative (laser and surgical procedures), and uveitis-glaucoma-hyphema syndrome (see Chapter 6).

Drug Induced

Steroids

Most common; possibly due to increased trabecular meshwork (TM) glycosaminoglycans. Steroid-related intraocular pressure elevation correlates with potency and duration of use; 30% of population develop increased intraocular pressure after 4–6 weeks of topical steroid use, intraocular pressure >30 mm Hg in 4%; 95% of patients with POAG are steroid responders; increased incidence of steroid response in patients with diabetes mellitus, high myopia, connective tissue disease, and family history of glaucoma.

Viscoelastic agents

Used during ophthalmic surgery, can transiently obstruct the TM (1–2 days).

Alpha-chymotrypsin

Used for intracapsular cataract extraction, produces zonular debris, which can block the TM.

Intraocular Tumor

Due to hemorrhage, angle neovascularization, direct tumor infiltration of the angle, or TM obstruction by tumor, inflammatory, or red blood cells.

Traumatic

Angle recession

If more than two-thirds of the angle is involved, 10% of patients develop glaucoma from scarring of angle structures.

Chemical injury

Toxicity to angle structures from direct or indirect (prostaglandin, ischemia-mediated) damage.

Hemorrhage

Red blood cells, ghost cells (degenerated red blood cells), or macrophages that have ingested red blood cells (hemolytic glaucoma) obstruct the TM; increased incidence in patients with sickle cell disease.

Siderosis or chalcosis

Toxicity to angle structures from iron or copper intraocular foreign body.

Uveitic

Due to outflow obstruction from inflammatory cells, trabeculitis, scarring of the TM, or increased aqueous viscosity.

Symptoms Asymptomatic; may have pain, photophobia, decreased vision.

Signs Normal or decreased visual acuity, increased intraocular pressure, optic nerve cupping, nerve fiber layer defects, visual field defects; may have blood in Schlemm's canal evident on gonioscopy (due to elevated episcleral venous pressure) or other signs of underlying etiology:

Intraocular Tumor

Iris mass, focal iris elevation, hyphema, hypopyon, anterior chamber cells and flare, pseudo-hypopyon, leukocoria, segmental cataract, invasion of angle, extrascleral extension, sentinel episcleral vessels.

Traumatic

Anterior chamber cells and flare, other signs of trauma including red blood cells in anterior chamber or vitreous, angle recession, iridodialysis, cyclodialysis, sphincter tears, iridodonesis, phacodonesis, cataract, corneal blood staining, corneal scarring, scleral blanching or ischemia, intraocular foreign body, iris heterochromia, retinal tears, choroidal rupture.

Uveitic

Ciliary injection, anterior chamber cells and flare, keratic precipitates, miotic pupil, peripheral anterior synechiae, posterior synechiae, iris heterochromia, iris atrophy, iris nodules, fine angle vessels, decreased corneal sensation, corneal edema, corneal scarring, ghost vessels, cataract, low intraocular pressure due to decreased aqueous production, cystoid macular edema.

Figure 11-35 • Gonioscopy of angle recession demonstrating deepened angle with blue–gray face of ciliary body evident.

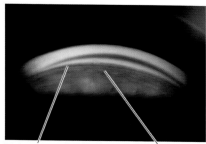

Trabecular meshwork   Angle recession

Evaluation
- Complete ophthalmic history and eye exam with attention to cornea, tonometry, anterior chamber, gonioscopy, iris, lens, and ophthalmoscopy.
- Check visual fields.
- B-scan ultrasonography if unable to visualize the fundus.
- Consider ultrasound biomicroscopy to evaluate angle and ciliary body.
- Consider orbital radiographs or head and orbital CT scan to rule out intraocular foreign body.
- Consider uveitis workup.
- May require medical or oncology consultation.

Management

- Treatment of increased intraocular pressure (see Primary Open-Angle Glaucoma section); laser trabeculoplasty is usually not effective; may require trabeculectomy or glaucoma drainage implant to lower pressure adequately.
- Treat underlying problem.

DRUG INDUCED
- Taper, change, or stop steroids.
- Consider releasing viscoelastic through paracentesis site on first postoperative day if intraocular pressure >30 mm Hg and there is no vitreous in the anterior chamber.

Continued

Management—Cont'd

INTRAOCULAR TUMOR
- Treatment for tumor with radiation, chemotherapy, or surgery should be performed by a tumor specialist.

TRAUMATIC
- May require anterior chamber washout or pars plana vitrectomy for hemorrhage-related, uncontrolled elevation of intraocular pressure.

UVEITIC
- Do not use pilocarpine or prostaglandin analogue.
- Treat uveitis with topical cycloplegic (cyclopentolate 1% or scopolamine 0.25% tid) and topical steroid (prednisolone acetate 1%, rimexolone [Vexol], loteprednol etabonate [Lotemax, Alrex], or fluorometholone [FML] qd to q1h depending on the amount of inflammation; beware of increased intraocular pressure with steroid use due to steroid response or recovery of ciliary body to normal aqueous production; consider tapering or changing steroid if steroid response exists); steroids are not effective in Fuchs' heterochromic iridocyclitis.

Prognosis Poorer than primary open-angle glaucoma because usually due to chronic process; depends on etiology, extent of optic nerve damage, and subsequent intraocular pressure control; typically good for drug-induced if identified and treated early.

Normal (Low) Tension Glaucoma

Definition Similar optic nerve and visual field damage as in POAG, but with normal intraocular pressure ($\leq$21 mm Hg).

Epidemiology Higher prevalence of vasospastic disorders including migraine, Raynaud's phenomenon, ischemic vascular disease, autoimmune disease, and coagulopathies; also associated with history of poor perfusion of the optic nerve from hypotension, shock, myocardial infarction, or massive hemorrhage.

Symptoms Asymptomatic; may have decreased vision or constricted visual fields in late stages.

Signs Normal or decreased visual acuity, normal intraocular pressure ($\leq$21 mm Hg), optic nerve cupping, splinter hemorrhages at optic disc (more common than in POAG), peripapillary atrophy, nerve fiber layer defects, visual field defects.

Figure 11-36 • Normal tension glaucoma demonstrating optic nerve cupping and a splinter hemorrhage at the disc inferiorly at the 5 o'clock position.

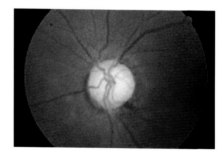

Differential Diagnosis POAG (undetected increased intraocular pressure or artifactually low intraocular pressure secondary to thin cornea [e.g., naturally occurring or after LASIK or PRK]), secondary glaucoma (steroid-induced, "burned out" pigmentary or postinflammatory glaucoma), intermittent angle-closure glaucoma, optic neuropathy, optic nerve anomalies, glaucomatocyclitic crisis (Posner–Schlossman syndrome).

Evaluation
- Complete ophthalmic history and eye exam with attention to cornea, tonometry, anterior chamber, gonioscopy, iris, lens, and ophthalmoscopy.
- Check visual fields.
- Check corneal pachymetry.
- Consider diurnal curve (intraocular pressure measurement q2h for 10–24 hours) and tonography.
- Consider evaluation for other causes of optic neuropathy: check color vision, lab tests (CBC, ESR, Venereal Disease Research Laboratory [VDRL] test, fluorescent treponemal antibody absorption [FTA-ABS] test, antinuclear antibody [ANA]), neuroimaging, or cardiovascular evaluation if age less than 60 years old, decreased visual acuity without apparent cause, visual field defect not typical of glaucoma, visual field and disc changes do not correlate, rapidly progressive, unilateral or markedly asymmetric, or nerve pallor greater than cupping.

Management

- Choice and order of topical glaucoma medications depend on many factors, including patient's age, intraocular pressure level and control, and amount and progression of optic nerve cupping and visual field defects. Treatment options are presented in the Primary Open-Angle Glaucoma section.
- Follow patients every 6 months with complete eye exam and visual fields; no treatment if stable unless other risk factors are present for progression (disc hemorrhage, history of migraine, or female); treatment goal is intraocular pressure reduction of 30% from baseline (Collaborative Normal Tension Glaucoma Study conclusion).

Prognosis Poorer than primary open-angle glaucoma.

Refractive Error 523
Refractive Surgery Complications 526
Refractive Surgery Complications:
Evaluation/Management 533
Vertebrobasilar Insufficiency 535
Migraine 536
Convergence Insufficiency 538
Accommodative Excess 539
Functional Visual Loss 540
Transient Visual Loss 541
Amblyopia 542
Cortical Blindness 544
Visual Pathway Lesions 544

12

Visual Acuity, Refractive Procedures, and Sudden Vision Loss

Refractive Error

Definition The state of an eye in which light rays are not properly focused on the retina resulting in image blur.

Ametropia

A refractive error (e.g., myopia, hyperopia, or astigmatism).

Anisometropia

A difference in refractive error between the two eyes; usually 2D or more.

Astigmatism

Light rays are unequally focused producing two lines rather than a single point because the curvature of the cornea or, less commonly, the curvature of the lens varies in different meridians. If the cornea is steeper in the vertical meridian, it is referred to as "with-the-rule" astigmatism; if it is steeper in the horizontal meridian, it is called "against-the-rule" astigmatism. Astigmatism can also be designated regular (symmetric or asymmetric) or irregular. A cylindrical lens corrects regular astigmatism.

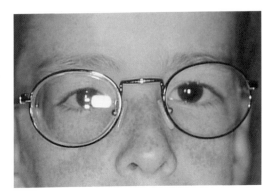

Figure 12-1 • Anisometropia with high myopia in the right eye (OD) (note minification from spectacle lens) and hyperopia in the left eye (OS) (note magnification from spectacle lens).

Emmetropia

No refractive error; light rays are focused on the retina, and thus no corrective lens is required for distance vision.

Hyperopia (Farsightedness)

Light rays are focused at a point behind the retina. A "plus" spherical lens is used to correct this refractive error.

Myopia (Nearsightedness)

Light rays from a distant object are focused at a point in front of the retina and those from a near object are focused on the retina. A "minus" spherical lens is used to correct this refractive error.

Presbyopia

Loss of accommodation of the crystalline lens with age; average age of the onset of symptoms is early 40s and this process continues through the early 60s. A "plus" spherical lens (i.e., bifocal "add") is used to correct this problem.

Etiology

Astigmatism

The curvature of the cornea or, less commonly, the curvature of the lens varies in different meridians. Acquired forms may be caused by disorders of the eyelids (tumor, chalazion, ptosis), cornea (pterygium, limbal dermoid, degenerations, ectasias, surgery), lens (cataract), and ciliary body (tumor).

Hyperopia

The refractive power of the cornea is too weak or the axial length of the eye is too short. Acquired forms may be caused by disorders that decrease the eye's refractive power (alteration in the lens [posterior lens dislocation, aphakia, diabetes], drugs [chloroquine, phenothiazines, antihistamines, benzodiazepines], poor accommodation [tonic pupil, drugs, trauma], corneal flattening [contact lens induced], intraocular silicone oil) or effective length (central serous retinopathy, retrobulbar masses, choroidal tumors).

Myopia

The refractive power of the eye is too strong or the axial length of the eye is too long. Acquired forms may be caused by disorders that increase the eye's refractive power (alteration in the lens [diabetes, galactosemia, uremia, cataracts, anterior lenticonus, anterior lens dislocation], drugs [sulfonamides, miotic agents], excessive accommodation, corneal steepening [keratoconus, congenital glaucoma, contact lens induced]) or effective length ([congenital glaucoma, posterior staphyloma, retinopathy of prematurity, scleral buckle surgery]). Myopia also increases in the dark (night myopia).

Presbyopia

Loss of lens elasticity or possibly reduced ciliary muscle effectivity. Premature presbyopia may occur with debilitating illness, diphtheria, botulism, mercury toxicity, head injury, cranial nerve III palsy, Adie's tonic pupil, and tranquilizers.

Epidemiology Hyperopia is normally present during infancy and early childhood and then declines between ages 8 and 13 years, resulting in emmetropia in most adults. The incidence of refractive errors in the US population is approximately 25% for myopia and 25% for hyperopia; 50% have some degree of astigmatism. After the age of 40 years old, 50% of people have hyperopia. Hyperopia is associated with shallow anterior chambers and narrow angles; myopia is associated with lattice degeneration and retinal detachment.

Symptoms Decreased vision when not wearing corrective lenses: distant objects are blurry and near objects are clear (myopia), distant and near objects are blurry (hyperopia), or near objects that are blurry become clearer when held further away (presbyopia); may have asthenopia (eye strain) due to sustained accommodative effort (overcorrected myopia, or undercorrected or uncorrected hyperopia; asthenopia may also be produced by convergence insufficiency or accommodative insufficiency [hypothyroidism, anemia, pregnancy, nutritional deficiencies, and chronic illness]). Hyperopia may be asymptomatic in children and young adults who can compensate enough with accommodation.

Signs Decreased uncorrected visual acuity that improves with pinhole testing, glasses, or contact lenses. Hyperopes may have normal uncorrected visual acuity.

Differential Diagnosis Normal eye exam except for decreased vision: amblyopia, retrobulbar optic neuropathy, other optic neuropathies (toxic, nutritional), nonorganic (functional) visual loss, rod monochromatism, cone degeneration, retinitis pigmentosa sine pigmento, cortical blindness.

Evaluation
- Complete ophthalmic history and eye exam with attention to pinhole visual acuity (corrects most low to moderate refractive errors to the 20/25 to 20/30 level), manifest (undilated) and cycloplegic (dilated) refraction, retinoscopy, pupils, keratometry, cornea, lens, and ophthalmoscopy.
- Consider potential acuity meter (PAM) testing, rigid contact lens overrefraction, and corneal topography (computerized videokeratography) if irregular astigmatism is suspected.

Management

- Glasses are the first-line of treatment and can correct virtually all refractive errors with the exception of irregular astigmatism.
- Contact lenses (soft or rigid). Numerous styles of contact lenses are available to correct almost any refractive error; rigid lenses can correct irregular astigmatism.
- Consider refractive surgery (see below).

Prognosis Good except for pathologic myopia (see Chapter 10).

Refractive Surgery Complications

Intraocular Refractive Procedures

Used to correct moderate to high degrees of myopia and hyperopia.

Clear Lens Extraction (Refractive Lens Exchange)

The noncataractous crystalline lens can be removed and replaced with an intraocular lens implant of appropriate power to correct the resulting aphakia. The main disadvantage of this method is loss of accommodation. This procedure is controversial for myopia because of the risk of retinal detachment in pseudophakic eyes; hyperopic eyes with nanophthalmos may develop choroidal effusions.

Phakic Intraocular Lens

A lens implant is placed in the anterior chamber, posterior chamber, or fixated to the iris with the optic centered over the pupil. Prophylactic peripheral iridotomies are performed prior to surgery to prevent postoperative pupillary block angle-closure glaucoma (see Chapter 6).

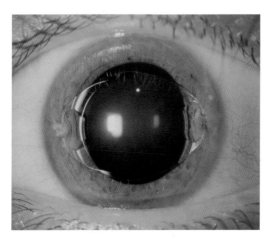

Figure 12-2 • Phakic intraocular lens demonstrating the Verisyse lens in the anterior chamber attached to the iris at the 3 o'clock and 9 o'clock positions.

Symptoms Postoperatively may have: photophobia, pain, decreased vision, glare, and halos.

Signs and Complications Corneal edema (endothelial cell loss), cataract, glaucoma, pupillary block, iridocyclitis, and endophthalmitis; may have residual refractive error. Additional complications of clear lens extraction include posterior capsular opacification, cystoid macular edema, retinal detachment, suprachoroidal hemorrhage, choroidal effusion, retained lens material, and iris damage.

Corneal Refractive Procedures

Incisional

Radial Keratotomy

This procedure corrects low-to-moderate myopia. Deep, radial, corneal incisions are created with a diamond knife to flatten the central cornea. The surgical effect depends on various factors including depth and number of incisions; size of optical zone; patient age and gender; design of diamond blade; and surgeon experience. Radial keratotomy can be combined with astigmatic keratotomy for compound myopia (myopia with astigmatism). It is rarely performed anymore.

Figure 12-3 • Eight-incision radial keratotomy demonstrating near full-thickness corneal incisions at 90–95% depth.

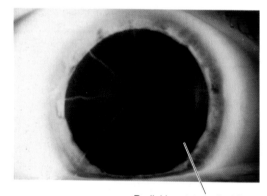

Radial keratotomy incisions

Astigmatic Keratotomy

This procedure corrects corneal astigmatism. Deep, midperipheral arcuate or straight incisions (parallel to the limbus) are made with a diamond knife on the steep corneal meridian to flatten it. As with RK, the surgical effect depends on depth and number of incisions; size of optical zone (usually 7 mm); patient age; and surgeon experience. The incisions must not be >90° or intersect with radial keratotomy (RK) incisions. This technique is useful after penetrating keratoplasty for high-to-moderate astigmatism.

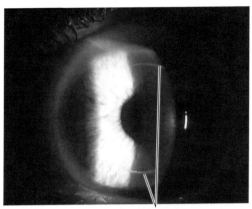

Figure 12-4 • Astigmatic keratotomy demonstrating a pair of 90% depth corneal incisions in the midperiphery of the vertical meridian.

Astigmatic keratotomy

Limbal Relaxing Incisions/Peripheral Corneal Relaxing Incisions

Similar to astigmatic keratotomy, this technique is used to correct low amounts of astigmatism usually in association with cataract surgery. Arcuate incisions, 500–600 microns deep, are placed at the 10–11 mm optical zone concentric to the limbus to correct 1–2D of astigmatism. Because ultrasound is not required, these relaxing incisions can be performed at the time of surgery or in the clinic. Corneal topography is recommended prior to performing this procedure.

Symptoms Postoperatively may have decreased vision (due to undercorrection, overcorrection, or irregular astigmatism), fluctuating vision, difficulty with night vision, halos, glare, starbursts, ghost images, double vision, and foreign body sensation.

Signs and Complications Corneal scarring, infection, or perforation. May have residual refractive error, regression or progression over time.

Excimer Laser

This ultraviolet laser (193 nm) ablates corneal tissue to correct myopia (central ablation), hyperopia (peripheral ablation), regular astigmatism (eliptical ablation), irregular astigmatism (topography-guided ablation), or reduce higher order aberrations (wavefront ablation).

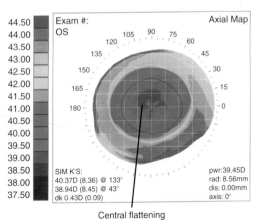

Figure 12-5 • Post-laser in-situ keratomileusis corneal topography map for a myopic excimer laser ablation. Note the blue central flattening on the map created by the photoablation of corneal stroma.

Central flattening

Photorefractive Keratectomy

This procedure uses excimer laser ablation to reshape the corneal stroma after epithelial removal (mechanical, alcohol, or laser). The visual recovery period is longer than with LASIK, but final visual outcomes are similar in low and moderate myopia. Patients may experience initial pain due to the epithelial defect, and decreased vision due to corneal haze.

Laser-Assisted Subepithelial Keratectomy and Epithelial-Laser In-Situ Keratomileusis

These procedures combine photorefractive keratectomy (PRK) and laser in-situ keratomileusis (LASIK) techniques. A flap composed of only epithelium is created with topical alcohol (LASEK) or a mechanical epithelial separator (epi-LASIK), the epithelial flap is carefully retracted, laser energy is applied to the stromal bed, and the epithelial flap is replaced or excised. This procedure may combine the advantages of PRK and LASIK by decreasing the incidence of pain and haze associated with PRK and risk of flap complications associated with LASIK.

Laser in Situ Keratomileusis

This procedure combines automated lamellar keratoplasty and photorefractive keratectomy (PRK) techniques. A mechanical microkeratome or femtosecond laser is first used to cut a partial-thickness hinged corneal flap that is then folded back. The programmed excimer laser energy is applied to the underlying stromal bed, and the flap is replaced. LASIK allows for faster visual recovery and minimal pain after surgery, but there is a higher risk of complications due to flap-related problems than with PRK.

Symptoms Postoperatively patients may have decreased vision (due to undercorrection, overcorrection, irregular astigmatism, or haze), fluctuating vision, difficulty with night vision, halos, glare, starbursts, ghost images, double vision, and variable discomfort (ranging from foreign body sensation to moderate pain).

Signs and Complications Corneal scarring, infection, or keratectasia, decentration (apparent on corneal topography), or dry eyes; may have residual refractive error, regression over time. Additional LASIK complications include flap striae, epithelial ingrowth, flap trauma, and diffuse lamellar keratitis (DLK, "sands of the Sahara"). Haze from surface ablation may be early (due to delayed epithelial healing) or late (≥3 months, due to deeper ablations and UV exposure).

Figure 12-6 • Photorefractive keratectomy demonstrating moderate central corneal haze 6 months after a treatment for high myopia.

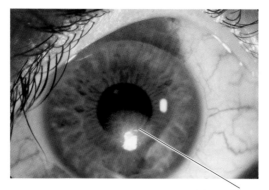

Corneal haze

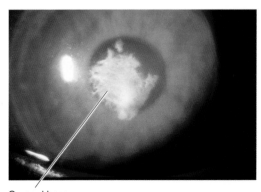

Corneal haze

Figure 12-7 • Dense (4+) central haze and scarring after photorefractive keratectomy in a corneal graft. The edge of the graft is visible as a fine white line at the right edge of the picture extending from the 1 o'clock to 5 o'clock positions.

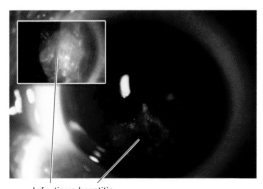

Infectious keratitis

Figure 12-8 • Atypical mycobacterial keratitis after laser in-situ keratomileusis demonstrating the infectious keratitis in the corneal flap interface.

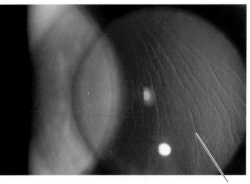

Flap wrinkles

Figure 12-9 • Laser in-situ keratomileusis flap striae demonstrating vertically curved wrinkles in the flap.

Figure 12-10 • Same patient as Figure 12-9 with laser in-situ keratomileusis flap striae demonstrating the curved striae that are enhanced with topical fluorescein and viewed with a blue light.

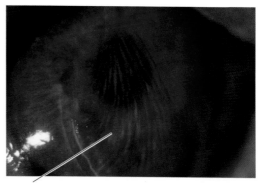

Flap wrinkles

Figure 12-11 • Epithelial ingrowth after laser in-situ keratomileusis proliferating from the inferior corneal flap edge. The gray puddy-like pseudopods represent epithelium in the corneal flap interface. Inset shows transillumination of the epithelial ingrowth.

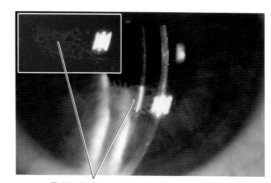

Epithelial ingrowth

Figure 12-12 • Grade 2 diffuse lamellar keratitis or "sands of the Sahara" after laser in-situ keratomileusis demonstrating characteristic appearance of white granular interface material distributed in a wavelike pattern.

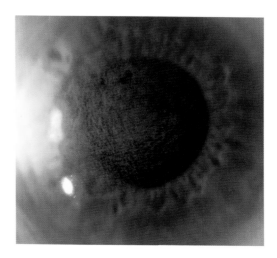

Implants

Intracorneal Inlays

This procedure combines a partial-thickness corneal flap (similar to LASIK) with a thin, contact lens-like, intrastromal implant that is placed in the central optical zone to correct refractive errors without removing corneal tissue. It may be most useful for treating presbyopia.

Intrastromal Corneal Ring Segments (Intacs)

Polymethylmethacrylate (PMMA) ring segment implants are placed into peripheral corneal channels at two-thirds depth outside the visual axis to correct low-to-moderate myopia by flattening the cornea without cutting or removing tissue from the central optical zone. These channels can be made manually or with a femtosecond laser. Also used to treat mild-to-moderate keratoconus by shifting and stabilizing the cone allowing for improved contact lens tolerance and best spectacle-corrected visual acuity.

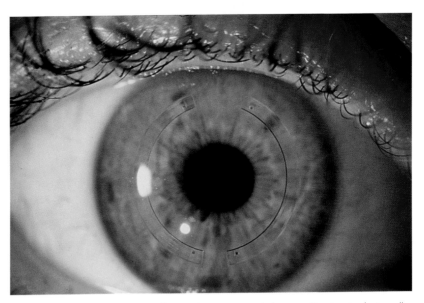

Figure 12-13 • Intacs (intrastromal corneal ring segments) demonstrating two implants well positioned in the cornea.

Symptoms Postoperatively may have decreased vision (due to undercorrection, overcorrection, or irregular astigmatism), fluctuating vision, difficulty with night vision, halos, glare, and foreign body sensation.

Signs and Complications Implant extrusion, implant decentration, infection, stromal deposits (intrastromal corneal ring segments), flap striae (intracorneal inlays), epithelial ingrowth (intracorneal inlays); may have residual refractive error.

Thermokeratoplasty

Conductive Keratoplasty

Radiofrequency energy is applied to the peripheral cornea to shrink collagen tissue and treat low-to-moderate hyperopia through central corneal steepening. A handheld contact probe with a 450 micron needle directly delivers energy in a ring pattern outside the visual axis. The number of spots determines the amount of central steepening (8 to 32 spots).

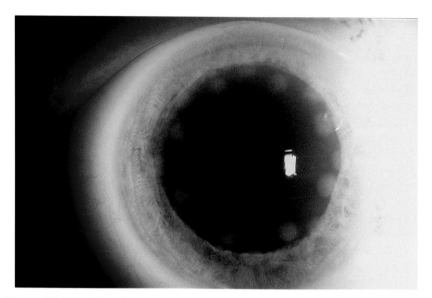

Figure 12-14 • Thermokeratoplasty treatment demonstrating a double ring, staggered pattern of eight spots each, visible as opaque white corneal spots in the area overlying the pupillary border.

Symptoms Postoperatively patients may have pain, foreign body sensation, decreased vision (irregular astigmatism, regression), glare, and halos.

Signs and Complications Corneal scarring in area of application, regression over time; may have residual refractive error.

Refractive Surgery Complications: Evaluation/Management

Evaluation

- Complete ophthalmic history and eye exam with attention to visual acuity, manifest and cycloplegic refractions, pupil size, keratometry, cornea, lens, and ophthalmoscopy.
- Corneal topography (computerized videokeratography).
- Consider rigid contact lens overrefraction if irregular astigmatism is suspected.

Management

- No treatment recommended unless patient is symptomatic and vision is decreased. Choice of treatment depends on type of refractive surgery performed.

- **Undercorrection or overcorrection:** modify topical medication regimen, glasses or contact lens; consider retreatment after corneal stabilization and failure of conservative management. Specific treatment must be tailored on an individual basis and is beyond the scope of this book, but should be performed by a cornea or refractive specialist.

- **Infectious keratitis:** culture (lift corneal flap), topical antiinfective agents (see Chapter 5); may require flap amputation.

- **Epithelial ingrowth:** lift corneal flap and scrape undersurface of flap and stromal bed; consider suturing flap; consider Nd:YAG laser treatment.

- **Diffuse lamellar keratitis:** frequent topical steroids (q1h initially) for grades 1 and 2 DLK; may require lifting flap and irrigating stromal bed to remove inflammatory debris (grades 3 and 4 DLK); consider short pulse of oral steroids.

- **Flap striae:** lift flap, refloat, and stretch; may require removing epithelium and suturing flap; consider heating flap with warm spatula. On postoperative day 1, striae often can be removed with massage or stretching at the slit lamp.

- **Decentration or irregular astigmatism:** rigid contact lens trial; retreatment with wavefront or topography-guided ablation.

- **Halo, glare, and starbursts:** consider topical miotic agent (pilocarpine 0.5–1%) or brimonidine (Alphagan-P 0.15%) qd to bid, polarized sunglasses, or retreatment with enlarged treatment zone.

- **Dry eye:** topical artificial tears (see Appendix) up to q1h; consider punctal plugs, topical cyclosporine 0.05% (Restasis) bid; may require a bandage contact lens for corneal surface irregularities.

- **Pain (surface ablation):** bandage contact lens, topical nonsteroidal antiinflammatory drug; consider topical dilute anesthetic drops, oral analgesic (Vicodin, Mepergan fortis, Toradol [20 mg then 10 mg every 4–6 hours], Neurontin [100 mg tid for 3 days] or Lyrica [75 mg tid for 5 days], Sumatriptan [100 mg once]), oral steroid (Prednisone taper [80, 60, 40, 20 mg qd for 4 days]); consider irrigating with chilled/frozen BSS solution for 30 seconds immediately after ablation.

- **Haze (surface ablation):** prevent postoperatively with topical steroid for 1–3 months, oral vitamin C 500 mg po bid for 1 month, sunglasses to decrease UV exposure, consider topical mitomycin C (MMC) 0.02% for 12–30 seconds immediately after ablation; treat existing haze with additional topical steroids, consider phototherapeutic keratectomy (PTK) with MMC.

Prognosis Usually good; depends on specific surgical technique and any complications. Hyperopia treatments tend to regress with time.

Vertebrobasilar Insufficiency (Vertebrobasilar Atherothrombotic Disease)

Definition Vertebrobasilar (posterior) circulation constitutes the arterial supply to the brain stem, cerebellum, and occipital cortex. Impaired blood flow to these areas may manifest in a myriad of symptoms. Transient ischemic attacks (TIAs) in this vascular territory are referred to as vertebrobasilar insufficiency (VBI).

Etiology Thrombus, emboli, hypertension, arrhythmias, arterial dissection, hypercoagulable states, and subclavian steel syndrome. Approximately one-fourth of strokes and TIAs occur in the vertebrobasilar distribution. MRI studies suggest that 40% of patients with vertebrobasilar TIAs have evidence of brainstem infarction.

Epidemiology Male predilection (2:1); occurs in elderly, usually in seventh to eighth decades.

Symptoms Vertigo is the hallmark of vertebrobasilar ischemia. Additionally, bilateral transient blurring or dimming of vision (seconds to minutes), photopsias (flashes of light), diplopia, unilateral weakness, sensory loss, ataxia, nystagmus, facial numbness, dysarthria, hoarseness, dysphagia, hearing loss, and vertigo; history of drop attacks (syncope) can occur.

Signs Usually none; may have small, paracentral, congruous, homonymous visual field defects.

Differential Diagnosis Amaurosis fugax, migraine, papilledema, temporal arteritis, labyrinthitis, vestibular neuronitis, benign paroxysmal positional vertigo.

Evaluation
- Complete ophthalmic history with attention to characteristics of attacks (monocular or bilateral, other symptoms, frequency, duration, etc.), neurologic exam, and eye exam with attention to motility, pupils, and ophthalmoscopy.
- Check visual fields.
- **Lab tests:** complete blood count (CBC), erythrocyte sedimentation rate (ESR), and blood glucose (hypoglycemia).
- Check blood pressure.
- Head and orbital magnetic resonance imaging (MRI).
- Cervical spine radiographs (cervical spondylosis).
- Medical consultation for complete cardiovascular evaluation, including electrocardiogram, echocardiogram, duplex and Doppler scans of carotid and vertebral arteries.
- Neurology consulation.

Management

- Usually no effective treatment.
- Aspirin (325 mg po qd).
- May require long-term anticoagulation.
- Treat underlying etiology.

Prognosis Usually poor.

Migraine

Definition A neurologic syndrome characterized by recurrent attacks lasting 4–72 hours often with unilateral throbbing moderate-to-severe headache, sensory changes, gastrointestinal symptoms, and mood disturbances. Five stages have been described: prodrome (premonitory symptoms 24–72 hours before other symptoms), aura (transient neurologic symptoms, usually visual), headache, resolution, and recovery. Often migraine is divided into the following categories: without aura, with aura, variant, and complicated. The formal migraine classification (according to the International Headache Society, second edition [IHS-2]) is:

Migraine without Aura (80%)

"Common" migraine; headache may or may not be preceded by a poorly defined prodrome of mood fluctuations (elation, hyperexcitability, food cravings, irritability, restlessness, depression, feeling of impending doom), excessive energy, fatigue, frequent yawning, and gastrointestinal disturbances (anorexia, nausea, and emesis).

Migraine with Aura

Aura (transient neurologic symptoms) develops over 5–20 minutes and lasts <60 minutes; most commonly visual (bilateral) consisting of scintillations, zigzag lines (fortification phenomenon), spreading scotomas, tunnel vision, micropsia, blurred vision, and altitudinal field loss; can also be vertigo, sensory or motor disturbances, fainting, confusion, or possibly auditory hallucinations. Headache, nausea, photophobia, phonophobia, emesis, irritability, and malaise usually follows immediately after or within an hour; other symptoms include diarrhea, vertigo, tremors, sweating, and chills. Subtypes include:

Typical aura with migraine headache (15–20%)

"Classic" migraine; gradual aura lasting less than 1 hour.

Typical aura with non-migraine headache

Headache does not satisfy criteria for migraine headache.

Typical aura without headache (5%)

"Acephalgic" migraine; aura (usually visual) without headache. Often occurs in older individuals with a history of classic migraine; 25% have a family history of migraine.

Hemiplegic migraine

Familial or sporadic; rare. Unilateral motor weakness or partial paralysis.

Basilar-type migraine (Bickerstaff syndrome)

Aura mimics vertebrobasilar artery insufficiency with brain stem or bilateral occipital lobe symptoms (i.e., blindness, diplopia, vertigo, difficulty with speech or coordination). Rare; typically occurs in teenage girls and young women.

Childhood periodic syndromes

Recurrent disorders in children with migraine features that are usually precursors of migraine. These include: cyclical vomiting (recurrent episodes of nausea and emesis [at least 5 within 5 days]), abdominal migraine (recurrent attacks of midline abdominal pain for up to 72 hours with nausea, emesis, anorexia, and/or pallor), and benign paroxysmal vertigo of childhood (recurrent vertigo attacks, commonly with emesis or nystagmus).

Retinal migraine

"Ocular" migraine; rare; monocular scotoma or visual loss for minutes to an hour due to retinal or optic nerve ischemia.

Complications of Migraine

This category includes: chronic migraine (headache for more than 15 days in a month), status migrainosus (headache lasting longer than 72 hours despite treatment, continuous or with brief interruptions [<4 hours]), persistent aura without infarction (aura lasting longer than 72 hours), migrainous infarction (stroke during a migraine or neurologic deficit lasting longer than 1 week with corresponding lesion on neuroimaging), and migraine-triggered seizures ("migralepsy"; seizure during or immediately after a migraine).

Etiology Although not completely elucidated, mounting evidence supports the role of neurogenic peptides in migraine formation, such as serotonin and dopamine, in the brain. These vasoactive neuropeptides stimulate an inflammatory cascade with the release of endothelial cells, mast cells, and platelets that produce vasodilation and a perivascular reaction. The susceptibility to headaches in migraineurs is due to a baseline state of hyperexcitability in the cerebral cortex, particularly the occipital area. The aura is caused by cortical spreading depression (a wave of neuronal excitation followed by suppression with blood vessel constriction and dilation); the headache is due to neurochemical release causing inflammation and blood vessel dilation. Dopamine stimulation may play a role, particularly in the prodrome. The serotonin receptor (5-HT) is believed to be the most important receptor in the headache pathway.

Epidemiology Affects approximately 18% of women and 6% of men in the US; can occur at any age; family history of migraine in 70%, or a history of motion sickness is common. Commonly triggered by foods, alcohol, caffeine withdrawal, drugs (nitroglycerine, reserpine, hydralazine, ranitidine, estrogen), hormonal changes (menstruation, ovulation, oral contraceptives, hormone replacement), sleep alteration, exertion, stress, fatigue, and head trauma (also fasting, strong odors, flickering lights, sun glare, smoky or noisy environments, altitude, and weather changes). Associated with epilepsy, familial dyslipoproteinemias, Tourette syndrome, hereditary essential tremor, ischemic stroke, depression, asthma, patent foramen ovale. Migraine often demonstrates maternal inheritance and occurs more frequently in patients with mitochondrial disorders. Familial hemiplegic migraine has been mapped to chromosomes 19p13 and 1q.

Symptoms May have prodrome, aura, headache, or other neurologic, gastrointestinal, or emotional symptoms (see above).

Signs Usually none; may have visual field defect, cranial nerve palsy, or other neurologic deficits.

Differential Diagnosis **Serious:** meningitis, subarachnoid hemorrhage, temporal arteritis, malignant hypertension, intracranial tumor, arteriovenous malformation, vertebrobasilar artery insufficiency, aneurysm, subdural hematoma, transient ischemic attack, occipital or temporal lobe seizure, cerebrovascular accident.

Others: tension or cluster headaches, trigeminal neuralgia, temporomandibular joint syndrome, cervical spondylosis, herpes zoster ophthalmicus, sinus or dental pathology, uveitis, angle-closure glaucoma, after lumbar puncture, nonorganic, caffeine withdrawal, carbon monoxide inhalation, and nitrite exposure.

Evaluation

- Complete ophthalmic history with attention to characteristics of attacks (precipitating factors, frequency, duration, associated symptoms, etc.), neurologic exam, and eye exam with attention to motility, pupils, tonometry, and ophthalmoscopy.
- Check visual fields.
- Check blood pressure and temperature.
- Consider lumbar puncture for suspected meningitis.
- Neuroimaging for complicated migraines or migraines with neurologic deficits.
- Medical or neurology consultation.

Management

- Rest in dark, quiet room.
- Pain relief: nonsteroidal antiinflammatory drugs (aspirin 325–500 mg po or ibuprofen 600 mg po qd), triptans (sumatriptan [Imitrex], rizatriptan [Maxalt], zolmitriptan [Zomig]), ergot alkaloids (ergotamine (1–3 mg po 1 tablet at onset of aura or headache, 1 more 15–20 minutes later) or dihydroergotamine [Migranal]); consider opioids (codeine, oxycodone). Triptans and ergots are vasoconstrictors and should not be used for complicated migraines.
- Consider antiemetics.
- Prevention: avoid triggers and precipitating agents (foods, alcohol, stress), reduce stress, regulate sleep and meals, exercise; consider biofeedback and relaxation techniques; β-blockers (propranolol 20–40 mg po bid to tid initially), tricyclic antidepressants (amitriptyline 25–75 mg po qd to bid initially), calcium-channel blockers (nifedipine 10–40 mg po or verapamil 80 mg po tid); consider antiepileptics (valproic acid [Depakote 500–1000 mg po qd], topiramate [Topamax 30–100 mg po qd], gabapentin [Neurontin]) or botulinum toxin (Botox) injections to the scalp and temple.
- Treatment should be monitored by an internist or neurologist.

Prognosis Good.

Convergence Insufficiency

Definition Decreased fusional convergence with near fixation, a remote near point of convergence and a low accommodation convergence/accommodation (AC/A) ratio.

Etiology Idiopathic but possibly innervational in origin; may be induced by drugs, trauma, or prismatic effect of glasses (base-out).

Epidemiology Prevelance is estimated at 3–5%; typically occurs in teenagers and young adults, rare before 10 years of age; slight female predilection. Common cause of asthenopia (eye strain); aggravated by anxiety, illness, or lack of sleep. Often associated with an exophoria or intermittent exotropia at near.

Symptoms Asthenopia, diplopia, blurred vision, headaches, difficulty reading.

Signs Inability to maintain fusion at near (patient closes one eye while reading to relieve visual fatigue), distant near point of convergence, reduced fusional convergence amplitudes; possible exophoria at near without exotropia (especially after prolonged reading).

Differential Diagnosis Presbyopia, refractive error (uncorrected hyperopia, overcorrected myopia), accommodative insufficiency.

Evaluation
- Complete ophthalmic history and eye exam with attention to manifest and cycloplegic refractions, motility (cover and alternate cover tests [exophoria at near]), near point of accommodation (normal is 5–10 cm, abnormal is 10–30 cm), fusional convergence amplitudes (normal is 30–35 prism diopters [PD] of base-out prism causes diplopia; abnormal is <20 PD), and 4 PD base-in prism test (differentiates convergence insufficiency [near vision improves] from accommodative insufficiency [near vision worsens]).

Management

- Correct any refractive error (undercorrect hyperopes, fully correct myopes).
- Orthoptic exercises: training of fusional convergence with pencil push-ups. (Bring pencil in from arms length toward nose while focusing on eraser. When diplopia [break point] develops, the exercise is repeated. Each attempt is designed to bring the pencil closer without diplopia. Alternatively, use base-out prisms (increase amount of prism diopters until blur point is reached, usually 4–6 PD, then increase further until break point is reached); exercises are repeated 15 times, 5 times a day; can also use major amblyoscope (stereograms).
- When no improvement is noted with exercises, base-in prism reading glasses are helpful.
- Very rarely, muscle surgery with bimedial rectus muscle resection.

Prognosis Usually good.

Accommodative Excess (Accommodative Spasm)

Definition A clinical state of excessive accommodation (lens focusing). Spasm of the near reflex is the triad of excess accommodation, excess convergence, and miosis.

Etiology Often triggered by stress or prolonged reading.

Symptoms Blurred distance vision, headache, brow ache, eye strain at near; may have diplopia.

Signs Abnormally close near point, miosis, and normal amplitude of accommodation; relief of symptoms with cycloplegia and cycloplegic refraction uncovers more hyperopia than on manifest refraction.

Differential Diagnosis Iridocyclitis, uncorrected refractive errors (usually hyperopes, but also astigmats and myopes), pseudomyopia (acquired myopia from systemic disorders, drugs, forward lens movement [see Myopia section above]).

Evaluation
• Complete ophthalmic history and eye exam with attention to manifest and cycloplegic refractions, pupils, and motility.

Management

• Stop offending medication if applicable.
• Correct any refractive error, including prescribing a reading aid if esotropia exists at near.
• Consider cycloplegic (scopolamine 0.25% qd to qid) to break spasm (only occasionally needed).
• Instruct patient to focus intermittently at distance during periods of prolonged near work.

Prognosis Good.

Functional Visual Loss

Definition Visual abnormality not attributable to any organic disease process (nonphysiologic).

Malingering
Fabrication of the existence or extent of a disorder for secondary gain.

Hysteria
Subconscious (not willful) expression of symptoms.

Epidemiology Twenty percent have coexistent organic disease. Malingering is usually associated with a financial incentive (i.e., legal action or compensation claim).

Symptoms Decreased vision (monocular or binocular, usually very vague about quality of symptoms), diplopia, metamorphopsia, oscillopsia.

Signs Decreased visual acuity (20/20 to no light perception), abnormal visual field (usually inconsistent or has characteristic pattern); may have voluntary nystagmus, gaze palsy, or blepharospasm. Malingerer is often uncooperative and combative, hysteric is often indifferent but cooperative; otherwise normal examination (especially pupils, optokinetic nystagmus response, fundus).

Differential Diagnosis Functional visual loss is a diagnosis of exclusion, must rule out organic disease, especially amblyopia, early keratoconus, anterior basement membrane dystrophy, early cataracts, central serous retinopathy, early Stargardt's disease, retinitis pigmentosa sine pigmento, rod monochromatism, cone degeneration, retrobulbar optic neuritis, optic neuropathy, and cortical blindness.

Evaluation
- Complete ophthalmic history and eye exam with attention to vision (distance and near, monocular and binocular, varying distance, fogging, red–green glasses with duochrome test or Worth 4 dot test, prism dissociation, stereopsis, startle reflex, proprioception, signing name, mirror tracking, optokinetic nystagmus response), retinoscopy, motility, pupils, and ophthalmoscopy.
- Check visual fields (monocular and binocular); beware tunnel vision, spiraling fields, crossing isopters.
- Consider corneal topography (computerized videokeratography).
- Consider electroretinogram, visual evoked response, fluorescein angiogram, or neuro-imaging in difficult cases or if unable to prove normal vision and visual field.

Management

- Reassurance.
- Offer a way out by instilling a topical medication in the office and then retesting, especially for children.
- Consider repeat examination several weeks later.
- Psychiatry consultation usually not necessary.

Prognosis No improvement in up to 30%.

Transient Visual Loss (Amaurosis Fugax)

Definition Unilateral transient visual loss due to ischemia. This is a type of TIA also called temporary monocular blindness (TMB).

Etiology Usually embolic from carotid artery or cardiac valvular disease; also due to arrhythmias, coagulation disorders, hyperviscosity syndromes, vasospasm, hypotension, and rarely an orbital mass.

Symptoms Monocular, brief, reversible dimming or loss of vision (typically 2–5 minutes).

Signs Usually none; may have visible emboli in retinal vessels.

Differential Diagnosis Vertebrobasilar artery insufficiency, migraine, temporal arteritis, papilledema, pseudopapilledema (optic nerve drusen).

Evaluation
- Complete ophthalmic history with attention to characteristics of visual loss (monocular or bilateral, other symptoms, frequency, duration, etc.), neurologic exam, and eye exam with attention to pupils and ophthalmoscopy.
- Check visual fields.
- Medical consultation for complete cardiovascular evaluation including electrocardiogram, echocardiogram, and carotid Doppler studies.

Management

- Aspirin (325 mg po qd).
- Treat underlying etiology.

Prognosis Depends on etiology; 1-year risk of cerebrovascular accident is 2%.

Amblyopia

Definition Unilateral or bilateral loss of best corrected vision in an otherwise anatomically normal eye.

Epidemiology Present in approximately 2% of general population.

Etiology

Strabismic

Most common form of amblyopia. Develops in a child when the visual input of a constantly deviated eye is inhibited in order to prevent diplopia and visual confusion.

Anisometropic

Due to unequal, uncorrected refractive errors between the two eyes which causes a constant defocusing of the image. Usually requires high degree of myopic anisometropia (> -6D) but mild degrees of hyperopic or astigmatic anisometropia (1–2D).

Isoametropic

Bilateral amblyopia due to large, but equal, uncorrected refractive errors. Usually requires hyperopic refractive errors >5D, myopic refractive errors > –10D, and astigmatic refractive errors >3D.

Deprivation

Uncommon; usually caused by congenital or acquired media opacities such as cataracts, corneal opacities, or ptosis. Often results in significant loss of vision.

Occlusion

Form of deprivation amblyopia resulting from excessive therapeutic patching during treatment of amblyopia.

Symptoms Variable decreased vision.

Signs Decreased visual acuity ranging from 20/20 to counting fingers (unilateral or bilateral) which often improves with neutral density filters (strabismic amblyopia) or single letter testing; may have strabismus, nystagmus, ptosis, cataract, corneal opacity, small relative afferent pupillary defect.

Differential Diagnosis Functional visual loss, optic neuropathy.

Evaluation
* Complete ophthalmic history and eye exam with attention to vision with neutral density filters and single letters, cycloplegic refraction, retinoscopy, pupils, motility, lids, cornea, lens, and ophthalmoscopy.

Management

* Correct any refractive error.
* Patching or occlusion therapy for children under 10 years old (full-time occlusion of preferred eye for no more than 1 week per year of age of child before reexamination) and continue until vision stabilizes. Discontinue if no improvement after 2–3 months of compliant, full-time patching. May require part-time occlusion to maintain visual level. Alternatively, may use cycloplegic (usually atropine 0.5% or 1% qd) to blur image and improve compliance.
* Protective eyewear with polycarbonate lenses to protect fellow eye if significant amblyopia exists after 10 years of age.
* Consider surgery in cases of deprivation (e.g., cataract extraction) or strabismus.

Prognosis Depends on extent and duration of amblyopia and age at which appropriate corrective therapy is initiated (the earlier the better, must be prior to 9 years of age); poor for deprivation amblyopia, better for strabismic amblyopia.

Cortical Blindness (Cortical Visual Impairment)

Definition   Rare syndrome of bilateral blindness with intact pupillary light response due to widespread damage to the occipital lobes.

Etiology   Cerebrovascular accident (bilateral occipital lobe infarction), rarely neoplasia.

Symptoms   Complete visual loss; rarely, denies blindness (Anton's syndrome), visual hallucinations.

Signs   Normal eye exam (including pupillary response) except for no light perception vision in both eyes; may demonstrate the Riddoch phenomenon (ability to perceive moving, but not static, objects) and "blind sight" (intact primitive mechanism that may allow navigation around objects).

Differential Diagnosis   Functional visual loss.

Evaluation
* Complete ophthalmic history, neurologic exam, and eye exam with attention to vision, pupils, and ophthalmoscopy.
* Head and orbital CT scan or MRI.
* Medical and neurology consultation.

Management

* No treatment recommended.
* Treat underlying etiology.

Prognosis   Poor.

Visual Pathway Lesions

Definition   Lesion of the visual pathway anywhere from the optic nerve to the occipital lobes (see Chapter 11 for Optic nerve lesions).

Etiology   Most commonly vascular or neoplastic; also due to trauma, infection, multiple sclerosis, sarcoidosis, and other rarer causes.

Symptoms   Asymptomatic or may notice decreased vision or visual field loss.

Signs   Normal or decreased visual acuity, visual field defect (usually a hemianopia or quadrantanopia [see Fig. 12-16]); may have relative afferent pupillary defect (if the lesion is anterior to the optic chiasm), may have associated endocrine abnormalities or other neurologic deficits.

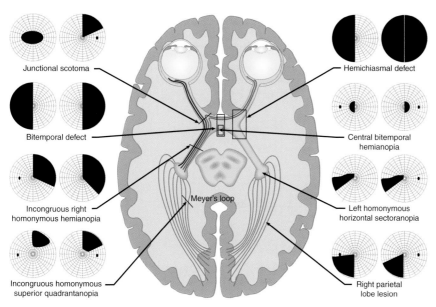

Figure 12-15 • Visual pathway and corresponding visual field defects.

Junctional scotoma

Hemichiasmal defect

Bitemporal defect

Central bitemporal hemianopia

Incongruous right homonymous hemianopia

Meyer's loop

Left homonymous horizontal sectoranopia

Incongruous homonymous superior quadrantanopia

Right parietal lobe lesion

Differential Diagnosis Amaurosis fugax, migraine, temporal arteritis, vertebrobasilar artery insufficiency, functional visual loss.

Evaluation
- Complete ophthalmic history, neurologic exam, and eye exam with attention to vision, pupils, and ophthalmoscopy.
- Check visual fields (defect helps localize the area of involvement).
- Head and orbital CT scan or MRI.
- Medical and neurology consultation.

Management

- Treat underlying etiology.

Prognosis Usually poor, but depends on etiology.

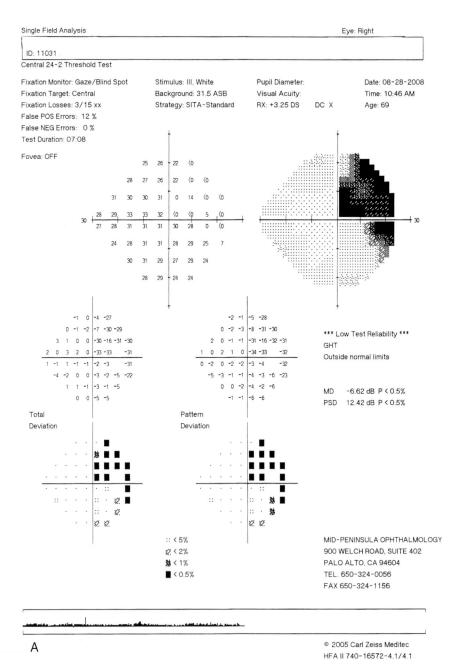

Figure 12-16 • Humphrey visual fields of a patient with a stroke demonstrating an incongruous right homonymous hemianopic field defect that is denser superiorly.

Continued

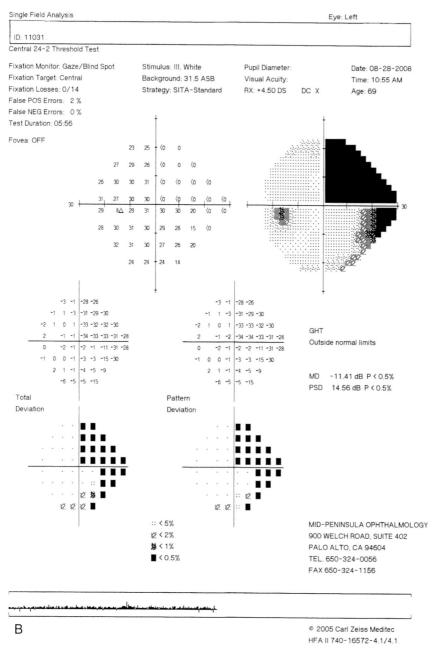

Single Field Analysis   Eye: Left

ID: 11031
Central 24-2 Threshold Test

Fixation Monitor: Gaze/Blind Spot   Stimulus: III, White   Pupil Diameter: Date: 08-28-2008
Fixation Target: Central   Background: 31.5 ASB   Visual Acuity: Time: 10:55 AM
Fixation Losses: 0/14   Strategy: SITA-Standard   RX: +4.50 DS   DC X   Age: 69
False POS Errors: 2 %
False NEG Errors: 0 %
Test Duration: 05:56

Fovea: OFF

GHT
Outside normal limits

MD   -11.41 dB P < 0.5%
PSD   14.56 dB P < 0.5%

Total Deviation

Pattern Deviation

:: < 5%
⬚ < 2%
⬚ < 1%
■ < 0.5%

MID-PENINSULA OPHTHALMOLOGY
900 WELCH ROAD, SUITE 402
PALO ALTO, CA 94604
TEL. 650-324-0056
FAX 650-324-1156

B

© 2005 Carl Zeiss Meditec
HFA II 740-16572-4.1/4.1

Figure 12-16—Cont'd

Ophthalmic History and Examination   549
AAO Suggested Routine Eye Examination
Guidelines   575
Differential Diagnosis of Common
Ocular Symptoms   575
Common Ophthalmic Medications   577
Color Codes for Topical Ocular
Medication Caps   586
Ocular Toxicology   586
List of Important Ocular Measurements   587
List of Eponyms   588
Common Ophthalmic Abbreviations   591
Common Spanish Phrases   593

APPENDIX

Ophthalmic History and Examination

History

As with any medical encounter, the initial part of the evaluation begins with a thorough history. The components of the history are similar to a general medical history but focus on the visual system:

- Chief complaint (CC)
- History of present illness (HPI)
- Past ocular history (POH)
- Eye medications
- Past medical and surgical histories (PMH/PSH)
- Systemic medications
- Allergies
- Family history (FH)
- Social history (SH)
- Review of systems (ROS)

Ocular Examination

The ocular examination is unique in medicine since most of the pathology is directly visible to the examiner; however, specialized equipment and instruments are necessary to perform a comprehensive examination. As with the general medical examination, there are multiple components to the eye examination, and they should be performed systematically.

Vision

Visual acuity

Visual acuity measures the ability to see an object at a certain distance. It is measured one eye at a time, with correction if the patient wears glasses or contact lenses, and usually recorded as a ratio comparing an individual's results with a standard.

Distance vision using a Snellen chart at 20 feet (or 6 meters) is the most common method for recording visual acuity (Table 1), and is denoted with VA, Va, or V and subscript of cc or sc (i.e., V_{cc} or V_{sc}) depending whether the acuity is measured with (cc) or without (sc) correction, respectively. An ocular occluder with pinholes (PH) can be used in an attempt to improve vision and estimate the eye's best potential vision. If pinhole testing improves vision, an uncorrected refractive error or cataract is typically present. Visual acuity worse than 20/400 is recorded either as counting fingers (CF at the test distance; e.g., CF at 6 inches) if the patient can identify the number of fingers the examiner holds up; hand motion (HM) if the patient can identify the movement of the examiner's hand; light perception with projection (LP and the quadrants) if the patient can identify the direction from which a light is shined into the eye; light perception without projection (LP) if the patient can only determine when a bright light is shined into the eye and not the direction the light is coming from; or no light perception (NLP) if the patient cannot perceive light from even the brightest light source. Near vision is similarly measured (monocularly with or without correction) and is denoted with N.

Other types of eye charts used to measure vision include the Bailie-Lovie or Early Treatment Diabetic Retinopathy Study (ETDRS) charts used in clinical trials (vision is measured at 2 and 4 meters). On ETDRS charts halving of the visual angle occurs every 3 lines as there are equal (0.1) logarithmic intervals between lines as well as consistent spacing between letters and rows, proportional to letter size. Unlike Snellen charts, the score is recorded by letter, not line. For preschool children and illiterate adults, other tests including the tumbling "E" chart, Landolt "C" chart, HOTV match test, and Allen card pictures can be used to assess visual acuity. For infants, vision is commonly evaluated by the ability to fix and follow (F&F) objects of interest or the presence of central steady maintained fixation (CSM).

Table A-1 – Measures of Visual Acuity: Central Visual Acuity Notations.

DISTANCE ACUITY NOTATIONS

DISTANCE SNELLEN

Feet	Meters	Decimal	logMAR	Loss of Central Vision (%)
20/10	6/3	2.00	−0.3	—
20/15	6/5	1.25	−0.1	—
20/20	6/6	1.00	0	—
20/25	6/7.5	0.80	0.10	5
20/30	6/10	0.63	0.20	10
20/40	6/12	0.50	0.30	15
20/50	6/15	0.40	0.40	25
20/60	6/20	0.32	0.50	35
20/70	6/22	0.29	0.55	40
20/80	6/24	0.25	0.60	45
20/100	6/30	0.20	0.70	50
20/125	6/38	0.16	0.80	60
20/150	6/50	0.125	0.90	70
20/200	6/60	0.10	1.00	80

Table A-1 – Measures of Visual Acuity: Central Visual Acuity Notations—Cont'd

DISTANCE ACUITY NOTATIONS

DISTANCE SNELLEN

Feet	Meters	Decimal	logMAR	Loss of Central Vision (%)
20/300	6/90	—	—	85
20/400	6/120	—	—	90
20/800	6/240	—	—	95

NEAR ACUITY NOTATIONS

NEAR SNELLEN			DISTANCE SNELLEN		
Inches	Centimeters	Jaeger Standard	American Point-Type	Equivalent	Loss (%)
14/14	35/35	1	3	20/20	—
14/18	35/45	2	4	20/25	0
14/21	35/53	3	5	20/30	5
14/24	35/50	4	6	20/40	7
14/28	35/70	5	7	20/45	10
14/35	35/88	6	8	20/50	50
14/40	35/100	7	9	20/60	55
14/45	35/113	8	10	20/70	60
14/60	35/150	9	11	—	80
14/70	35/175	10	12	—	85
14/80	35/200	11	13	—	87
14/88	35/220	12	14	20/100	90
14/112	35/280	13	21	—	95
14/140	35/350	14	23	—	98

Figure 1 • Eye charts for nonverbal patients or patients who cannot read English letters. Left, Tumbling E chart. Right, Eye chart with pictures.

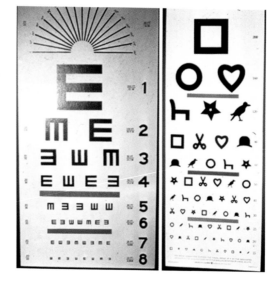

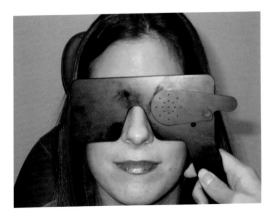

Figure 2 • Patient with pinhole occluder over her left eye.

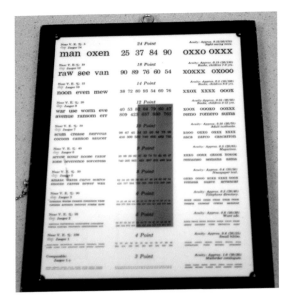

Figure 3 • Near vision chart.

Refraction

A subjective measurement of the refractive error performed with a phoropter or trial frame that allows the patient to decide which lens power gives the sharpest image. This test is used to determine the best spectacle-corrected visual acuity (BSCVA) and prescription for glasses. A manifest refraction is done before dilating the eyes and is denoted with M_R or M. A cycloplegic refraction is done after dilating the eyes with cycloplegic drops to prevent accommodation and is denoted with C_R or C. A cycloplegic refraction is particularly important when refracting children, hyperopes, and refractive surgery candidates, in whom a manifest refraction may not be accurate. The duochrome (red-green) test is a useful method to check the refraction for overcorrection or undercorrection. An autorefractor is an instrument that performs automated retinoscopy and measures refractive error; however, the values should be confirmed with a subjective refraction before prescribing lenses.

Figure 4 • Patient behind a phoropter undergoing manifest refraction.

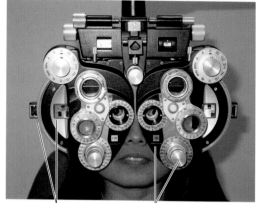

Sphere adjustment   Cylinder adjustment

Figure 5 • Patient undergoing autorefraction.

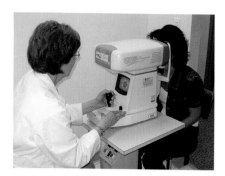

Retinoscopy

An objective measurement of the refractive error performed with a retinoscope; it is denoted with R.

Lensometer

A manual or automated instrument that measures the power of a spectacle or lens; the prescription the patient is wearing is denoted with W.

Glasses placed here

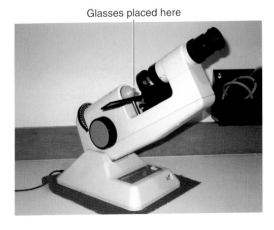

Figure 6 • A lensometer measures the power of spectacle lenses placed on the middle platform.

Potential Acuity Meter (PAM)

An instrument that measures the visual potential of the retina by projecting the eye chart onto the retina through corneal and/or lens opacities. This test is most commonly used to assess visual potential before cataract surgery when there is coexisting retinal pathology.

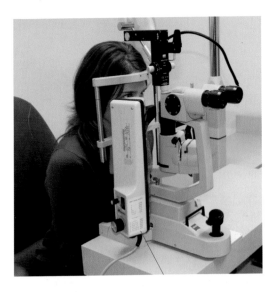

Figure 7 • Patient undergoing potential acuity meter testing. The eyechart is placed on the retina by the instrument mounted on a slit lamp. The eyechart can be focused and takes into account the patient's refractive error.

Contrast Sensitivity

Tested monocularly, usually with special charts (i.e., Pelli–Robson) having bar patterns on backgrounds with varying contrast. Reading can be plotted on a curve for different spatial frequencies.

Color Vision

Tested monocularly and most commonly with Ishihara pseudoisochromatic (red–green only) or Hardy–Rand–Ritter plates. More extensive evaluation is done using Farnsworth tests. Gross macular or optic nerve function can be assessed by asking the patient to identify the color of a red object such as an eyedrop bottle cap (all dilating drops have red caps). Red saturation can also be tested with the red cap by asking the patient whether the cap appears to be the same degree of brightness of red when the eyes are alternately tested.

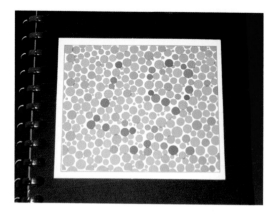

Figure 8 • Ishihara pseudoisochromatic chart with the number 42 evident.

Stereopsis

Stereo acuity is tested binocularly and is commonly done with titmus or randot tests. The titmus test uses polarized images of a fly (patient is asked to grasp or touch the wings), animals (three rows of five cartoon animals each are pictured, and the patient is asked to touch the animal that is popping up), and circles (nine groups of four circles each are pictured, and the patient is asked to touch the circle that is popping up) of increasing difficulty to quantitate the degree of stereopsis (40 seconds of arc is normal).

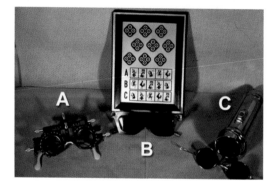

Figure 9 • Three specialized tests. (A) Trial frame. (B) Stereo vision tests with polarized glasses. (C) Worth 4 dot test.

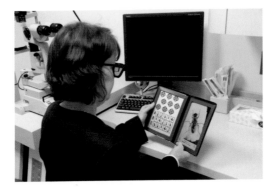

Figure 10 • Patient wearing polarized glasses and performing stereo acuity test. While the patient is wearing the glasses, the fly in the picture appears thee-dimensional.

4 diopter base-out prism test

This test is useful for detecting fusion or suppression in what appear to be "straight" eyes. It is an objective test that can be used on a cooperative young child who may not understand the stereo acuity test. It is also useful for the patient suspected of "faking" a negative stereo test. A 4 diopter base-out prism is placed over one eye, as the patient fixes on a distant target. A normal response is a small convergence movement by each eye. If the prism is placed over a suppressing eye, that eye will not move. A fusing eye will move toward the nose.

Worth 4 dot test

Assesses binocularity in cases of strabismus. The patient views 4 lights (1 red, 2 green, and 1 white) at distance and near while wearing special glasses with a red lens over the right eye and a green lens over the left eye. The size and location of a suppression scotoma can be determined depending on the number and pattern of lights perceived.

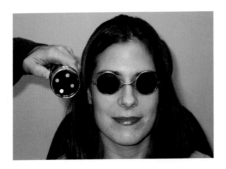

Figure 11 • Worth 4 dot test equipment showing patient with red-green glasses and hand held test light.

Ocular Motility

The alignment of the eyes in primary gaze is observed, and the movement of the eyes is assessed as the patient looks in all directions of gaze by following an object that the examiner moves. Normal motility (extraocular movements) is often recorded as intact (EOMI) or full. If misalignment, gaze restriction, or nystagmus is present, then other tests are performed. Several methods are used to distinguish and measure ocular misalignment.

Figure 12 • Patient undergoing ocular motility testing. *Note:* Her eyes are following the pencil.

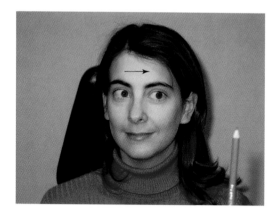

Cover Tests

Assess ocular alignment by occluding an eye while the patient fixates on a target. Measurements are made for both distance and near with and without glasses.

Cover-uncover test

Distinguishes between a tropia and a phoria. One eye is covered and then uncovered. If the unoccluded eye moves when the cover is in place, a tropia is present. If the covered eye moves when the cover is removed, a phoria is present.

Figure 13 • Patient undergoing cover-uncover test to determine if she has a phoria or tropia.

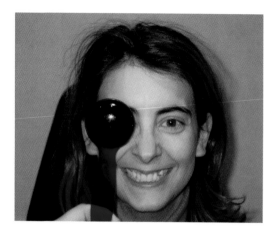

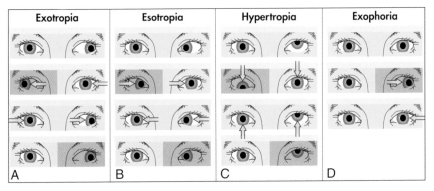

Exotropia	Esotropia	Hypertropia	Exophoria

A   B   C   D

Figure 14 • Cover test for tropias and phorias. (A) For exotropia, covering the right eye drives inward movement of the left eye to take up fixation; uncovering the right eye shows recovery of fixation by the right eye and leftward movement of both eyes; covering up the left eye discloses no shift of the preferred right eye. (B) For esotropia, covering the right eye drives outward movement of the left eye to take up fixation; uncovering the right eye shows recovery of fixation by the right eye and rightward movement of both eyes; covering the left eye shows no shift of the preferred right eye. (C) For hypertropia, covering the right eye drives downward movement of the left eye to take up fixation; uncovering the right eye shows recovery of fixation by the right eye and upward movement of both eyes; covering the left eye shows no shift of the preferred right eye. (D) For exophoria, the left eye deviates outward behind a cover and returns to primary position when the cover is removed. An immediate inward movement denotes a phoria, a delayed inward movement denotes an intermittent exotropia (reproduced with permission from Diamond G, Eggers H: *Srasbismus and Pediatric Ophthalmology*, 1993, London, Mosby).

Alternate cover test (prism and cover test)

Measures the total ocular deviation (tropia and phoria). The occluder is alternately placed in front of each eye until dissociation occurs, and then hand-held prisms are held in front of an eye until no movement occurs.

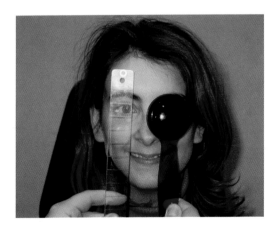

Figure 15 • Patient undergoing alternate cover test in which the total ocular deviation is determined by holding prisms over the eye until no movement occurs.

Corneal Light Reflex Tests

Assess ocular alignment by observing the relative position of the corneal light reflections from a light source directed into the patient's eyes; can be used in patients who cannot cooperate for cover tests. The position of the corneal light reflexes can be used to measure the ocular deviation.

Hirschberg's Method

The amount of decentration of the light reflex is used to estimate ocular deviation (1 mm of decentration corresponds to 7° or 15 prism diopters [PD]). Light reflections at the pupillary margin (2 mm decentration), mid-iris (4 mm decentration), and limbus (6 mm decentration) correspond to deviations of approximately 15° or 30 PD, 30° or 45 PD, and 45° or 60 PD, respectively.

Figure 16 • Hirschberg's method of estimating deviation (reproduced with permission from von Noorden GK; *Von Noorden-Maumenee's Atlas of Strabismus,* ed 3, 1977, St. Louis, Mosby).

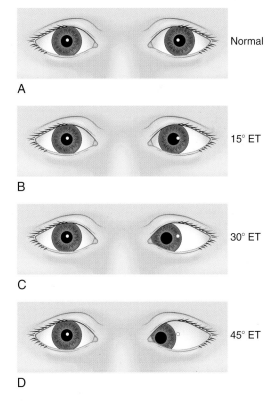

Modified Krimsky's Method

Prisms are placed in front of the fixating eye to center the light reflection in the deviated eye.

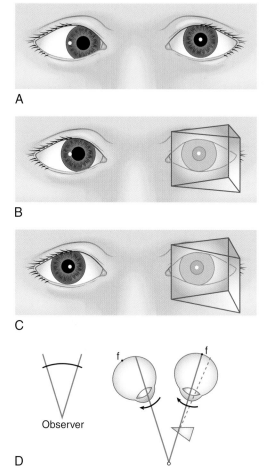

A

B

C

D

Figure 17 • Modified Krimsky's method of estimating deviation (reproduced with permission from von Noorden GK; *Von Noorden-Maumenee's Atlas of Strabismus*, ed 3, 1977, St. Louis, Mosby).

Observer

Forced Ductions

Determine whether limited ocular motility is due to a restrictive etiology. Under topical anesthesia the eye is grasped at the limbus with forceps and rotated into the deficient direction of gaze. Resistance to movement indicates restriction. The forceps should be placed on the same side of the limbus in which the eye is being moved to avoid an inadvertent corneal abrasion should the forceps slip.

Optokinetic Testing

Assesses patients with nystagmus and other eye movement disorders. A rotating drum (or strip) with alternating black and white lines is slowly moved both horizontally and vertically in front of the patient and the resultant eye movements are observed.

Figure 18 • Patient undergoing OKN testing.

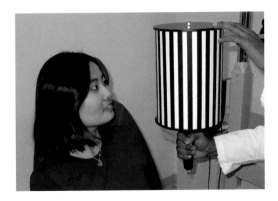

Pupils

The size, shape, and reactivity of the pupils are assessed while the patient fixates on a distant target. Both the direct and consensual responses are observed. The swinging flashlight test is done to identify a relative afferent pupillary defect (see RAPD in Chapter 7), particularly if anisocoria or poor reaction to light is present. If the pupils react to light, then they will react to accommodation, so this does not need to be tested; however, if one or both pupils do not react to light, then the reaction to accommodation should be assessed since some conditions may cause light-near dissociation.

The reactivity of each pupil is graded on a scale of 1+ (sluggish) to 4+ (brisk). Normal pupils should be equal, round, and briskly reactive to light. The most common abbreviation for denoting this pupillary response is "pupils equal round and reactive to light" (PERRL or PERRLA if accommodation is also tested). A preferred method that provides more information is to note the size of the pupils before and after the light stimulus is applied (i.e., P 4 → 2 OU). If anisocoria is present, the pupils should be measured in both normal lighting conditions and dim conditions (mesopic or scotopic).

Visual Fields

Confrontation visual fields are evaluated monocularly with the patient and examiner sitting opposite one another and looking into the examiner's opposite eye (used as a control) while being asked to identify the number of fingers presented or the movement of a finger in each quadrant. Normal fields are recorded as visual fields full to confrontation (VFFC or VF full).

Figure 19 • Patient undergoing confrontation visual field testing.

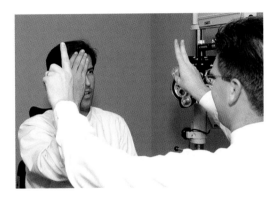

Amsler Grid

A 10 cm × 10 cm grid composed of 5 mm squares that evaluates the central 10° of the visual field. This test is most commonly used to assess central visual distortion in patients with age-related macular degeneration and other macular pathology.

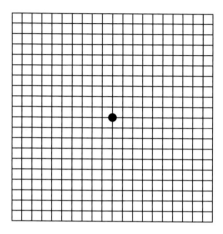

Figure 20 • Amsler grid.

Tangent Screen

A manual test that is performed with the patient seated 1 m in front of a 2 m × 2 m square black cloth over which the examiner presents test objects (spheres of various size and color).

Goldmann Visual Field

A manually operated machine used to perform static and kinetic perimetry centrally and peripherally.

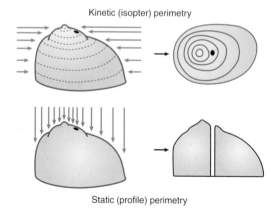

Kinetic (isopter) perimetry

Static (profile) perimetry

Figure 21 • Kinetic and static perimetry (reproduced with permission from Bajandas FJ, Kline LB: *Neuro-Ophthalmology Review Manual*, ed 3, 2004, Thorofare, NJ, Slack).

Figure 22 • Patient undergoing Goldmann visual field examination.

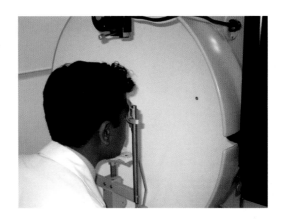

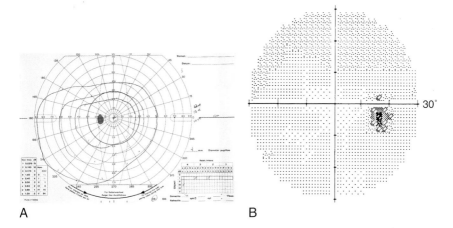

A   B

Figure 23 • Normal (A) Goldman and (B) Humphrey visual field.

Humphrey Visual Field

A computerized static perimetry test with various programs to screen for and evaluate glaucomatous, neurologic, and lid-induced visual field defects.

External Examination

Orbit, eyelid, and lacrimal structures are evaluated for symmetry, position, and any abnormalities. Palpation and auscultation are performed when indicated.

Exophthalmometry

Measurement of the distance the corneal apex protrudes from the lateral orbital rim to assess for proptosis or enophthalmos. The exophthalmometer is adjusted to rest against the lateral orbital rims, and with the patient looking in primary gaze, the level of each corneal apex is viewed in the exophthalmometer mirrors; these measurements along with the base number (width of the orbital rims) are recorded.

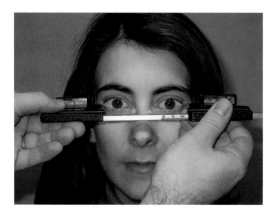

Figure 24 • Patient undergoing exophthalmometry test to measure for proptosis or enophthalmos.

Schirmer's Test

Special strips of 5 × 35 mm Whatman #41 filter paper are placed in the lower eyelids to absorb tears and measure tear production to evaluate dry eyes (see Dry Eye Disease in Chapter 4).

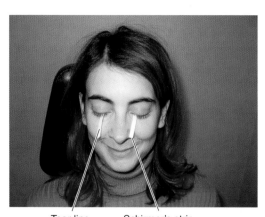

Figure 25 • Patient undergoing Schirmer's testing for dry eyes. This patient's tears have wet the strips sufficiently, indicating that she does not have dry eyes.

Tear line   Schirmer's strip

Jones' Dye Tests

Two tests that evaluate lacrimal drainage obstruction (see Nasolacrimal Duct Obstruction in Chapter 3).

Other Cranial Nerve Examination

CN5 is tested to assess facial and corneal sensation, and CN7 is tested to assess facial movement including eyelid closure, when warranted.

Slit Lamp Examination

This specialized biomicroscope allows detailed examination of the eye. The height, width, and angle of the light beam can all be controlled, and various filters can be changed to enhance visualization. A thin beam directed through the clear ocular media (cornea, anterior chamber, lens, and vitreous) acts as a scalpel of light illuminating a cross-sectional slice of optical tissue. This property of the slit-lamp allows precise localization of pathology. The technique of retroillumination (coaxial alignment of the light beam with the oculars) uses the red reflex from the retina to backlight the cornea and lens, making some abnormalities more easily visible. Furthermore, anterior segment lesions can be accurately measured by recording the height of the slit-beam from the millimeter scale on the control knob. Although the posterior segment can be evaluated with the aid of additional lenses, the SLE typically focuses on the anterior segment.

Portable, hand-held, slit-lamp devices facilitate examination at the bedside. If a slit-lamp instrument is not available, a penlight examination can be done with a magnifying lens to briefly assess the anterior segment. Similarly, a direct ophthalmoscope or indirect ophthalmoscope and lens can also be focused on the anterior segment structures for examination.

Figure 26 • Patient undergoing slit-lamp examination.

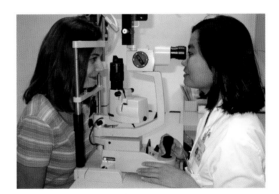

Components of the Slit Lamp Examination

Lids, Lashes, and Lacrimal Glands The lids, lashes, puncta, and Meibomian gland orifices are inspected. The medial canthus or lid margin can be palpated to express discharge or secretions from the inferior punctum or Meibomian glands, respectively. The lacrimal gland can also be inspected and palpated.

Conjunctiva and Sclera The patient is asked to look in the horizontal and vertical directions to observe the entire bulbar conjunctiva, and the lids are everted to observe the tarsal conjunctival surface. The caruncle and plica semilunaris are also inspected. The upper eyelid can be double everted to evaluate the superior fornix, and a moistened cotton-tipped applicator can be used to sweep the fornix to remove suspected foreign bodies.

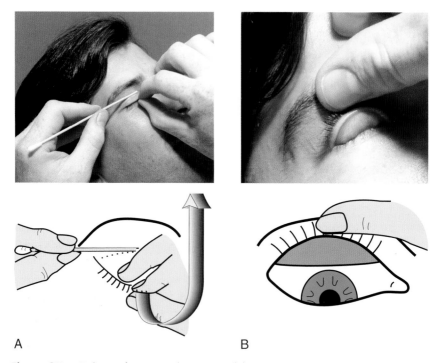

Figure 27 • Technique for everting the upper eyelid.

Cornea All five layers of the cornea are inspected. The tear film is evaluated for break-up time and height of the meniscus. The cobalt blue filter allows better visualization of corneal iron lines.

Anterior Chamber The anterior chamber is evaluated for depth – graded on a scale from 1+ (shallow) to 4+ (deep) – and the presence of cells and flare (see Chapter 6). Normally, the AC is deep and quiet (D&Q).

Iris and Lens The iris and lens are inspected. The lens is better evaluated after pupillary dilation. If the eye is pseudophakic, the position and stability of the intraocular lens implant are noted, and the condition of the posterior capsule is assessed. The anterior vitreous (AV) can also be observed without the use of additional lenses. For aphakic eyes, the integrity of the anterior hyaloid face is evaluated, and any vitreous prolapse into the AC or strands to anterior structures is noted.

Dyes

Fluorescein, rose bengal, and lissamine green can be used to evaluate the health and integrity of the conjunctival and corneal epithelium. The integrity of wounds is assessed with the Seidel test (see Laceration in Chapter 5).

Gonioscopy

Evaluation of the anterior chamber angle structures with special mirrored contact lenses that are placed on the cornea. Various grading systems exist to specify the degree to which the angle is open. Indentation gonioscopy is used to determine whether angle-closure is due

Figure 28 • Goldmann gonioscopy lens.

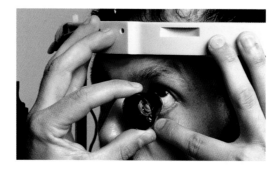

Figure 29 • Shaffer's angle grading system (reproduced with permission from Fran M, Smith J, Doyle W: Clinical examination of glaucoma. In: Yanoff M, Duker JS [eds]: *Ophthalmology*, ed 2, 2004, St. Louis, Mosby).

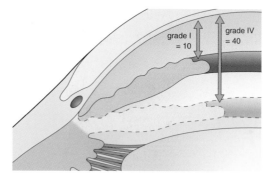

to apposition (opens with indentation of the central cornea which pushes aqueous peripherally) or synechiae (does not open with indentation).

Fundus contact and noncontact lenses

Numerous lenses can be used to examine the retina and optic nerve. Although performed with a slit-lamp, these findings are recorded as part of the fundus examination (see below).

Tonometry

Various instruments can be used to measure the intraocular pressure (IOP). Most commonly, IOP is measured as part of the slit lamp examination (SLE) with the Goldmann applanation tonometer (a biprism that creates optical doubling) that is attached to the slit-lamp. Topical anesthetic drops and fluorescein drops (either individually or in a combination drop) are instilled into the eye, the tonometer head is illuminated with a broad beam and cobalt blue filter, the tip contacts the cornea, the dial is adjusted until the mirror-image semicircular mires slightly overlap so that their inner margins just touch each other, and the pressure measurement in mm Hg is obtained by multiplying the dial reading by 10 (i.e., "2" equals 20 mm Hg). If marked corneal astigmatism exists, to obtain an accurate reading the tonometer tip must be rotated so that the graduation marking corresponding to the flattest corneal meridian is aligned with the red mark on the tip holder. Central corneal thickness also affects pressure readings. It is important to record the time when the pressure is measured. If a slit-lamp is not available, portable hand-held devices such as the Tono-Pen, Perkins, or Shiotz tonometers can be used. Estimating IOP by digital palpation (finger tension) is highly inaccurate.

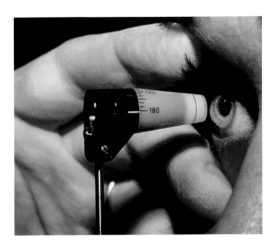

Figure 30 • Goldmann applanation tonometer.

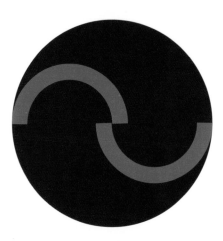

Figure 31 • Applanation tonometer mires as viewed through a slit lamp. When the mires overlap, as in this figure, the intraocular pressure can be determined.

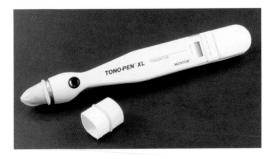

Figure 32 • Hand-held tonometer (Tono-Pen).

Specialized Tests

Pachymetry

Measurement of corneal thickness by an optical or ultrasound pachymeter. Ultrasound instruments are used to measure central corneal thickness by applanation and therefore require topical anesthesia. This is most commonly performed in order to adjust IOP measured by applanation tonometry and to screen refractive surgery candidates. Optical devices are computerized to generate a thickness map of the entire cornea, which can be helpful in evaluating corneal ectasia and edema.

Figure 33 • Patient undergoing pachymetry testing.

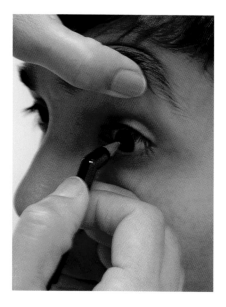

Keratometry

Measurement of corneal curvature and power using a keratometer, which evaluates two paracentral points on the anterior corneal surface. Mires are projected onto the cornea and by turning the instrument knobs to align the reflected images, a direct reading is obtained. Automated machines often combine keratometry with other measurements such as refractive error or biometry.

Figure 34 • Patient undergoing manual keratometry.

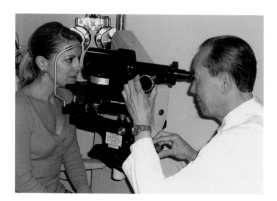

Corneal Topography

Computerized videokeratography (CVK) measures the curvature or elevation of the entire corneal surface providing more information than keratometry. These instruments produce topographic maps, and some can measure the posterior corneal surface as well as corneal thickness. Many contain software to help identify early corneal irregularities.

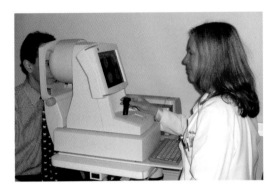

Figure 35 • Patient undergoing corneal topography. Note the corneal topographic map on the screen.

Wavefront Aberrometry

Measurement of the total aberrations of the eye (cornea and lens) including the higher order aberrations (HOAs). Zernicke or Fourier analysis is used to determine the aberrations and generate a map. This technology is utilized in wavefront refractive surgical procedures.

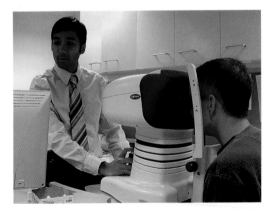

Figure 36 • Patient undergoing wavefront aberrometry.

Specular Microscopy

Evaluation of the corneal endothelial cells by specular light reflection. The instrument measures cell count and morphology.

Figure 37 • A specular microscope measures corneal endothelial cell count and morphology.

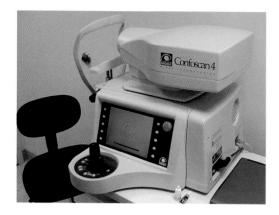

Fundus Examination

The optic nerve and retina can be examined with or without pupillary dilation and with a variety of instruments and lenses. Direct ophthalmoscopy (DO) and indirect ophthalmoscopy (IO) are performed with a direct or indirect ophthalmoscope, respectively. The direct ophthalmoscope provides monocular high magnification (15×) with a narrow field of view, whereas the indirect ophthalmoscope produces a wide binocular field of view at lower magnification (2–3×). The image obtained through the indirect lenses used for IO and slit-lamp examination are flipped and inverted, and this must be taken into account when drawing retinal diagrams. An easy way to correct for this image reversal is to turn the retinal diagram upside-down and then draw the pathology as it is seen through the lens; when the diagram is viewed right side up, the picture will then be correct. A dilated fundus examination is often denoted as DFE, and the appearance of the disc, vessels, macula, and periphery are noted. A normal retinal examination is commonly abbreviated as d/v/m/p wnl. The dimensions and location of lesions are compared to the size of the disc; thus measurements are recorded as multiples of disc diameters (DD) or areas (DA).

Figure 38 • Patient undergoing direct ophthalmoscopic examination.

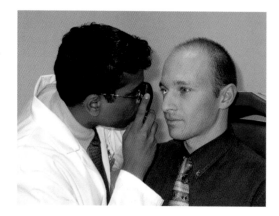

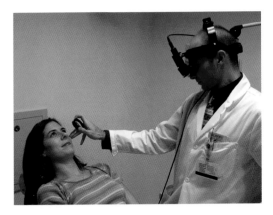

Figure 39 • Patient undergoing indirect ophthalmoscopic examination.

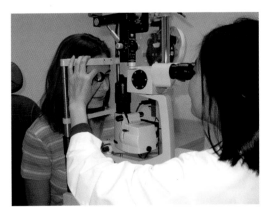

Figure 40 • Patient undergoing slit-lamp fundus examination with a high magnification lens to evaluate the macula.

Components of the fundus examination

Disc The optic nerve is inspected with particular attention to the cup-to-disc ratio (C/D), appearance of the neural rim (normally sharp and flat), and color (orange–yellow). The presence/absence of disc edema is also important.

Vessels The retinal vessels are observed as they emerge from the optic cup and followed as they branch toward the periphery. Spontaneous venous pulsations can sometimes be seen at the nerve head. Any anomalous pattern or abnormality of the vasculature is recorded. This includes color (important for diseases such as hypertension where the vessels can take on an appearance of copper wires), tortuosity, caliber, and any changes where arteries and veins cross (i.e., AV nicking).

Macula The macula, especially the fovea, is evaluated. Usually a bright light reflex is seen at the center of the fovea, especially in younger patients. In eyes with a suspected macular hole or cyst, the Watzke–Allen test can be performed by shining a thin vertical slit-beam over the center of the fovea and asking the patient if the light beam appears discontinuous or narrower in the middle (see Macular Hole in Chapter 10).

Peripheral Retina The retinal periphery is most easily examined through a widely dilated pupil. The patient is asked to look in all directions of gaze so that the entire retina (360°) can be viewed with indirect ophthalmoscopy. Visualization and differentiation of pathology near the ora serrata and far retinal periphery are aided with scleral depression.

Figure 41 • Patient undergoing scleral depression in combination with binocular indirect ophthalmoscopic examination to evaluate the far peripheral retina.

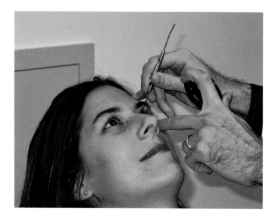

Specialized Tests

Ultrasonography

Measurement of the acoustic reflectivity of ocular interfaces. Two modes:

A-scan (Amplitude)

Produces a 1-dimensional display that is primarily used to determine axial length measurement (biometry) for IOL calculations, but it can also be helpful to differentiate the internal structure of ocular masses. Methods include immersion (more accurate) or contact (less accurate due to corneal indentation and misalignment errors). Biometry measurement is based upon reflectivity from the internal limiting membrane.

Figure 42 • Patient undergoing immersion A-scan ultrasonography.

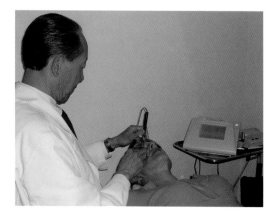

B-scan (Brightness)

Produces a 2-dimensional image of the posterior segment, and is obtained when the fundus cannot be directly visualized.

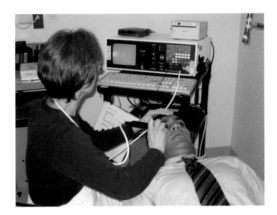

Figure 43 • Patient undergoing a B-scan ultrasonography evaluation.

Partial Coherence Laser Interferometry (IOLMaster)

Measurement of the optical reflectivity from the retinal pigment epithelium to determine axial length. Non-contact modality with accuracy equivalent to or better than immersion A-scan. The IOLMaster instrument also performs keratometry, anterior chamber depth, and white-to-white measurements as well as IOL calculations.

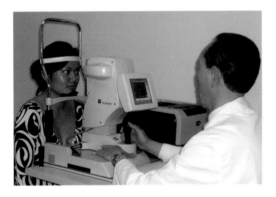

Figure 44 • Patient undergoing IOLMaster evaluation.

Optical Coherence Tomography

A noninvasive, noncontact imaging modality that provides high-resolution, cross-sectional images of the eye by measurement of the optical reflectivity of ocular structures. Optical coherence tomography (OCT) is useful for diagnosing and following anterior segment, macular and optic nerve pathology. Time domain OCT (TDOCT) relies on movement of a mirror and thus requires a longer period of time to acquire images. Spectral (SDOCT) or fourier domain OCT offers dramatically increased speed as no movement of the mirror is required. In addition, SDOCT offers improved resolution. By using OCT perpendicular to the cornea, anterior segment structures can also be imaged with excellent detail.

Figure 45 • Patient undergoing Stratus time-domain optical coherence tomography evaluation of her nerve fiber layer for glaucoma.

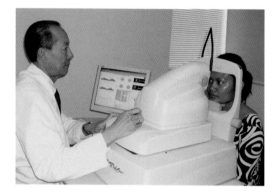

Reference

Wilson FM, Gurland JE: *Practical Ophthalmology: A manual for beginning residents,* ed 5, San Francisco, 2005, American Academy of Ophthalmology.

AAO Suggested Routine Eye Examination Guidelines

Ages 0-2: screening during regular pediatric appointments.

Ages 3-5: screening every 1–2 years during regular primary care appointments.

Ages 6–19: schedule examinations as needed.

Ages 20–29: one examination.

Ages 30–39: two examinations.

Ages 40–65: examination every 2–4 years.

Ages 65 and over: examination every 1–2 years.

(More frequent examinations may be recommended if any of the following risk factors exist: history of eye injury, diabetes, family history of eye problems, African Americans older than 40 years of age.)

Differential Diagnosis of Common Ocular Symptoms

Blurred vision

There are many causes of blurred or decreased vision, so to narrow the differential diagnosis, it is important to characterize further the visual loss in terms of rapidity of onset, duration, central versus peripheral vision, distance versus near vision, monocular versus binocular, and other associated symptoms (i.e., none, pain, red eye, tearing, flashes of light, headache, other neurologic symptoms):

- **Sudden loss of vision:** ophthalmic artery occlusion, retinal vascular occlusion (central will cause profound loss, branch will cause visual field defect), wet macular degeneration (usually central loss, peripheral vision preserved), macular hole (usually central loss, peripheral vision preserved), retinal detachment, vitreous hemorrhage, hyphema, acute angle closure (painful), central corneal epithelial defect (blurry vision and very painful; i.e., abrasion, recurrent erosion, herpes simplex keratitis).

Table A-2 – Common Causes and Associated Findings of a Red Eye

Diagnosis	Vision	Redness	Pain	Discharge	Cornea	Intraocular pressure	Pupil
Conjunctivitis	Normal	Diffuse, superficial	Itch or foreign body	Watery, sticky, or purulent	May have punctate staining	Normal	Normal
Subconjunctival hemorrhage	Normal	Bright red confluent	None	None	Normal	Normal	Normal
Corneal abrasion	May be blurred	Diffuse or ciliary flush	Sharp, foreign body	Tearing	Staining defect	Normal	Normal
Episcleritis	Normal	Often sectoral	Irritation	None	Normal	Normal	Normal
Scleritis	Normal	Deep, violaceous	Tender, deep ache	None	Normal	Normal	Normal
Angle-closure glaucoma	Decreased	Ciliary flush	Severe	None	Cloudy, edema	Very high	Mid dilated
Uveitis	May be blurred	Ciliary flush	Ache, photophobia	None	May have keratic precipitates	Normal, low, or high	Normal

- **Gradual loss of vision:** optic neuropathy, optic neuritis (pain with eye movements), glaucoma, dry macular degeneration, macular edema, diabetic retinopathy, central serous retinopathy, chronic retinal detachment, uveitis (mild pain/photophobia), cataract (may also cause glare from bright lights), corneal edema, corneal dystrophy, change in refractive error.
- **Transient loss of vision (<24 hours):** amaurosis fugax (transient ischemic attack), vertebrobasilar insufficiency, migraine, papilledema, presyncopal episode.
- **Visual field defect:** stroke, optic neuropathy, branch retinal vascular occlusion, chronic glaucoma, retinal detachment.

Eye Pain

Patients with ocular discomfort must be asked about the character of their pain:

- **Superficial/foreign-body sensation/itch/burn:** usually due to anterior ocular structures, including corneal or conjunctival foreign body, pingueculitis, inflamed pterygium, corneal abrasion, recurrent erosion, keratitis, dry eye disease, conjunctivitis, blepharitis, trichiasis.
- **Deep/ache:** uveitis, angle closure, scleritis, myositis, optic neuritis, cranial nerve palsy, orbital lesion (idiopathic orbital inflammation, cellulitis, mass).

Tearing

Dry eye, trichiasis, ectropion, conjunctivitis, nasolacrimal duct obstruction, dacryocystitis, keratitis, corneal or conjunctival foreign body, blepharitis.

Discharge

Conjunctivitis, nasolacrimal duct obstruction, dacryocystitis, canaliculitis, corneal ulcer, blepharitis.

Flashes of light

Retinal tear/detachment, posterior vitreous detachment, migraine, optic neuritis.

Red Eye

The common causes and associated findings of a red eye are listed in Table A-2.

Common Ophthalmic Medications

Anti-Infectives

Antibiotics

Aminoglycosides

amikacin (Amikin) 10 mg/mL up to q1h

amikacin 25 mg/0.5 mL subconjunctival

amikacin 0.4 mg/0.1 mL intravitreal

amikacin 15 mg/kg/day IV in 2–3 divided doses

gentamicin (Genoptic, Gent-AK, Gentacidin, Garamycin) 0.3% qid fortified tobramycin 13.6 mg/mL up to q1h

tobramycin (Tobrex, AK-Tob, Tobralcon, Tobrasol) 0.3% qid to q1h

neomycin-polymyxin B-gramicidin 0.025 (Neosporin, AK-Spore) qid to q1h

Fluoroquinolones

ciprofloxacin (Ciloxan) 0.3% solution or ointment qid to q1h

ciprofloxacin (Cipro) 500–750 mg PO bid

gatifloxacin (Zymar) 0.3% qid to q1h

levofloxacin (Quixin) 0.5% (Iquix) 1.5% qid to q1h

levofloxacin (Levaquin) 500 mg PO qd

moxifloxacin (Vigamox) 0.5% tid to q1h

norfloxacin (Chibroxin, Noroxin) 0.3% qid to q1h

ofloxacin (Ocuflox) 0.3% qid to q1h

ofloxacin (Floxin) 200–400 mg PO q12h

Penicillins

amoxicillin/clavulanate (Augmentin) 250 mg PO q8h or 500 mg PO bid

ampicillin 500 μg/0.1 mL intravitreal

ampicillin 50–150 mg/0.5 mL subconjunctival

ampicillin (Polycillin) 4–12 g/day IV in 4 divided doses

methicillin 200–300 mg/kg/day IV in 4 divided doses

penicillin G 12–24 million/units/day IV in 4 divided doses

ticarcillin (Ticar) 200–300 mg/kg/day IV in 3 divided doses

Cephalosporins

cefazolin 100 mg/0.5 mL subconjunctival

cefazolin 2.25 mg/0.1 mL intravitreal

cefazolin (Ancef) 50–100 mg/kg/day IV in 3–4 divided doses

cefotaxime (Claforan) 25 mg/kg IV q8–12h

ceftazidime 2.25 mg/0.1 mL intravitreal

ceftazidime 100 mg/0.5 mL subconjunctival

ceftazidime (Fortaz) 2 g IV q8h

ceftriaxone 100 mg/0.5 mL subconjunctival

ceftriaxone (Rocephin) 2 gm IV q12h

cephalexin (Keflex) 500 mg PO bid

fortified cefazolin 50–100 mg/mL up to q1h

fortified ceftazidime 50–100 mg/mL up to q1h

Macrolides

azithromycin (Azasite) 1% bid for 2 days then qd for 5 days

azithromycin (Zithromax) 250–600 mg PO Z-Pak

erythromycin (Ilotycin, AK-Mycin, Romycin) 0.5% qd to qid

erythromycin 0.5 mg/0.1 mL intravitreal

erythromycin 100 mg/0.5 mL subconjunctival

Peptides

bacitracin (AK-Tracin) qd to qid

neomycin-polymyxin B-bacitracin (AK-Spore, Neosporin, Ocutricin) qid to q2h

polymyxin B-bacitracin (Polysporin, AK-Poly Bac, Polycin B) qid to q4h

polymyxin B-oxytetracycline (Terak, Terramycin) qid to q4h

trimethoprim-polymyxin B (Polytrim) qid to q1h

fortified vancomycin 25–50 mg/mL up to q1h

vancomycin 1 mg/0.1 mL intravitreal

vancomycin 25 mg/0.5 mL subconjunctival

vancomycin 1 gm IV q12h

Sulfonamides

sulfacetamide sodium (AK-Sulf, Bleph-10, Cetamide, Ophthacet, Sodium Sulamyd, Sulf-10) 10% (Sodium Sulamyd, Vasosulf) 30% solution (AK-Sulf, Bleph-10, Cetamide, Sodium Sulamyd) 10% ointment, qid to q2h

trimethoprim/sulfamethoxazole (Bactrim) 1 double-strength tablet PO bid

Tetracyclines

doxycycline 20–200 mg PO qd

minocycline 25–100 mg PO qd

tetracycline 250–500 mg PO qd

tetracycline (Achromycin) 1% qid to q2h

Miscellaneous Antibiotics

chloramphenicol (Chloroptic, AK-Chlor, Ocuchlor, Chloromycetin) 0.5% gtts, 1.0% ung qid to q4h

clindamycin (Cleocin) 50 mg/mL up to q1h

clindamycin (Cleocin) 15–50 mg/0.5 mL subconjunctival

clindamycin (Cleocin) 200 μg/0.1 mL intravitreal

clindamycin (Cleocin) 300 mg PO qid

clindamycin (Cleocin) 600–900 mg IV q8h

Antibiotic/Steroid Combinations

gentamicin-prednisolone acetate 0.6% (Pred-G) solution or ointment qid to q2h

neomycin-polymyxin B-dexamethasone (AK-Trol, Maxitrol, Dexacidin, Dexasporin) qid to q2h

neomycin-dexamethasone 0.05% (NeoDecadron) qid to q2h

neomycin-polymyxin B-prednisolone acetate (Poly-Pred Liquifilm) qid to q2h

neomycin-polymyxin B-hydrocortisone (AK-Spore HC, Cortisporin) qid to q2h

oxytetracycline-hydrocortisone acetate (Terra-Cortril) qid

sulfacetamide sodium 10%-prednisolone acetate 0.2% (Blephamide) solution or ointment qid to q4h

sulfacetamide sodium 10%-flurometholone 1% (FML-S) qid to q4h

sulfacetamide sodium 10%-prednisolone phosphate 0.25% (Isopto Cetapred, Vasocidin) qid to q4h

sulfacetamide sodium 10%-prednisolone phosphate 0.25% (Cetapred) ointment qid to q4h

sulfacetamide sodium 10%-prednisolone acetate 0.5% (Ak-Cide, Metimyd) solution or ointment qid to q4h

tobramycin 0.3%-dexamethasone 0.1% (Tobradex) solution or ointment qid to q2h

tobramycin 0.3%-loteprednol etabonate 0.5% (Zylet) qid to q2h

Antiamoebics

chlorhexidine 0.02% up to q1h

polyhexamethylene biguanide (PHBG, Baquacil) 0.02% up to q1h

propamidine isethionate (Brolene) 0.1% up to q1h

hexamidine (Desomedine) 0.1% up to q1h

paromomycin (Humatin) 10 mg/mL up to q1h

Antifungals

amphotericin B 0.1–0.5% up to q1h

amphotericin B 0.25–1.0 mg/kg IV over 6 hours

amphotericin B 5 mg/0.1 mL intravitreal

clotrimazole 1% up to q1h

fluconazole (Diflucan) 800 mg PO loading dose, 400 mg/day maintenance

fluconazole (Diflucan) 0.2% up to q1h

flucytosine (Ancobon) 50–150 mg/kg/day IV in 4 divided doses

ketoconazole 1–2% up to q1h

ketoconazole (Nizoral) 200–400 mg PO qd to tid

metronidazole 0.75% ointment qd

miconazole 1% up to q1h

miconazole 25 µg/0.1 mL intravitreal

miconazole 30 mg/kg/day IV

natamycin (Natacyn) 5% up to q1h

voriconazole 1% up to q 1h

Antivirals

acyclovir (Zovirax) 200–800 mg; for herpes simplex virus: 200–400 mg PO bid to five times a day; for herpes zoster virus: 800 mg PO five times a day for 7–10 days

famciclovir (Famvir) 250–500 mg; for herpes simplex virus: 250–500 mg PO qd to tid; for herpes zoster virus: 500 mg PO tid for 7 days.

foscarnet (Foscavir) induction: 90–120 mg/kg IV bid for 14–21 days; maintenance: 90–120 mg/kg IV qd

ganciclovir (Cytovene) induction: 5 mg/kg IV bid for 14–21 days; maintenance: 5 mg/kg IV qd

idoxuridine (Herplex, Stoxil) 0.1% solution, 0.5% ointment qd to 5 times a day

trifluridine (Viroptic) 1% qd to 9 times a day

valacyclovir (Valtrex) 500–1000 mg; for herpes simplex virus: 500–1000 mg PO qd to tid; for herpes zoster virus: 1 g PO tid for 7 days

vidarabine (Vira-A) 3% qd to 5 times a day

Antiinflammatories

NSAIDs

bromfenac (Xibrom) 0.09% qd to bid

celecoxib (Celebrex) 100 mg PO bid

diclofenac sodium (Voltaren) 0.1% qd to qid

diclofenac sodium (Voltaren) 75 mg PO bid

diflunisal (Dolobid) 250–500 mg PO bid

flurbiprofen sodium (Ocufen) 0.03% for prevention of intraoperative miosis

indomethacin (Indocin) 50 mg PO bid to tid

ketorolac tromethamine (Acular) 0.5% (Acular LS) 0.4% qd to qid

naproxen (Naprosyn) 250 mg PO bid

nepafenac (Nevanac) 0.1% qd to tid

suprofen (Profenal) 1% for prevention of intraoperative miosis

Immunomodulator

cyclosporine (Restasis) 0.05% bid

Steroids

dexamethasone alcohol (Maxidex) 0.1% qd to q1h

dexamethasone sodium phosphate (Decadron, AK-Dex) 0.05–0.1% qd to q1h

difluprednate (Durezol) 0.05% qd to q1h

fluorometholone acetate (Flarex, Eflone) 0.1% qd to q1h

fluorometholone alcohol (Fluor-Op, FML) 0.1% (FML Forte) 0.25% qd to q1h

fluorometholone alcohol (FML S.O.P.) 0.1% ointment qd to q1h loteprednol etabonate (Lotemax) 0.5% (Alrex) 0.2% qd to q1h

medrysone (HMS) 1% qd to q1h

prednisolone acetate (Pred Mild) 0.12% (Econopred) 0.125% (AK-Tate, Pred Forte, Econopred Plus) 1% qd to q1h

prednisolone sodium phosphate (Inflamase Mild, AK-Pred) 0.125% (Inflamase Forte, AK-Pred) 1% qd to q1h

prednisone 60–100 mg PO qd followed by taper; co-therapy (to prevent peptic ulcer disease) with famotidine (Pepcid), lansoprazole (Prevacid), omeprazole (Prilosec), or ranitidine (Zantac)

rimexolone (Vexol) 1% qd to q1h

Ocular Hypotensive (Glaucoma) Medications
Alpha-Adrenergic Receptor Agonists (Purple Cap)

Mechanism of action: inhibit aqueous production, may enhance uveoscleral outflow.

apraclonidine (Iopidine) 0.5% tid or 1.0% bid

brimonidine (Alphagan-P) 0.15% (Alphagan) 0.2% tid.

Side effects: superior lid retraction, miosis, blanching of conjunctival vessels, dry mouth, dry nose, tachyphylaxis, lethargy, headache, allergic reactions

dipivefrin (Propine) 0.1% bid

epinephrine (Glaucon, Epifrin, Epitrate) 0.25%, 0.5%, 1%, 2% bid

Side effects: cystoid macular edema in aphakic eyes, hypertension, tachycardia, adrenochrome deposits in conjunctiva (epinephrine)

Beta-Blockers (Yellow or Blue Cap)

Mechanism of action: inhibit aqueous production by blocking β_2-receptors on non-pigmented ciliary epithelium.

betaxolol (Betoptic S) 0.25% (Betoptic) 0.5% bid

carteolol (Ocupress) 1.5%, 3% bid

levobetaxolol (Betaxon) 0.5% bid

levobunolol (Betagan) 0.25–0.5% qd or bid

metipranolol (OptiPranolol) 0.3% bid

timolol (Timoptic, Betimol) 0.25%, 0.5% bid or (Istalol) 0.5% qd

timolol gel (Timoptic-XE) 0.25%, 0.5% qd

Side effects: bradycardia, bronchospasm (contraindicated in asthmatics), hypotension, depression, lethargy, decreased libido, impotence.

Cholinergic Agonists (Miotics; Green Cap)

Mechanism of action: enhance trabecular outflow, may enhance uveoscleral outflow.

carbachol (Isopto Carbachol, Miostat [intraocular 0.01%]) 0.75%, 1.5%, 2.25%, 3% tid

echothiophate (Phospholine iodide) 0.03%, 0.0625%, 0.125%, 0.25% bid pilocarpine (Pilocar, Ocusert, Isopto Carpine, Pilopine HS gel) 0.5%, 1%, 2%, 3%, 4%, 6% qid (qhs for gel)

Side effects: miosis, induced myopia, accommodative spasm, brow ache, pupillary block, angle-closure

Carbonic Anhydrase Inhibitors (Orange Cap)

Mechanism of action: inhibit aqueous production.

acetazolamide (Diamox; 125 to 250 mg tablets, 500 mg Sequels) up to 1 g PO qd in divided doses

brinzolamide (Azopt) 1% tid

dorzolamide (Trusopt) 2% tid

methazolamide (Neptazane) 25–50 mg PO bid to tid

Side effects: lethargy, depression, aplastic anemia, thrombocytopenia, agranulocytosis, Stevens–Johnson syndrome, paresthesias, renal stones, diarrhea, nausea (especially for oral medications), transient myopia, loss of libido, metallic taste. Remember that these agents are sulfonamide derivatives; beware in sulfa allergic patients.

Prostaglandin Analogues (Turquoise/Teal Cap)

Mechanism of action: enhance uveoscleral outflow.

bimatoprost (Lumigan) 0.03% qd

latanoprost (Xalatan) 0.005% qd

travoprost (Travatan) 0.004% qd

unoprostone isopropyl (Rescula) 0.15% bid (docosanoid compound related to prostaglandin analogues)

Side effects: iris and eyelid pigmentation, iritis, conjunctival hyperemia, cystoid macular edema, hypertrichosis, reactivation of HSV keratitis, flu-like symptoms

Hyperosmotics

Mechanism of action: shrink vitreous by creating osmotic gradient.

glycerin (Osmoglyn) 50% 8 oz PO

mannitol (Osmitrol) up to 2 g/kg IV of 20% solution over 30-60 minutes

isosorbide (Ismotic) up to 2 g/kg PO of 45% solution

Side effects: backache, headache, mental confusion, heart failure, ketoacidosis (glycerin in diabetic patients), nausea, emesis

Combinations

brimonidine 0.2%-timolol 0.5% (Combigan) bid

dorzolamide 2%-timolol 0.5% (Cosopt) bid

Allergy Medications

azelastine hydrochloride (Optivar) 0.05% bid

cetirizine (Zyrtec) 5–10 mg PO qd

cromolyn sodium (Crolom, Opticrom) 4% qd to q4h

desloratadine (Clarinex) 5 mg PO qd

emedastine (Emadine) 0.05% qid

epinastine hydrochloride (Elestat) 0.05% bid

fexofenadine (Allegra) 60 mg PO bid; 180 mg PO qd

ketorolac tromethamine (Acular) 0.5% qid

ketotifen fumarate (Zaditor, Alaway) 0.025% bid

levocabastine (Livostin) 0.05% qid

lodoxamide tromethamine (Alomide) 0.1% qd to qid

loratadine (Claritin) 10 mg PO qd

loteprednol etabonate (Alrex) 0.2% qid

naphazoline (Naphcon, Vasocon) qd to qid

naphazoline-antazoline (Vasocon A) qd to qid

naphazoline-pheniramine (Naphcon-A, Opcon-A, Ocuhist) qid

nedocromil sodium (Alocril) 2% bid

olopatadine hydrochloride (Patanol) 0.1% bid or (Pataday) 0.2% qd

pemirolast potassium (Alamast) 0.1% bid

Mydriatics/Cycloplegics

atropine sulfate (Atropisol, Isopto Atropine) 0.5%, 1%, 2% qd to qid

cyclopentolate (Cyclogyl) 0.5%, 1%, 2% qd to qid

eucatropine 5–10% qd to qid

homatropine (Isopto Homatropine) 2%, 5% qd to qid

hydroxyamphetamine hydrobromide 1%/tropicamide 0.25% (Paremyd) qd to qid (onset within 15 minutes, recovery begins within 90 minutes)

phenylephrine (Neo-Synephrine, Mydfrin) 2.5%, 5%, 10% for pupillary dilation

scopolamine (Isopto Hyoscine) 0.25% qd to qid

tropicamide (Mydriacyl) 0.5%, 1% for pupillary dilation

Anesthetics

bupivacaine (Marcaine) 0.25–0.75% for peribulbar/retrobulbar injection

chloroprocaine (Nesacaine) 1–2% solution

cocaine 1–10% for topical anesthesia, pupil testing (Horner's syndrome)

fluorescein (Fluress [with benoxinate 0.4% anesthetic]) 0.25–2% for examination of conjunctiva, cornea, and intraocular pressure

lidocaine (Xylocaine) 0.5–4% for topical anesthesia (preservative-free for intracameral anesthesia)

mepivacaine (Carbocaine) 1–2% solution

proparacaine (Ophthaine) 0.5% for topical anesthesia

procaine (Novocain) 0.5–2% solution

tetracaine (Pontocaine) 0.5% for topical anesthesia

Miscellaneous

acetylcholine (Miochol; 1:100 [20 mg]) 0.5–2 mL intracameral for miosis during surgery

acetylcysteine (Mucomyst) 10–20% up to q4h

aminocaproic acid (Amicar) 50–100 mg/kg PO q4h up to 30 g/day

dapiprazole (Rev-Eyes) 0.5% for reversing pupillary dilation

edrophonium (Tensilon) 10 mg IV

hydroxyamphetamine (Paredrine) 1% for pupil testing (Horner's syndrome)

methacholine (Mecholyl) 2.5% for pupil testing (Adie's pupil)

sodium chloride (Adsorbonac, Muro 128) 2.5%, 5% solution or ointment qd to qid

Artificial Tear Gel Formulations

GenTeal gel	Moisture Eyes
Tears Again	Refresh PM
HypoTears	Tears Naturale
Lacrilube	

Artificial Tear Solution Formulations

Tear Name	Preservative	Viscosity
Cellufresh	Free	Low
Refresh	Free	Low
Refresh Plus	Free	Low
Tears Naturale	Free	Low
GenTeal Mild	Free	Low
HypoTears PF	Free	Low
Moisture Eyes	Present (BAK)	Low
GenTeal	Present (sodium perborate)	Low
HypoTears	Present (BAK)	Low
Murine Tears	Present (BAK)	Low
Refresh Tears	Present (Purite)	Low
Tears Naturale	Present (Polyquad)	Low
Tears Naturale II	Present (Polyquad)	Low
TheraTears	Present (sodium perborate)	Low
Visine Tears	Present (BAK)	Low
Bion Tears	Free	Medium
OcuCoat PF	Free	Medium
Refresh Endura	Free	Medium
Systane	Present (Polyquaternium-1)	Medium
Blink	Present (OcuPure)	Medium
Optive	Present (Purite)	Medium
Soothe	Present (Polyhexamethylene biguanide)	Medium
Refresh Celluvisc	Free	High
Refresh Liquigel	Present (Purite)	High
Ultra Tears	Present (BAK)	High

Color Codes for Topical Ocular Medication Caps

(Based on the American Academy of Ophthalmology recommendations to the FDA to aid patients in distinguishing among drops and thus minimize the chance of using an incorrect medication)

Class	Color
Antiinfectives	Tan
Steroids	Pink
Nonsteroidal antiinflammatories	Gray
Mydriatics/cycloplegics	Red
Miotics	Green
β-Blockers	Yellow or blue
α-Adrenergic agonists	Purple
Carbonic anhydrase inhibitors	Orange
Prostaglandin analogues	Turquoise

Ocular Toxicology

Table A–3 – Ocular Toxicology

Ocular structure	Effect	Drug
Extraocular muscles	Nystagmus, diplopia	Anesthetics, sedatives, anticonvulsants, propranolol, antibiotics, phenothiazines, pentobarbital, carbamazepine, monoamine oxidase inhibitors
Lid	Edema	Chloral hydrate
	Discoloration	Phenothiazines
	Ptosis	Guanethidine, propranolol, barbiturates
Conjunctiva	Hyperemia	Reserpine, methyldopa
	Allergy	Antibiotics, sulfonamides, atropine, antivirals, glaucoma medications
	Discoloration	Phenothiazines, chlorambucil, phenylbutazone
Cornea	Keratitis	Antibiotics, phenylbutazone, barbiturates, chlorambucil, steroids
	Deposits	Chloroquine, amiodarone, tamoxifen, indomethacin, gold
	Pigmentation	Vitamin D
Increased intraocular pressure	Open-angle	Anticholinergics, caffeine, steroids
	Narrow-angle	Anticholinergics, antihistamines, phenothiazines, tricyclic antidepressants, Haldol, Topamax
Lens	Opacities/cataract	Steroids, phenothiazines, ibuprofen, allopurinol, long-acting miotics
	Myopia	Sulfonamides, tetracycline, Compazine, autonomic antagonists, Cymbalta
Retina	Edema	Chloramphenicol, indomethacin, tamoxifen, carmustine
	Hemorrhage	Anticoagulants, ethambutol
	Vascular damage	Oral contraceptives, oxygen, aminoglycosides, talc, carmustine, interferon
	Pigmentary degeneration	Phenothiazines, indomethacin, nalidixic acid, ethambutol, Accutane, chloroquine, hydroxychloroquine
Optic nerve	Neuropathy	Ethambutol, isoniazid, sulfonamides, digitalis, imipramine, streptomycin, busulfan, cisplatin, vincristine, chloramphenicol, disulfiram
	Papilledema	Steroids, vitamin A, tetracycline, phenylbutazone, amiodarone, nalidixic acid, isotretinoin

List of Important Ocular Measurements

Volumes	Orbit = 30 mL Globe = 6.5 mL Vitreous = 4.5 mL Anterior chamber = 250 μL Conjunctival sac = 35 μL
Densities	Rods = 120 million Cones = 6 million Retinal ganglion cells = 1.2 million
Distances	Corneal thickness (central) = 0.5–0.6 mm Anterior chamber depth = 3.15 mm
Diameter of	Cornea (horizontal) = 10 mm (infant), 11.5 mm (adult) Lens = 9.5 mm Capsular bag = 10.5 mm Ciliary sulcus = 11.0 mm Optic disc = 1.5 mm Macula = 5 mm Fovea = 1.5 mm Foveal avascular zone (FAZ) = 0.5 mm Foveola = 0.35 mm

Distance from limbus to	Ciliary body = 1 mm
	Ora serrata = 7–8 mm
	Rectus muscle insertions:
	   Medial = 5.5 mm
	   Inferior = 6.5 mm
	   Lateral = 6.9 mm
	   Superior = 7.7 mm

Length of	Pars plicata = 2 mm
	Pars plana = 4 mm
	Optic nerve = 45–50 mm
	   Intraocular = 0.7–1 mm
	   Intraorbital = 25–30 mm
	   Intracanalicular = 7–10 mm
	   Intracranial = 10–12 mm

Length of orbital entrance	Width = 35 mm Height = 40 mm
Extent of monocular visual field	Nasal = 60° Temporal = 100° Superior = 60° Inferior = 70°
Miscellaneous	Visual field background illumination = 31.5 apostilb Photopic maximum sensitivity = 555 nm Scotopic maximum sensitivity = 507 nm Fibers crossing in chiasm = 52% (nasal fibers) Basal tear secretion = 2 μL/min

List of Eponyms

Adie's pupil: Tonic pupil that demonstrates cholinergic supersensitivity

Alexander's law: Jerk nystagmus, usually increases in amplitude with gaze in direction of the fast phase

Argyll Robertson pupil: Small, irregular pupils that do not react to light but do respond to accommodation; occurs in syphilis

Arlt's line: Horizontal palpebral conjunctival scar in trachoma

Arlt's triangle: (Ehrlich–Türck line) base-down triangle of central keratic precipitates in uveitis

Bergmeister's papilla: Remnant of fetal glial tissue at optic disc

Berlin nodules: Clumps of inflammatory cells in anterior chamber angle in granulomatous uveitis

Berlin's edema: (Commotio retinae) whitening of retina in the posterior pole from disruption of photoreceptors after blunt trauma

Bielschowsky phenomenon: Downdrift of occluded eye as increasing neutral density filters are placed over fixating eye in dissociated vertical deviation (DVD)

Bitot's spot: White, foamy-appearing area of keratinizing squamous metaplasia of bulbar conjunctiva in vitamin A deficiency

Bonnet's sign: Hemorrhage at arteriovenous crossing in branch retinal vein occlusion

Boston's sign: Lid lag on downgaze in thyroid disease

Brushfield spots: White–gray spots on peripheral iris in Down's syndrome

Busacca nodules: Clumps of inflammatory cells on front surface of iris in granulomatous uveitis

Coats' ring: White granular corneal stromal opacity containing iron from previous metallic foreign body

Cogan's sign: Upper eyelid twitch when patient with ptosis refixates from downgaze to primary position; nonspecific finding in myasthenia gravis; also refers to venous engorgement over lateral rectus muscle in thyroid disease

Collier's sign: Bilateral eyelid retraction associated with midbrain lesions

Czarnecki's sign: Segmental pupillary constriction with eye movements due to aberrant regeneration of cranial nerve III

Dalen–Fuchs nodules: Small, deep, yellow retinal lesions composed of inflammatory cells seen histologically between retinal pigment epithelium and Bruch's membrane in sympathetic ophthalmia (also in sarcoidosis, Vogt–Koyanagi–Harada syndrome)

Dalrymple's sign: Widened palpebral fissure secondary to upper eyelid retraction in thyroid disease

Depression sign of Goldberg: Focal loss of nerve fiber layer after resolution of cotton-wool spot

Ehrlich–Türck line: (See Arlt's triangle)

Elschnig pearls: Cystic proliferation of residual lens epithelial cells on capsule after cataract extraction

Elschnig spot: Yellow patches (early) of retinal pigment epithelium overlying area of choroidal infarction in hypertension, eventually becomes hyperpigmented scar with halo

Enroth's sign: Eyelid edema in thyroid disease

Ferry's line: Corneal epithelial iron line at edge of filtering bleb

Fleischer ring: Corneal basal epithelial iron ring at base of cone in keratoconus

Fischer–Khunt spot: (Senile scleral plaque) blue–gray area of hyalinized sclera anterior to horizontal rectus muscle insertions in elderly individuals

Fuchs' spots: Pigmented macular lesions (retinal pigment epithelial hyperplasia) in pathologic myopia

Globe's sign: Lid lag on upgaze in thyroid disease

Guiat's sign: Tortuosity of retinal veins in arteriosclerosis

Gunn's dots: Light reflections from internal limiting membrane around disc and macula

Gunn's sign: Arteriovenous nicking in hypertensive retinopathy

Haab's striae: Breaks in Descemet's membrane (horizontal or concentric with limbus) in congenital glaucoma (versus vertical tears associated with birth trauma)

Hassall–Henle bodies: Peripheral hyaline excrescences on Descemet's membrane due to normal aging

Henle's layer: Obliquely oriented cone fibers in fovea

Herbert's pits: Scarred limbal follicles in trachoma

Hering's law: Equal and simultaneous innervation to yoke muscles during conjugate eye movements

Hirschberg's sign: Pale round spots (Koplik spots) on conjunctiva and caruncle in measles

Hollenhorst plaque: Cholesterol embolus usually seen at vessel bifurcations, associated with amaurosis fugax and retinal artery occlusions

Horner–Trantas dots: Collections of eosinophils at limbus in vernal conjunctivitis

Hudson–Stahli line: Horizontal corneal epithelial iron line at inferior one-third of cornea due to normal aging

Hutchinson's pupil: Fixed, dilated pupil in comatose patient due to uncal herniation and compression of cranial nerve III

Hutchinson's sign: Involvement of tip of nose in herpes zoster ophthalmicus (nasociliary nerve involvement)

Hutchinson's triad: Three signs of congenital syphilis – interstitial keratitis, notched teeth, and deafness

Kayes' dots: Subepithelial infiltrates in corneal allograft rejection

Kayser–Fleischer ring: Limbal copper deposition in Descemet's membrane that occurs in Wilson's disease

Khodadoust line: Corneal graft endothelial rejection line composed of inflammatory cells

Klein's tags: Yellow spots at base of macular hole

Koeppe nodules: Clumps of inflammatory cells at pupillary border in granulomatous uveitis

Krukenbergspindle: Bilateral, central, vertical corneal endothelial pigment deposits in pigment dispersion syndrome

Kunkmann–Wolffian bodies: Small white peripheral iris spots that resemble Brushfield spots but occur in normal individuals

Kyreileis' plaques: White–yellow vascular plaques in toxoplasmosis

Lander's sign: Inferior preretinal nodules in sarcoidosis

Lisch nodules: Iris melanocytic hamartomas in neurofibromatosis

Loops of Axenfeld: Dark limbal spots representing scleral nerve loops

Mittendorf's dot: White spot (remnant of hyaloid artery) at posterior lens surface

Mizuo–Nakamura phenomenon: Loss of abnormal macular sheen with dark adaptation in Oguchi's disease

Morgagnian cataract: Hypermature cortical cataract in which liquified cortex allows nucleus to sink inferiorly

Munson's sign: Protrusion of lower lid with downgaze in keratoconus

Panum's area: Zone of single binocular vision around horopter

Parry's sign: Exophthalmos in thyroid disease

Paton's sign: Conjunctival microaneurysms in sickle cell disease

Paton's lines: Circumferential peripapillary retinal folds due to optic nerve edema

Pseudo–von Graefe sign: Lid elevation on adduction or downgaze due to aberrant regeneration of cranial nerve III

Pulfrich phenomenon: Perception of stereopsis (elliptical motion of a pendulum) due to difference in nerve conduction times between eyes and cortex, seen in multiple sclerosis

Purkinje images: Reflected images from front and back surfaces of cornea and lens

Purkinje shift: Shift in peak spectral sensitivity from photopic (555 nm, cones) to scotopic (507 nm, rods) conditions

Riddoch phenomenon: Visual field anomaly in which a moving object can be seen whereas a static one cannot

Roth spots: Intraretinal hemorrhages with white center in subacute bacterial endocarditis, leukemia, severe anemia, collagen vascular diseases, diabetes mellitus, and multiple myeloma

Rizutti's sign: Triangle of light on iris from oblique penlight beam focused by cone in keratoconus

Salus' sign: Retinal vein angulation (90°) at arteriovenous crossing in hypertension and arteriosclerosis

Sampaoelesi's line: Increased pigmentation anterior to Schwalbe's line in pseudoexfoliation syndrome

Sattler's veil: Superficial corneal edema (bedewing) caused by hypoxia (contact lens)

Scheie's line: Pigment on lens equator and posterior capsule in pigment dispersion syndrome

Schwalbe's line: Angle structure representing peripheral edge of Descemet's membrane

Schwalbe's ring: Posterior embryotoxon (anteriorly displaced Schwalbe's line)

Seidel test: Method of detecting wound leak by observing aqueous dilute concentrated fluorescein placed over the suspected leakage site

Shafer's sign: Anterior vitreous pigment cells (tobacco-dust) associated with retinal tear

Sherrington's law: Contraction of muscle causes relaxation of antagonist (reciprocal innervation)

Siegrist streak: Linear chain of hyperpigmented spots over sclerosed choroidal vessel in chronic hypertension or choroiditis

Soemmering's ring cataract: Residual peripheral cataractous lens material following capsular rupture and central lens resorption from trauma or surgery

Spiral of Tillaux: Imaginary line connecting insertions of rectus muscles

Stocker's line: Corneal epithelial iron line at edge of pterygium

Sugiura's sign: Perilimbal vitiligo associated with Vogt–Koyanagi–Harada syndrome

Tenon's capsule: Fascial covering of eye

Uhthoff's symptom: Decreased vision/diplopia secondary to increased body temperature (e.g., exercise or hot shower), occurs after recovery in optic neuritis

van Trigt's sign: Venous pulsations on optic disc (normal finding)

Vogt's sign: White anterior lens opacities (glaukomflecken) caused by ischemia of lens epithelial cells from previous attacks of angle-closure

Vogt's striae: Deep stromal vertical stress lines at apex of cone in keratoconus

Von Graefe's sign: Lid lag on downgaze in thyroid disease

Vossius ring: Ring of iris pigment from pupillary ruff deposited onto anterior lens capsule after blunt trauma

Watzke–Allen sign: Patient with macular hole perceives break in light when a slit-beam is focused on the fovea

Wessely ring: Corneal stromal infiltrate of antigen-antibody complexes

White lines of Vogt: Sheathed or sclerosed vessels seen in lattice degeneration

Wieger's ligament: Attachment of hyaloid face to back of lens

Weiss ring: Ring of adherent peripapillary glial tissue on posterior vitreous surface after posterior vitreous detachment

Willebrandt's knee: Inferonasal optic nerve fibers that decussate in chiasm and loop into contralateral optic nerve before traveling back to optic tract

Common Ophthalmic Abbreviations

(How To Read an Ophthalmology Chart)

AC	anterior chamber
AFX	air fluid exchange
AK	astigmatic keratotomy
ALT	argon laser trabeculoplasty
AMD	age-related macular degeneration
APD (RAPD) (relative)	afferent pupillary defect
ASC	anterior subcapsular cataract
AV	arteriovenous
BCVA (BSCVA)	best (spectacle) corrected visual acuity
BVO or BRVO	branch retinal vein occlusion
C or C_R	cycloplegic refraction
CB	ciliary body
C/D	cup/disc ratio
CE (ECCE, ICCE, PE)	cataract extraction (extracapsular, intracapsular, phacoemulsification)
C/F	cell/flare
CF	count fingers
CL (DCL, SCL, EWCL)	contact lens (disposable, soft, extended wear)
CME	cystoid macular edema
CNV/CNVM	choroidal neovascular membrane
CRA	chorioretinal atrophy
C/S	conjunctiva/sclera

CS	cortical spoking (cataract)
CSME	clinically significant macular edema
CVO or CRVO	central retinal vein occlusion
CWS	cotton-wool spot
D	diopter(s)
DD	disc diameter(s)
DFE (NDFE)	(non)dilated fundus examination
DME	diabetic macular edema
DR (BDR, NPDR, PDR)	diabetic retinopathy (background, nonproliferative, proliferative)
E (ET)	esophoria (esotropia)
EL	endolaser
EOG	electro-oculogram
EOM	extraocular muscles/movements
ERG	electroretinogram
ERM	epiretinal membrane
FA	fluorescein angiogram
FAZ	foveal avascular zone
FB	foreign body
FBS	foreign body sensation or fasting blood sugar
GA	geographic atrophy
H	Hertel exophthalmometry measurement or hemorrhage
HM	hand motion
HT	hypertropia
I/L	iris/lens
ILM	internal limiting membrane
IO	inferior oblique muscle
IOFB (IOMFB)	intraocular (metallic) foreign body
IOL (ACIOL, PCIOL)	intraocular lens (anterior chamber, posterior chamber)
IOP	intraocular pressure
IR	inferior rectus muscle
IRMA	intraretinal microvascular abnormalities
K	keratometry
KP	keratic precipitates
L/L/L	lids/lashes/lacrimal
LF	levator function
LP	light perception/projection
LR	lateral rectus muscle
M or M_R	manifest refraction
MA	macro/micro aneurysm
MCE	microcystic corneal edema
MP	membrane peel
MR	medial rectus muscle
MRD	margin to reflex distance
NLP	no light perception
NS (NSC)	nuclear sclerosis (nuclear sclerotic cataract)
NV (NVD, NVE, NVI)	neovascularization (of the disc, elsewhere [retina], iris)
NVG	neovascular glaucoma
OD	right eye
ON	optic nerve
OS	left eye
OU	both eyes
P	pupil(s)
PC	posterior chamber/capsule
PCO	posterior capsular opacification
PD	prism diopters/pupillary distance
PEE	punctate epithelial erosion
PERRL(A)	pupils equal round reactive to light (& accommodation)
PF	palpebral fissure

PH	pinhole vision
PI	peripheral iridectomy/iridotomy
PK or PKP	penetrating keratoplasty
PPL	pars plana lensectomy
PPV	pars plana vitrectomy
PRP	panretinal photocoagulation
PRK	photorefractive keratectomy
PSC	posterior subcapsular cataract
PTK	phototherapeutic keratectomy
PVS	posterior vitreous separation
PVD	posterior vitreous detachment
R	retinoscopy
RD (RRD, TRD)	retinal detachment (rhegmatogenous, tractional)
RGP	rigid gas permeable contact lens
RK	radial keratotomy
RPE	retinal pigment epithelium
(R)PED	(retinal) pigment epithelial detachment
SB	scleral buckle
SLE	slit-lamp examination
SO	superior oblique muscle
SPK (SPE)	superficial punctate keratopathy (epitheliopathy)
SR	superior rectus muscle
SRF	subretinal fluid
SRNVM	subretinal neovascular membrane
SS	scleral spur
T (T_a, T_p, T_t)	tonometry (applanation, palpation, Tonopen)
TH	macular thickening/edema
TM	trabecular meshwork
V (VA, V_{cc}, V_{sc})	vision (visual acuity, with correction, without correction)
VH	vitreous hemorrhage
VF (GVF, HVF)	visual field (Goldmann, Humphrey)
W	wearing (refers to current glasses prescription)
X (XT)	exophoria (exotropia)

Common Spanish Phrases

Introduction

I am doctor …	Yo soy el doctor/la doctora …
Ophthalmologist	Oftalmólogo/oculista
I don't speak Spanish	No hablo español
I speak a little Spanish	Hablo un poco de español
Please	Por favor
Come in, enter	Pase(n), entre
Come here	Venga acá
Sit down (here)	Siéntese (aquí)

History

What is your name?	¿Cómo se llama usted?
Do you understand me?	¿Me comprende? or ¿Me entiende?
How are you?	¿Cómo está usted?
How old are you?	¿Cuántos años tiene usted?
Where do you live?	¿Dónde vive usted?
What is your telephone number?	¿Cuál es su número de teléfono?
Tell me	Dígame

Do you have?	¿Tiene usted? or ¿Tiene?
glasses	pejuelos/lentes/gafas
for distance	para ver de lejos
for reading	para leer
bifocals	bifocales
sunglasses	espejuelos obscuros/gafas de sol
contact lenses	lentes de contacto
prescription	receta/prescripción
insurance	seguro médico
allergies	alergias
Do you take?	¿Toma usted? or ¿Toma?
medications	medicinas
pills, tablets, capsules	pastillas/píldoras, tabletas, cápsulas
Do you use?	¿Usa usted? or ¿Usa?
drops	gotas
ointment	pomada
How much?	¿Cuánto?
Do you have problems?	¿Tiene problemas?
reading	al leer
with distance	al ver de lejos
with the cornea	con la cornea
with the retina	con la retina
Do you have?	¿Tiene usted? or ¿Tiene?
blurred vision	visión borrosa
diplopia	visión doble
excessive tearing	muchas lágrimas
How long?	¿Por cuánto tiempo?
How long ago?	¿Hace cuánto tiempo?
Does your eye hurt?	¿Le duele el ojo?
never	nunca
once	una vez
many times	muchas veces
What did you say?	¿Qué dijo? or ¿Cómo?
Please repeat	Repita, por favor
Again	Otra vez
Excuse me	Con permiso, dispénseme

Examination

Cover one eye	Tápese un ojo
Can you read this?	¿Puede leer ésto?
the letters/numbers	las letras/números
Better or worse?	¿Mejor o peor?
Which is better, one or two?	¿Cuál es mejor, uno o dos?
Put your chin here	Ponga la barbilla aquí
Put your forehead against the bar	Ponga la frenta pegada a la barra
Look at the light	Mire la luz
Lie down	Acuéstese, boca arriba
Look up	Mire para arriba
Look down	Mire para abajo
Look to the right	Mire para la derecha
Look to the left	Mire para la izquierda

Diagnosis

You have …	Tiene …
normal eyes	ojos normales
myopia	miopía
hyperopia	hiperopía

presbyopia	presbiopía
strabismus	estrabismo
cataracts	cataratas
glaucoma	glaucoma
infection	infección
inflammation	inflamación
a retinal detachment	un desprendimiento de retina

Treatment

I'll be right back	Ahorita vengo or Regreso enseguida
I will put a patch/shield on the eye	Le voy a poner un parche/protector sobre el ojo
You need (do not need) …	Usted necesita (no necesita) …
an operation	una operación
new glasses	espejuelos nuevos
Don't worry	No se preocupe
Everything is OK (very good)	Toda está bien (muy bien)
I am giving you a prescription for	Le doy una prescripción para
drops/ointment	gotas/pomada
Take/put/use …	Ome/ponga/use …
one drop bid/tid/qid	una gota dos/tres/cuatro veces al día
ointment at bedtime	omada por la noche antes de acostarse
in the right/left eye	en el ojo derecho/izquierdo
in both eyes	en los dos ojos
Do not bend over	No baje la cabeza
Do not strain	No haga fuerza
Do not touch/rub the eye	No se toque/frote el ojo
Do not get your eyes wet	No se moje los ojos
Do you understand the instructions?	¿Entiende las instrucciones?
I want to check your eye again tomorrow	Quiero examinarle el ojo otra vez mañana
I am giving you an appointment	le doy una cita
in 1 week	para dentro de una semana
in 3 months	para dentro de tres meses
Return when necessary	vuelva cuando lo necesite
Thank you	Gracias
Goodbye	Adiós

Suggested Readings

The following subspecialty textbooks provide more detailed information regarding conditions discussed in this book, as well as less common entities.

Abelson MB: *Allergic diseases of the eye*, Philadelphia, 2001, WB Saunders.

Arffa RC: *Grayson's diseases of the cornea*, ed 4, St Louis, 1998, Mosby.

Foster CS, Vitale A: *Diagnosis and treatment of uveitis*, Philadelphia, 2002, WB Saunders.

Gass JDM: *Stereoscopic atlas of macular diseases*, ed 4, St Louis, 1997, Mosby.

Grant WM, Schuman JS: *Toxicology of the eye*, ed 4, Springfield, 1993, Charles C Thomas.

Guyer DR, Yannuzzi LA, Chang A, Shields JA, Green WR: *Retina-vitreous-macula*, Philadelphia, 1999, WB Saunders.

Kline LB, Bajandas F: *Neuro-ophthalmology review manual*, ed 5, Thorofare, NJ, 2001, SLACK.

Krachmer JH, Mannis MJ, Holland EJ: *Cornea*, St Louis, 1997, Mosby.

Mackie IA: *External eye disease*, Boston, 2003, Butterworth-Heinemann.

Mannis MJ, Macsai M, Huntley AC: *Eye and skin disease*, Philadelphia, 1996, Lippincott-Raven.

Miller NR: *Walsh & Hoyt's clinical neuro-ophthalmology*, ed 5, Baltimore, 1999, Williams & Wilkins.

Nelson LB, Calhoun JH, Harley RD: *Pediatric ophthalmology*, ed 4, Philadelphia, 1998, WB Saunders.

Nussenblatt RB, Whitcup SM, Palestine AG: *Uveitis: fundamentals and clinical practice*, ed 2, Philadelphia, 2003, Mosby.

Pepose JS, Holland GN, Wilhelmus KR: *Ocular infection and immunity*, St Louis, 1996, Mosby.

Ritch R, Shields MB, Krupin T: *The glaucomas*, ed 2, St Louis, 1996, Mosby.

Rootman J: *Diseases of the orbit*, ed 2, Philadelphia, 2002, JB Lippincott.

Ryan SJ: *Retina*, ed 3, St Louis, 2001, Mosby.

Shields JA, Shields CL: *Intraocular tumors: a text and atlas*, Philadelphia, 1992, WB Saunders.

Smolin G, Thoft RA: *The cornea: scientific foundations and clinical practice*, ed 3, Boston, 1994, Little, Brown.

Spencer WH: *Ophthalmic pathology: an atlas and textbook*, ed 4, Philadelphia, 1996, WB Saunders.

Tabbara JH, Mannis MJ, Holland EJ: *Infections of the eye*, ed 2, Boston, 1995, Little, Brown.

Tabbara JH, Nussenblatt RB: *Posterior uveitis: diagnosis and management*, Philadelphia, 1994, Butterworth-Heinemann.

von Noorden GK: *Atlas of strabismus*, ed 4, St Louis, 1983, Mosby.

Walsh TJ: *Neuro-ophthalmology: clinical signs and symptoms*, ed 4, Philadelphia, 1997, Lea & Febiger.

Watson P, Hazleman B, Pavesio C: *Sclera and systemic disorders*, Philadelphia, 2003, Butterworth-Heinemann.

Yanoff M, Fine BS: *Ocular pathology: a text and atlas*, ed 5, Philadelphia, 2002, JB Lippincott.

Subject Index

Note: Page numbers suffixed by 'f' refer to figures; those suffixed by 't' refer to tables.

A

Abbreviations, 591–593
Abducens nerve palsy, 45–46, 45f
Aberrometry, wavefront, 570, 570f
Abetalipoproteinemia, 459
Abrasion
    corneal, 175–176, 175f, 176f
        contact lens-related, 185
    eyelid, 70
Acanthamoeba keratitis, 188, 197–198, 198f,
        201, 203
    treatment, 202
Accommodative convergence-to-accommoda-
        tion (AC/A) ratio, 38, 39, 40, 41
Accommodative esotropia, 38–39, 39f
Accommodative excess, 539–540
Acetazolamide, 583
    for angle-closure glaucoma, 235
    for central retinal artery occlusion, 338
    for congenital glaucoma, 509
    for cystoid macular edema, 385
    for idiopathic intracranial hypertension, 486
    for primary open-angle glaucoma, 516
Acetylcholine, 585
Acetylcysteine, 585
    for corneal burns, 178
    for dry eyes, 140
    for filamentary keratitis, 192
    for herpes zoster virus keratitis, 203

Achromatopsia, 448
Acid burn, corneal, 177–178
Acne rosacea, 84–85, 84f
    blepharitis/meibomitis and, 74
Acquired anophthalmia, 31–32, 31f
Acquired nevus, 103, 103f
Acquired nonaccommodative esotropia, 39–40
Acquired retinal arterial macroaneurysm,
        365–366, 365f
Acquired retinoschisis, 400
Actinic corneal degeneration, 208
Actinic keratosis, 112, 112f
Actinomyces israelii canaliculitis, 120, 121
Acute idiopathic blind spot enlargement
        syndrome, 432
Acute macular neuroretinopathy, 426
Acute posterior multifocal placoid pigment
        epitheliopathy, 426, 427t, 428, 428f
Acute retinal necrosis, 414–415, 414f
Acute retinal pigment epitheliitis, 428–429
Acute syphilitic posterior placoid
        chorioretinitis, 423
Acyclovir, 581
    for anterior uveitis, 253
    for Bell's palsy, 96
    for dacryoadenitis, 127
    for herpes simplex virus infection
        of cornea, 196, 202–203
        of eyelid, 75

Acyclovir (*Continued*)
  for herpes zoster virus infection
    of cornea, 203
    of eyelid, 77
    of retina, 414, 421
Adalimumab
  for anterior uveitis, 254
  for posterior uveitis, 442
Adduction deficit, myasthenia gravis, 67f
Adenocarcinoma, pleomorphic, of lacrimal
    gland, 129
Adenoid cystic carcinoma, 129
Adenoma, pleomorphic, of lacrimal gland, 128–129
Adenoviral conjunctivitis, 145, 145f
Adie's pupil, 272–274, 273f, 588
Adult foveomacular vitelliform dystrophy,
    448, 449f
Afferent nystagmus, 47
Age-related macular degeneration, 367–374
  exudative (wet), 367, 370–374, 370f, 371f,
    372, 372f
  non-exudative (dry), 368–370, 368f, 369f
Alagille's syndrome, 283
Albinism, 464, 464f
Albright's syndrome, 29
Alexander's law, 588
Alkali burn, corneal, 177–178, 177f
Alkaptonuria, 171
Allergic conjunctivitis
  acute, 146–147, 147f
  chronic, 148–149, 149f
Allergy medications, 583–584
  see also specific drugs
Alpha-adrenergic receptor agonists, 582
  see also specific drugs
Alpha-chymotrypsin, secondary open-angle
    glaucoma due to, 518
Alport's syndrome
  anterior lenticonus, 294, 294f
  congenital cataract, 298
Alström's disease, 459
Alternate cover test, 558, 558f
Alveolar rhabdomyosarcoma, 23
Amaurosis fugax, 541–542, 577
Amblyopia, 542–543
Ametropia, 523
  see also Refractive errors
Amikacin, 577
  maculopathy due to, 392

Aminocaproic acid, 585
  for hyphema, 241
Aminoglycosides, 577–578
  allergic conjunctivitis due to, 147
  maculopathy due to, 392
  see also specific drugs
Amoxicillin-clavulanate, 578
  for acquired anophthalmia, 32
  for dacryoadenitis, 127
  for dacryocystitis, 123
  for intraorbital foreign body, 8
  for Le Fort fractures, 8
  for orbital cellulitis, 15
  for preseptal cellulitis, 13
Amoxicillin-sulbactam, for dacryocystitis,
    123
Amphotericin B, 580
  for *Aspergillus* canaliculitis, 121
  for candidiasis, 415
  for endophthalmitis, 247
  for infectious keratitis, 202
  for mucormycosis, 15, 60
Ampicillin, 578
Ampicillin-sulbactam
  for dacryoadenitis, 127
  for orbital cellulitis, 15
  for preseptal cellulitis, 13
Amsler grid, 562, 562f
  for age-related macular degeneration,
    369, 372
Amyloidosis
  conjunctival, 154, 154f
  of eyelid, 119f, 190–120
  vitreous, 319–320, 319f
Analgesics
  for corneal abrasion, 175
  for migraine, 538
  see also specific drugs
Ancylostoma caninum, 418
Anemia, retinopathy of, 354–355, 355f
Anesthetics, 584
  see also specific drugs
Aneurysm
  Leber's miliary, 350–351, 351f
  retinal arterial, 365–366, 365f
Aneurysmal bone cyst, 29
Angioid streaks, 379–381, 380f
Angioma, optic nerve, 501
Angiomatosis, encephalotrigeminal, 466, 466f

Angiomatosis retinae, 465, 465f
Angiomatous proliferation, retinal, 374–375, 375f
Angle cleavage syndromes, 282–285
Angle-closure glaucoma, 576t
  primary, 233–236
    acute, 233, 234, 235
    chronic, 234, 235
    subacute, 234, 235
  secondary, 236–238
    acute, 236, 237, 237f
    chronic, 236, 237
    neovascular, 265–266
    phacomorphic, 314, 315f
    pigmentary, 268
  see also Glaucoma
Angle recession, 258, 258f, 259f, 260
  glaucoma, 518, 519f
Aniridia, 280, 281f
Anisocoria, 271–272, 271f
Anisometropia, 523, 524f
  see also Refractive errors
Anisometropic amblyopia, 542
Ankyloblepharon, 99
Ankylosing spondylitis, 249
Anophthalmia
  acquired, 31–32, 31f
  congenital, 19–20, 20f
Anterior basement membrane dystrophy,
    218, 218f
Anterior chamber, 233–255
  blood in, 240–241, 240f
  cells and flare in, 241–243, 242f
  hypotony, 238–239, 239f
  paracentesis, for central retinal artery
    occlusion, 338
  slit lamp examination, 566
  white blood cells in, 242, 243–244, 243f
  see also specific disorders
Anterior ischemic optic neuropathy, 488–491,
    489f, 490f
  arteritic see Arteritic ischemic optic
    neuropathy
Anterior scleritis, 169, 170f
Anterior subcapsular cataract, 302, 305f
Anterior uveitis, 248–254
  granulomatous, 251–252
  HLA-B27-associated, 249
  infectious, 248
  noninfectious, 249–251

Antiamebic agents, 580
  see also specific drugs
Antibiotic(s), 577–580
  allergic conjunctivitis due to, 147
  steroid combinations, 580
  see also specific drugs
Antifungal agents, 580–581
  see also specific drugs
Antihistamines, for allergic conjunctivitis,
    152, 153t
Antiinfective drugs, 577–581
  see also specific drugs
Anti-inflammatories, 581–582
  see also specific drugs
Antiviral agents, 581
  allergic conjunctivitis due to, 147
  see also specific drugs
Anton's syndrome, 544
A-pattern strabismus, 41–42
Apert's syndrome, 21
Aphakia, 308–309, 308f
Aphthous oral ulcers, Behçet's disease,
    433f
Applanation tonometer, 567, 568f
Apraclonidine, 582
  for angle-closure glaucoma, 235
  for primary open-angle glaucoma, 516
Aqueous-deficient dry eye, 137
Aralen, maculopathy due to, 392–394
Arcus juvenilis, 206
Arcus senilis, 206–207, 207f
Argyll Robertson pupil, 274–275, 588
Argyrosis, corneal, 227, 227f
Arlt's line, 588
Arlt's triangle, 588
Arteritic ischemic optic neuropathy, 488, 489,
    490–491
  in central retinal artery occlusion, 338
Arteritis, giant cell, 288
Artery occlusion
  ophthalmic, 339–340
  retinal
    branch, 334–336, 334f, 335f
    central, 336–339, 337f
Arthritis
  juvenile rheumatoid, 250, 254
  psoriatic, 249
Artificial tear(s)
  for Bell's palsy, 96

Artificial tear(s) (*Continued*)
    for coloboma, 100
    for conjunctival degenerations, 155
    for corneal burns, 178
    for corneal erosion, 180
    for distichiasis, 101
    for dry eyes, 140
        following refractive surgery, 534
    for ectropion, 90
    for euryblepharon, 102
    for exposure keratopathy, 62, 66
    for floppy eyelid syndrome, 97
    formulations, 585
    for infectious keratitis, 203
    for keratitis, 192
    for microblepharon, 102
    for ocular cicatricial pemphigoid, 157
    for peripheral ulcerative keratitis, 182
    for Stevens–Johnson syndrome, 158
    for superficial punctuate keratitis, 189
    for thyroid ophthalmology, 17
    for trichiasis, 98
    for viral conjunctivitis, 152
A-scan ultrasonography, 573, 573f
Ascorbic acid, for macular degeneration, 369
Aspergillus canaliculitis, 120, 121
Aspirin
    for anterior ischemic optic neuropathy, 491
    avoidance, vitreous hemorrhage, 325
    for branch retinal vein occlusion, 342
    for migraine, 538
    for transient visual loss, 542
    for vertebrobasilar insufficiency, 535
Asteroid hyalosis, 320–321, 321f
Asthenopia, 36, 40
Astigmatic keratotomy, 527, 528f
Astigmatism, 523, 524
    following refractive surgery, 534
    see also Refractive errors
Astrocytic hamartoma, 471, 501
    in tuberous sclerosis, 467, 468f
Ataxia telangiectasia, 465
Atopic keratoconjunctivitis, 146, 146f, 153
Atovaquone, for toxoplasmosis, 425
Atrophia bulbi, 32–33, 32f
Atropine, 584
    allergic conjunctivitis due to, 147
    for amblyopia, 543
    for angle-closure glaucoma, 237

for anterior chamber cells/flare, 243
for anterior uveitis, 253
for choroidal hemorrhage, 407
for endophthalmitis, 246, 247
for hyphema, 241
for hypopyon, 244
for hypotony, 239
for infectious keratitis, 202
for microspherophakia, 295, 318
for neovascular glaucoma, 266
for open globe, 134
for rubeosis iridis, 265
for uveitis-glaucoma-hyphema syndrome, 255
Autoimmune disease, anterior uveitis, 249–250, 251–252
Automated lamellar keratoplasty, 529
Autorefraction, 553, 553f
Avellino dystrophy, 219
Avulsion
    eyelid, 70, 70f
    optic nerve, 491, 492f
    of vitreous base, 330
Axenfeld's anomaly, 283, 283f
Azathioprine
    for intermediate uveitis, 412
    for posterior scleritis, 436
    for posterior uveitis, 442
    for sarcoidosis, 437
    for serpiginous choroidopathy, 438
    for sympathetic ophthalmia, 439
Azelaic acid, for acne rosacea, 85
Azelastine, 583
    for allergic conjunctivitis, 153t
Azithromycin, 579
    for blepharitis/meibomitis, 75
    for conjunctivitis, 151
    for toxoplasmosis, 425
    for trichiasis, 98

B
Bacillus infection, endophthalmitis, 244
Bacitracin, 579
    for blepharitis/meibomitis, 75
    for chalazion, 80
    for conjunctivitis, 152
    for contact dermatitis, 81
    for contact lens solution hypersensitivity/ toxicity, 185
    for entropion, 93

for eyelid abrasion, 70
for eyelid laceration, 72
for floppy eyelid syndrome, 97
for foreign body in conjunctiva/sclera, 131
for herpes zoster virus infection of eyelid, 77
for keratitis, 192
    herpetic, 203
for orbital cellulitis, 15
for phlyctenule, 144
for preseptal cellulitis, 13
for trichiasis, 98
Baclofen, for nystagmus, 49
Bacterial conjunctivitis
    acute, 144, 145f
    chronic, 148, 148f
    neonatal, 150–151, 151f, 153
    treatment, 151
    see also specific bacterial infections
Bacterial keratitis, 196–197, 196f, 202
Band keratopathy, 207, 207f
Bardet–Biedl syndrome, 460–461, 460f
Bartonella henselae, 412, 413
Basal cell carcinoma, eyelid, 110–111, 111f
Bassen–Kornzweig syndrome, 459
Batten disease, 461
Baylisascaris procyonis, 418
Bear tracks, 474, 474f
Behçet's disease, 250, 254, 432–433, 432f, 433f
Behr's syndrome, 494
Bell's palsy, 94–96, 95f
    ectropion in, 89
Benedikt's syndrome, 51
γ-Benzene hexachloride, for pediculosis, 78
Bergmeister's papilla, 588
Berlin nodules, 289, 588
Berlin's edema, 328–329, 329f, 588
Best's disease, 448–451, 450f
Beta-blockers, 582
    for congenital glaucoma, 509
    for primary open-angle glaucoma, 516
    see also specific drugs
Beta carotene, for macular degeneration, 369
Betaxolol, 582
    for congenital glaucoma, 509
    for primary open-angle glaucoma, 516
Bevacizumab
    for age-related macular degeneration, 373
    for angioid streaks, 381
    for branch retinal vein occlusion, 342

for punctuate inner choroidopathy, 431
for radiation retinopathy, 367
for retinopathy of prematurity, 350
Bielschowsky phenomenon, 588
Bietti's crystalline retinopathy, 446, 446f
Bietti's nodular dystrophy, 208
Bilateral acoustic neurofibromatosis, 117–118
Bilateral acquired parafoveal telangiectasia,
    353–354, 354f
Bilateral diffuse uveal melanocytic proliferation
    syndrome, 480
Bilateral perifoveal telangiectasis with capillary
    obliteration, 354
Bimatoprost, 583
    for primary open-angle glaucoma, 516
Birdshot choroidopathy, 427t, 429–430, 429f
Birth trauma, corneal, 176, 176f, 177f
Bitot's spot, 588
Blepharitis, 73–75, 74f
    acquired anophthalmia and, 31
    sebaceous cell carcinoma and, 113
Blepharochalasis, 82
Blepharophimosis, 99, 99f
Blepharospasm, 93–94
Blindness *see* Visual loss
Blind spot enlargement syndrome, 432
Blood, in anterior chamber, 240–241, 241f
Blood abnormalities, retinopathies associated
    with, 354–357
Blurred vision, differential diagnosis, 575,
    576t, 577
Bone cyst, aneurysmal, 29
Bonnet's sign, 588
Boston's sign, 588
Botryoid rhabdomyosarcoma, 23
Botulinum toxin
    for Bell's palsy, 96
    for blepharospasm, 94
Bourneville's disease, 467–468, 468f
Branch retinal artery occlusion, 334–336,
    334f, 335f
Branch retinal vein occlusion, 340–342, 341f
Brimonidine, 582
    allergic conjunctivitis due to, 147
    for congenital glaucoma, 509
    for corneal laceration in open globe, 134
    for orbital compartment syndrome, 5
    for primary open-angle glaucoma, 516
    for refractive procedure complications, 534

Brimonidine-timolol, 583
Brinzolamide, 583
  for congenital glaucoma, 509
  for primary open-angle glaucoma, 516
Bromfenac, 581
  for cystoid macular edema, 385
Brown–McLean syndrome, 193
Brown's syndrome, 42–43, 43f
Brows see Eyebrows
Bruch's membrane, angioid streaks in,
     379–381, 380f
Brushfield spots, 288, 288f, 588
B-scan ultrasonography, 573, 574f
Bull's eye maculopathy, 393, 393f,
     394, 395f
  in Stargardt's disease, 453, 454f
Bupivacaine, 584
Burn, corneal, 177–178, 177f
Busacca nodules, 289, 289f, 588
Butterfly pattern dystrophy, 451

C

Calcifying epithelioma of Malherbe, 109
Calcium deposits, corneal, 226
Calcium phosphate deposits, on contact
     lenses, 187f
Canalicular laceration, 71–73, 72f
Canaliculitis, 120–121, 120f
Cancer see Carcinoma; Metastasis; Tumors;
     specific types/sites
Candida infection
  canaliculitis, 120, 121
  endophthalmitis, 244, 245, 415, 415f
  phlyctenule and, 143
Candidiasis, 415, 415f
Canthaxanthine, maculopathy due to,
     392, 392f
Capillary hemangioma
  eyelid, 109, 109f
  retina, 471–472, 472f
Capsaicin, for postherpetic neuralgia, 77
Capsular cataract, 296
Carbachol, 582
Carbogen treatment, central retinal artery
     occlusion, 338
Carbonic anhydrase inhibitors, 583
  for congenital glaucoma, 509
  for primary open-angle glaucoma, 516
  see also specific drugs

Carcinoma
  adenoid cystic, 129
  basal cell, 110–111, 111f
  retinopathy associated with,
       480–481
  sebaceous cell, 113–114, 113f
  squamous cell see Squamous cell
       carcinoma
Carotid-cavernous fistula, 10–11, 11f
Carteolol, 582
  for primary open-angle glaucoma, 516
Caruncle, tumors, 167–168, 168f
Cataract(s), 300–306
  cholesterol, 303, 304f
  Christmas tree, 303, 304f
  congenital see Congenital cataract(s)
  cortical, 300, 300f
  cortical degeneration in, 300–301
  hypermature, 301, 314, 314f
  mature, 300, 301f
  Morgagnian, 301, 301f
  nuclear sclerotic, 301–302, 302f
  secondary, 306–308, 307f
  senile, 303, 305
  subcapsular see Subcapsular cataract
  sugar, 303
  sunflower, 304, 304f
Cat-eye syndrome, 281
Cat-scratch disease, 412
Cavernous hemangioma
  conjunctival, 165, 165f
  orbital, 26, 26f
  retinal, 472–473, 472f, 473f
Cavernous sinus, 59f
  syndrome, 59
Cefaclor
  for orbital cellulitis, 15
  for preseptal cellulitis, 13
Cefazolin, 578
  for infectious keratitis, 202
Cefotaxime, 578
Ceftazidime, 578
  for cavernous sinus syndrome, 60
  for endophthalmitis, 246
  for open globe, 134
Ceftriaxone, 578
  for dacryoadenitis, 127
  for orbital cellulitis, 15
Cefuroxime, for preseptal cellulitis, 13

Celecoxib, 581
  for anterior uveitis, 254
  for posterior uveitis, 442
  for scleritis, 171
Cellophane maculopathy, 388–390, 389f, 390f
Cellulitis
  orbital, 13–15, 14f
  preseptal, 12–13, 12f
Central areolar choroidal dystrophy, 442–443, 443f
Central cloudy dystrophy, 219, 220f
Central crystalline dystrophy, 220, 220f
Central retinal artery occlusion, 336–339, 337f
Central retinal vein occlusion, 342–345, 343f
Central serous chorioretinopathy, 381–383, 382f
Central visual acuity see Visual acuity
Cephalexin, 578
  for acquired anophthalmia, 32
  for eyelid laceration, 72
Cephalosporins, 578
  see also specific drugs
Cetirizine, 583
Cevimeline, for dry eyes, 140
Chalazion, 79–80, 79f
  sebaceous cell carcinoma and, 113
Chalcosis, 226, 518
Chalcosis lentis, 304, 304f
Chandler's syndrome, 285, 285f
Charts, eye, 550, 550f, 551f, 552f
Chemical injury
  corneal, 177–178, 177f
  open-angle glaucoma due to, 518
Chemosis, 141, 141f
Cherry-red spot, 336, 337f
  in lipid storage diseases, 397–398, 398f
Chiasmal syndromes, 505–509, 505f, 506f–507f
Children
  orbital floor fracture, 6
  orbital tumors see Orbit
  periodic syndromes and migraine, 536–537
  see also entries beginning juvenile; specific disorders
Chlamydia infection
  conjunctivitis, 148, 148f, 152
    neonatal, 150
  phlyctenule and, 143
Chlamydial conjunctivitis, 148, 148f, 152
Chlorambucil
  for anterior uveitis, 254
  for Behçet's disease, 433
  for posterior uveitis, 442

  for sarcoidosis, 437
  for sympathetic ophthalmia, 439
Chloramphenicol, 579
Chlorhexidine, 580
  for infectious keratitis, 202
Chloroma, 25
Chloroprocaine, 584
Chloroquine, maculopathy due to, 392–394
Chlorpromazine
  corneal deposits, 228
  maculopathy due to, 394
Chocolate cyst, 21
Cholesterol
  cataract, 303, 304f
  deposits, corneal, 228–229
  granuloma, 29
Cholinergic agonists, 582–583
  see also specific drugs
Chondrosarcoma, 30
Chorioretinal coloboma, 409–410, 410f
Chorioretinal dystrophies, 442–448
  central areolar choroidal dystrophy,
    442–443, 443f
  choroideremia, 443–444, 443f
  congenital stationary night blindness see
    Congenital stationary night blindness
  crystalline retinopathy of Bietti, 446, 446f
  gyrate atrophy, 446–447, 447f
  progressive cone dystrophy, 447–448, 447f
Chorioretinal folds, 408–409, 409f
Chorioretinal scars
  in toxocariasis, 423, 424f
  in toxoplasmosis, 424, 425f
Chorioretinitis
  luetic, 422–423, 423f
  vitiliginous, 427t, 429–430, 429f
Chorioretinitis sclopetaria, 331, 331f
Chorioretinopathy, central serous, 381–383,
    382f
Choristoma
  conjunctival, 159
  corneal, 214
  epibulbar osseous, 159
  orbital, 21, 21f
Choroidal detachment, 407, 407f
Choroidal effusion, 407
Choroidal granuloma, tuberculosis, 426, 426f
Choroidal hemangioma, 468–470, 469f
Choroidal hemorrhage, 407

Choroidal malignant melanoma, 475–477, 476f, 477f
Choroidal metastasis, 477–478, 478f
Choroidal neovascularization
    in exudative age-related macular degeneration, 367, 369, 370f, 371f, 372–374, 372f
    in myopic degeneration, 377, 379
    retinal angiomatous proliferation, 374–375, 375f
Choroidal nevus, 470, 470f
Choroidal osteoma, 470–471, 471f
Choroidal rupture, 328, 328f
Choroidal tumors
    benign, 468–471
    malignant, 475–478
Choroidal vasculopathy, polypoidal, 375–377, 376f, 377f
Choroideremia, 443–444, 443f
Choroidopathy
    birdshot, 427t, 429–430, 429f
    Pneumocystis carinii, 419–420, 420f
    punctuate inner, 427t, 430–431, 431f
    serpiginous, 427t, 437–438, 438f
Christmas tree cataract, 303, 304f
Chronic angle-closure glaucoma *see* Angle-closure glaucoma
Chronic progressive external ophthalmoplegia, 61–62, 62f
Chrysiasis, 227
α-Chymotrypsin, secondary open-angle glaucoma due to, 518
Cialis, maculopathy due to, 396
Cicatricial ectropion, 89, 90
Cicatricial entropion, 91, 92f, 93
Cicatricial pemphigoid, 156–157, 156f
Cidofovir, for cytomegalovirus retinitis, 417
Ciliary body, trauma, 258–259, 258f, 259f
Ciprofloxacin, 578
    corneal deposits, 227, 227f
Citrate, for corneal burns, 178
Clarithromycin, for toxoplasmosis, 425
Claude's syndrome, 51
Clear lens extraction, 526
Climatic droplet keratopathy, 208
Clindamycin, 579
    for acne rosacea, 85
    for toxoplasmosis, 425
Clinically significant macular edema, 361, 363t
Clofazimine, for leprosy, 79

Clotrimazole, 580
    for infectious keratitis, 202
Coats' disease, 350–351, 351f
Coats' ring, 588
Cobblestone degeneration, 399, 399f
Cobblestones, conjunctival, 142, 143f, 147, 147f, 149f
Cocaine, topical anesthesia in pupil testing, 584
Coccidioides infection, phlyctenule and, 143
Cockayne's syndrome, 460
Cogan–Reese syndrome, 286, 286f
Cogan's microcystic dystrophy, 218, 218f
Cogan's sign, 588
Cogan's syndrome, 203, 205
Colchicine, for Behçet's disease, 433, 442
Collier's sign, 588
Coloboma
    chorioretinal, 409–410, 410f
    eyelid, 99–100, 100f
    iris, 281, 281f
    lens, 293, 293f
    optic nerve, 497, 497f
Color-coded medication caps, 586
Color vision test, 555, 555f
Combined hamartoma of retinal pigment epithelium and retina, 475, 475f, 501
Commotio retinae, 328–329, 329f, 588
Computerized video keratography, 570, 570f
Concretions, conjunctival, 148f, 154
Conductive keratoplasty, 533
Cone dystrophy, progressive, 447–448, 447f
Confrontation visual field testing, 561, 561f
Congenital anomalies
    conjunctival tumors, 158–159
    corneal, 214–217
    of eyelid, 99–103
        ectropion, 89, 90
        entropion, 91, 93
        ptosis, 86–88, 87f
    of iris, 269–270, 280–282
    of lens *see* Lens
    nasolacrimal duct obstruction, 123, 124, 125
    of optic nerve *see* Optic nerve
    orbital, 19–21
    see also specific disorders
Congenital anophthalmia, 19–20, 20f
Congenital cataract(s), 296–300
    types, 296–297
        capsular, 296

lamellar, 296, 296f
lenticular, 296, 296f
nuclear, 296, 296f
polar, 294f, 297, 297f
sutural, 297, 297f
zonular, 296, 296f
Congenital fibrosis syndrome, 46–47
Congenital glaucoma, 509–509
Congenital hereditary endothelial dystrophy,
    223, 223f
Congenital hereditary stromal dystrophy, 220
Congenital hypertrophy of retinal pigment
    epithelium, 473–474, 474f
Congenital parafoveal telangiectasia, 353
Congenital ptosis, 86–88, 87f
Congenital rubella syndrome, 298, 422, 422f
Congenital stationary night blindness, 444–448
    fundus albipunctatus, 444–445, 445f
    Kandori's flecked retina syndrome, 445
    Nougaret's disease, 444
    Oguchi's disease, 445–446, 445f
    Riggs type, 444
    Schubert–Bornschein type, 444
Congenital toxoplasmosis, 424–425, 425f
Congenital varicella syndrome, 298
Conjunctiva
    in amyloidosis, 154, 154f
    chemosis, 141, 141f
    cobblestones, 142, 143f
    concretions, 148f, 154
    degeneration, 153–155
    dermolipoma, 159
    follicles, 141, 141f
    foreign body, 131, 132f
    granuloma, 142
    hyperemia, 142, 142f
    inflammation, 141–144
    laceration, 131, 133f
    in metabolic diseases, 225t
    papillae, 142, 143f
    phlyctenule, 143–144, 143f
    pinguecula, 154, 154f
    slit lamp examination, 565
    toxicology, 586t
    trauma, 131–134, 132f, 134f
    tumors, 158–168
        congenital, 158–159
        cysts, 159, 159f
        epithelial, 159–161

        melanocytic, 161–164
        stromal, 165–167
Conjunctival intraepithelial neoplasia, 160, 160f
Conjunctival membranes, 142
Conjunctival pseudomembrane, 142, 142f
Conjunctival vessels
    microaneurysm, 136
    telangiectasia, 135–136, 135f
Conjunctivitis, 144–153
    acute, 144–147
    adenoviral, 145, 145f
    allergic see Allergic conjunctivitis
    bacterial see Bacterial conjunctivitis
    chronic, 144, 148–153
    differential diagnosis, 576t
    in erythema multiforme major, 142, 157–158,
        158f
    in floppy eyelid syndrome, 96–97, 97f
    follicular, 141f
    giant papillary, 149, 149f, 152, 187
    inclusion, 148
    infectious
        acute, 144–146
        chronic, 148–149
        neonatal, 150–151, 151f, 153
    in Kawasaki's disease, 150, 153, 250
    ligneous, 150, 150f, 153
    management, 151–153, 153t
    membranes in, 142, 142f
    in ocular cicatricial pemphigoid, 156
    in Parinaud's oculoglandular syndrome, 150,
        150f, 152
    in pediculosis, 146
    viral, 145–146, 145f, 146f
    see also Keratoconjunctivitis
Contact dermatitis, 80–82, 81f
Contact lens(es)
    abnormalities caused by, 183–189
        corneal abrasion, 185
        corneal hypoxia, 185
        corneal neovascularization, 185–186, 186f
        corneal warpage, 186–187, 186f
        dendritic keratitis, 185
        giant papillary conjunctivitis, 149, 149f,
            152, 187
        infectious keratitis, 188
        sterile corneal infiltrates, 188
        superficial punctuate keratitis, 188–189
    daily wear, 184

Contact lens(es) (*Continued*)
    damaged, 187
    deposits on, 187, 187f
    extended wear, 184
    fundus, 567
    gas-permeable, 184, 184f
    poor fit, 188
    for refractive errors, 526
    rigid, 183–184, 183f, 184f
    soft, 184, 184f
    solution hypersensitivity/toxicity, 185
Contrast sensitivity, 554
Contusion
    eyelid, 69–70, 70f
    orbital, 3–4, 3f
Convergence insufficiency, 40–41, 538–539
Convergence-retraction nystagmus, 48
Copper
    deposits
        corneal, 226, 226f
        glaucoma due to, 518
        intralenticular, 304, 304f
    for macular degeneration, 369
Corectopia, 261, 261f
    in iris atrophy, 285, 285f
    in iris nevus syndrome, 286, 286f
Cornea
    congenital anomalies, 214–217
    curvature, measurement, 569, 569f
    delle, 189, 189f
    deposits, 226–230
    ectasias, 211–214
    edema, 193–194, 193f
    endothelial cell evaluation, 570, 571f
    graft rejection/failure, 194–196, 195f
    light reflex tests, 559–560, 559f, 560f
    in metabolic diseases, 225–226, 225t
    nerves, enlarged, 230–231, 230f
    pannus, 205–206, 206f
    precipitates, 190–191, 191f
    slit lamp examination, 566
    staphyloma, 172, 172f
    sterile infiltrates, contact lens-related, 188
    thickness, measurement, 568–569, 569f
    topography, 213–214, 213f, 570, 570f
    toxicology, 586t
    traumatic injury, 175–180
        abrasion, 175–176, 175f, 176f
        abrasion, differential diagnosis, 576t
        birth-related, 176, 176f, 177f

    burns, 177–178, 177f
    contact lens-related *see* Contact lens(es)
    foreign body, 178–179, 178f
    laceration, 179–180, 179f
    recurrent erosion, 180
    tumors, 231–232
    ulcers *see* Infectious keratitis
    verticillata, 229–230, 229f
    warpage, contact lens-related, 186–187, 186f
    see also Keratitis; Keratopathy
Corneal degenerations, 206–210
    see also specific types
Corneal dystrophies, 218–225
    anterior (epithelial and Bowman's membrane),
        218–219
    posterior (endothelial), 223–225
    stromal, 219–223
Corneal intraepithelial neoplasia,
    231–232, 231f
Corneal refractive procedures, 527–533
    excimer laser, 528–529
        complications, 529, 529f, 530f, 531f
        postoperative symptoms, 529
    implants, 532
    incisional, 527–528, 527f, 528f
        complications, 528
        postoperative symptoms, 528
    thermokeratoplasty, 533, 533f
Cornea plana, 214
Corneoscleral laceration, 131, 133, 133f
Cortical blindness, 544
Cortical cataract, 300, 300f
Cortical degeneration, 300–301
Corticosteroids *see* Steroids
Corynebacterium diphtheriae infection
    conjunctivitis, 142
    keratitis, 196
Costeff syndrome, 494
Cotton-wool spots, 333
Cover tests, 557–558, 557f, 558f
Cover-uncover test, 557, 557f
Cranial nerve examination, 564
Cranial nerve palsies
    fourth nerve, 53–55, 53f, 54f, 55f
    multiple, 58–60
    seventh *see* Bell's palsy
    sixth nerve, 56–58, 56f, 57f
    third nerve, 50–53, 50f, 52f
Craniofacial disorders, 20–21
Craniosynostoses, 20–21

Crocodile shagreen, 207, 208f
Crohn's disease, 249
Cromolyn sodium, 584
  for allergic conjunctivitis, 153t
  for giant papillary conjunctivitis, 187
  for superior limbic keratoconjunctivitis, 152
Crouzon's syndrome, 21
Cryptophthalmos, 100
Crystalline keratopathy, 197f
Crystalline retinopathy of Bietti, 446, 446f
Cutaneous melanoma
  of eyelid, 114, 114f
  retinopathy and, 481
Cyclical esotropia, 40
Cyclodialysis, 258, 258f, 260
Cyclopentolate, 584
  for cells/flare, 243
  for corneal abrasion, 176
  for corneal burns, 178
  for corneal foreign body, 179
  for corneal graft rejection/failure, 195
  for corneal laceration, 134, 179
  for hypopyon, 244
  for hypotony, 239
  for keratitis, 192
  for lens-induced secondary glaucoma, 315
  for peripheral ulcerative keratitis, 182
  for uveitis-related glaucoma, 520
Cyclophosphamide
  for anterior uveitis, 254
  for Behçet's disease, 433
  for ocular cicatricial pemphigoid, 157
  for posterior uveitis, 442
Cycloplegic refraction, 552–553
Cycloplegics, 584
  see also specific drugs
Cyclosporine, 581
  for anterior uveitis, 254
  for atopic/vernal keratoconjunctivitis, 153
  for Behçet's disease, 433
  for birdshot choroidopathy, 430
  for blepharitis/meibomitis, 75
  for dry eyes, 140
  for intermediate uveitis, 412
  for posterior scleritis, 436
  for posterior uveitis, 442
  for refractive procedure complications, 534
  for serpiginous choroidopathy, 438
  for Vogt–Koyanagi–Harada syndrome, 440
Cylindroma, 129

Cyst(s)
  aneurysmal bone, 29
  chocolate, 21
  conjunctival, 159, 159f
  Cysticercus cellulosae, 416, 416f
  dermoid see Dermoid
  epidermal inclusion, 107–108, 107f
  iris, 287, 287f
  Moll's gland, 107, 107f
  sebaceous (pilar), 108, 109f
  sudoriferous, 107, 107f
Cysteine deposits, corneal, 227
Cysticercosis, 416, 416f
Cysticercus cellulosae, 416, 416f
Cystinosis, 227
Cystoid degeneration, peripheral, 400
Cystoid macular edema, 383–385, 384f
Cytomegalovirus retinitis, 416–418, 417f
Cytoxan, for intermediate uveitis, 412
Czarnecki's sign, 588

D

Dacryoadenitis, 125–127, 126f
Dacryocystitis, 121–123, 122f
Dalen–Fuchs' nodules, 438, 439f, 588
Dalrymple's sign, 588
Dapiprazole, 585
Dapsone
  for anterior uveitis, 254
  for leprosy, 79
  for ocular cicatricial pemphigoid, 157
  for posterior uveitis, 442
Deep filiform dystrophy, 223
Deferoxamine, maculopathy due to, 394
Delle, 189, 189f
Demodex infection, eyelid, 73, 78
Demodicosis, 78
De Morsier syndrome, 500
Dendritic keratitis, contact lens-related, 185
Depression sign of Goldberg, 588
Deprivation amblyopia, 543
Dermatitis, contact, 80–82, 81f
Dermatochalasis, 88, 89f
Dermoid
  conjunctival, 159
  limbal, 214, 215f
  orbital, 21, 21f
Dermolipoma, conjunctival, 159
Descemet's membrane, birth trauma, 176,
    176f, 177f

Desferal, maculopathy due to, 394
Desloratadine, 584
Devic's syndrome, 487
Dexamethasone, 581
    for atopic/vernal keratoconjunctivitis, 153
    for candidiasis, 415
    for endophthalmitis, 246
    for macular edema in diabetic retinopathy, 362
    for open globe, 134
Diabetes insipidus diabetes mellitus optic atrophy
        and deafness (DIDMOAD), 494
Diabetes mellitus
    cataracts in, 303
    insulin-dependent (type I), 357–358
    non-insulin-dependent (type II), 357–358
    optic neuropathy in, 489
Diabetic retinopathy, 332f, 333f, 357–363, 358f,
        359f, 360f, 363t
    nonproliferative, 358, 358f, 359f
    proliferative, 360, 360f, 361–362, 362f, 363t
Diclofenac sodium, 581
    for anterior uveitis, 254
    for corneal abrasion, 175
    for cystoid macular edema, 385
    for posterior uveitis, 442
Dicloxacillin, for eyelid laceration, 72
Differential diagnosis
    of common ocular symptoms, 575, 576t, 577
    see also specific disorders
Diffuse lamellar keratitis, following refractive
        procedures, 529, 531f, 534
Diffuse scleritis, 169, 170f
Diffuse unilateral subacute neuroretinitis,
        418–419, 418f
Diflunisal, 581
    for anterior uveitis, 254
    for posterior uveitis, 442
    for scleritis, 171
Diphenhydramine
    for allergic conjunctivitis, 152
    for contact dermatitis, 81
Dipivefrin, 582
    for primary open-angle glaucoma, 516
Direct ophthalmoscopy, 571, 571f
Discharge, differential diagnosis, 577
Disciform keratitis, 199, 199f, 203
Dislocated lens see Ectopia lentis
Dissociated nystagmus, 48
Dissociated strabismus complex, 43

Distance vision chart, 550, 550f
Distichiasis, 100–101, 101f
Dog hook-worm, 418
Dominant drusen, 451–452, 452f
Dominant optic atrophy, 493
Dorsal midbrain (Parinaud's) syndrome, 65, 66
Dorzolamide, 583
    for congenital glaucoma, 509
    for orbital compartment syndrome, 5
    for primary open-angle glaucoma, 516
Dorzolamide-timolol, 583
Dosages, drug, 577–585
    see also specific drugs
Dot/blot hemorrhage, 332, 333f
Double elevator palsy, 44–45, 44f
Downbeat nystagmus, 48
Down's syndrome, 298
Doxycycline, 579
    for acne rosacea, 84
    for blepharitis/meibomitis, 75
    for chalazion, 80
    for corneal burns, 178
    for corneal erosion, 180
    for peripheral ulcerative keratitis, 182
    for toxoplasmosis, 425
Doyne's honeycomb dystrophy, 451–452, 452f
Drug
    deposits, corneal, 227–228, 227f
    therapy see Medications
Drug-induced conditions
    anterior uveitis, 250
    cataracts, 305, 305f
    maculopathies, 392–397
    nystagmus, 48
    optic neuropathy, 494
    secondary open-angle glaucoma, 517–518, 519
    Stevens–Johnson syndrome, 157–158, 158f
Drusen
    dominant, 451–452, 452f
    in macular degeneration, 368, 368f
    optic nerve, 498, 499f
Dry eye disease, 136–140, 138f, 139f, 140t
    aqueous-deficient, 137
    evaporative, 137
Dry macular degeneration, 368–370, 368f, 369f
Duane's retraction syndrome, 45–46, 45f
Dural sinus fistula, 10–11
Dyes, 566
Dysconjugate nystagmus, 48

Dyslipoproteinemias, 228–229
Dysthyroid orbitopathy, 15–18, 16f

E

Eales' disease, 352, 352f
Echothiophate, 582
Ectasia
    corneal, 211–214
    scleral, 172, 172f
Ectopia lentis, 316–318, 316f, 317f, 318f
Ectopia lentis et pupillae, 316
Ectopic lashes, 100–101, 101f
Ectopic pupil *see* Corectopia
Ectropion, 89–91, 90f
Edema
    Berlin's, 328–329, 329f
    corneal, 193–194, 193f
    cystoid macular, 383–385, 384f
    eyelid *see* Eyelid
    retinal, in Behçet's disease, 432, 432f
Edrophonium, 585
Efferent nystagmus, 47
Ehlers–Danlos syndrome, 212
Ehrlich–Türck line, 588
Elderly
    arcus senilis, 206–207, 207f
    asteroid hyalosis, 320–321, 321f
    bilateral diffuse uveal melanocytic
        proliferation syndrome, 480
    lentigo maligna melanoma, 114
    macular degeneration *see* Age-related macular
        degeneration
    ophthalmic artery occlusion, 339–340
    pleomorphic adenocarcinoma, lacrimal gland,
        129
    sebaceous cyst, 108, 109f
    seborrheic keratosis, 104, 105f
    senile cataract, 303, 305
    senile scleral plaque, 172–173, 173f
    squamous cell carcinoma *see* Squamous cell
        carcinoma
    vertebrobasilar insufficiency, 535–536
    White limbal girdle of Vogt, 209–210, 210f
    see also Branch retinal artery occlusion;
        Central retinal artery occlusion
Elschnig pearls, 307, 307f, 588
Elschnig spots, 363, 364f, 588
Embryonal rhabdomyosarcoma, 23
Embryotoxon, posterior, 282f, 283

Emedastine, 584
    for allergic conjunctivitis, 153t
Emmetropia, 524
Encephalotrigeminal angiomatosis, 466, 466f
Endophthalmitis, 244–248, 435
    endogenous, 245, 245f, 247, 435
    postoperative, 244, 246, 435
    posttraumatic, 244, 247
Endotheliitis, 199, 200, 203
Enhanced S-cone syndrome, 456
Enroth's sign, 588
Entropion, 91–93, 92f
Enucleation
    adult, 31–32, 31f
    for choroidal malignant melanoma, 476
    infantile, 20
    orbital asymmetry and, 20
Eosinophilic granuloma, 23
Ephelis, 103
Epiblepharon, 101, 101f
Epibulbar osseous choristoma, 159
Epicanthus, 101–102, 102f
Epidemic keratoconjunctivitis, 145, 145f
Epidermal inclusion cyst, 107–108, 107f
Epi-laser in-situ keratomileusis, 529
Epinastine hydrochloride, 584
    for allergic conjunctivitis, 153t
Epinephrine, 582
    deposits, 227, 580
Epiretinal membrane, 388–390, 389f, 390f
Episcleritis, 168–169, 168f, 576t
Epithelial basement membrane dystrophy,
    218, 218f
Epithelial ingrowth, following refractive
    procedures, 529, 531f, 534
Epithelial keratitis, 198, 199f, 200, 200f, 202
Eponyms, 586–589
Epstein-Barr virus infection, dacryoadenitis
    and, 125, 127
Ergot alkaloids, for migraine, 538
Erythema multiforme major, 142, 157–158, 158f
Erythromycin, 579
    for acne rosacea, 84
    for blepharitis/meibomitis, 75
    for chalazion, 80
    for conjunctivitis, 152
    for contact dermatitis, 81
    for contact lens solution hypersensitivity/
        toxicity, 185

Erythromycin (*Continued*)
  for dacryocystitis, 123
  for entropion, 93
  for eyelid abrasion, 70
  for floppy eyelid syndrome, 97
  for herpes zoster virus infection of eyelid, 77
  for keratitis, 192
    herpetic, 203
  for ocular cicatricial pemphigoid, 157
  for orbital cellulitis, 15
  for phlyctenule, 144
  for phthiriasis, 78
  for preseptal cellulitis, 13
  for Stevens–Johnson syndrome, 158
  for trichiasis, 98
Esotropia, 35, 37
  accommodative, 38–39, 39f
  acquired nonaccommodative, 39–40
  A-pattern, 41–42
  cover test, 558f
  cyclical, 40
  infantile, 37–38, 38f
  muscle surgery, 39, 39t
  V-pattern, 42, 42f
Essential iris atrophy, 285, 285f
Etanercept
  for anterior uveitis, 254
  for posterior uveitis, 442
Eucatropine, 584
Euryblepharon, 102
Evaporative eye disease, 137
Examination, ocular, 549–575
  external, 564f, 576t, 563–564
  of fundus, 571–572, 571f, 572f, 573f
  motility assessment, 556–560, 557f, 558f,
    559f, 560f, 561f
  routine, guidelines, 575
  slit lamp *see* Slit lamp examination
  tests
    color vision, 555, 555f
    contrast sensitivity, 554
    corneal light reflex, 559–560, 559f, 560f
    cover, 557–558, 557f, 558f
    forced ductions, 560
    4 diopter base-out prism, 556
    keratometry, 569, 569f
    optical coherence tomography (OCT),
      574, 575f
    optokinetic, 560, 561f

    pachymetry, 568–569, 569f
    partial coherence laser interferometry
      (IOL Master), 574, 574f
    refraction, 552–553, 553f
    retinoscopy, 553
    specular microscopy, 570, 571f
    stereo acuity, 555, 555f, 556f
    tonometry, 567, 568f
    ultrasonography, 573, 573f, 574f
    visual acuity, 549–550, 550f–552f
    visual field, 561–563, 561f, 562f, 563f
    wavefront aberrometry, 570, 570f
    Worth 4 dot, 556, 556f
Excimer laser, corneal refractive procedures,
    528–529, 528f, 529f, 530f, 531f
Exercises, orthoptic, for convergence
    insufficiency, 539
Exfoliation, lens, 310–311, 310f
Exophoria, cover test, 558f
Exophthalmometry, 563, 564f
Exotropia, 35, 40–41, 40f
  A-pattern, 41–42
  basic, 40
  cover test, 558f
  muscle surgery, 41, 41t
  V-pattern, 42, 42f
  X-pattern, 42
Exposure keratopathy, 189–190, 190f, 200
Extraocular muscles, toxicology, 586t
Exudative (serous) retinal detachment,
    404–405, 405f
  central serous chorioretinopathy, 381, 382f
  Coats' disease, 350, 351f
  idiopathic uveal effusion syndrome,
    433, 434f
  optic nerve pit, 499, 500f
  posterior scleritis, 435, 435f
  retinoblastoma, 479, 479f
  toxemia of pregnancy, 365f
  Vogt–Koyanagi–Harada syndrome,
    439–440, 440f
Exudative macular degeneration *see* Age-related
    macular degeneration
Eyebrows
  loss of, 82–83, 83f
  white (poliosis), 83, 83f
Eye charts, 550, 550f, 551f, 552f
Eye drops, toxic conjunctivitis, 147
Eye examination *see* Examination, ocular

Eyelashes
    ectopic, 100–101, 101f
    lice infestation, 78, 78f
    loss of, 82–83, 83f
    misdirected, 97–98, 98f
    slit lamp examination, 565
    white (poliosis), 83, 83f
Eyelid
    amyloidosis, 119f, 190–120
    blepharospasm, 93–94
    congenital anomalies *see* Congenital anomalies
    edema
        blepharochalasis, 82
        in contact dermatitis, 80
        in dacryoadenitis, 126, 126f
        in mechanical ectropion, 89
        in traumatic injury, 69
    floppy eyelid syndrome, 96–97, 97f
    hematoma, 69
    infections, 73–79
        blepharitis *see* Blepharitis
        demodicosis, 78
        herpes simplex virus, 75–76, 76f
        herpes zoster virus, 76–77, 76f
        leprosy, 79
        molluscum contagiosum, 77–78, 77f
        phthiriasis/pediculosis, 78, 78f
    inflammation, 79–85
        in acne rosacea *see* Acne rosacea
        blepharochalasis, 82
        chalazion *see* Chalazion
        in contact dermatitis, 80–82, 81f
    lower, defects, 71
    malpositions, 85–93
        dermatochalasis, 88, 89f
        ectropion, 89–91, 90f
        entropion, 91–93, 92f
        ptosis *see* Ptosis
    neurofibroma, 117, 117f
    sarcoidosis, 118
    slit lamp examination, 565
    toxicology, 586t
    trauma, 69–73
        abrasion, 70
        avulsion, 70, 70f
        contusion, 69–70, 70f
        laceration, 71–72, 71f, 72f
    tumours *see* Eyelid tumors
    upper

        defects, 71
        everting, 565, 566f
        vitiligo, 83, 83f
Eyelid tumors, 103–116
    benign, 103–110
        nonpigmented, 106–109
        pigmented, 103–106
        vascular, 109–110
    malignant, 110–116
        metastatic, 115–116, 115f
Eye pain, differential diagnosis, 577

F

Fabry's disease, 225t, 229f, 298, 304
Facial nerve palsy *see* Bell's palsy
Famciclovir, 581
    for anterior uveitis, 253
    for dacryoadenitis, 127
    for herpes simplex virus infection
        of cornea, 203
        of eyelid, 75
    for herpes zoster virus infection
        of cornea, 203
        of eyelid, 77
        of retina, 414, 421
Familial exudative vitreoretinopathy,
        454–455, 455f
Familial high-density lipoprotein deficiency, 229
Farber's disease, 398
Farnsworth tests, 555
Farsightedness, 524–525, 524f, 525
    see also Refractive errors; Refractive procedures
Ferguson–Smith syndrome, 112
Ferry line, 228, 589
Fexofenadine, 584
Fibro-osseous tumors, 29, 30
Fibrous dysplasia, 29
Fibrous histiocytoma, 28
Fibrovascular stalk, persistent hyperplastic
        primary vitreous, 321, 322f
Filamentary keratitis, 190, 190f
Fischer–Khunt spot, 589
Fish-eye disease, 229
Fistulas
    carotid-cavernous, 10–11, 11f
    dural sinus, 10–11
Flame-shaped hemorrhage, 332, 332f
Flap striae, following refractive procedures, 529,
        530f, 531f, 534

Flare, anterior chamber, 241–243, 242f
Flashes of light, differential diagnosis, 577
Fleck dystrophy, 221, 221f
Fleischer ring, 228, 228f, 587
Floppy eyelid syndrome, 96–97, 97f
Fluconazole, 580
    for *Candida albicans* canaliculitis, 121
    for candidiasis, 415
Flucytosine, 580
Fluocinolone acetonide, for macular edema in
        diabetic retinopathy, 362
Fluorescein, 566, 584
    for pediculosis, 78
Fluorometholone, 581
    for allergic conjunctivitis, 152
    for contact dermatitis, 81
    for epidemic keratoconjunctivitis, 152
    for episcleritis, 169
    for infectious keratitis, 203
    for peripheral ulcerative keratitis, 183
    for superior limbic keratoconjunctivitis, 188
    for Thygeson's superficial punctuate
        keratitis, 192
    for uveitis-related glaucoma, 520
Fluoroquinolones, 578
    for infectious keratitis, 188
    see also specific drugs
Flurbiprofen sodium, 581
Folate, for optic neuropathy, 496
Folinic acid, for toxoplasmosis, 425
Follicles, 141, 141f
Follicular conjunctivitis, 141f
Fomivirsen, for cytomegalovirus retinitis, 418
Forced ductions, 560
Foreign body
    cataract due to, 305, 305f
    conjunctival, 131, 132f
    corneal, 178–179, 178f
    intralenticular, 305, 305f
    intraorbital, 8–9, 8f
    scleral, 131
Foscarnet
    for acute retinal necrosis, 415
    for cytomegalovirus retinitis, 417, 418
    for herpes zoster virus infection of eyelid, 75
    for progressive outer retinal necrosis
        syndrome, 422
Foster–Kennedy syndrome, 483, 489
4 diopter base-out prism test, 556

Fourth cranial nerve palsy, 53–56, 53f, 54f, 55f
Fractures, orbital, 5–8, 5f, 6f
    apex, 7
    floor (blow-out), 5–6, 5f, 6f
        pediatric, 6
    Le Fort, 7–8
    medial wall (nasoethmoidal), 6
    roof, 7
    tripod, 7
François–Neetans dystrophy, 221, 221f
Freckle, 103
Fuchs' endothelial dystrophy, 223, 223f, 224
Fuchs' heterochromic iridocyclitis, 250, 251f
Fuchs' spots, 589
Fumagillin, for infectious keratitis, 202
Functional visual loss, 540–541
Fundus albipunctatus, 444–445, 445f
Fundus contact/noncontact lens, 567
Fundus examination, 571–573, 571f, 572f, 573f
Fundus flavimaculatus, 453–454, 454f
Fungal infections
    keratitis, 197, 197f, 202
    orbital, 13, 14, 14f, 15
    see also specific infections
Furosemide, for idiopathic intracranial
        hypertension, 486
Furrow degeneration, 208

G
Galactosemia, 298
γ -benzene hexachloride, for pediculosis, 78
Ganciclovir, 581
    for acute retinal necrosis, 415
    for cytomegalovirus retinitis, 417, 418
    for progressive outer retinal necrosis
        syndrome, 422
Gangliosidosis
    type I, 225t, 398, 398f
    type II, 225t, 398
Garamycin, maculopathy due to, 392
Gardner's syndrome, 108
Gatifloxacin, 578
    for central retinal artery occlusion, 338
    for conjunctival laceration, 131
    for conjunctivitis, 151
    for corneal burns, 178
    for corneal laceration, 134, 179
    for hypotony, 239
    for infectious keratitis, 202, 203

Gaze-evoked nystagmus, 48
Gaze palsy
  horizontal, 63–65
  in myasthenia gravis, 67, 67f
  vertical, 65–66
Gelatinous droplike dystrophy, 218–219
Gentamicin, 577
  for acquired anophthalmia, 31
  maculopathy due to, 392
Gentamicin-prednisolone acetate, 580
Geographic helicoid peripapillary choroidopa-
    thy, 254, 427t, 437–438, 438f
Ghost vessels, corneal, 204f
Giant cell arteritis, 288
Giant papillary conjunctivitis, 149, 149f, 152, 187
Giant retinal tear, 330, 330f
Gillespie's syndrome, 280
Glasses
  prescription determination, 552–553, 553f
  for refractive errors, 526
Glaucoma
  angle-closure see Angle-closure glaucoma
  congenital, 509–509
  lens-induced, 314–315, 314f
  malignant, 236, 237, 238
  medications, 582–583
    see also specific drugs
  normal tension, 520–521, 521f
  open-angle see Open-angle glaucoma
  pseudoexfoliative, 312–314, 313f
Glaucomatocyclitic crisis, 250
Glaukomflecken, 234, 234f, 237
Glioblastoma multiforme, 501, 501f
Glioma, optic nerve, 502, 502f
Globe
  open see Open globe
  subluxation, 9–10, 9f
Globe's sign, 589
Glycerin, 583
  for angle-closure glaucoma, 235
Gold deposits, corneal, 227
Goldenhar's syndrome, 159, 214
Goldmann applanation tonometer, 567, 568f
Goldmann–Favre syndrome, 456
Goldmann gonioscopy lens, 567f
Goldmann visual field, 562, 562f, 563f
Gonioscopy, 566–567, 567f
Gonococcal conjunctivitis, 144
  neonatal, 150, 151f, 152

Gout, 229
Gradenigo's syndrome, 57
Graft rejection/failure, corneal transplant,
    194–196, 195f
Granular dystrophy, 221, 221f
Granuloma, 142
  cholesterol, 29
  choroidal, tuberculosis, 426, 426f
  eosinophilic, 23
  pyogenic, 167, 167f
  Toxocara canis, 423, 424f
Granulomatous uveitis, 251–252, 252f
Graves' ophthalmology, 15–18, 16f
Guiat's sign, 589
Gunn's dots, 589
Gunn's sign, 589
Gyrate atrophy, 446–447, 447f

H

Haab's striae, 215, 215f, 589
Haemophilus aegyptius infection, keratitis, 196
Haemophilus influenzae infection
  dacryocystitis, 121
  endophthalmitis, 244
  keratitis, 196
  orbital cellulitis, 13
  preseptal cellulitis, 12
Hagberg–Santavuori syndrome, 461
Hallgren's syndrome, 461
Halo nevus, 103
Halos, after refractive procedures, 527, 528, 529,
    532, 533
Hamartoma
  astrocytic see Astrocytic hamartoma
  conjunctival, 158
  retinal pigment epithelium and retina, 475,
    475f, 501
Hand-held tonometer, 567, 568f
Hand–Schüller–Christian disease, 23
Harada's disease, 439–440, 440f
Hardy–Rand–Ritter plates, 555
Hassall–Henle bodies, 589
Headache, migraine see Migraine
Hemangioma
  capillary see Capillary hemangioma
  cavernous see Cavernous hemangioma
  choroidal, 468–470, 469f
Hemangiomatosis, racemose, 467, 467f
Hematoma, eyelid, 69

Hemiretinal vein occlusion, 342, 343f
Hemorrhage
    choroidal, 407
    open-angle glaucoma due to, 518
    orbital, 4–5, 4f
    retinal *see* Retinal hemorrhage
    subconjunctival, 134, 135f, 576t
    vitreous, 324–325, 325f
Henle's layer, 589
Herbert's pits, 589
Hereditary benign intraepithelial
        dyskeratosis, 232
Hereditary chorioretinal dystrophies
        see Chorioretinal dystrophies
Hereditary macular dystrophies *see* Macular
        dystrophy
Hereditary vitreoretinal degenerations, 454–457
Hering's law, 589
Herpes simplex virus infection
    acute retinal necrosis, 414–415, 414f
    anterior uveitis, 248
    canaliculitis, 120, 121
    conjunctivitis, 145, 146f, 152
        neonatal, 145, 146f
    dacryoadenitis, 125, 127
    of eyelid, 75–76, 76f
    keratitis, 198–199, 199f
        treatment, 202–203
    retinal necrosis, 414, 421
    Stevens–Johnson syndrome, 157
Herpes zoster virus infection
    acute retinal necrosis, 414–415, 414f
    anterior uveitis, 248
    canaliculitis, 120, 121
    conjunctivitis, 146, 146f
    dacryoadenitis, 125, 127
    episcleritis, 168
    of eyelid, 76–77, 76f
    keratitis, 199–200, 200f
        treatment, 203
Heterochromia iridis, 269, 269f
Heterochromia iridium, 269, 269f
Hexamidine, 580
    for infectious keratitis, 202
Hidrocystoma, 107, 107f
Hirschberg's method, 559, 559f
Hirschberg's sign, 589
Histiocytic tumors, 23
Histiocytoma, fibrous, 28

Histoplasma capsulatum, 420
Histoplasmosis, 420–421, 420f
History, ophthalmic, 549
HLA-B27-associated anterior uveitis, 249
Hollenhorst plaque, 334, 334f, 589
Homatropine, 584
    for acute retinal necrosis, 415
    for anterior uveitis, 253
Homocystinuria, 316
Honeycomb dystropy, 219, 219f
Hordeolum, 79–80
Horizontal motility disorders, 63–65
Horizontal strabismus, 37–42
Horner's syndrome, 275–277, 276f
Horner–Trantas dots, 147, 147f, 589
Horseshoe-shaped retinal tear, 330, 330f
House-Brackmann facial nerve grading
        system, 95t
Hudson–Stahli line, 228, 589
Human immunodeficiency virus retinopathy,
        419, 419f
Humphrey visual field, 563, 563f
Hunter's syndrome, 225, 225t
Hurler syndrome, 225t
Hutchinson's pupil, 589
Hutchinson's sign, 589
Hutchinson's triad, 589
Hyaloid face, detached, 323f
Hydrops, 211, 211f
Hydroxyamphetamine, 584
    for pupil testing, 585
Hydroxychloroquine
    maculopathy due to, 392–394, 393f
    for sarcoidosis, 437
Hydroxypropyl methylcellulose, for
        dry eyes, 140
Hyperemia, 142, 142f
Hyperlipoproteinemia, 228
Hyperlysinemia, 316
Hypermature cataract, 301, 314, 314f
Hyperopia, 524–525, 524f, 525
    see also Refractive errors; Refractive
        procedures
Hyperosmotics, 583
    see also specific drugs
Hypertelorism, 20, 83
Hypertension, idiopathic intracranial,
        485–486, 485f
Hypertensive retinopathy, 363–364, 364f

Hypertropia, 35, 36f
  cover test, 558f
Hyperuricemia, 229
Hyphema, 240–241, 240f
Hypocalcemia, 303
Hypoplasia, optic nerve, 497, 498f
Hypopyon, 243–244, 243f
  in endophthalmitis, 245f
Hypotensive medications, 582–583
  see also specific drugs
Hypotony, ocular, 238–239, 239f
Hypotropia, 36
Hysteria, 540

I

Ibuprofen, for migraine, 538
Icterus, scleral, 172, 172f
Idiopathic central serous choroidopathy,
  381–383, 382f
Idiopathic intracranial hypertension, 485–486,
  485f
Idiopathic juxtafoveal retinal telangiectasia,
  352–354
  type 1A, 353
  type 1B, 353, 353f
  type 2, 353–354, 354f
  type 3, 354
Idiopathic orbital inflammation, 18–19, 18f
Idiopathic uveal effusion syndrome, 433, 434f
Idoxuridine, 581
Immunoglobulin deposits, corneal, 228
Immunomodulator *see* Cyclosporine
Inclusion conjunctivitis, 148
Indirect ophthalmoscopy, 571, 572f
Indomethacin, 581
  for anterior uveitis, 254
  for cystoid macular edema, 385
  for episcleritis, 169
  for posterior uveitis, 442
  for scleritis, 171
    posterior, 436
Infantile esotropia, 37–38, 38f
Infectious keratitis, 196–203, 204f
  bacterial, 196–197, 196f, 202
  contact lens–related, 188
  following laser in-situ keratomileusis,
    530f, 534
  fungal, 197, 197f
  parasitic, 197–198, 198f

perforated, 197f
  viral *see* Viral keratitis
  see also specific pathogens
Inflammatory bowel disease, 249
Infliximab
  for anterior uveitis, 254
  for posterior uveitis, 442
Intacs (intrastromal corneal ring segments),
  214, 532, 532f
Interferon-alpha
  maculopathy due to, 394
  for optic neuritis, 488
Intermediate uveitis, 411–412, 411f
Internuclear ophthalmoplegia, 63, 63f
Interstitial keratitis, 200, 203–205, 204f
Interstitial nephritis, 250
Intracorneal inlays, 532
Intracranial hypertension, idiopathic,
  485–486, 485f
Intraocular infection *see* Endophthalmitis
Intraocular lens, phakic, 526, 526f
Intraocular lymphoma, 434, 479
Intraocular pressure
  elevated
    primary open-angle glaucoma, 510
    steroid-related, 517
    toxicology, 586t
  low, 238–239, 239f
  measurement, 567, 568f
Intraocular refractive procedures *see* Refractive
  procedures
Intraocular tumor, in open-angle glaucoma,
  518, 520
Intraorbital foreign body, 8–9, 8f
Intraretinal hemorrhage, 331–333, 333f
Intrastromal corneal ring segments (Intacs),
  214, 532, 532f
Intrauterine infections, 298
Inverted follicular keratosis, 108
Involutional ectropion, 89, 91
Involutional entropion, 92, 93
IOL Master, 574, 574f
Iridocorneal endothelial syndromes, 285–287
Iridocyclitis *see* Anterior uveitis
Iridodialysis, 258, 259f, 305f
  management, 260
Iris
  anatomy, 257f
  atrophy, 285, 285f

Iris (*Continued*)
  congenital anomalies, 269–270, 280–282
  in mesodermal dysgenesis syndromes, 282–285
  neovascularization
    glaucoma, 265–266
    rubeosis iridis, 264–265, 264f
  peripheral anterior synechiae, 263–264, 263f
  pigmentary glaucoma, 268
  slit lamp examination, 566
  trauma, 257–261
    angle recession *see* Angle recession
    cyclodialysis, 258, 258f, 260
    iridodialysis *see* Iridodialysis
    sphincter tears *see* Sphincter tears
  tumors, 287–291
    cysts, 287, 287f
    juvenile xanthogranuloma, 290
    malignant melanoma, 290–291, 290f
    metastatic, 291, 291f
    nevi, 288, 288f
    nodules, 288–289, 288f, 289f
    of pigment epithelium, 290
  see also specific disorders
Iris heterochromia, 269–270, 269f
Iris nevus syndrome, 286, 286f
Iris pigment dispersion syndrome, 266–267,
    267f
Iritis *see* Anterior uveitis
Iron deposits, corneal, 228, 228f
Irvine-Gass syndrome, 383
Ischemic optic neuropathy *see* Anterior ischemic
    optic neuropathy
Ishihara pseudoisochromatic chart, 555, 555f
Isoametropic amblyopia, 543
Isoniazid
  for dacryoadenitis, 127
  for tuberculosis, 426
Isosorbide, 583
  for angle-closure glaucoma, 235
Itraconazole
  for *Aspergillus* canaliculitis, 121
  for infectious keratitis, 202

J

Jansen vitreoretinal dystrophy, 457
Jaundice, scleral icterus, 172, 172f
Jones' dye tests, 124, 564
Juvenile optic atrophy, 493
Juvenile pilocytic astrocytoma, 502

Juvenile retinoschisis, 400, 401, 402f, 403
Juvenile rheumatoid arthritis, 250, 254
Juvenile xanthogranuloma, 22, 165, 290
Juxtafoveal retinal telangiectasia, idiopathic
    see Idiopathic juxtafoveal retinal
    telangiectasia

K

Kandori's flecked retina syndrome, 445
Kaposi's sarcoma, 116, 116f, 165, 165f
Kawasaki's disease, 150, 153, 250
Kaye's dots, 589
Kayser–Fleischer ring, 226, 226f, 589
Kearns–Sayre syndrome, 60, 62, 62f, 460, 460f
Keratectomy
  laser-assisted subepithelial, 529
  photorefractive, 529, 529f
Keratic precipitates, 190–191, 191f, 251f, 252f
Keratitis
  dendritic, contact lens-related, 185
  diffuse lamellar, following refractive
      procedures, 529, 531f, 534
  disciform, 199, 199f, 203
  epithelial, 198, 199f, 200, 200f, 202
  filamentary, 190, 190f
  infectious (corneal ulcer) *see* Infectious keratitis
  interstitial, 200, 203–205, 204f
  mucus plaque, 200, 203
  necrotizing interstitial, 199
  peripheral ulcerative, 180–183, 254
  staphylococcal marginal, 180–181, 182–183, 182f
  stromal, 200
  superficial punctuate *see* Superficial punctuate
      keratitis
Keratoacanthoma, 112–113, 113f
Keratoconjunctivitis
  atopic, 146, 146f, 153
  epidemic, 145, 145f
  superior limbic, 149, 149f, 152, 188
  vernal, 143f, 147, 147f, 153
Keratoconjunctivitis sicca *see* Dry eye disease
Keratoconus, 211, 211f, 213f
  posterior, 216, 216f
Keratoglobus, 212, 212f
Keratolysis, marginal, 180, 181, 181f
Keratometry, 569, 569f
Keratomileusis
  epi-laser in-situ, 529
  laser in-situ, 528f, 529, 530f, 531f

Keratopathy
    band, 207, 207f
    climatic droplet, 208
    crystalline, 197f
    exposure, 189–190, 190f, 200
    Labrador, 208
    lipid, 208, 208f
    mucus plaque, 200
    neurotrophic, 200
    pseudophakic bullous, 193–194, 193f
    vortex, 229–230, 229f
Keratoplasty, conductive, 533
Keratosis
    actinic, 112, 112f
    inverted follicular, 108
    seborrheic, 104, 105f
Keratotomy
    astigmatic, 527, 528f
    radial, 527, 527f
Ketoconazole, 580
    for infectious keratitis, 202
Ketorolac tromethamine, 581, 584
    for allergic conjunctivitis, 153t
    for cystoid macular edema, 385
Ketotifen fumarate, 584
    for allergic conjunctivitis, 153t
Khodadoust line, 589
Kjer optic atrophy, 493
Klein's tags, 386, 386f, 589
Koeppe nodules, 289, 289f, 589
Krill's disease, 428–429
Krukenberg spindle, 229, 589
Kunkmann–Wolffian bodies, 589
Kyrieleis' plaques, 589

L

Labrador keratopathy, 208
Laceration
    canalicular, 71–73, 72f
    conjunctival, 131, 133f
    corneoscleral, 131, 179–180, 179f
        open globe and, 131, 133, 133f
    eyelid, 71–72, 71f, 72f
Lacrimal gland
    inflammation, 125–127, 126f
    slit lamp examination, 565
    tumors, 128–129, 128f
Lacrimal sac, infection, 121–123, 122f
Lactic acidosis, 61

Lamellar cataract, 296, 296f
Lander's sign, 590
Langerhans' cell histiocytoses, 23
Laser-assisted subepithelial keratectomy, 529
Laser in-situ keratomileusis, 528f, 529,
        530f, 531f
Laser peripheral iridotomy, for angle-closure
        glaucoma, 235, 237
Laser photocoagulation
    for angioid streaks, 381
    for bilateral acquired parafoveal
        telangiectasia, 354
    for branch retinal vein occlusion, 342
    for central retinal vein occlusion, 345
    for central serous chorioretinopathy, 383
    for choroidal hemangioma, 469
    for congenital optic nerve anomalies, 501
    for diabetic retinopathy, 361–362
    for Eales' disease, 352
    for macular degeneration, 373
    for myopic degeneration, 379
    for ocular ischemic syndrome, 347
    punctuate inner choroidopathy, 431
    for radiation retinopathy, 367
    for retinal ischemia in neovascular
        glaucoma, 266
    for retinoblastoma, 480
    for retinopathy of prematurity, 350
    for sarcoidosis, 437
    for serpiginous choroidopathy, 438
    for sickle cell retinopathy, 357
    for unilateral congenital parafoveal
        telangiectasia, 353
Laser trabeculoplasty, 516
    for pigmentary glaucoma, 268
Lashes see Eyelashes
Latanoprost, 583
    for primary open-angle glaucoma, 516
Latent nystagmus, 37, 43, 47
Lateral canthotomy, 4–5
Lattice degeneration, 398–399, 399f
Lattice dystrophy, 221, 222f
Laurence–Moon syndrome, 460–461, 460f
Leber's congenital amaurosis, 458, 458f
Leber's hereditary optic neuropathy,
        493, 494f
Leber's idiopathic stellate neuroretinitis,
        412–414, 413f
Leber's miliary aneurysms, 350–351, 351f

Lecithin-cholesterol acyltransferase deficiency, 229
Lefler–Wadsworth–Sidbury dystrophy, 452–453
Le Fort fractures, 7–8
Lens
    aphakia, 308–309, 308f
    cataract *see* Cataract(s)
    congenital anomalies, 293–300
        cataract *see* Congenital cataract(s)
        coloboma, 293, 293f
        lenticonus, 294, 294f
        lentiglobus, 294
        microspherophakia, 294, 317
        Mittendorf dot, 295, 295f
    dislocated *see* Ectopia lentis
    exfoliation, 310–311, 310f
    pseudoaphakia, 309–310, 309f
    pseudoexfoliation syndrome, 311–312, 312f
        glaucoma associated with, 312–314, 313f
    slit lamp examination, 566
    toxicology, 586t
Lens-induced secondary glaucoma, 314–315, 314f
Lensometer, 553, 554f
Lenticonus, 294, 294f
Lenticular cataract, 296, 296f
Lentiglobus, globe-shaped, 294
Lentigo maligna melanoma, 114
Leprosy, 79
Lesions, visual pathway, 544–545, 545f, 546f–547f
Letterer–Siwe disease, 23
Leukemia, 24
Leukemic retinopathy, 355–356, 355f
Leukocoria, 279–280, 279f
Levitra, maculopathy due to, 396
Levobetaxolol, 582
Levobunolol, 582
    for primary open-angle glaucoma, 516
Levocabastine, 584
    for allergic conjunctivitis, 153t
Levofloxacin, 578
    for infectious keratitis, 202
Lice infestation, 78, 78f
    eyelashes, 78, 78f
Lidocaine, 584
    for endophthalmitis, 247
Light flashes, differential diagnosis, 577
Light reflex tests, corneal, 559–560, 559f, 560f

Ligneous conjunctivitis, 150, 150f, 153
Limbal dermoid, 214, 215f
Limbal relaxing incisions, 528
Lindane, for pediculosis, 78
Lipid deposits, corneal, 228–229
Lipid keratopathy, 208, 208f
Lipidoses, 225, 225t
Lipid storage diseases, 397–398
Lisch nodules, 289, 289f, 590
Lissamine green, 566
Listeria infection, keratitis, 196
Lodoxamide tromethamine, 584
    for allergic conjunctivitis, 153t
    for giant papillary conjunctivitis, 187
Loops of Axenfeld, 590
Loratadine, 584
Loteprednol etabonate, 582, 584
    for allergic conjunctivitis, 152, 153t
    for uveitis-related glaucoma, 520
Louis–Bar syndrome, 465
Lowe's oculocerebrorenal syndrome, 298
Luetic chorioretinitis, 422–423, 423f
Lyme disease, 248
Lymphangiectasis, 166, 166f
Lymphangioma, 21–22, 22f, 110
Lymphogranuloma venereum, 148
Lymphoid tumors
    conjunctival, 166, 166f
    orbital, 29–30, 30f
Lymphoma
    conjunctival, 166–167, 166f, 167f
    intraocular, 434, 479
    metastatic eyelid lesions, 115–116, 115f
    orbital, 29–30, 30f

M
Macroaneurysm, retinal arterial, 365–366, 365f
Macrolides, 579
    see also specific drugs
Macula
    cherry-red spot *see* Cherry-red spot
    examination, 572, 572f
Macular degeneration, age-related *see* Age-related macular degeneration
Macular dystrophy, 222, 222f, 448–454
    adult foveomacular vitelliform, 448, 449f
    Best's disease, 448–451, 450f
    butterfly pattern, 451

dominant drusen, 451–452, 452f
North Carolina, 452–453
pseudoinflammatory, 453
Sjögren reticular pigment, 453
Stargardt's disease, 453–454, 454f
Macular edema, cystoid, 383–385, 384f
Macular hole, 385–388, 386f
Macular Photocoagulation Study, 373, 374t
Macular pucker, 388–390, 389f, 390f
Macular star
   in hypertensive retinopathy, 363, 364f
   in Leber's idiopathic stellate neuroretinitis,
     412, 413, 413f, 414
Maculopathy
   Bull's eye, 393, 393f, 394, 395f
   cellophane (pucker), 388–390, 389f, 390f
   toxic (drug), 392–397
Madarosis, 82–83, 83f
Magnesium silicate (talc), maculopathy
   due to, 396
Malattia leventinese, 451–452, 452f
Malignant melanoma
   choroidal, 475–477, 476f, 477f
   conjunctival, 164, 164f
   cutaneous, retinopathy associated with, 481
   eyelid, 114, 114f
   iris, 290–291, 290f
Malingering, 540
Mannitol, 583
Map-dot-fingerprint dystrophy, 218, 218f
Marcus Gunn pupil, 277–279, 278f
Marfan's syndrome, ectopia lentis, 316, 317f
Marginal keratolysis, 180, 181, 181f
Maroteaux–Lamy syndrome, 225t
Marshall syndrome, 456
Masquerade syndromes, posterior uveitis,
   434–435
Mast cell stabilizer, for allergic conjunctivitis,
   153t
Mature cataract, 300, 301f
Maxillary fractures, 5–8
Measurements, ocular see Examination, ocular
Medications
   ocular toxicology and, 586t
   ophthalmic, 577–585
     allergy, 583–584
     anesthetics, 584
     anti-infectives, 577–581
     anti-inflammatories, 581–582

     mydriatics/cycloplegics, 584
     ocular hypotensive (glaucoma), 582–583
     see also Drug-induced conditions; specific
       drugs
Medroxyprogesterone, for corneal burns, 178
Medrysone, 582
Meesman dystrophy, 218, 219f
Megalocornea, 215, 215f
Meibomitis, 73–75, 74f
Meige's syndrome, 93
Melanin deposits, corneal, 229
Melanocytoma, optic nerve, 502, 503f
Melanocytosis, oculodermal, 104, 104f, 163,
   163f
Melanoma, malignant see Malignant
   melanoma
Melanosis
   primary acquired, 163, 163f
   secondary acquired, 163–164, 164f
Mellaril, maculopathy due to, 397, 397f
Membranes, conjunctival, 142
Meningioma, 28, 28f
   optic nerve, 503, 503f, 504f
Mepivacaine, 584
Mercury deposits, corneal, 227
Merkel cell tumor, 115, 115f
Mesodermal dysgenesis syndromes, 282–285
Metabolic diseases
   as cause of cataracts, 298
   ocular involvement, 225–226, 225t
Metaherpetic ulcer, 199, 203
Metallic foreign body, corneal, 178–179, 178f
Metastasis
   choroidal, 477–478, 478f
   eyelid, 115–116, 115f
   iris, 291, 291f
   orbital, 31
Methacholine, for pupil testing, 585
Methazolamide, 583
   for primary open-angle glaucoma, 516
Methicillin, 578
Methotrexate
   for anterior uveitis, 254
   for intermediate uveitis, 412
   for intraocular lymphoma, 434
   for posterior uveitis, 442
   for sarcoidosis, 437
   for sympathetic ophthalmia, 439
Methoxyflurane, maculopathy due to, 394, 395f

Methylprednisolone
   for anterior ischemic optic neuropathy, 490
   for arteritic ischemic optic neuropathy, 338
   for optic neuritis, 488
   for traumatic optic neuropathy, 492
Metipranolol, 582
   for primary open-angle glaucoma, 516
Metronidazole, 580
   for acne rosacea, 85
Miconazole, 580
   for infectious keratitis, 202
Microaneurysm, conjunctival vessels, 136
Microblepharon, 102
Microcornea, 216, 216f
Microhyphema, anterior chamber, 240, 242
Microphthalmos, 20
Microscopy, specular, 570, 571f
Microspherophakia, 294, 295, 317
Microsporidia keratitis, 198, 198f, 202
Migraine, 536–538
   with aura, 536
      childhood periodic syndromes, 536–537
      complications, 537
      retinal, 537
      without aura, 536
Milia, 108, 108f
Millard–Gubler syndrome, 57
Miller's syndrome, 280
Minocycline, 579
   for acne rosacea, 84
   for blepharitis/meibomitis, 75
   for chalazion, 80
Miotic agents
   allergic conjunctivitis due to, 147
Mitochondrial encephalopathy with lactic acido-
      sis and stroke-like episodes (MELAS), 61
Mitomycin C, for prevention of corneal haze, 534
Mittendorf dot, 295, 295f, 590
Mixed cell tumor, of lacrimal gland, 129
Mizuo–Nakamura phenomenon, 590
Möbius' syndrome, 46
Modified Krimsky's method, 559, 560f
Moll's gland cyst, 107, 107f
Molluscum contagiosum, 77–78, 77f, 148
Monocular elevation deficiency, 44–45, 44f
Mooren's ulcer, 180, 181f
Moraxella catarrhalis infection
   conjunctivitis, 144
   keratitis, 196

Morgagnian cataract, 301, 301f, 590
Morning glory syndrome, 498, 498f
Morquio syndrome, 225t
Motility disorders
   horizontal, 63–65
   vertical, 65–66
Motor nystagmus, 47
Mouchetée dystrophy, 221, 221f
Moxifloxacin, 578
   for central retinal artery occlusion, 338
   for conjunctival laceration, 131
   for conjunctivitis, 151
   for corneal abrasion, 175
   for corneal burns, 178
   for corneal edema, 194
   for corneal foreign body, 179
   for corneal laceration, 134, 179
   for ectasias, 214
   for hypotony, 239
   for infectious keratitis, 202, 203
   for peripheral ulcerative keratitis, 183
   for superficial punctuate keratitis, 189
Mucocele, 26–27, 27f
Mucolipidosis, 225, 225t, 398
Mucopolysaccharidoses, 225, 225t, 398
Mucormycosis, 14f, 15, 60
Mucus plaque keratitis, 200, 203
Muir–Torre syndrome, 113
Multifocal choroiditis and panuveitis, 427t,
      430, 430f
Multiple evanescent white dot syndrome, 427t,
      431–432, 431f
Multiple myeloma, 228
Mumps, dacryoadenitis and, 125, 127
Munson's sign, 211f, 213, 590
Myasthenia gravis, 58, 67–68, 67f
Mycobacterium infection
   dacryoadenitis, 127
   phlyctenule and, 143
Mycobacterium leprae, 79
Mycobacterium tuberculosis, 248, 426
Mycophenolate mofetil
   for anterior uveitis, 254
   for posterior uveitis, 442
Mycoplasma infection, Stevens–Johnson
      syndrome, 157
Mydriatics, 584
   see also specific drugs
Myelinated nerve fibres, 390–391, 391f

Myeloma, multiple, 228
Myoclonic epilepsy with ragged red fibers
        (MERRF), 61
Myopia, 524, 524f, 525
    see also Refractive errors; Refractive procedures
Myopic degeneration, 377–379, 377f, 378f
Myotonic dystrophy
    cataracts, 303
    chronic progressive external
        ophthalmoplegia, 61

N

Nafcillin, for orbital cellulitis, 15
Nanophthalmos, 20
Naphazoline, 584
    for allergic conjunctivitis, 153t
    for conjunctival degenerations, 155
    episcleritis, 169
Naphazoline-antazoline, 584
Naphazoline-pheniramine, 584
Naproxen, 581
    for anterior uveitis, 254
    for posterior uveitis, 442
Nasoethmoidal fracture, 6
Nasolacrimal duct obstruction, 123–125, 124f
Natamycin, 581
    for endophthalmitis, 247
    for infectious keratitis, 202
Nearsightedness, 524, 524f, 525
    see also Refractive errors; Refractive procedures
Near vision chart, 550, 552f
Nebcin, maculopathy due to, 392
Necrotizing interstitial keratitis, 199
Necrotizing scleritis, 169, 170f, 171
Nedocromil, 584
    for allergic conjunctivitis, 153t
Neisseria gonorrhoeae infection
    conjunctivitis, 142, 144, 1525
        neonatal, 150, 151f
    dacryoadenitis, 125, 127
Nematode infection, 418–419, 418f
    phlyctenule and, 143
Neodymium:yttrium-aluminum-garnet
        (Nd:YAG) laser
    for central retinal artery occlusion, 338
    for cystoid macular edema, 385
    for persistent hyperplastic primary
        vitreous, 322
    for posterior capsular opacification, 307, 307f, 308

Neomycin
    allergic conjunctivitis due to, 147
    for infectious keratitis, 202
Neomycin-dexamethasone, 580
Neomycin-polymyxin B-bacitracin, 580
Neomycin-polymyxin B-dexamethasone, 580
    for nasolacrimal duct obstruction, 125
Neomycin-polymyxin B-gramicidin, 578
Neomycin-polymyxin B-hydrocortisone, 580
Neonatal conjunctivitis, 150–151,
        151f, 153
Neovascular glaucoma, 265–266
Nepafenac, 581
    for corneal abrasion, 175
    for cystoid macular edema, 385
Nephritis, interstitial, 250
Neurilemoma, 27, 27f
Neuritis, optic *see* Optic neuritis
Neuroblastoma, 24, 25f
Neurofibromatosis, 116–118, 117f, 466, 466f
    type 1, 116–117, 117f
    type 2, 117–118
Neuronal ceroid lipofuscinosis, 461
Neuropathy, optic *see* Optic neuropathy
Neuroretinitis, 412–414, 413f
    diffuse unilateral subacute, 418–419, 418f
Neuroretinopathy, acute macular, 426
Neurotrophic keratopathy, 200
Nevus
    acquired, 103, 103f
    caruncle, 167, 168f
    choroidal, 470, 470f
    conjunctival, 161, 162f
    eyelid, 103, 103f
    iris, 288, 288f
Nevus flammeus, 110
Nevus of Ota, 104, 104f, 163, 163f
Niacin, maculopathy due to, 395
Niemann–Pick disease, 225t, 398
Night blindness, congenital stationary *see*
        Congenital stationary night blindness
Nocardia asteroides canaliculitis, 120, 121
Nodular scleritis, 169, 170f
Nodules
    Berlin, 289
    Busacca, 289, 289f
    iris, 288–289, 288f, 289f
    Koeppe, 289, 289f
    Lisch, 289, 289f

Nolvadex, maculopathy due to, 396–397

Non-exudative macular degeneration, 368–370, 368f, 369f

Nonproliferative diabetic retinopathy, 358, 358f, 359f

Nonsteroidal anti-inflammatory drugs, 581
  for allergic conjunctivitis, 153t
  see also specific drugs

Norfloxacin, 578

North Carolina macular dystrophy, 452–453

Nothnagel's syndrome, 51

Nougaret's disease, 444

Nuclear cataract, 296, 296f

Nuclear sclerotic cataract, 301–302, 302f

Nutritional supplements
  for abetalipoproteinemia, 459
  for age-related macular degeneration, 369
  for blepharitis/meibomitis, 75
  for dry eyes, 140
  for optic neuropathy, 496
  for retinitis pigmentosa, 463

Nystagmus, 47–50
  acquired, 48–49
  congenital, 47–48
  physiologic, 49
  see also specific types

O

Occlusion amblyopia, 543

Occlusion therapy
  amblyopia, 543
  strabismus, 37

Occlusio pupillae, 262, 262f

Ochronosis, 171

Ocular albinism, 464, 464f

Ocular cicatricial pemphigoid, 156–157, 156f

Ocular examination *see* Examination, ocular

Ocular hypotensive medications, 582–583
  see also specific drugs

Ocular ischemic syndrome, 346–347

Ocular measurements, 587

Ocular motility assessment, 556–560, 557f, 558f, 559f, 560f, 561f

Ocular toxicology, 586t

Oculocutaneous albinism, 464

Oculodermal melanocytosis, 104, 104f, 163, 163f

Oculopharyngeal muscular dystrophy, 61

Ofloxacin, 578

Oguchi's disease, 445–446, 445f

Olopatadine hydrochloride, 584
  for allergic conjunctivitis, 153t

Omega-3 fatty acids, for abetalipoproteinemia, 459

One-and-a-half syndrome, 63–65, 64f

Open-angle glaucoma
  primary, 509–517, 511f, 512f–515f, 517f
    mechanism, 510
  secondary, 517–520, 519f
    associated with pseudoexfoliation syndrome, 312–314, 313f, 517

Open globe, 131, 133, 133f, 134
  Seidel test, 179, 179f

Ophthalmia neonatorum, 150–151, 151f, 153

Ophthalmic abbreviations, 591–593

Ophthalmic artery occlusion, 339–340

Ophthalmic history, 549
  see also Examination, ocular

Ophthalmoplegia
  chronic progressive external, 61–62, 62f
  internuclear, 63, 63f

Opioids, for migraine, 538

Opsoclonus, 48

Optical coherence tomography, 574, 575f

Optic atrophy
  complicated hereditary infantile (Behr's syndrome), 494
  dominant (Kjer/juvenile), 494
  recessive (Costeff syndrome), 494
  X-linked, 494

Optic chiasm, disorders, 505–509, 505f, 506f–507f

Optic disc
  depression (pit) in, 499, 500f
  edema
    due to raised intracranial pressure *see* Papilledema
    in meningioma, 503, 503f
  examination, 572
  tilted, 500

Optic nerve
  congenital anomalies, 496–501, 497f
    aplasia, 497
    coloboma, 497, 497f
    drusen, 498, 499f
    dysplasias, 497–500
    hypoplasia, 497, 498f
    morning glory syndrome, 498, 498f

pits, 499, 500f
types, 497–500
damage, in primary open-angle glaucoma, 510
examination, 571–572
in metabolic diseases, 225t
toxicology, 586t
trauma, 491–493, 492f
tumors, 501–504
  see also specific tumors
Optic neuritis, 486–488
  Devic's syndrome, 487
  papillitis, 486
  retrobulbar, 486
Optic neuropathy, 491–496, 495f
  anterior ischemic *see* Anterior ischemic
    optic neuropathy
  compressive, 493, 496
  hereditary, 493–494, 494f, 496
  infectious, 494, 496
  infiltrative, 494, 496
  ischemic, 494
  nutritional, 494, 496
  toxic, 495, 496
  traumatic, 491–493, 492f
Optokinetic testing, 558–559, 559f
Orbit, 3–33
  congenital anomalies, 19–21
  fistulas, 10–11, 11f
  fractures of *see* Fractures, orbital
  globe subluxation, 9–10, 9f
  infections, 12–15
    cellulitis, 13–15, 14f
  inflammation, 15–19
    idiopathic, 18–19, 18f
    thyroid-related, 15–18, 16f
  pseudotumor of, 18–19
  trauma
    blunt, 3–8, 5f, 6f
    contusion, 3–4, 3f
    hemorrhage, 4–5, 4f
    penetrating, 8–9, 8f
  tumours *see* Orbital tumors
Orbital apex syndrome, 59–60
Orbital compartment syndrome, 4–5
Orbital floor fracture, 5–6, 5f, 6f
  pediatric, 6
Orbital tumors, 21–31
  adult, 26–31
    benign, 26–29

malignant, 29–31
metastatic, 31
pediatric, 21–25
  benign, 21–23
  malignant, 23–25
Orthoptic exercises, for convergence
    insufficiency, 539
Osteogenesis imperfecta, 172
Osteoma, 29
  choroidal, 470–471, 471f
Osteosarcoma, 30
Oxytetracycline-hydrocortisone
    acetate, 580

P
Pachymetry, 568–569, 569f
Pain, eye, differential diagnosis, 577
Pain management
  for corneal abrasion, 175
  migraine, 538
  see also specific analgesics
Pannus, 205–206, 206f
Panum's area, 590
Papillae, conjunctival, 142, 143f, 147, 147f
Papilledema, 483–484, 484f
  in idiopathic intracranial hypertension,
    485–486, 485f
Papillitis, 486
Papilloma
  caruncle, 167, 168f
  conjunctival, 159–160, 160f
  squamous, 105, 105f
  viral, 105–106, 106f
Parafoveal telangiectasia
  bilateral acquired, 353–354, 354f
  unilateral congenital, 353
  unilateral idiopathic, 353, 353f
Paraneoplastic syndromes, 480–481
Parasitic keratitis, 197–198, 198f, 202
Parinaud's oculoglandular syndrome, 65, 66,
    150, 150f, 152
Parks-Bielschowsky three-step test, 55, 55f
Paromomycin, 580
  for infectious keratitis, 202
Parry's sign, 590
Pars plana vitrectomy
  for candidiasis, 415
  for cystoid macular edema, 385
  for epiretinal membrane, 390

Pars plana vitrectomy (*Continued*)
　for macular hole, 387
　for vitreous hemorrhage, 325
Pars planitis, 411–412, 411f
Partial coherence laser interferometry, 574, 574f
Patch, occlusive *see* Occlusion therapy
Pathologic myopia, 377–379, 377f, 378f
Patient history, 549
　see also Examination, ocular
Paton's lines, 590
Paton's sign, 590
Paving stone degeneration, 399, 399f
Pediculosis, 78, 78f
　conjunctivitis and, 146
Pegaptanib sodium, for age-related macular
　degeneration, 373
Pellucid marginal degeneration, 212, 212f, 213f
Pemirolast potassium, 584
　for allergic conjunctivitis, 153t
Pemphigoid, ocular cicatricial, 156–157, 156f
Penetrating trauma
　in open globe, 131, 133, 133f, 134
　orbital, 8–9, 8f
Penicillin(s), 578
　see also specific drugs
Penicillin G
　for *Actinomyces israelii* canaliculitis, 121
　for Argyll Robertson pupil, 275
　for cavernous sinus syndrome, 60
　for dacryoadenitis, 127
　for luetic chorioretinitis, 423
Penicillin V
　for *Actinomyces israelii* canaliculitis, 121
　for eyelid laceration, 72
Penthrane, maculopathy due to, 394, 395f
Peptide antibiotics, 579
　see also specific drugs
Perennial conjunctivitis, 148
Perifoveal telangiectasis, bilateral with capillary
　obliteration, 354
Periodic alternating nystagmus, 48–49
Peripapillary atrophy, myopic degeneration, 377,
　377f, 378f
Peripheral anterior synechiae, 263–264, 263f
Peripheral corneal relaxing incisions, 528
Peripheral cystoid degeneration, 400
Peripheral retinal degenerations,
　398–400, 399f
Peripheral ulcerative keratitis, 180–183, 254

Permethrin
　for acne rosacea, 85
　for pediculosis, 78
Persistent fetal vasculature syndrome, 321–322,
　322f
Persistent hyperplastic primary vitreous,
　321–322, 322f
Persistent pupillary membrane, 281–282, 282f
Peters' anomaly, 284, 284f, 285
Phacoanaphylactic endophthalmitis, 251, 254
Phacolytic glaucoma, 314, 314f
Phacomorphic glaucoma, 314, 315f
Phakic intraocular lens, 526, 526f
Phakomatoses, 465–468
Phenylephrine, 584
　for cataract, 306
　congenital, 299
Phlyctenule, 143–144, 143f
Phoria, 35
　cover tests, 557–558, 557f, 558f
Phospholine iodide, for primary open-angle
　glaucoma, 516
Photic retinopathy, 391, 391f
Photocoagulation *see* Laser photocoagulation
Photorefractive keratectomy, 529, 529f, 530f
Phthiriasis, 78, 78f
Phthisis bulbi, 32–33, 32f
Phycomycetes infection, orbital cellulitis, 13
Phycomycosis, 14f, 15, 60
Physostigmine, for pediculosis, 78
Pigmentary glaucoma, 268
Pigment dispersion syndrome, 266–267, 267f
Pilar cyst, 108, 109f
Pilocarpine, 583
　for angle-closure glaucoma, 235
　for dry eyes, 140
　for pigmentary glaucoma, 268
　for primary open-angle glaucoma, 516
　for refractive procedure complications, 534
Pilomatrixoma, 109
Pinguecula, 154, 154f
Pinhole occluder, 550, 552f
Pink eye, 145
Pits, optic disc, 499, 500f
Plaquenil, maculopathy due to, 392–394, 393f
Plateau iris syndrome, 233
Pleomorphic adenoma/adenocarcinoma,
　lacrimal gland, 128–129
Pleomorphic rhabdomyosarcoma, 24

Pneumocystis carinii choroidopathy, 419–420, 420f
Polar cataract, 294f, 297, 297f
Poliosis, 83, 83f
Polyhexamethylene biguanide, 580
    for infectious keratitis, 202
Polymyxin B, for acquired anophthalmia, 31
Polymyxin B-bacitracin, 579
    for corneal abrasion, 175
Polymyxin B-oxytetracycline, 579
Polymyxin B-trimethoprim
    for conjunctival foreign body, 131
    for conjunctivitis, 152
    for corneal abrasion, 175
    for corneal edema, 194
    for corneal foreign body, 179
    for ectasias, 214
    for infectious keratitis, 203
    for ocular cicatricial pemphigoid, 157
    for peripheral ulcerative keratitis, 182, 183
    for Stevens–Johnson syndrome, 158
    for superficial punctuate keratitis, 189
Polypoidal choroidal vasculopathy, 375–377,
        376f, 377f
Port wine stain, 110
Posner–Schlossman syndrome, 250
Posterior capsular opacification, 306–308, 307f
Posterior embryotoxon, 282f, 283
Posterior polymorphous dystrophy, 224–225, 224f
Posterior scleritis, 169, 435–436, 435f, 436f
Posterior subcapsular cataract, 302, 303f, 305
Posterior uveitis, 414–442, 441f
    in Behçet's disease, 432–433, 432f, 433f
    differential diagnosis, 434–440
    in idiopathic uveal effusion syndrome,
        433–434, 434f
    infections, 414–426
        acute retinal necrosis, 414–415, 414f
        candidiasis, 415, 415f
        cysticercosis, 416, 416f
        cytomegalovirus, 416–418, 417f
        diffuse unilateral subacute neuroretinitis,
            418–419, 418f
        histoplasmosis, 420–421, 420f
        human immunodeficiency virus, 419, 419f
        Pneumocystis carinii, 419–420, 420f
        progressive outer retinal necrosis syndrome,
            421–422, 421f
        rubella, 422
        syphilis, 422–423, 423f

        toxocariasis, 423–424, 424f
        toxoplasmosis, 424–425, 425f
        tuberculosis, 426, 426f
    management, 441–442
    masquerade syndromes, 434–435
    white dot syndromes, 426, 427t, 428–432
Posterior vitreous detachment, 323–324, 323f
Postherpetic neuralgia, 76, 77
Postoperative anterior uveitis, 251
Postoperative endophthalmitis, 244, 246
Posttraumatic endophthalmitis, 244, 247
Potential acuity meter, 554, 554f
Pre-Descemet's dystrophy, 223
Prednisolone acetate, 582
    for acute retinal necrosis, 415
    for allergic conjunctivitis, 152
    for angle-closure glaucoma, 235, 237
    for anterior uveitis, 253
    for Behçet's disease, 433
    for candidiasis, 415
    for cells/flare, 243
    for choroidal hemorrhage, 407
    for contact lens-induced corneal
        neovascularization, 186
    for corneal burns, 178
    for corneal edema, 194
    for corneal graft rejection/failure, 195
    for endophthalmitis, 246, 247
    for giant papillary conjunctivitis, 187
    for hyphema, 241
    for hypopyon, 244
    for idiopathic orbital inflammation, 19
    for infectious keratitis, 202, 203
    for intermediate uveitis, 412
    for interstitial keratitis, 205
    for lens-induced secondary glaucoma, 315
    for neovascular glaucoma, 266
    for open globe, 134
    for peripheral ulcerative keratitis, 183
    for progressive outer retinal necrosis
        syndrome, 422
    for rubeosis iridis, 265
    for Stevens–Johnson syndrome, 158
    for superior limbic keratoconjunctivitis, 188
    for sympathetic ophthalmia, 439
    for toxocariasis, 424
    for uveitis-glaucoma-hyphema syndrome, 255
    for uveitis-related glaucoma, 520
    for Vogt–Koyanagi–Harada syndrome, 440

Prednisolone phosphate, 582
    for herpes simplex virus keratitis, 203
Prednisone, 582
    for acute retinal necrosis, 414
    for anterior ischemic optic neuropathy, 490
    for anterior uveitis, 254
    for arteritic ischemic optic neuropathy, 338
    for Behçet's disease, 433
    for Bell's palsy, 96
    for birdshot choroidopathy, 429
    for cells/flare, 243
    for compressive optic neuropathy, 496
    for contact dermatitis, 82
    for corneal graft rejection/failure, 195
    for cystoid macular edema, 385
    for diplopia in Graves' ophthalmology, 17
    for idiopathic intracranial hypertension, 486
    for idiopathic orbital inflammation, 19
    for intermediate uveitis, 412
    for myasthenia gravis, 68
    for optic neuritis, 488
    for optic neuropathy in Graves'
        ophthalmology, 17
    for peripheral ulcerative keratitis, 183
    for posterior scleritis, 436
    for posterior uveitis, 441
    for progressive outer retinal necrosis
        syndrome, 422
    for sarcoidosis, 437
    for scleritis, 171
    for serpiginous choroidopathy, 438
    for Stevens–Johnson syndrome, 158
    for sympathetic ophthalmia, 439
    for Tolosa–Hunt syndrome, 60
    for toxocariasis, 424
    for Vogt–Koyanagi–Harada syndrome, 440
Pregnancy, toxemia of, 364–365, 365f
Premature infants, retinopathy, 348–350, 349f
Preretinal hemorrhages, 331, 332f
    sickle cell retinopathy, 356, 357f
Presbyopia, 524, 525
    see also Refractive errors
Preseptal cellulitis, 12–13, 12f
Presumed ocular histoplasmosis syndrome,
        420–421, 420f
Primary acquired melanosis, 163, 163f
Primary intraocular lymphoma, 479
Primary open-angle glaucoma see Open-angle
        glaucoma

Primary orbital meningioma, 28
Procaine, 584
Progressive cone dystrophy, 447–448, 447f
Progressive iris atrophy, 285, 285f
Progressive outer retinal necrosis syndrome,
        421–422, 421f
Progressive supranuclear palsy, 65, 66
Proliferative diabetic retinopathy, 360, 360f,
        361–362, 362f, 363t
Proliferative vitreoretinopathy, 410
Propamidine isethionate, 580
    for infectious keratitis, 202
Proparacaine, 584
Propionibacterium acnes endophthalmitis, 244
Prostaglandin analogues, 583
    see also specific drugs
Pseudoaphakia, 309–310, 309f
Pseudo divergence excess, 41
Pseudoepitheliomatous hyperplasia, 112, 232
Pseudoexfoliation glaucoma, 312–314, 313f
Pseudoexfoliation syndrome, 311–312, 312f
Pseudoinflammatory macular dystrophy, 453
Pseudomembrane, conjunctival, 142, 142f
Pseudomonas infection
    dacryocystitis, 121
    keratitis, 188, 196, 196f
Pseudophakic bullous keratopathy, 193–194, 193f
Pseudotumor, orbital, 18–19
Pseudotumor cerebri, 485–486, 485f
Pseudo-von Graefe sign, 590
Psoriatic arthritis, 249
Pterygium, 154–155, 155f
Ptosis, 85–88
    acquired, 85–86, 86f
    congenital, 86–88, 87f
    in myasthenia gravis, 67, 67f
Pucker maculopathy, 388–390, 389f, 390f
Pulfrich phenomenon, 590
Punctuate inner choroidopathy, 427t,
        430–431, 431f
Pupil(s)
    Adie's, 272–274, 273f
    Argyll Robertson, 274–275
    displaced see Corectopia
    examination, 278f, 279, 561
    leukocoria, 279–280, 279f
    Marcus Gunn, 277–279, 278f
    seclusio pupillae, 262, 262f
    size inequality, 271–272, 271f

Pupillary block
  primary angle-closure glaucoma, 233
  secondary angle-closure glaucoma, 236
Pupillary membrane, persistent, 281–282, 282f
Purkinje images, 590
Purkinje shift, 590
Purtscher's retinopathy, 329, 329f
Pyogenic granuloma, 167, 167f
Pyrazinamide
  for dacryoadenitis, 127
  for tuberculosis, 426
Pyrethrins liquid, for pediculosis, 78
Pyridostigmine, for myasthenia gravis, 68
Pyrimethamine, for toxoplasmosis, 425

Q

Quinamm, maculopathy due to, 395, 395f
Quinine, maculopathy due to, 395, 395f

R

Raccoon intestinal worm, 418
Racemose hemangiomatosis, 467, 467f
Radial keratotomy, 527, 527f
Radiation retinopathy, 366–367, 366f
Ragged red fibres, 61, 459
Ranibizumab
  for age-related macular degeneration, 373
  for angioid streaks, 381
Ranitidine, 582
  for anterior uveitis, 254
  for Behçet's disease, 433
  for birdshot choroidopathy, 429
  for corneal graft rejection/failure, 195
  for idiopathic intracranial hypertension, 486
  intermediate uveitis/pars planitis, 412
  for ischemic optic neuropathy, 488, 491
  in migraine etiology, 537
  for myasthenia gravis, 68
  for orbital pseudotumor, 19
  for peripheral ulcerative keratitis, 183
  for posterior scleritis, 436
  for posterior uveitis, 414, 441
  for sarcoidosis, 437
  for scleritis, 171
  for Stevens–Johnson syndrome, 158
  for sympathetic ophthalmia, 439
  for Tolosa–Hunt syndrome, 60
  for toxoplasmosis, 425
  for Vogt–Koyanagi–Harada syndrome, 440

Reactive lymphoid hyperplasia, 29–30, 30f
Recessive optic atrophy, 494
Red blood cells, in anterior chamber, 242–243
Red eye, common causes/associated findings, 576t
Refraction, 552–553, 553f
Refractive errors, 523–526
  measurement, 552–553, 553f
  types, 523–524
Refractive lens exchange, 526
Refractive procedures, 526–533
  corneal see Corneal refractive procedures
  intraocular, 526–527
    complications, 527
    postoperative symptoms, 527
    types, 526, 526f
Refsum's disease, 461
Reis–Bückler dystrophy, 219, 219f
Reiter's syndrome, 249
Relative afferent pupillary defect, 277–279, 278f
Restrictive strabismus, 46, 46f
Reticulum cell sarcoma, 479
Retina
  in metabolic diseases, 225t
  peripheral, examination, 572, 573f
  toxicology, 586t
  trauma to, 328–331
Retinal angiomatous proliferation, 374–375, 375f
Retinal arterial macroaneurysm, 365–366, 365f
Retinal artery occlusion
  branch, 334–336, 334f, 335f
  central, 336–339, 337f
Retinal degenerations, peripheral, 398–400, 399f
Retinal detachment, 259f, 403–406
  exudative (serous) see Exudative (serous) retinal detachment
  with proliferative vitreoretinopathy, 410, 410f
  rhegmatogenous, 403–404, 404f
  traction see Traction retinal detachment
Retinal dialysis, 330
Retinal edema, in Behçet's disease, 432, 432f
Retinal hamartoma, 475, 475f, 501
  astrocytic see Astrocytic hamartoma
Retinal hemorrhage, 331–333, 332f, 333f
  in Behçet's disease, 432, 432f
  in cytomegalovirus retinitis, 416, 417f
Retinal migraine, 537

Retinal necrosis
  acute, 414–415, 414f
  progressive outer, 421–422, 421f
Retinal pigment epithelium
  congenital hypertrophy of, 473–474, 474f
  hamartoma, 475, 475f, 501
Retinal tears, 330–331, 330f
Retinal telangiectasia, idiopathic juxtafoveal *see*
        Idiopathic juxtafoveal retinal telangiectasia
Retinal tumors
  benign, 471–475
  malignant, 475, 479–480
Retinal vein occlusion
  branch, 340–342, 341f
  central, 342–345, 343f
Retinal vessels, examination, 572
Retinitis
  cytomegalovirus, 416–418, 417f
  herpetic, 414–415, 414f
  in nematode infection, 418–419, 418f
Retinitis pigmentosa, 459–464, 462f, 463f
  forms
    associated with systemic abnormalities,
        459–462
    atypical, 459
Retinitis pigmentosa inversus, 459
Retinitis pigmentosa sine pigmento, 459
Retinitis punctata albescens, 459
Retinoblastoma, 479–480, 479f, 480f
Retinopathy
  of anemia, 354–355, 355f
  carcinoma-associated, 480–481
  cutaneous melanoma-associated, 481
  diabetic *see* Diabetic retinopathy
  human immunodeficiency virus, 419, 419f
  hypertensive, 363–364, 364f
  leukemic, 355–356, 355f
  photic, 391, 391f
  of prematurity, 348–350, 349f
  Purtscher's, 329, 329f
  radiation, 366–367, 366f
  rubella, 422, 422f
  sickle cell, 356–357, 357f
  solar, 391, 391f
  Valsalva, 331, 332f
  venous stasis, 346, 346f
Retinoschisis, 400–403, 401f
  juvenile, 400, 401, 402f, 403
  types, 400

Retinoscopy, 553
Retrobulbar hemorrhage, 4, 4f
Retrobulbar neuritis, 486
Rhabdomyosarcoma, 23–24, 24f
Rhegmatogenous retinal detachment, 403–404,
        404f
Rheumatoid arthritis, juvenile, 250, 254
Rhinophyma, 84, 84f, 85
Riddoch phenomenon, 590
Rieger's anomaly, 283
Rieger's syndrome, 283, 283f
Rifampin
  for dacryoadenitis, 127
  for leprosy, 79
  for tuberculosis, 426
Riggs' congenital stationary night
        blindness, 444
Riley-Day syndrome, 273
Rimexolone, 582
Rizutti's sign, 213, 590
Rod monochromatism, 448
Rose bengal, 566
Roth spots, 333, 355f, 590
Rubella, congenital, 298, 422, 422f
Rubeosis iridis, 264–265, 264f
Rush disease, 350
Rust ring, 178, 178f

S

Saccadomania, 48
Salus' sign, 590
Salzmann's nodular degeneration, 208, 209f, 210
Sampaoelesi's line, 590
Sandhoff syndrome, 225t, 398
Sanfilippo's syndrome, 225, 225t
Sarcoidosis, 118, 254, 436–437, 437f
Sarcoma
  chondrosarcoma, 30
  Kaposi's, 116, 116f
  orbital rhabdomyosarcoma, 23–24, 24f
  reticulum cell, 479
Sattler's veil, 590
Scheie's line, 590
Scheie syndrome, 225t
Schirmer's test, 564, 564f
Schnyder's central crystalline dystrophy,
        220, 220f
Schubert–Bornschein type congenital stationary
        night blindness, 444

Schwalbe's line, 590
Schwalbe's ring, 590
Schwannoma, 27, 27f
Sclera
    discoloration, 171–173
    inflammation of see Scleritis
    laceration, 131
        open globe and, 131, 133, 133f
        slit lamp examination, 565
        traumatic injury, 131, 133–134, 133f
Scleral ectasia, 172, 172f
Scleral icterus, 172, 172f
Scleral plaque, senile, 172–173, 173f
Scleritis, 169–171, 170f, 576t
    anterior, 169, 170f
    posterior, 169, 435–436, 435f, 436f
Sclerocornea, 216, 217f
Scleromalacia perforans, 169, 170f, 171
Scopolamine, 584
    for accommodative excess, 540
    for angle-closure glaucoma, 237, 238
    for anterior uveitis, 253
    for candidiasis, 415
    for cells/flare, 243
    for corneal burns, 178
    for corneal edema, 194
    for corneal graft rejection/failure, 195
    for corneal laceration, 178
    for endophthalmitis, 246
    for hyphema, 241
    for hypopyon, 244
    for hypotony, 239
    for infectious keratitis, 202, 203
    for intermediate uveitis, 412
    for interstitial keratitis, 205
    for keratitis, 192
    for lens-induced secondary glaucoma, 315
    for microspherophakia, 295, 318
    for open globe, 134
    for progressive outer retinal necrosis
        syndrome, 422
    for sympathetic ophthalmia, 439
    for toxocariasis, 424
    for uveitis-glaucoma-hyphema syndrome,
        255
    for uveitis-related glaucoma, 520
Sea-fans, 356, 357f
Seasonal conjunctivitis, 146
Sebaceous cell carcinoma, 113–114, 113f

Sebaceous cyst, 108, 109f
Seborrheic keratosis, 104, 105f
Seclusio pupillae, 262, 262f
Secondary acquired melanosis, 163–164, 164f
Secondary cataract, 306–308, 307f
Secondary open-angle glaucoma see Open-angle
        glaucoma
Sector retinitis pigmentosa, 459
See-saw nystagmus, 49
Seidel test, 590
    for open globe, 179, 179f
Senile cataract, 303, 305
Senile scleral plaque, 172–173, 173f
Sensory deprivation nystagmus, 47
Septo-optic dysplasia, 500
Serous retinal detachment see Exudative
        (serous) retinal detachment
Serpiginous choroidopathy, 254, 427t,
        437–438, 438f
Seventh cranial nerve palsy see Bell's palsy
Shafer's sign, 590
Shaffer's angle grading system, 567f
Sherrington's law, 590
Sickle cell retinopathy, 356–357, 357f
Siderosis
    corneal, 228, 230
    glaucoma due to, 518
Siegrist streaks, 363, 364f, 590
Sildenafil, maculopathy due to, 396
Silver deposits, corneal, 227, 227f
Silver nitrate
    ophthalmia neonatorum due to, 150
    for superior limbic keratoconjunctivitis, 188
Sixth cranial nerve palsy, 56–58, 56f, 57f
Sjögren reticular pigment dystrophy, 453
Sjögren syndrome, 137
Skew deviation, 65, 66
Slit lamp examination, 565–567, 565f, 566f,
        567f
    of fundus, 571, 572f
Sly syndrome, 225t
Snail track degeneration, 400
Snellen chart, 550, 550f–551f
Snowflake degeneration, 456
Sodium ascorbate, for corneal burns, 178
Sodium chloride, 585
Soemmering's ring cataract, 590
Solar retinopathy, 391, 391f
Sorsby's dystrophy, 453

Spanish phrases, 593–595
Spasm, accommodative, 539–540
Spasmus nutans, 48
Spastic entropion, 92, 93
Spectral domain optical coherence
    tomography, 574
Specular microscopy, 570, 571f
Sphenoid meningioma, 28, 28f
Spheroidal corneal degeneration, 208
Sphincter tears, 259, 259f
    management, 260
Spiral of Tillaux, 591
Spitz nevus, 103
Spondyloarthropathies, 249
Squamous cell carcinoma
    conjunctival, 161, 161f
    corneal, 231–232, 232f
    eyelid, 111–112, 112f
Squamous papilloma, 105, 105f
Staphylococcus infection
    conjunctivitis, 144
    dacryoadenitis, 125, 127
    dacryocystitis, 121
    endophthalmitis, 244, 245, 245f
    eyelid, 73, 79
    keratitis, 196
        marginal, 180–181, 182–183, 182f
    orbital cellulitis, 13
    phlyctenule and, 143
    preseptal cellulitis, 12
Staphyloma, scleral, 172, 172f
Stargardt's disease, 453–454, 454f
Steele–Richardson–Olszewski syndrome, 65, 66
Stelazine deposits, corneal, 228
Stereopsis, 555, 555f, 556f
Steroidal anti-inflammatory drugs, for allergic
    conjunctivitis, 152, 153t
Steroids, 581–582
    antibiotic combinations, 580
    secondary open-angle glaucoma due to, 517
    see also specific drugs
Stevens–Johnson syndrome, 142, 157–158, 158f
Stickler vitreoretinal dystrophy, 457–458, 457f
Stocker's line, 154, 228, 591
Strabismus, 35–47, 554, 554f
    amblyopia and, 542
    in congenital fibrosis syndrome, 46–47
    horizontal, 37–42
    restrictive, 46, 46f

types of deviation, 35–36
    vertical, 42–45
        muscle surgery, 43, 44f
Strabismus fixus, 47
Streptococcus infection
    conjunctivitis, 142, 144
    dacryocystitis, 121
    keratitis, 196, 196f, 197f
    orbital cellulitis, 13
    postoperative endophthalmitis, 244
    Stevens–Johnson syndrome, 157
Stromal keratitis, 200
Sturge–Weber syndrome, 465–466, 466f
Stye, 79–80
Subcapsular cataract
    anterior, 302, 305f
    posterior, 302, 303f, 305
Subconjunctival hemorrhage, 134, 135f, 576t
Subretinal fibrosis and uveitis syndrome, 430,
    430f
Subretinal hemorrhage, 333
Sub-Tenon's steroid injection see Triamcinolone
    acetate
Sudoriferous cyst, 107, 107f
Sugar cataracts, 303
Sugiura's sign, 591
Sulfacetamide, 579, 580
    for Nocardia asteroides canaliculitis, 121
Sulfacetamide-fluorometholone, 580
Sulfacetamide-prednisolone acetate, 580
    for blepharochalasis, 82
Sulfacetamide-prednisolone phosphate, 580
Sulfadiazine, for toxoplasmosis, 425
Sulfite oxidase deficiency, 317
Sulfonamides, 579
    see also specific drugs
Sunflower cataract, 304, 304f
Superficial punctuate keratitis, 138f, 188–189,
    191, 191f
    Thygeson's, 191–192, 192f
Superior limbic keratoconjunctivitis, 149, 149f,
    152, 188
Superior oblique tendon sheath syndrome,
    42–43, 43f
Suprofen, 581
Surgery, refractive see Refractive procedures
Sutural cataract, 297, 297f
Swinging flashlight test, 277, 278f, 279, 559
Sympathetic ophthalmia, 438–439, 439f

Synchesis scintillans, 324
Syphilis, 248, 422–423, 423f
    episcleritis and, 168

T

Tacrolimus
    for anterior uveitis, 254
    for contact dermatitis, 81
    for posterior uveitis, 442
Tadalafil, maculopathy due to, 396
Taenia solium, 416
Talc, maculopathy due to, 396
Tamoxifen, maculopathy due to, 396–397
Tangent screen, 562
Tangier's disease, 229
Tapeworm, 416, 416f
Tay–Sachs disease, 225t, 398, 398f
Tearing, differential diagnosis, 577
Tears, ocular, 259f
    see also specific types
Tea tree oil
    for acne rosacea, 85
    for blepharitis/meibomitis, 75
Telangiectasia
    conjunctival vessels, 135–136, 135f
    idiopathic juxtafoveal retinal *see* Idiopathic
        juxtafoveal retinal telangiectasia
    perifoveal, 354
Telecanthus, 102, 103f
Tenon's capsule, 591
Terrien's marginal degeneration, 209,
        209f, 210
Tests *see* Examination, ocular
Tetanus booster
    for eyelid laceration, 72
    for intraorbital foreign body, 9
Tetracaine, 584
Tetracycline(s), 579
    for acne rosacea, 84
    for Argyll Robertson pupil, 275
    for blepharitis/meibomitis, 75
    for chalazion, 80
    for luetic chorioretinitis, 423
    see also specific drugs
Thermokeratoplasty, 533, 533f
Thiamine, for optic neuropathy, 496
Thiel–Behnke dystrophy, 219, 219f
Thioridazine, maculopathy due to, 397, 397f
Third cranial nerve palsy, 50–53, 50f, 52f

Thorazine
    corneal deposits, 228
    maculopathy due to, 394
Thygeson's superficial punctuate keratitis,
        191–192, 192f
Thyroid-related ophthalmology, 15–18, 16f
Ticarcillin, 578
"Tigroid" fundus, myopic degeneration, 377,
        378f
Tilted optic disc, 500
Time domain optical coherence tomography,
        574, 575f
Timolol, 582
    for angle-closure glaucoma, 235
    for central retinal artery occlusion, 338
    for congenital glaucoma, 509
    for corneal laceration in open globe, 134
    for orbital compartment syndrome, 5
    for primary open-angle glaucoma, 516
Tobramycin, 578
    for corneal abrasion, 175
    for corneal edema, 194
    for corneal foreign body, 179
    for ectasias, 214
    for infectious keratitis, 202, 203
    maculopathy due to, 392
    for peripheral ulcerative keratitis, 182, 183
    for superficial punctuate keratitis, 189
Tobramycin-dexamethasone, 580
    for blepharitis/meibomitis, 75
    for chalazion, 80
Tobramycin-loteprednol etabonate, 580
Tolosa–Hunt syndrome, 18, 59, 60
Tonometry, 567, 568f
Toothpaste sign, 74
Topical anesthetics, 584
    see also specific drugs
Torre's syndrome, 108
Toxemia of pregnancy, 364–365, 365f
Toxic anterior segment syndrome, 245, 251
Toxic cataract, 305, 305f
Toxic conjunctivitis, 147, 149
Toxic (drug) maculopathies, 392–397
Toxicology, ocular, 586t
Toxocara canis, 423
    granuloma, 423, 424f
Toxocariasis, 423–424, 424f
Toxoplasma gondii, 424, 425
Toxoplasmosis, 424–425, 425f

Trabecular meshwork, tears, 259f
Trabeculoplasty, laser, 516
    for primary open-angle glaucoma, 516
Trabulectomy, 516, 517f
Trachoma, 141f, 148, 148f
Traction retinal detachment, 405–406, 406f
    proliferative diabetic retinopathy, 360, 361f
Transient visual loss, 541–542, 577
Translation guide, English-Spanish, 593–595
Trauma
    anterior uveitis due to, 251
    cataract due to, 305, 305f
    ectopia lentis due to, 317, 317f
    open-angle glaucoma due to, 518, 520
    penetrating
        in open globe, 131, 133, 133f, 134
        orbital, 8–9, 8f
    see also specific sites
Traumatic optic neuropathy, 491–493, 492f
Travoprost, 583
    for primary open-angle glaucoma, 516
Treponema pallidum infection
    dacryoadenitis, 127
    luetic chorioretinitis, 422–423, 423f
Triamcinolone acetate
    for anterior uveitis, 254
    for Behçet's disease, 433
    for birdshot choroidopathy, 430
    for branch retinal vein occlusion, 342
    for cells/flare, 243
    for chalazion, 80
    for corneal graft rejection/failure, 195
    for cystoid macular edema, 385
    for intermediate uveitis, 412
    for macular edema in diabetic retinopathy, 362
    for posterior scleritis, 436
    for posterior uveitis, 441
    for presumed ocular histoplasmosis
        syndrome, 421
    for radiation retinopathy, 367
    for sarcoidosis, 437
    for serpiginous choroidopathy, 438
    for sympathetic ophthalmia, 439
    for toxocariasis, 424
    for Vogt–Koyanagi–Harada syndrome, 440
Trichiasis, 97–98, 98f
Trifluridine, 581
    for anterior uveitis, 253
    for canaliculitis, 121

for herpes simplex virus infection
    of conjunctiva, 152
    of cornea, 202, 203
    of eyelid, 75
Trimethoprim-polymyxin B, 579
Trimethoprim-sulfamethoxazole, 579
    for dacryocystitis, 123
    for Nocardia asteroides canaliculitis, 121
    for orbital cellulitis, 15
    for preseptal cellulitis, 13
    for toxoplasmosis, 425
Tripod fracture, 7
Triptans, for migraine, 538
Trochlear nerve palsy, 53–56, 53f, 54f, 55f
Trophic ulcer, 199, 203
Tropia, 35
    cover tests, 557–558, 557f, 558f
Tropicamide, 584
    for cataract, 306
        congenital, 299
True divergence excess, 41
Tuberculosis, 248, 426, 426f
    episcleritis and, 168
Tuberous sclerosis, 467–468, 468f
Tumors
    caruncle, 167–168, 168f
    choroidal see Choroidal tumors
    corneal, 231–232
    histiocytic, 23
    intraocular, in open-angle glaucoma, 518, 520
    lacrimal gland, 128–129, 128f
    lymphoid see Lymphoid tumors
    optic nerve see Optic nerve
    retinal see Retinal tumors
    see also specific tumors/sites
Tyrosine deposits, corneal, 229
Tyrosinemia, 229

U

Uhthoff's symptoms, 591
Ulcer, corneal see Infectious keratitis
Ulcerative colitis, 249
Ulcerative keratitis, peripheral, 180–183, 254
Ultrasonography, 573, 573f, 574f
Unilateral congenital parafoveal telangiectasia, 353
Unilateral fibrosis syndrome, 44, 46
Unilateral idiopathic parafoveal telangiectasia,
    353, 353f
Unoprostone isopropyl, 583

Upbeat nystagmus, 49
Urate deposition, corneal, 229
Usher's syndrome, 461–462
Uveitis, 576t
    anterior *see* Anterior uveitis
    intermediate, 411–412, 411f
    open-angle glaucoma and, 518, 519, 520
    posterior *see* Posterior uveitis
Uveitis-glaucoma-hyphema syndrome, 255

V

Valacyclovir, 581
    for anterior uveitis, 253
    for herpes simplex virus infection
        of cornea, 203
        of eyelid, 75
    for herpes zoster virus infection
        of cornea, 203
        of eyelid, 77
        of retina, 414, 421
Valsalva retinopathy, 331, 332f
Vancomycin, 579
    for cavernous sinus syndrome, 60
    for endophthalmitis, 246
    for infectious keratitis, 202
    for open globe, 134
van Trigt's sign, 591
Vardenafil, maculopathy due to, 396
Varicella, congenital syndrome, 298
Vasoconstrictors, for allergic conjunctivitis, 153t
Vein occlusion
    branch retinal, 340–342, 341f
Venous stasis retinopathy, 346, 346f
Vernal keratoconjunctivitis, 143f, 147, 147f, 153
Verruca vulgaris, 105–106, 106f
Vertebrobasilar insufficiency (vertebrobasilar
        atherothrombotic disease), 535–536
Vertical motility disorders, 65–66
Vertical retraction syndrome, 47
Vertical strabismus *see* Strabismus
Verticillata, cornea, 229–230, 229f
Vestibular nystagmus, 49
Viagra, maculopathy due to, 396
Vidarabine, 581
    for herpes simplex virus infection
        of cornea, 202
        of eyelid, 75
    for herpes zoster virus infection of eyelid, 75
Viral conjunctivitis, 145–146, 145f, 146f, 152

Viral keratitis, 198–201, 199f, 200f
    treatment, 202–203
Viral papilloma, 105–106, 106f
Viscoelastic agents, secondary open-angle
        glaucoma due to, 517
Visual acuity
    measurement, 549–550, 550f–552f
    notations, 550, 550f–551f
Visual field
    defect, differential diagnosis, 577
    testing, 561–563, 561f, 562f, 563f
Visual loss
    cortical blindness and, 544
    functional, 540–541
    gradual, differential diagnosis, 577
    sudden, differential diagnosis, 575
    transient, 541–542
        differential diagnosis, 577
Visual pathway lesions, 544–545, 545f,
        546f–547f
Vitamin A
    for abetalipoproteinemia, 459
    deficiency, dry eye and, 137, 138f
    for retinitis pigmentosa, 463
Vitamin B1, for optic neuropathy, 496
Vitamin B6, for gyrate atrophy, 447
Vitamin B12, for optic neuropathy, 496
Vitamin C, for macular degeneration, 369
Vitamin E
    for abetalipoproteinemia, 459
    for macular degeneration, 369
Vitamin K, for abetalipoproteinemia, 459
Vitiliginous chorioretinitis, 427t, 429–430, 429f
Vitiligo, 83, 83f
Vitravene, for cytomegalovirus retinitis, 418
Vitreoretinal degenerations, hereditary, 454–457
Vitreoretinopathy
    familial exudative, 454–455, 455f
    proliferative, 410
Vitreous disorders, 319–326
    amyloidosis, 319–320, 319f
    asteroid hyalosis, 320–321, 321f
    hemorrhage, 324–325, 325f
    inflammation, 326
    persistent hyperplastic primary vitreous,
        321–322, 322f
    posterior detachment, 323–324, 323f
    snowballs, 411, 411f
    synchysis scintillans, 324

Vitritis, 326
Vogt–Koyanagi–Harada syndrome, 254, 439–440, 440f
Vogt's sign, 591
Vogt's striae, 213, 591
Voluntary nystagmus, 49
Von Graefe's sign, 591
Von Hippel lesion, 501
Von Hippel–Lindau disease, 465, 465f
Von Recklinghausen's disease, 116–117, 117f, 466, 466f
Voriconazole, 581
    for infectious keratitis, 202
Vortex keratopathy, 229–230, 229f
Vossius ring, 591
V-pattern strabismus, 42, 42f

W

Waardenburg's syndrome, 83, 102
Wagner vitreoretinal dystrophy, 456
Watzke–Allen sign, 591
Wavefront aberrometry, 570, 570f
Weber's syndrome, 51
Wegener's granulomatosis, 181f, 254
Weill–Marchesani syndrome, 294, 317
Weiss ring, 591
    posterior vitreous detachment, 323, 323f
Wernicke–Korsakoff syndrome, 56
Wessely ring, 591

Wet macular degeneration see Age-related macular degeneration
Whipple's disease, 249
White blood cells, in anterior chamber, 242, 243–244, 243f
White cells, in anterior chamber, 243–244, 243f
White dot syndromes, 426–432, 427t
    multiple evanescent, 427t, 431–432, 431f
    see also specific disorders
White limbal girdle of Vogt, 209–210, 210f
White lines of Vogt, 591
Wieger's ligament, 591
Willebrandt's knee, 591
Wilson's disease, 226, 304, 304f
Wolfram's syndrome, 494
Worms, subretinal, 418–419, 418f
Worth 4 dot test, 556, 556f
Wyburn–Mason syndrome, 467, 467f

X

Xanthelasma, 106, 106f
Xanthogranuloma, juvenile, 22, 165, 290
X-linked optic atrophy, 494
X-pattern strabismus, 42

Z

Zinc, for macular degeneration, 369
Zonular cataract, 296, 296f
Zygomatic fracture, 7, 8